Pediatric Rehabilitation

Third Edition

Pediatric Rehabilitation

Third Edition

Gabriella E. Molnar, MD, FAAPMR

Gabriella E. Molnar, MD, FAAPMR
Emeritus Clinical Professor
Department of Physical Medicine and Rehabilitation
University of California, Davis, School of Medicine
Emeritus Director
Department of Pediatric Rehabilitation
Oakland Children's Hospital
Oakland, California

Michael A. Alexander, MD, FAAP, FAAPMR
Clinical Professor and Chief
Department of Pediatric Rehabilitation
Jefferson Medical College of Thomas Jefferson University
A.I. duPont Hospital for Children
Wilmington, Delaware

HANLEY & BELFUS, INC. / Philadelphia

Publisher: HANLEY & BELFUS, INC.
                 Medical Publishers
                 210 South 13th Street
                 Philadelphia, PA 19107
                 (215) 546-7293; 800-962-1892
                 FAX (215) 790-9330
                 Web site: http://www.hanleyandbelfus.com

Disclaimer: Although the information in this book has been carefully reviewed for correctness of dosage and indications, neither the authors nor the editors nor the publisher can accept any legal responsibility for any errors or omissions that may be made. Neither the publisher nor the editors make any warranty, expressed or implied, with respect to the material contained herein. Before prescribing any drug, the reader must review the manufacturer's current product information (package inserts) for accepted indications, absolute dosage recommendations, and other information pertinent to the safe and effective use of the product described.

Library of Congress Cataloging-in-Publication Data

Pediatric rehabilitation / edited by Gabriella E. Molnar, Michael A.
  Alexander. — 3rd ed.
      p.   cm.
  Includes bibliographical references and index.
  ISBN 1-56053-306-4 (alk. paper)
  1. Physically handicapped children—Rehabilitation.   I. Molnar,
Gabriella E., 1926–   . II. Alexander, Michael A. (Michael Allen),
1947–   .
  [DNLM: 1. Rehabilitation—in infancy & childhood.
  2. Rehabilitation—in infancy & childhood.   WS 368 P371 1999]
RJ138.P38   1999
617'.03'083—dc21
DNLM/DLC
for Library of Congress   98-31219
                                                           CIP

PEDIATRIC REHABILITATION, 3rd edition   ISBN 1-56053-306-4

Last digit is the print number: 9   8   7   6   5   4   3   2   1

Contents

Contributors

Christine Aguilar, MD
Associate Director, Department of Pediatric Rehabilitation, Oakland Children's Hospital, Oakland, California

Michael A. Alexander, MD, FAAP, FAAPMR
Clinical Professor and Chief, Department of Pediatric Rehabilitation, Jefferson Medical College of Thomas Jefferson University, A.I. duPont Hospital for Children, Wilmington, Delaware

Hillary B. Berlin, MD
Head, Section of Pediatric Rehabilitation, Schneider Children's Hospital, New Hyde Park; Assistant Professor of Rehabilitation Medicine and Pediatrics, Albert Einstein College of Medicine, Bronx, New York

Jane Crowley, PsyD
Rehabilitation Psychologist, Department of Physical Medicine and Rehabilitation, A.I. duPont Hospital for Children, Wilmington, Delaware

Jessie K. M. Easton, MD, MPH
Clinical Professor, University of South Dakota School of Medicine, Sioux Falls, South Dakota

Deborah Gaebler-Spira, MD
Associate Professor, Departments of Pediatrics and Physical Medicine and Rehabilitation, Northwestern University Medical School, Rehabilitation Institute of Chicago, Chicago, Illinois

Robert Haining, MD
Director, Department of Pediatric Rehabilitation, Oakland Children's Hospital, Oakland, California

Joyce Harvey, RN, MSN, PNP
Clinical Nurse Specialist, Pediatric Rehabilitation, Children's Hospital, Oakland, California

Joy P. Hill, MA
Rehabilitation Clinical Specialist, Therapeutic Services and Rehabilitation, A.I. duPont Hospital for Children, Wilmington, Delaware

Ellen S. Kaitz, MD, FAAPMR
Clinical Assistant Professor, Department of Physical Medicine and Rehabilitation, Ohio State University College of Medicine; Pediatric Physiatrist, Children's Hospital, Columbus, Ohio

Judy Kerr, RN, MSN, CRRN
Nurse Manager, Children's Hospital, Oakland, California

Elizabeth L. Koczur, MPT
Staff Physical Therapist, A.I. duPont Hospital for Children, Wilmington, Delaware

Linda E. Krach, MD
Clinical Assistant Professor, Department of Physical Medicine and Rehabilitation, University of Minnesota Medical School–Minneapolis; Medical Director of Rehabilitation and Co-Director, Pediatric Brain Injury Service, Gillette Children's Specialty Health Care, St. Paul, Minnesota

Robert L. Kriel, MD
Professor, Departments of Neurology, Pediatrics, and Pharmacy Practice, University of Minnesota Medical School–Minneapolis; Co-Director, Pediatric Brain Injury Service, Gillette Children's Specialty Health Care, and Pediatric Neurologist, Hennepin County Medical Center, Minneapolis, Minnesota

Richard Lytton, MA, CCC-SLP
Speech Language Pathologist/Program Manager, Therapeutic and Rehabilitation Services, A.I. duPont Hospital for Children, Wilmington, Delaware

Dennis J. Matthews, MD
Associate Professor and Chairman, Department of Rehabilitation Medicine, University of Colorado Health Sciences Center and Children's Hospital, Denver, Colorado

Craig M. McDonald, MD
Associate Professor, Departments of Physical Medicine and Rehabilitation and Pediatrics, University of California, Davis, School of Medicine; Director of Pediatric Rehabilitation and Neuromuscular Disease Clinics, University of California, Davis, Medical Center; and Director of Spinal Cord Injury and Spina Bifida Programs, Shriners Hospital for Children–Northern California, Sacramento, California

Michelle A. Miller, MD, FAAPMR
Clinical Assistant Professor, Department of Physical Medicine and Rehabilitation, Ohio State University College of Medicine; Pediatric Physiatrist, Children's Hospital, Columbus, Ohio

Gabriella E. Molnar, MD, FAAPMR
Emeritus Clinical Professor, Department of Physical Medicine and Rehabilitation, University of California, Davis, School of Medicine; Emeritus Director, Department of Pediatric Rehabilitation, Oakland Children's Hospital, Oakland, California

Kevin P. Murphy, MD
Medical Director, Pediatric Rehabilitation, Polinsky Medical Rehabilitation Center; Associate Professor, University of Minnesota–Duluth School of Medicine, Duluth, Minnesota

Virginia Simson Nelson, MD, MPH
Clinical Associate Professor, Department of Physical Medicine and Rehabilitation, University of Michigan Medical School; Chief, Pediatric and Adolescent Physical Medicine and Rehabilitation, C.S. Mott Children's Hospital, Ann Arbor, Michigan

Denise Peischl, BSE
Rehabilitation Engineer, A.I. duPont Hospital for Children, Wilmington, Delaware

Bruce Rens, BA, EdS, NCSP
School Psychologist, Children's Care Hospital and School; Adjunct Professor, Dordt College, Sioux Falls, South Dakota

Anne R. Robbins, PsyD
Rehabilitation Psychologist, Department of Physical Medicine and Rehabilitation, A.I. duPont Hospital for Children, Wilmington, Delaware

Cheryl Smith, PhD
Dysphagia Program Coordinator, Therapeutic Services and Rehabilitation, A.I. duPont Hospital for Children; Adjunct Associate Professor, University of Delaware, Wilmington, Delaware

Kerstin M. Sobus, MD
Medical Director, Child Evaluation and Treatment Program, University of North Dakota, Grand Forks; Altru Health System, Manvel, North Dakota

Beverly M. Steele, DNSc, RN, CS-FNP
Pediatric Nurse Practitioner, Department of Physical Medicine, The Duluth Clinic, Duluth, Minnesota

Carrie Strine, OTR/L
Therapeutic Services and Rehabilitation, A.I. duPont Hospital for Children, Wilmington, Delaware

Patricia Taggart, MBA, PT
Adjunct Assistant Professor, Department of Physical Therapy, Samuel Merritt College; Director, Rehabilitation Care, Oakland Children's Hospital, Oakland, California

Jack Uellendahl, CPO
Director of Prosthetics and Orthotics, Rehabilitation Institute of Chicago, Chicago, Illinois

Pamela Wilson, MD
Assistant Clinical Professor, Department of Rehabilitation Medicine, University of Colorado Health Sciences Center and Children's Hospital, Denver, Colorado

Preface

The field of pediatric rehabilitation has seen significant changes since the publication of the second edition of this book in 1992. Caring for children with physical disabilities became recognized as a well-defined area within the specialty of physical medicine and rehabilitation. The number of physiatrists who devote their practice entirely or partly to pediatric rehabilitation, or are now in training for a future career in this area, has increased. The editors were induced to embark on preparing this third edition in response to many requests received during the last few years. Advances in medical diagnosis, treatment methods, and rehabilitation engineering also made this endeavor necessary.

In conceptualizing and preparing the new edition, we used several principles. Our aims were (1) to provide an update on the interim medical developments and (2) to present a text that reads and looks different from the previous editions by the infusion of a group of new contributors. Further changes include an additional chapter on sports for children with disabilities, more figures and tables, and a brief summary of adult outcome in each chapter on specific disabilities. Finally, a new format has allowed the inclusion of more material.

The purpose of this volume is to provide a readily available comprehensive reference book for physiatrists, pediatricians, and other medical specialists, as well as for physical, occupational, and speech therapists, nurses, psychologists, and other allied health professionals involved in the multidisciplinary team for the rehabilitation of children with special disabilities. An extensive bibliography serves to guide further reading and is a source of additional details on each subject.

The editors wish to express appreciation to all contributing authors for their participation and commitment to this project and their willingness to share their expertise and knowledge, and for the many hours of hard work devoted to preparing such comprehensive reviews.

As are the previous editions, this book is dedicated to disabled children and their families. We are grateful for their trust and confidence, for the opportunities to share their experience in growing up with disability, and for allowing us to provide care and guidance in preparation for adulthood.

Gabriella E. Molnar, MD
Michael A. Alexander, MD

Chapter 1

History and Examination

Michael A. Alexander, MD
Gabriella E. Molnar, MD

The physiatric history and examination of a child require a blend of medical diagnostic skills to establish or confirm the diagnosis and a knowledge of child development and behavior to evaluate functional assets and difficulties for the intervention phase of rehabilitation.

Setting the Tone

To ensure the best cooperation, especially in the preschool age, the environment should be child-friendly. Exposure to crying and upset children should be avoided in the waiting room or other areas. If the family brings the child's siblings, someone should take care of them for a while so that the parents can focus on the interview without distraction. The examination room should have a small table and chair with an assortment of toys for different ages to make the child comfortable and relaxed. The examiner's attire also influences the child. A good rule is to "lose the white coat." The child is not impressed by it, and, in fact, may be intimidated from past medical visits. Pictures of cartoon characters or animals on the wall, small toys, and decals on instruments help to create a playful atmosphere and alleviate the child's fears.

The visit starts by asking the parents to tell in their own words why they came and what specific questions they have. Concerns stated by the referral source should be shared with them. Many parents are unsure about what information the visit can provide. This is the opportunity to explain what pediatric rehabilitation is and what it can offer the child and family. The examiner also should explain that it is part of the examination to watch the child so that the parents will not feel offended by the examiner's wandering gaze. Because observation of spontaneous behavior is one of the most informative aspects of evaluating youngsters with a disability, examination begins from the moment the child is in the physician's view. Questions about

history and illnesses should be asked in simple terms so that the family can understand them and provide proper information. It is also important to clarify insurance coverage and whether additional tests can be performed on the same day or must await approval.

History

Prenatal and Perinatal History

The prenatal and perinatal history includes the preconceptual period and the parents' age and health before and since the birth of the child. Maternal factors during gestation may lead to fetal malformations. Examples of these associations include febrile illnesses,[1] anticonvulsants[2] with spina bifida, maternal diabetes with caudal regression syndrome and sacral agenesis, and rubella, thalidomide, or fetal alcohol syndromes. Feeble or eventually lost fetal movements may be the earliest sign of a motor disability of prenatal origin. Prenatal care, unusual weight gain or loss, hypertension, or any other gestational problems should be explored. Mode and duration of delivery, use of anesthesia, induction, intrapartum complications, and expected and actual date of birth should be noted. History of previous pregnancies, deliveries, and fetal loss is necessary. Prenatal cerebral damage seems to be increased in infants of mothers with previous spontaneous abortions.[3]

A detailed neonatal history is essential, including birth weight, Apgar scores, onset and success of breast-feeding, and the infant's age at discharge. Weak lip seal and sucking force and inadequate feeding may be preliminary signs of oral motor dysfunction. If the infant needed admission to the neonatal intensive care unit (NICU), what were the problems, medications, and supportive measures? Neonatal seizures may signal pre- or perinatal brain damage. Prematurity, particularly very low birth weight, is a frequent cause of cerebral palsy. Large birth weight may lead to intrapartum trauma, brachial plexus palsy, or, on rare occasions, spinal cord injury, particularly with breech or other fetal malposition. When extended hospitalization was required, one should note the infant's age, weight, and condition on discharge, including means of feeding and need for ventilatory or other supportive measures at home, which may predict subsequent, persistent, or recurrent problems.

Developmental History

The developmental history should cover all major aspects of function and behavior. For details of developmental milestones and testing, the reader is referred to chapter 2. This discussion presents only guidelines for the purpose of diagnostic interpretations. Discrepancies between different areas of functioning provide clues about the nature of medical diagnosis and developmental disability.

Delayed accomplishments, primarily in motor function, suggest a neuromuscular deficit. One of the earliest signs that parents report is lack of spontaneous movements when the infant is held or placed in the crib. They may add that the baby feels limp or stiff, suggesting hypotonia or spasticity. In all cases of motor dysfunction it is important to clarify whether the dysfunction was a steady, continuing delay from an early age, suggesting a static disease, or an arrest or regression noted at a particular point. However, the relatively fast pace of early motor development may mask slow deterioration due to progressive neurologic disease for a while.

Developmental history and subsequent assessment must take into consideration the interactive effect of coexistent deficits. A significant cognitive dysfunction by itself may delay gross and fine motor development.[4] It also tends to enhance the functional consequences of a neuromuscular disability. Slow development in personal and adaptive tasks that require both motor and cognitive abilities may be related to impairment in either area. A combination of both can create the impression that the motor deficit is more severe than it actually is.

A history of delay in communication development raises several differential diagnostic possibilities: (1) true language dysfunction affecting receptive or expressive domains or both; (2) oral motor dysfunction interfering with speech production; and (3) significant hearing loss. In a child with motor disability language dysfunction may result from diffuse or focal cerebral lesions, such as head injury or cerebral palsy, particularly when cognitive function is also affected.

The ability to follow simple and, at a later point, complex commands indicates preserved receptive language even in the absence of verbalization. Parents report a variety of responses, such as smiling, cooing, crying, pointing, or vocalization with inflection as a substitute for speech. Oral motor dysfunction is also associated with cerebral palsy, most often with spastic quadriparesis or dyskinetic disorders due to suprabulbar or pseudobulbar palsy. Bulbar palsy in medullary involvement affects speech production, for example, in spinal muscular atrophy or spina bifida with syringobulbia. There is a close association between anatomic structures and neurologic control for speech and oral feeding. Concurrent oral motor dysfunction with feeding difficulties is an additional sign of bulbar or pseudobulbar pathology and confirms the suspicion of speech production deficit. In such cases, history of early feeding is most relevant. For example, was there a good lip seal and strong suction on breast-feeding? When bottle-fed, the infant can handle 4 oz in about 10 minutes, and feedings every 3–4 hours are generally adequate. The need for longer and more frequent feeding to maintain weight gain, especially during the first few months; coughing; nasal regurgitation of liquids; difficulty with drinking from a cup; and difficulty with introduction of solid food due to chewing problems are early symptoms of oral motor dysfunction and a possible subsequent deficit in speech production. Augmentative communication training should be initiated early in such cases. Hearing is an essential factor for speech development. Early cooing and babbling are innate characteristics of infants and involve the same vocal components regardless of the language spoken in their environment. Infants with hearing loss start to fall behind after 6–8 months of age when learning of auditory-dependent vocalization begins. Parents may notice a decrease even in spontaneous babbling at that age. All neonates and infants at high risk for developmental disability or recurrent ear infections should have an initial and, if warranted, repeated hearing evaluations. Correction of hearing deficit should be provided as soon as possible after it is detected.[5]

For infants and young children the history is obtained from parents or caretakers. While gathering information from one person about another, the examiner gains an understanding of both and establishes rapport with parents and child. Early school-aged children can provide some information about themselves and should be encouraged to do so. Preadolescents and particularly adolescents generally prefer to give an account of their problems and achievements.

Adolescents often wish to have privacy without the parent present at least for part of the visit.

General Health History

The examiner should determine whether the patient is an essentially well child with an impairment or a sick child who has been hospitalized several times. In the latter case one should explore in detail the frequency, reasons, tests, and treatments. Even if one has access to records, the parents should be asked to tell the child's history in their own words. Their account provides an insight into their knowledge and participation in the child's care. One should ask how many visits they make to medical centers and therapists and how much time is spent in transit for the child's care.

History of allergies to medications or other substances should be noted. An early history of allergies to different and often inconsistent formulas may indicate that the child in fact had feeding difficulties, which were attributed to allergy. Multiple exposures to Latex and any signs of allergy should be determined, particularly in spina bifida or after repeated surgeries. Any medications that the child takes regularly, including diet supplements or aerosols, should be recorded with dosage and schedule. The risk and incidence of seizures are higher in static and progressive diseases of the central nervous system. Overt or suspicious signs, type and frequency of seizures, anticonvulsants, and their effectiveness and possible side effects should be recorded.

Nutrition with special consideration for the child's disability should be reviewed. Feeding difficulties or behavior problems may lead to inadequate consumption of calories and essential nutrients. Dietary intake may be lower than required for the increased energy expenditure on physical activities in children with motor disability. In contrast, caloric intake may be excessive when physical activity level is restricted and lead to obesity, most often in wheelchair users with spina bifida[6] or muscular dystrophy. Dietary information and guidance are fundamental for regulation of neurogenic bowel incontinence. Family eating patterns should be taken into consideration. Injuries, burns, fractures, and spinal cord and head trauma are followed by a catabolic state. Monitoring of weight, nutrition, and fluid intake is essential during inpatient rehabilitation for major injuries. Caloric requirements for children are calculated from age-appropriate standards, which take into consideration growth (Table 1–1). In children with motor disability, upward or downward adjustment in height and weight may be

TABLE 1–1. Selected Physiologic Guidelines in Childhood

1. Calorie and fluid requirements (3,7,12,18,22,23,37,60)*

Age	Cal/kg	Protein gm/kg	Water ml/kg
Infancy	120	2.2	120–150
1 yr	110	2.0–2.2	120–135
2–3 yr	100	1.8–2.0	100–125
4–6 yr	85–90	1.5–1.6	90–100
7–10 yr	80–85	1.5	75–100
11–14 yr	60–70	1.2	50–70
15–18 yr	50–60	0.8–1.0	40–60

2. Blood pressure and heart rate (68, 72)

Age	In Seated Position		At Rest
	Systolic	Diastolic	Heart Rate/Min
Infancy	80	55	125
1 yr	90	55	120
2–5 yr	90–94	55	100–110
6–9 yr	95–98	55–60	90–100
10–13 yr	98–109	60–65	85–90
14–18 yr	110–115	63–68	70–80

3. Vital Capacity (39)

Newborn	5 Years	10 Years	15 Years
100 cc	1300 cc	2300 cc	4000 cc

4. Urinary output (7, 60): 2 ml/kg/hr in infants and young children

5. Bladder capacity (8, 36, 47): newborn = 16-25 ml; 1–14 years = (age in years + 2) × 30 ml

* Numbers in parentheses refer to references.

needed, depending on their level of physical activity and individual growth trend. Specific recommendations are available for children with spina bifida to avoid obesity.[7,8]

History of respiratory complications, past or present, should be explored in certain disabilities. Central ventilatory dysfunction (CVD) is a complication of Arnold-Chiari malformation in spina bifida.[9] Syringobulbia may cause similar symptoms. Nightmares, insomnia, and night sweating are complaints associated with hypercapnia and may be reported in advanced stages of muscular dystrophy or atrophy. Hypercapnia and sleep apnea may occur in diseases of the central nervous system. Intercostal muscle paralysis in high thoracic paraplegia with spinal cord injury or spina bifida, spinal muscular atrophy, or advanced muscle diseases leads to inefficient pulmonary ventilation and handling of secretions. With severe spastic or dyskinetic cerebral palsy, the respiratory musculature may lack coordination. Such children are prone to recurrent bouts of pulmonary infections. Coexistent feeding difficulties with minor aspirations or restrictive pulmonary disease due to spinal deformities are additional adverse factors. Restricted mobility of the spine and thoracic cage may be present in ankylosing spondylitis or severe systemic-onset juvenile rheumatoid arthritis. Detailed information about home management and use and frequency of equipment must be included in the history. Exercise dyspnea may be a sign of pulmonary compromise or deconditioning due to high energy cost of physical activities in children with a motor disability. Cardiac decompensation with right-sided failure, a potential complication of pulmonary dysfunction, is more likely to occur in older children or young adults with the above disabilities. Myopathic conduction defects and arrhythmias are often symptom-free in the absence of heart failure. Consultation with pulmonary and/or cardiology specialists should be arranged when history reveals suspicious symptoms.

Visual and hearing impairments are more frequent in childhood disabilities. Inquiry about these aspects of function should not be overlooked in taking the history. The necessity of regular hearing assessment was mentioned earlier. The same applies to visual function. Prenatal infections, anoxic or infectious encephalopathy, metabolic diseases, meningitis, hydrocephalus, and head injury warrant exploration of visual and auditory function. With the development of new antibiotics, acquired hearing deficit due to antibiotic use is not a significant concern. Like all children, handicapped youngsters are prone to having a variety of childhood illnesses. In some cases, however, acute symptoms and febrile illnesses may be directly related to complications of a specific disability. Vomiting, headache, irritability, or lethargy may be prodromal signs of decompensating hydrocephalus in spina bifida, cerebral palsy,[2] or an intercurrent unrelated illness. Recurrent headaches are also a manifestation of autonomic dysreflexia in spinal cord injury, along with bowel or bladder distention. Fever may represent central hyperpyrexia in severe head injury or hyperthermia due to sudorimotor paralysis in high thoracic spinal cord injury. However, such conclusions can be reached only after other causes of fever have been excluded. In neurogenic bladder, urinary tract infection should always be investigated as a possible cause of febrile illness. A history of the usual pattern of the amount and frequency of voiding is essential in neurogenic bladder dysfunction. Systematic daily recording is a guide for bladder training. Fluid intake, in accordance with pediatric norms, needs to be monitored at home, and records of both bladder and bowel dysfunction should be available on the medical visit (see Table 1–1).

Immunization history is part of all pediatric visits. Often a disabled child in good health has not received the recommended vaccinations because of excessive concern on the part of the family or pediatrician. But it also may mean that the child has always looked ill when scheduled for immunization.

History of Behavior

The examiner should ask about the child's behavior in terms of temperament and personality. The parents may state that the child was always a good baby, but this report may mean that the youngster never cried and slept more than expected for age. In other cases, parents may report excessive crying and restlessness while the child is awake and during sleep. Some children may show excessive mood swings from lethargy to hyperactivity, whereas others are even-tempered and react appropriately. One should ask the parents whether the child is friendly, outgoing, and sociable or shy and withdrawn, particularly in group situations. Parental guidance may be needed to encourage interactive behavior by the child. Compliance or problems with obedience, daily activity level, attention span, sleeping and eating habits, and special interests and dislikes are revealing information. Separation from the parents may be a problem for children with disability. The parents may be uncomfortable to leave the child with relatives or other caretakers. In this context it is important to point out the need and methods to foster the child's independence.

Educational and Social History

Very young children may be enrolled in an early intervention program, home- or center-based. Frequency, length of sessions, components of training, the child's tolerance and cooperation in the program, and its effectiveness, as perceived by the parents, should be clarified. The same applies when the slightly older child attends a preschool program. In school-aged children, information about the type of class—mainstream, integrated, or special education—is important. Academic expectations are different in each of these educational pathways and should be taken into consideration when report card grades are interpreted. Individualized education program (IEP) meetings and environmental accommodations are other pertinent details. The child may have special interests and strengths that should be further developed or difficulties in certain subjects, which may require additional help and adjustment of the

IEP. Review of educational status is a consistent part of follow-up visits, and assistance should be offered when problems arise.

Opportunities to meet and play with other children in addition to school or home contacts, visits and sleepovers with friends and participation in various recreational activities are formative experiences that prepare all youngsters for social functioning and adulthood. Asking the parents to describe the child's daily schedule, including regular and occasional activities on weekdays and weekends, yields a valuable insight into these aspects of the entire family's lifestyle. Time spent in school, therapy, homework, play, and leisure activities with family members, friends, or alone should be noted. Housing, employment of the parents, siblings and their ages, and social support of the family provide further understanding of the physical and social environment. Some families with a disabled child experience social isolation. Information about or referral to community resources is helpful in all cases.

Family History

In motor or other developmental disabilities a detailed family history must be obtained to rule out the possibility of an inheritable genetic disease. Health and function of the parents, siblings, and other family members on the maternal and paternal side should be explored through several preceding generations. One should ask specifically whether there are other children in the family with developmental delay or adults with known motor disability, limb deficiency, or other malformations. Historical information is at times incomplete until further questioning brings to light additional facts. Family albums and pictures of relatives may be helpful to detect dysmorphic facial or other features. Consanguinity is an increased risk for genetic disease, including diseases with a recessive autosomal inheritance pattern. In some autosomal dominant conditions mild variants of a disease may be missed until a thorough investigation of suspected family members is carried out. Congenital myotonic dystrophy and facioscapulohumeral dystrophy are examples. Affected males with familial history on the maternal side are typical of X-linked conditions. Multifactorial inheritance, such as spina bifida, creates a complex situation with or without known familial history.[2,7] Referral for genetic work-up is necessary whenever a genetic condition is known or suspected. Pregnant mothers of affected children should be referred for genetic counseling; prenatal diagnostic tests for detection are also available.

Examination

This chapter provides only general guidelines for the format and structure of the pediatric rehabilitation examination at different ages. Specific details of diagnostic signs and interpretation of findings are discussed in subsequent chapters about different disabilities.

Observation

As emphasized previously, the examination begins as soon as the family and child enter the examination room, before the child is actually touched or asked to perform. Sometimes it may be the most informative phase of the examination.

Specific behaviors to observe and note include (1) reaction to separation from the parents (in young children); (2) apparent visual and auditory awareness; (3) temperament (calm or hyperactive, compliant or difficult); (4) spontaneous exploration and interest in toys, games, or books in the room; (5) style, concentration, attention span, or distractibility during play; (6) level and manner of motor activities; (7) attempts to engage the parents and the examiner in conversation, vocabulary, complexity of language, and quality of speech; and (8) interaction with parents or examiner (appropriate, shy, or demanding). Observations of the parents' response and their way of handling the child's behavior are also revealing.

Examination by Age

For infants and young children the examiner must create an atmosphere of trust. Friendly advances during history taking or while the child is at play allay initial fears and anxiety. At this age most, if not all, of the examination can be accomplished with the child in the parent's lap if the child remains fearful. Interactive play in this phase of the examination can incorporate developmental testing by offering toys for grasping or raisins to test pincer grasp. Hearing, vision, cranial nerves, and postural abnormalities also can be observed.

As the parent gradually undresses the child, gentle touch and tickling or funny sounds with a smile help to maintain relaxation and to facilitate hands-on examination. Inspection and palpation of body parts and gentle movements to examine tone are performed at this point. The examiner should be prepared to improvise if the child shows increasing anxiety.

The actual hands-on examination, consisting of bodily handling and manipulation, is the last stage; anxiety-provoking or painful tests are deferred to the end. If the examination requires placement of the child on a table, the mother can sit at the end and let the child's head rest in her lap. With anxious children performance of gross motor activities, such as sitting, crawling, standing, or walking also can be conducted through the parent. One should note the quality of movements, postures, weakness, incoordination, asymmetry, or reflex abnormalities that reflect a motor deficit. Range of motion, deep tendon reflexes, or primitive reflexes that need physical manipulation should be examined after evaluation of active mobility. Tests that require instrumentation, such as sensation, fundoscopy, otoscopy, and oral function, conclude the examination.

Giving choices involves the preschool child in the examination. For example, the examiner may ask, "Should we look at your arm or leg now?" On the other hand, questions such as "Can I look at your arm?" should be avoided because if the child says "no," confrontation results. Parents can often bring out many capabilities of their children without the examiner touching them.

School-aged and Adolescent Patients

The customary method of systematic medical examination is applicable. Children with cognitive deficit need to be approached according to their mental rather than chronologic age. Children in this age group, particularly adolescents, are usually embarrassed about walking in underwear in front of their parents. Shorts or a bathing suit is more acceptable. Adolescents need to be seen with and without their parents. Their concerns may be different from those of the family and should be addressed with respect for their privacy.

The scope of the examination is expanded to reflect the growing child's increasing functional needs in activities of daily living (ADLs) and other areas of competence. A comprehensive examination includes screening in educational achievements, reading, writing, and arithmetic. Formal psychological or pychoeducational testing follows in case of deficits.

Growth

Parameters of physical growth should be routinely measured on each visit and plotted on the standard growth chart. Height and weight are obtained at all ages, and head circumference is measured in children under 3 years and thereafter in children with deviations. Serial monitoring is necessary in hydrocephalus, regardless of etiology, and microcephaly, which reflects defective brain growth. In spina bifida and other disabilities that require full-time wheelchair use, arm span measurement is recommended instead of height.[7] Extremity length and girth are recorded in children with localized growth disturbance due to neurogenic weakness, epiphyseal fracture, or arthritis. In growth disturbances that involve one side of the body, one must determine whether the condition represents hemihypertrophy or hemiatrophy. Hemihypertrophy unrelated to neurologic causes requires investigation for renal tumor.

Inspection

General appearance and special features may help to establish a diagnostic entity. Dysmorphic facial features, epicanthal folds, increased intercanthal distance, external ear anomalies, and malformations of the toes or fingers suggest a prenatal disorder, possibly teratogenic or genetic, and at times an identifiable syndrome.[10] Blue sclerae are a sign of osteogenesis imperfecta. Asymmetric face and palpebral fissures and pupils may indicate facial palsy or Horner syndrome, whereas craniofacial asymmetry and vertical strabismus develop in torticollis. Dolichocepaly is typical in premature infants and children. A bald spot or area of short, thinning hair over the posterior skull is a sign of weak neck muscles, most likely associated with generalized weakness. Extraocular, facial, and tongue muscle weakness may represent cranial nerve dysfunction, myopathy, or other neurologic disease. Involuntary eye movements and nystagmus are noted in cerebellar or other CNS disorders.

The skin should be inspected for telangiectasias, nevi, or other lesions. Café-au-lait spots or pigmented skin areas are seen in neurofibromatosis. In children with ataxia, telangiectasic skin lesions are usually present over the flexor surface of the knees and elbows. Malar rash suggests a rheumatic disease. Adenomatous rash, seizures, and hemiplegia are present in tuberous sclerosis. Hairy patches, dimples, or other skin lesions over the spine are frequent signs of spina bifida occulta.[7] A small sinus, dermal tract, or pylonidal cyst in the gluteal crease also may accompany occult spina bifida. Sudden weakness in such cases may indicate an infection penetrating into the spinal canal or a neurologic complication related to underlying malformation in or around the spinal cord. In children with sensory deficit the entire area must be routinely examined for skin lesions, pressure abrasions, ulcerations, and infections. Foot deformities, varus or valgus deformity, or claw toes lead to abnormal weight distribution and callus formation consistent with the pathologic posture. Calluses over the dorsum of the feet and knees, the so-called "housemaid's knee," develop in older children whose preferred mode of locomotion is crawling. Multiple scars, bruises, and abrasions in various stages of healing may indicate frequent falls or child abuse.

Asymmetry in the size of skeletal muscles should be noted in terms of location and distribution. Anterior axillary and upper chest muscle atrophy may represent absent pectoralis muscle or wasting due to an old brachial plexus injury. Congenital clubfeet or multiple joint deformities are manifestations of prenatal muscle weakness due to spina bifida, arthrogryposis, or myotonic dystrophy or may be idiopathic. A hypertrophic, "muscle-bound" appearance is a sign of myotonic dystrophy. Deformed, fusiform, dimpled joints are seen in arthrogryposis. Lower extremity joint positions reflect the distribution of muscle weakness in newborns with spina bifida. Hypertrophy of the calf muscles is an early sign of Duchenne muscular dystrophy. Hypertrophic musculature of the shoulder girdles and upper extremities is a convincing indication of functional crutch walking or effective wheelchair locomotion. An enlarged limb with bruit detectable by palpation or auscultation may signal an arteriovenous shunt and increased blood flow in the extremity.

Flaring of the ribs or the so-called bell-shaped chest suggests ineffective intercostal muscle function in children with motor unit disease or high spinal cord dysfunction. In scoliosis the thoracic cage is asymmetric.

Palpation

In infants and young children the fontanelles and cranial sutures should be palpated for patency, tension, and size with the child in sitting position and while the child is quiet and not crying. A tense fontanel in a vigorously crying child does not necessarily mean increased intracranial pressure. In case of ventriculoperitoneal shunt, the reservoir should be located and checked for ease of emptying and speed of refill.

The skin should be felt for texture, temperature, and absent or excessive perspiration. Sudorimotor paralysis in spinal cord injury eliminates sweating below the level of the lesion, and compensatory excessive perspiration occurs above the level of the lesion with high environmental temperature. Vasomotor dysfunction with coldness to touch and paleness or slight cyanosis of the skin may be present in severe upper motor neuron impairment. It is seen in the lower extremities of some children with cerebral palsy. Subcutaneous abnormalities may be palpable, such as hard calcific deposits in dermatomyositis or neurofibromatous nodules along the course of peripheral nerves. When arthritis is suspected, each joint should be felt for the cardinal signs of inflammation, warmth, discomfort, and swelling due to synovial thickening and effusion.

Much can be learned from palpation of muscles. Tone and bulk are reduced in lower motor neuron paralysis, and in longstanding denervation the muscle tissue feels less resilient and fibrotic. The pseudohypertrophic calf muscles in Duchenne muscular dystrophy have a typical rubbery, doughy, hard consistency. A fibrotic nodule is usually palpable in the sternocleidomastoid muscle in congenital torticollis. In an infant who has an isolated knee extension contracture, a palpable nodule in the quadriceps indicates fibrotic muscle changes at the site of previous repeated intramuscular injections. Localized pain and swelling accompany injuries to soft tissue or bone. Osteoporotic fractures in lower motor neuron lesions with sensory deficit show swelling but are painless. Tenderness in many muscle groups with weakness, fatigue, or skin rash is suspicious for myositis due to collagen disease or parasitic or viral infections.

Organ Systems

Although the primary health care of children with disabilities remains the responsibility of the pediatrician, the pediatric physiatrist should perform a selective general physical examination. The emphasis is placed on organ systems that are at increased risk in certain handicaps and may affect both overall health and successful rehabilitation.

Vital signs, including blood pressure and heart rate, are obtained in all patients. Table 1–1 shows selected physiologic parameters by age in children. In myopathies and collagen diseases cardiac auscultation should be performed because of the possibility of associated heart disease. In a child with developmental delay the presence of a heart murmur may suggest an undiagnosed syndrome. Blood pressure monitoring is particularly important in spinal cord injury, neurogenic bladder, Guillain-Barré syndrome, and residual poliomyelitis, as well as in children receiving stimulant medications.

In disabilities that cause ineffective ventilation and involve the risk of minor aspirations, auscultation of the lungs must be a routine procedure. Myopathies, thoracic spinal cord dysfunction due to injury or malformation, severe spastic quadriparetic cerebral palsy, and any disability with oral motor dysfunction are such indications.

Abdominal and rectal examinations are essential in children with neurogenic bladder and bowel dysfunction to evaluate bladder distention, bowel or rectal impaction, and anal sphincter tone. Stool consistency, intermittent or continuous bladder incontinence, and gross appearance and microscopic examination of the urine should be noted. Umbilical movements in response to eliciting superficial abdominal reflexes help to delineate the spinal cord level in thoracic lesions. Absent abdominal muscles result in loose skin folds resembling a prune; hence the name prune-belly syndrome.

Neuromuscular System

Examination of neuromuscular function consists of testing reflexes, tone, active motion, strength, and coordination. Limited understanding and cooperation in infants and young children requires adaptation of traditional methods of testing. After 4–5 years of age the standard examination is generally applicable.

In infancy reflex testing includes age-appropriate responses that reflect early immaturity and subsequent maturation of the central nervous system. These primitive reflexes and postural responses and their implications are discussed in Chapter 2.

In newborns and young infants, state of alertness, activity, and comfort influence muscle tone.[11-14] If the baby is anxious, upset, restless, or crying, this part of the examination should be postponed. Valid assessment may require several attempts. In the first few months of life flexor tone predominates. Hypotonia or hypertonicity signals neurologic abnormalities. Increased tone is the symptom of corticospinal or basal ganglion damage. Myopathy, cerebellar dysfunction, and lower motor neuron lesions due to anterior horn disease, neuropathy, or spina bifida result in hypotonia. However, a hypotonic stage usually precedes the appearance of increased tone in perinatal anoxic brain damage.[15] This stage of hypotonicity tends to last longer in dyskinetic cerebral palsy than in spastic types. On passive motion of hypotonic muscles or extremities no resistance is felt. The infant with generalized hypotonia is limp and floppy with handling and, in severe cases, may feel like a "rag-doll"—a descriptive term for this finding. In hypotonia related to motor unit disease or lower motor neuron lesion, deep tendon reflexes are diminished or absent. In contrast, they are present or increased in floppy infants during the transient hypotonic phase of central

nervous system damage.[15] Spastic hypertonicity and related postures are influenced by position in space and the effect of gravity. The child should be examined in supine, prone, and vertical positions to elicit typical postures. Examples include increased scissoring, extension, and plantarflexion of the legs when a child with spastic cerebral palsy is suddenly lifted into vertical suspension. Resistance to both slow and fast stretching of muscle should be tested to differentiate rigidity from spasticity.[16] In infants and young children one may use a number of developmental reflexes to examine active movements and strength.[17] The Moro reflex includes shoulder abduction followed by forward flexion of the arm. Eliciting palmar or plantar grasp reflexes demonstrates finger or toe flexor function. Asymmetric responses in the upper extremities may suggest Erb or Klumpke paralysis or hemiplegia. Unilateral or bilateral absence of protective extension response is likewise suggestive of weakness in the respective extremity. A 4-month-old infant elevates the head and trunk on extended arms in the prone position. Scapular winging during this activity is a sign of a weak serratus anterior muscle.[18] In older children the wheelbarrow maneuver demonstrates the same finding.[18] Lifting up under the axilla elicits spontaneous active shoulder depression. When these muscles are weak, the shoulders slide upward, virtually touching ears. These signs suggest myopathy with proximal weakness.

Young children often adopt ingenious substitutions or vicarious movements to cope with weakness of particular muscles. With weakness of the deltoid they may fling the arm forward by momentum or substitute the long head of the biceps for shoulder flexion. In advanced shoulder and elbow weakness they may "walk up" the arm on the torso, using their fingers to get the hand to the mouth. Combat crawl is a usual way of crawling in lower extremity paralysis. Deformities around a joint reflect an imbalance of strength in muscles acting on the joint. The deformity or deviation is in the direction of overpull. Such imbalance may be spastic or paralytic.

Visual observation during performance of functional activities to detect muscle weakness should consider the child's age and the achievements expected for the child's developmental stage. Walking on tiptoes, squatting and rising without using the arms for assistance, and straight sitting up from the supine position without rolling to the prone position or to the side are mastered by children around 3 years of age.[19] Thus, inability of younger children to perform these activities in a mature pattern should not be interpreted as weakness of the plantarflexors, hip and knee extensors, or abdominal muscles. Testing for the Trendelenburg sign and grading the triceps surae by having the child rise on the toes of one leg must be deferred until 4 years of age when children develop adequate balance.

The standard technique of manual muscle testing can be used after school age except in children who have serious behavioral problems or mental retardation.[20-23] The customary grading system of scores from 0–5 or zero to normal is used. Above fair grade the wide range of normal variations in growth patterns should be considered in judging good vs. normal strength. Because children are adept in using substitution movements, the examiner must pay special attention and adhere to precise technical conduct of testing individual muscles. Side-to-side comparison may detect even mild neurologic weakness, although disuse atrophy or mild bilateral neurologic weakness may escape detection. Quantitative strength determination with comparison of both sides is helpful to demonstrate unilateral disuse atrophy in such strong muscles as the quadriceps. This determination is particularly advisable in teenage athletes after knee injury. Resumption of training for competition before virtually equal bilateral quadriceps strength is regained predisposes to recurrent injuries. Testing of strength in upper motor neuron lesions requires the well-known considerations for position in space and orientation of head and major joints, which may affect recruitment of motor units and produce synergistic movement patterns.

A common sign of central movement disorders is impaired coordination. Proprioceptive sensory loss or parietal lobe syndrome may contribute to incoordination. Movement abnormalities associated with cerebellar dysfunction, basal ganglion disease, dyskinetic disorders, or spastic incoordination present with specific distinguishing signs. Detection of coordination deficit is based mostly on observation of gross and fine motor function in children less than 2–3 years of age. Concurrent mild delay of motor development is not unusual. After 3 years of age the examination becomes more specific for testing the quality of performance in complex and more advanced developmental skills. Around 3 years of age the child can walk along a straight line, unsteadily placing one foot in front of the other. In comparison, facility at tandem walking at 5 years of age is a good illustration of continuing refinement of motor skills with age. The pediatric physiatrist may be asked to evaluate the appropriateness of coordination in children without an overt physical disability.[24] Clumsiness of handwriting and drawing, difficulties in physical education or sports, and other subtle signs may be present. Such children may have a motor incompetence of apraxic nature, sometimes related to visuomotor perceptual deficit.[25] It also may be associated with learning and behavioral dysfunction. A number of tests are available for examining motor proficiency and dexterity in children without physical disability.[26,27] Tasks to evaluate youngsters with minor neurologic dysfunction include imitation of gestures,[28] hopping,[29] hand-clapping,[30] and pegboard performance.[31-32]

Musculoskeletal System

Examination of the musculoskeletal system includes inspection and palpation of bones and soft tissues, measurement of active and passive joint range of motion, and assessment of stance and gait.[33-36] It is complementary to neuromuscular assessment. As in previous parts of this chapter, only developmental variations are discussed.

Bone configuration and joint mobility change during the growing years.[37-38] Full-term infants may lack as much as 25° of elbow extension because of predominant flexor tone. In contrast, joint hyperextensibility and hypotonia allow increased passive motion in preterm infants. The scarf sign is a good illustration of excessive joint mobility in premature babies. Holding the infant's hand, the examiner draws one arm across the chest, like a scarf, toward the contralateral shoulder. In premature infants the elbow crosses the midline, indicating hypotonic laxity of the shoulder and elbow joints. Full-term neonates have incomplete hip extension with an average limitation of 30° as a result of early flexor tone predominance.[37,38] The limitation decreases to less than 10° by 3–6 months. At birth and during early infancy, hip external rotation exceeds internal rotation.[37,39] With the resolution of early hip flexion attitude, internal rotation gradually increases. Differences between bilateral hip abduction, apparent shortening of one leg, and asymmetric gluteal and upper thigh skin folds are highly suggestive of congenital or acquired hip dysplasia or dislocation.[38] Alignment of the femoral neck in neonates is consistent with prenatal coxa valga and increased anteversion. Femoral inclination is 160°, and the angle of anteversion is 60°. Respective adult measurements of 125 and 10–20° develop postnatally accelerated by weight bearing. Persistent fetal configuration in nonambulatory children with physical disabilities enhances the effect of neurogenic muscle imbalance on the hip joint and contributes to acquired hip dislocation in spina bifida and cerebral palsy. The popliteal angle is 180° in the hypotonic preterm infant compared with 90° in full-term neonates. A combination of increased flexor tone and retroversion of the proximal tibia causes this limitation of knee extension in mature newborns. By 10 years tibial retroversion resolves spontaneously. An early varus configuration of the tibia contributes to the physiologic bowleg appearance in infancy and corrects itself by 2–3 years of age. A systematic review of skeletal development with examination of the spine and extremities is presented in chapter 19.

The most significant developmental changes of posture and gait in childhood are described in Table 2–5 of Chapter 2. Normal variations of stance and gait should not be mistaken for pathology in the growing child.[35,40,41] Gait abnormalities evident on clinical observation include (1) asymmetric stride length and stance phase in hemiparesis; (2) toe walking and scissoring with lower extremity spasticity; (3) crouch posture and gait in diplegic cerebral palsy; (4) Trendelenburg gait in motor unit diseases and hip dislocation; (5) gastrocnemius limp with lack of push-off in L4–L5 weakness due to spina bifida; and (6) various types of gait deviations associated with involuntary movements, such as ataxia, tremor, or dyskinesias, in dysfunction of the central nervous system.

Sensory Examination

A complete examination of all peripheral sensory modalities is possible only in older children.[42] Nevertheless, some modalities can be tested in infants and young children and provide significant information. An infant who cries and squirms to move away from pinprick obviously perceives pain.[43] A sleepy infant may be slow to respond and requires repeated stimuli. Withdrawal of the leg from painful stimuli may represent the triple flexion spinal withdrawal reflex in thoracic spinal cord lesion and should not be mistaken for active movement and presence of sensation. Comparing the infant's reaction to pinprick on the arms or face differentiates actual sensory perception in such cases. Older infants respond to touch and vibration by turning toward or moving away from the stimulus. Presence of superficial reflexes signals an intact afferent and efferent reflex arc. The neurosegmental levels are T8–T12 for abdominal reflexes, L1–L2 for the cremasteric reflex, and S4–S5 for the anocutaneous reflex. In spina bifida absence of these reflexes generally coincides with sensory deficit in the respective dermatomes. In young children who cannot

be tested for proprioceptive function, ataxia and incoordination may suggest absence of this sensation. Testing of position sense is usually reliable by school age.

Cortical sensory function is impaired in parietal lobe damage.[42,44] The most frequent childhood example is hemiparetic cerebral palsy. Disproportionately poor spontaneous function, neglect, and visual monitoring during use of the arm and hand are suspicious signs. Objective evaluation is generally feasible after 5–6 years of age, using the same technique as in adults for stereognosis, two-point discrimination,[45] and topagnosia with single or double sensory stimulation. Testing for graphesthesia may be attempted by using a circle or square. Around 8 years of age the traditional number identification gives more accurate information. Cutaneous sensation and proprioception must be intact, and adequate cognitive ability is a prerequisite for testing cortical sensory function.

The child's age and ability to cooperate need to be considered in the examination of special senses. Moving a bright light or attractive object across the visual field is used to test vision in infants. At 1 month the infant will follow to midline and at 3 months from side to side through a 180° arc. The Stycar test and the illiterate E chart are used for screening preschool children at risk for visual deficit.[46,47] At an early age, unilateral impairment or loss of vision and visual field defects, such as hemianopsia, are more likely to remain undetected than bilateral deficits. A child with strabismus or suspicion of diminished vision should see an ophthalmologist as soon as the problems are discovered. Early treatment with eye patching or corrective lenses is necessary to prevent amblyopia ex anopsia.[48,49] Central dysfunction of visual attentiveness, discrimination, and information processing may be misinterpreted as diminished vision and requires both ophthalmologic and neuropsychologic investigation.

Screening of auditory function is a routine procedure in the neonatal nursery, pediatric office, and school. The examination of handicapped infants and children also should include simple screening of hearing, eliciting the blink or startle reflex. Responses by hand clapping to speech of conversational loudness or whisper, perception of finger rubbing near the ear, and reaction to tuning fork, bell, or cricket toy are methods of testing. Absent, lost, or delayed speech, articulation deficits, inattentiveness to sound, a history of recurrent otitis media, head injury, or failure to pass the screening test indicates a need for complete evaluation of auditory function.[43,48,50,51]

Functional Evaluation

The pediatric rehabilitation examination is meaningless if the physiatrist does not construct from it a coherent picture of the child's functional achievements. This evaluation both complements and integrates the variety of information derived from all phases of the examination.

The developmental diagnostic evaluation is a convenient, functionally oriented assessment tool for infants and preschool children.[19,52] Language, fine motor and adaptive skills, gross motor abilities, and personal-social behavior are the four major areas of function in the organizational framework of developmental testing. The same functional domains are considered in the evaluation of older children and adolescents. However, in these age groups the examination includes a wider range of developmental expectations and abilities to function in school and society. ADLs and gross mobility skills need to be assessed in this context. In addition to speech, testing of language function includes other modes of communication—reading, writing, spelling, and, if indicated, augmentative communication. Drawing, design construction, arithmetic problems, and questions about handling hypothetical situations in daily life offer a brief, preliminary insight into cognitive and learning abilities. A number of specific assessment instruments were designed for various childhood disabilities[53–56] (see Table 2–2). These instruments are useful functional assessment tools for their designated conditions and appropriately complement the customary developmental evaluation.

Informing Interview

Informing the family about the findings of the examination and their implications is an important responsibility of the physician. Factual information must be imparted with a caring attitude. Informing the parents about a newly established diagnosis should be considered as crisis intervention. A diagnostic label is insufficient without explanation of its meaning. The parents need to know the estimated prognosis, including the uncertainties of early prognostication, particularly in central nervous system dysfunction with the possibility of multiple handicaps. Future needs in care and functional rehabilitation should be outlined. One should emphasize the need to avoid focusing on the physical disability alone and to consider the child's developmental and social needs. Effective counseling and communication skills are essential for establishing a partnership between the physician and family to ensure the successful outcome of a comprehensive rehabilitation program.

References

1. Milunski A, Ulcickas M, et al: Maternal heat exposure and neural tube defects. JAMA 1992;268:882.
2. Aicardi J: Diseases of the nervous system in childhood. Clin Dev Med 1992;11:118.
3. Nelson KB, Ellenberg JH: Antecedent of cerebral palsy: Multivariant analysis of risk. N Engl J Med 1986;315:81.
4. Molnar GE: Motor deficit in retarded infants and young children. Arch Phys Med Rehab 1974;55:393.
5. Northern J, Downs M: Hearing in Children, 4th ed. Baltimore, Williams & Wilkins, 1991.
6. Mita K, Akataki K, et al: Assessment of obesity in children with spina bifida. Dev Med Child Neurol 1993;35:305.
7. Shurtleff DB (ed): Myelodysplasias and Extrophies: Significance, Prevention and Treatment. New York, Grune and Stratton, 1986.
8. Roberts D, Sheperd RW, et al: Anthropometry and obesity in myelomeningocele. J Pediatr Child Health 1991;27:83.
9. Hays R, Jordan R, et al: Central respiratory dysfunction in myelodysplasia: An independent determination of survival. Dev Med Child Neurol 1989;31:366.
10. Jones KL: Smith's Recognizable Patterns of Human Malformation, 5th ed. Philadelphia, WB Saunders, 1997.
11. Baird HW, Gordon EC: Neurologic evaluation of infants and children. Clin Dev Med 1983;84/85.
12. Brazelton TB: Neonatal behavioral assessment scale. Clin Dev Med 1984;88.
13. Dubowitz V, Dubowitz L: The neurological assessment of the preterm and full-term infant. Clin Dev Med 1981;79.
14. Fenichel GM: Neonatal Neurology. New York, Churchill Livingstone, 1980.
15. Dubowitz V: The floppy infant. Clin Dev Med 1980;76.
16. Young RR, Delwaide PJ: Spasticity. Parts I and II. N Engl J Med 304:28,96,1981.
17. Johnson EW: Examination for muscle weakness in infants and small children. JAMA 1958;168:1306.
18. Swaiman KF: Pediatric Neurology: Principles and Practice, 2nd ed. St. Louis, Mosby, 1994.
19. Gesell AL, Halverson HM, Thompson H, et al: The First Five Years of Life. New York, Harper and Row, 1946.
20. Cole TM, Barry DT, Tobis JS: Measurement of musculoskeletal function. In Kottke FJ, Lehman JF (eds): Krusen's Handbook of Physical Medicine and Rehabilitation, 4th ed. Philadelphia, WB Saunders, 1990.
21. Daniels L, Worthingham C: Muscle Testing Techniques of Manual Examination, 5th ed. Philadelphia, WB Saunders, 1986.
22. Kendall FP, McCreary EK: Muscles, Testing and Function, 3rd ed. Baltimore, Williams & Wilkins, 1983.
23. Pact V, Sirotkin-Roses M, Beatus J: The Muscle Testing Handbook. Boston, Little, Brown, 1984.
24. Touwen BCL: Examination of the child with minor neurologic dysfunction. Clin Dev Med 1980;71.
25. Rapin I: Children with Brain Dysfunction: Neurology, Cognition, Language and Behavior. New York, Raven Press, 1982.
26. Lin JP, Brown JK, Walsh EG: The maturation of motor dexterity, or why Johnny can't go any faster. Dev Med Child Neurol 1996;38:244.
27. Broadhead GD, Bruininks RH: Factor structure consistency of the Bruininks-Oseretsky Test–Short Form. Rehabil Let 1983;44:13.
28. Berges J, Lezine I: The imitation of gestures. Clin Dev Med 1965;18.

29. Denckla MB: Development of Coordination in Normal Children. Dev Med Child Neurol 1974;16:729.
30. Denckla MB: Development of speed in repetition and successive finger movements in normal children. Dev Med Child Neurol 1973;15:635.
31. Gardner RA: Normative Data (Revised) Examiner Manual for the Purdue Pegboard Test. Chicago, Science Research Associates, 1978.
32. Wilson BC, Iacovillo JM, Wilson JJ, Risucci D: Purdue Pegboard performance in normal preschool children. J Clin Neuropsychol 1982;4:125.
33. Inman VT, Ralston JH, Todd F: Human Walking. Baltimore, Williams & Wilkins, 1981.
34. Lehman JF, DeLateur BJ: Gait analysis, diagnosis and management. In Kottke JF, Lehman JF (eds): Krusen's Handbook of Physical Medicine and Rehabilitation, 4th ed. Philadelphia, WB Saunders, 1990.
35. Sutherland DM, Olshen R, Cooper L, Woo-Sam J: The development of mature gait. J Bone Joint Surg 1980;62A:336.
36. Broughton NS: A Textbook of Pediatric Orthopedics. Philadelphia, WB Saunders, 1997.
37. Steindler A: Kinesiology of the Human Body. Springfield, IL, Charles C Thomas, 1955.
38. Tachdjian MO: Pediatric Orthopedics, 2nd ed. Philadelphia, WB Saunders, 1990.
39. Forero N, Okamura, LA Larson, MA: Normal ranges of hip motion in neonates. J Pediatr Orthop 1086;9:391.
40. Staheli LT: In-toeing and out-toeing in children. J Fam Pract 1983;16;1005.
41. Sutherland DM: Gait Disorders in Childhood and Adolescence. Baltimore, Williams & Wilkins, 1984.
42. Brown SB: Neurologic examination of the older child. In Swaiman YF, Wright FS (eds): The Practice of Pediatric Neurology. St. Louis, Mosby, 1982.
43. Brown SB: Neurologic examination during the first 2 years of life. In Swalman KF, Wright FS (eds): The Practice of Pediatric Neurology. St. Louis, Mosby, 1982.
44. Rapin I: Children with Brain Dysfunction: Neurology, Cognition, Language and Behavior. New York, Raven Press, 1982.
45. Hermann RP, Novak CB, MacKinnon SE: Establishing normal values of moving two-point discrimination in children and adolescents. Dev Med Child Neurol 1996; 38:255.
46. Savitz R, Valadian I, Reed R: Vision Screening of the Pre-School Child. Children's Bureau Publication no. 414.
47. Sheridan MD: Manual for the STYCAR Vision Tests, 3rd ed. Windsor, 1976.
48. Lewis M, Taft LT (eds): Developmental Disabilities. Theory, Assessment and Intervention. New York, SP Medical and Scientific Books, 1982.
49. Martin LJ: Pediatric ophthalmology. In Behnnan RE, Vaughan VC (eds): Nelson's Textbook of Pediatrics, 12th ed. Philadelphia, WB Saunders, 1983.
50. Milstein JM: Abnormalities of hearing. In Swaiman KF, Wright FS (eds): The Practice of Pediatric Neurology, 2nd ed. St. Louis, Mosby, 1982.
51. Rapin I: Children with hearing impairment. In Swaiman KF, Wright FS (eds): The Practice of Pediatric Neurology, 2nd ed. St. Louis, Mosby, 1982.
52. Gesell AL, Ilg FL: The Child from Five to Ten, New York, Harper and Row, 1946.
53. Gross Motor Measures Group. Hamilton, Ontario, Chedoke-McMasters Hospital, 1993.
54. Hally SM, Coster B, et al: Pediatric Evaluation of Disability Inventory (PEDI): Development, Standardization and Administration Manual: New England Medical Center Hospital. Boston, PEDI Research Group, 1992.
55. Sousa YC, Tezrow RW, et al: Developmental guidelines for children with myelodysplasia. Phys Ther 1983; 63:21.
56. Pruitt S, Vami YW: Functional states in limb deficiency: Development of outcome measures for preschool children. Arch Phys Med Rehabil 1998;79:405.

Growth and Development

Gabriella E. Molnar, MD
Kerstin M. Sobus, MD

Considerations for growth and development are essential components in the diagnostic armamentarium of pediatric physiatrists. Deviations from normal are used to project short-term and long-term prognoses, on which both functional and preventive interventions are based. Changes produced by continuing growth and development call for adjustments of therapeutic goals and their mode of delivery. During childhood, the customary patient-physician relationship is extended to a three-way communication, including both the parents and the child.

Growth

Growth is an increase in physical size and dimensions relative to maturity. Growth occurs at different rates, most rapidly in infancy and prepubescence through adolescence. Body proportions also change during growth. In the newborn, the head is relatively large, the face is round, the abdomen is prominent, and compared with adults the trunk and extremities are short. Specific body parts grow at selective rates during certain ages: head growth is fastest in infancy; trunk growth is fastest in infancy and adolescence; and extremities growth is fastest from 1 year through puberty.[1] With changing body proportion, there is a shift in the center of gravity from the xiphoid process in the newborn to the sacral promontory in late childhood.[2] Body posture also changes over time with growth in skeletal height and development of musculature. The typical 2- to 3-year-old has a mild lumbar lordosis with protuberant abdomen. By early school age, increased strength, particularly of the abdominal muscles, leads to a more mature pelvic alignment and decreased lordosis. Changing body size and proportions in a child or adolescent with physical disability may alter orthotic needs or ambulatory potential.

The rate of growth, rather than the absolute size of an individual child, is a sensitive indicator of health or disease. All parameters of growth should be serially measured in a consistent manner and recorded on the standard growth chart for immediate comparison. Values outside the ±2 standard deviation (SD) range on the normal distribution curve or a continued and unexplained shift in growth trend indicates a need for evaluation. Transient shifts in growth parameters may occur in the first 4–18 months of life but should reach a stable rate by 1.5 years of age. Genetic factors influence ultimate height and weight and generally exert their effect after 6 months of age.[3]

Certain childhood illnesses or disabilities may affect growth. Infants with neurologic impairment and oral motor dysfunction are at significant risk for failure to thrive because of their inability to meet caloric needs for growth by oral intake. They require supplemental feeding, and the appropriateness of caloric and fluid intake needs to be monitored. Some endocrine dysfunctions or systemic skeletal diseases may lead to generalized growth retardation.[4,5] As a group, children with cerebral palsy tend to have a shift to the left in height and weight. Growth delays are also seen in children with Down's syndrome, who are typically at or near the 3rd percentile for the general population. Their average adult height is 4.5 feet for women and 5 feet for men.[6] Normative charts are available for children with Down's syndrome.[6]

Some neurologic lesions affect growth, resulting in asymmetry. Limb shortening or atrophy may be seen with brachial plexus palsy sustained at birth, congenital varicella syndrome, or myelodysplasia.[7,8] To a lesser extent, upper motor neuron lesions present from birth or acquired in early childhood are also associated with underdevelopment of an extremity, for example, hemiplegia.

With an awareness of growth trends, the clinician can anticipate and plan for changes needed in orthoses, wheelchairs, and other adaptive

TABLE 2–1.   Growth from Birth to Maturity

Head Circumference		Weight		Height/Stature		Sitting Height		
							Girls	Boys
Birth	35 cm	Birth (full term)	3400 gm	Birth	50 cm			
4 months	41 cm	5 months	Double	12 months	75 cm	Newborn	34 cm	35 cm
12 months	47 cm	12 months	Triple	4 years	100 cm	5 years	61 cm	62 cm
Maturity	57 cm	Until adolescent growth spurt	2 kg (annually)	Early school age	5 cm (annually)	10 years	73 cm	74 cm
				Prepubescence/ adolescence	5–8 cm (annually)	18 years	88 cm	92 cm

Data from references 1, 4, 9, and 10.

devices. Timing for treatment of leg length discrepancy and scoliosis can be decided with cognizance of adolescent growth trends.

Table 2–1 provides a brief guide for growth in head circumference, sitting height, height, and weight. Figures 2–1 and 2–2 are examples of the standard growth charts for girls from birth to 3 years of age and for boys aged 2 to 18 years.[1,4,9–11]

Head Circumference

The average head circumference is 34–35 cm at birth. It increases by approximately 12 cm during the first year, representing more than half of the total growth until maturity.[1,12] Head circumference is measured with a tape placed firmly over the glabella and supraorbital ridges anteriorly and on the maximal protuberance of the occiput posteriorly. Head circumference should be obtained up to 3 years of age and thereafter if central nervous system pathology is suspected.

A rapid increase in head size during the first year of life reflects the growth and maturation of the brain. Excessive enlargement of head circumference may be caused by hydrocephalus with elevated intracranial pressure or a space-occupying lesion, particularly in infancy and early childhood because the fontanels are open until 12–18 months and the calvarial sutures do not unite firmly until about puberty. Disproportionately enlarging head because of hydrocephalus is most common with myelodysplasia. It can also develop in premature infants with intracranial hemorrhage. Microcephaly is an indication of lack of brain growth after a severe anoxic encephalopathy or cerebral atrophy associated with a degenerative or genetic disease of the central nervous system. Concern for possible central nervous system abnormality should always arise and be investigated when head circumference falls outside the ±2 SD from the mean or *crosses percentiles* because of deceleration or acceleration of head growth.[1,13,14]

Height

The average length of a full-term newborn is 50 cm. Length increases by 50% in the first 12 months. The average growth is 12 cm in the second year and 6–8 cm annually from 3 to 5 years.[1] Adult height can be estimated by doubling body length at 2 years. Skeletal age is another means to predict eventual height and is discussed in detail in Chapter 19. Girls attain maximal growth velocity before menarche and cessation 2 years thereafter. Boys grow fastest in late puberty concurrent with the appearance of facial hair on the cheeks and chin.[15] Accurate serial measurements are important. Recumbent length is much more precise than standing height in children under 5 years and for those who have difficulties with standing. The child should lie on a flat, firm surface and soles of the feet are held firmly at a fixed point of reference considered the zero mark. A movable upright crosses the table overhead and is guided down firmly against the vertex. For children with marked deformity of the spine or lower extremities, height prediction can be obtained by measuring arm span. With significant bilateral lower extremity atrophy due to lower motor neuron lesions or malformations of the legs, sitting height may be a better indicator of general growth than total height (see Table 2–1).

Weight

The average full-term neonate weighs approximately 3400 gm, with a range of 2500–4600 gm in 95% of cases. Newborns below 2500 gm are categorized as low-birth-weight infants. This category includes those who are small for gestational age and premature infants delivered at less than 37 weeks of gestation. A full-term infant usually doubles birth weight by 5 months and triples birth weight by 1 year. During the second year of life, average weight gain is 2.5 kg, and it is 2 kg annually from 3–5 years. Weight should be measured consistently,

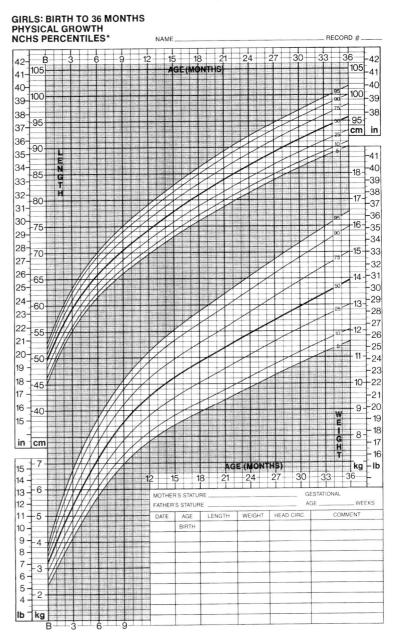

FIGURE 2–1. Growth chart—girls, birth to 36 months. (Adapted from Hamill PVV, Drizd TA, Johnson CL, et al: Physical growth: National Center for Health Statistics percentiles. Am J Clin Nutr 1979;32: 607. Copyright Ross Laboratories, 1982, with permission.)

especially in an infant or child who falls outside of the normal range or has a shift in relative values.[1] Preferably infants and young children should be weighed in underwear because variance can occur with seasonal changes in full clothing.

Development

Development is the acquisition and refinement of advancing skills.[16] The neurophysiologic basis for achieving new developmental milestones is an ascending process of central nervous system maturation.[13,17,18] Under normal circumstances, the acquisition of new skills proceeds along a predictable sequence and timetable. Individual variations may occur within certain limits, more likely in the timing than in the sequence of obtaining specific milestones.[16] Central nervous system abnormalities are manifested by developmental delays beyond the accepted normal deviations. The area or areas of delay provide general guidelines for the suspected nature and diagnosis of a presenting developmental disability. Psychosocial factors and parenting practices may also influence development, particularly in the case of a high-risk infant.

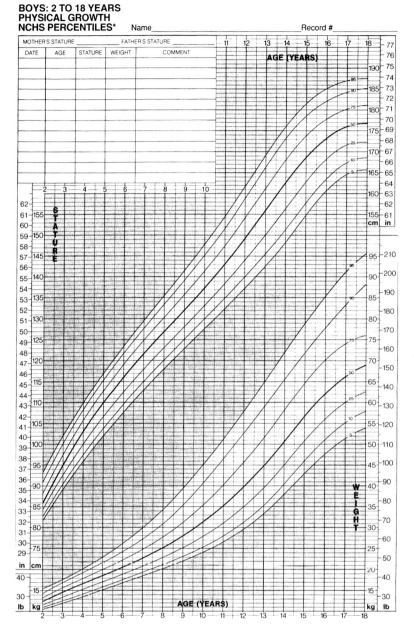

FIGURE 2–2. Growth chart—boys, 2–18 years. (Adapted from Hamill PVV, Drizd TA, Johnson CL, et al: Physical growth: National Center for Health Statistics percentiles. Am J Clin Nutr 1979; 32:607. Copyright Ross Laboratories, 1982, with permission.)

Developmental Assessment

Developmental evaluation is a comparison of the child's behavior relative to age-specific normative data. The young child should be examined in a nonthreatening environment, which may be difficult in a *doctor's office*. The evaluation should include observed behaviors and those reported at home or other familiar settings. It is best performed with the child wearing regular clothing and before formal physical examination that requires undressing and therefore might make the child upset, crying, or uncooperative. Developmental evaluation is complementary to a standard neurologic evaluation, which intends to identify and localize signs of specific central nervous system lesions. In infants and children with physical disabilities, it is important to note not only the accomplishment of a task, but also the quality of motor performance. A child's style of coping with difficult tasks also gives some insight into personality and temperament. Evaluation and detection of infants and children who may be at risk or delayed is necessary for referral to early intervention or preschool programs. These services have specific guidelines for qualification and require an assessment of age equivalence.

Gesell and Amatruda[19] pioneered in categorizing development milestones in four distinct areas of function:

1. Gross motor behavior—preambulatory skills, walking, and advanced physical activities

2. Fine motor–adaptive behavior—prehension, manipulatory hand skills, and application of sensorimotor abilities to tasks of daily life

3. Language behavior—vocalization, comprehension, expression in spoken or other modes of communication

4. Personal–social behavior—acquisition of societal and cultural standards of behavior

The Test of Developmental Diagnosis by Gesell and Amatruda yields a developmental quotient in each of the four areas.[19–22] The quotients represent the proportion of achievements compared with normal expectations. Selected milestones that were found to be most reliable and useful among the Gesell test items provide the basis for the Denver Developmental Screening Test. As its name indicates, this test is intended as a method of screening and should be followed by additional, more detailed and specific diagnostic testing when deviations are present.[23,24]

Over the years, many other assessment instruments have been developed for infants and children. Some of them examined all areas of development, whereas others concentrated on selective aspects of function. A number of assessment instruments have also been established for children with certain physical disabilities, which include testing of tone and reflexes, functional independence, hand function, and activities of daily living. Some assessments can be used at all ages in childhood, whereas others are age-specific. Table 2–2 is a list of the pediatric assessment instruments indicating functional areas tested, age range, and applicability to selected aspects of function, dysfunction, or disability.

The standard developmental tests are able to identify children who fail to achieve normal motor milestones but cannot be used to evaluate the quality of motor performance or monitor progress during therapy in children with physical disabilities. The Gross Motor Functional Measure (GMFM) is a standardized and validated observational test to demonstrate changes over time in children with cerebral palsy.[25] *Functional* in the test is defined as the child's degree of achievement of a motor behavior when instructed to perform or placed in a particular position. The test dimensions include activities in prone and supine progressing to lying, rolling, sitting, crawling, kneeling, standing, walking, running, and jumping. All items are achievable by 5-year-olds with normal motor development.[25–29] Other testing instruments designed to evaluate the child with physical disability are the Functional Independence Measure for Children (WEEFIM), the Pediatric Evaluation of Disability Inventory (PEDI), and the TUFTS Assessment of Motor Performance (TAMP).[30–32] Special testing aimed to evaluate children with specific

TABLE 2–2. Pediatric Assessment Instruments

Assessment Test	Postural Control/ Gross Motor	Fine Motor Prehension	ADL	Adaptive Behavior	Language Communication	Reflex Development	Diagnosis/ Application	Age Range
	Functional Areas Tested							
1. Developmental Diagnosis–Gesell[19]	X	X		X	X		Developmental delay	1–36 months
2. Denver Developmental Screening Test[23,24]	X	X		X	X		Developmental delay	1 month– 6 years
3. Bayley Scales of Infant Development[48]	X	X		X	X	X	Developmental delay	2–30 months
4. Peabody Motor Scales[49]	X	X		X			Motor delay	0–83 months
5. Vineland Adaptive Behavior Scales[50]	X		X	X			Developmental disability, mental retardation	0–19 years
6. Bruininks-Oseretsky Test of Motor Proficiency[51]	X	X					Motor proficiency, able bodied	4.5–14.5 years
7. Gross Motor Function Measures (GMFM)[25]	X						Cerebral palsy	Childhood
8. The Motor Control Assessment (MCA)[52]	X					X	Motor disability	2–17 years
9. Movement Assessment of Infants (MAI)[53]	X					X	Motor delay, cerebral palsy	0–12 months

(Table continued on following page.)

TABLE 2–2.   Pediatric Assessment Instruments *(Continued)*

	Functional Areas Tested							
Assessment Test	**Postural Control/ Gross Motor**	**Fine Motor Prehension**	**ADL**	**Adaptive Behavior**	**Language Communication**	**Reflex Development**	**Diagnosis/ Application**	**Age Range**
10. Early Intervention Developmental Profile[54]	X	X		X			Developmental delay	0–36 months
11. Miller Assessment for Preschoolers (MAP)[55]	X	X		X			Developmental delay	3–6 years
12. Sensory Integration and Praxis Test *(Southern California Integration Test)*[56]		X		X			Learning impairment	4–9 years
13. Scales for Rating the Physical Demands of Daily Life[57]	X	X	X				Childhood-onset disability	Adults
14. Hawaii Early Learning Profile (HELP)[58]	X	X	X	X	X		Developmental disability	3–6 years
15. Pediatric Assessment of Self-care Activities[59]	X		X	X			Motor disability	All ages in childhood
16. Jebsen Test of Hand Function[60,61]		X					Disabled, able bodied	≥ 6 years
17. Erhardt Developmental Prehension Test[62]		X					Hand function	Neonate–6 years
18. Functional Activities Score[33,34]	X	X	X				Spina bifida	All ages
19. Spina Bifida: Neurologic Scale[35]	X			X		X	Spina bifida	2 years–adult
20. Child Amputee Prosthetic Project Functional Status Inv (CAPP-FSI)[36,37]		X	X				Limb deficiency	Childhood
21. Prosthetic Upper Extremity Functional Index (PUFI)[38]		X	X				Upper limb deficiency	Childhood
22. Functional Independence Measure of Children (WEEFIM)[30]	X		X	X			Motor disability	0–18 years
23. Pediatric Evaluation of Disability Inventory (PEDI)[31]	X		X	X			Motor disability	6 months–7 years
24. TUFTS Assessment of Motor Performance (TAMP)[32]	X	X	X	X			Motor disability	≥ 3 years
25. Gross Motor Function Classification System (GMFCS)[29]	X						Cerebral palsy	Childhood
26. Standard Recording of Central Motor Deficit[39–41]	X	X		X	X		CNS deficit	Childhood
27. Bobath Test Chart of Motor Ability[63]	X					X	Cerebral palsy	Childhood
28. Cerebral Palsy Assessment Chart[42,43]	X					X	Cerebral palsy	Childhood
29. Milani-Comparetti Motor Development Screening Test[44,45]	X					X	Cerebral palsy, motor delay	2–24 months
30. Reflex Testing Methods for Evaluation of CNS Development (Fiorentino)[46]	X					X	Cerebral palsy	Infancy–6 years
31. Test for Gross Motor and Reflex Development[47]	X					X	Cerebral palsy, motor delay	2–24 months

ADL, Activities of daily living; CNS, central nervous system.

physical disabilities is available for spina bifida and for limb deficiency (see Table 2–2).[33–38] WEEFIM is a discipline-free test of disability for assessing functions in mobility, locomotion, self-care, sphincter control, communication, and social cognition.[30] The WEEFIM seeks to measure the overall cost or caregiver assistance needed to accomplish daily tasks so that a certain quality of life is achieved and sustained. The test is useful in tracking outcomes over time across health, developmental, and community settings and for use in program evaluation of overall rehabilitation outcomes. The test is appropriate for children from 6 months to 12 years of age.[30] The PEDI is a discriminative tool for young children from 6 months to 7.5 years developmental age for detecting functional limitations and disability in age-appropriate independence and an instrument for monitoring progress and program evaluation of pediatric rehabilitation services or therapeutic educational settings.[31] The test includes three content domains—self-care, mobility, and social function—and evaluates functional skill level, caregiver assistance, and use of mechanical modifications or device within domain. [31]

Examination of muscle tone and reflex development may give the first indication of an underlying central nervous system dysfunction, such as cerebral palsy in infants and young children. A number of tests are available for this particular aspect of development.[39–47]

Infantile Reflex Development

In neonates and young infants, motor behavior is influenced by primitive reflexes as a result of the immature central nervous system. These reflexes generate predictable and stereotypic movements and postures. During the first 6–8 months of life as central nervous system maturation progresses, these reflexes become gradually suppressed.[63] Concurrently, more sophisticated postural responses emerge between 2 and 14 months of age that are used and incorporated into volitional motor behavior.[64] Tables 2–3 and 2–4 show the timetables of these two processes.

The relationship between reflexes, postural responses, and evolution of volitional motor control has been demonstrated by Twitchell[65,66] and by Milani-Comparetti and Gidoni[44,45] in the development of prehension and gross motor milestones. Obligatory or persistent primitive reflexes are the earliest markers of abnormal neurologic maturation.[63–67] Appearance of postural responses is useful in evaluation of readiness for specific motor milestones, for example, rolling, sitting, or standing.[68]

Cognitive Development

Cognitive development refers to increasing ability of the child to interpret sensory events; register and retrieve information from memory; and manipulate schemata, images, symbols, and concepts in thinking, reasoning, problem solving, and the acquisition of knowledge and beliefs about the environment.[69] Piaget was a psychologist who developed the cognitive-developmental theory by studying how children come to know what they know and the process by which they acquire the ability to reason logically.[70] He viewed the child as going through stages in which the mind is described as undergoing a series of evolutionary reorganizations. Piaget described four stages of cognitive development. The *sensorimotor stage* from birth to 18 months is a stage that spans transition from immature reflex and sensorimotor responses to purposeful activity by the formation of increasingly complex sensory and motor abilities. These skills allow infants to organize and exercise some control over their environment. The next phase, called the *preoperational stage*, starts when the child begins to learn language and ends at 6–7 years of age. During this period, children develop the tools for representative schemes symbolically through language, imitation, imagery, symbolic play, and drawing. They acquire the capacity to deal with objects and events not present in the immediate situation. Between ages 6–7 and 11 years is the stage of *concrete operational thought*, at which time children enter formal education. During this period, they develop logical thinking and can manipulate groups of categories, classification systems, and hierarchies. The final stage, achieved at 11–12 years, is *formal operational thought*, which is characterized by the ability to conceptualize about many simultaneous interacting variables, to use abstract reasoning, and to develop hypothetical theories.[70,71]

Personality Development

Theories of childhood personality development are as diverse as the advice given to parents over the years on how to raise children. The biologic theories note the evolutionary history of the species and the maturation of the individual. These theories are primarily influenced by the ideas of Darwin. The cognitive theories focus on activities of the learner, the process of thought, and the development and function of the mind.[72]

The *psychoanalytic theory* encompasses Freud's work on human motivation and sexual development. Erickson modified Freud's theory into

TABLE 2–3.   Reflex Development*

Reflex	Stimulus	Response	Age of Suppression	Clinical Significance
Moro	Sudden neck extension	Shoulder abduction, shoulder, elbow, and finger extension followed by arm flexion adduction	4–6 months	Persists in CNS pathology, static encephalopathy
Startle	Sudden noise, clapping	Same as Moro reflex	4–6 months	Persists in CNS pathology, static encephalopathy
Rooting	Stroking lips or around mouth	Moving mouth, head toward stimulus in search of nipple	4 months	Diminished in CNS pathology, may persist in CNS pathology
Positive supporting	Light pressure or weight bearing on plantar surface	Legs extend for partial support of body weight	3–5 months Replaced by volitional weight bearing with support	Obligatory or hyperactive abnormal at any age, early sign of lower extremity spasticity, may be associated with scissoring
Asymmetric tonic neck	Head turning to side	Extremities extend on face side, flex on occiput side	6–7 months	Obligatory response abnormal at any age, persists in static encephalopathy
Symmetric tonic neck	Neck flexion Neck extension	Arms flex, legs extend Arms extend, legs flex	6–7 months	Obligatory response abnormal at any age, persists in static encephalopathy
Palmar grasp	Touch or pressure on palm or stretching finger flexors	Flexion of all fingers, hand fisting	5–6 months	Diminished in CNS suppression, absent in LMN paralysis; persists/hyperactive in spasticity
Plantar grasp	Pressure on sole distal to metatarsal heads	Flexion of all toes	12–14 months when walking is achieved	Diminished in CNS suppression, absent in LMN paralysis, persists or hyperactive in spasticity
Automatic neonatal walking	On vertical support plantar contact and passive tilting of body forward and side to side	Alternating automatic steps with support	3–4 months	Variable activity in normal infants, absent in LMN paralysis
Placement or placing	Tactile contact on dorsum of foot or hand	Extremity flexion to place hand or foot over an obstacle	Before end of first year	Absent in LMN paralysis or with lower extremity spasticity
Neck righting or body derotational	Neck rotation in supine	Sequential body rotation from shoulder to pelvis toward direction of face	4 months Replaced by volitional rolling	Nonsequential leg rolling suggests increased tone
Tonic labyrinthine	Head position in space, strongest at 45° from horizontal		4–6 months	Hyperactive/obligatory abnormal at any age, persists in CNS damage/static encephalopathy
	Supine Prone	Predominant extensor tone Predominant flexor tone		

* *Primitive reflexes:* Present at birth, suppressed at certain ages in normal development.
CNS, Central nervous system; LMN, lower motor neuron.
Data from references 44, 45, 63–67, 77, 78.

stages that describe emotional development across the life span.[72] His theory of stages conceptualizes personality development as a progressive resolution of conflict between needs and social demands. Personality evolves according to steps predetermined by the individual's readiness to react with a widening social world. During the first 18 months, infants develop a relationship with their caregiver, usually their mother, as their basic needs are met. They attain feelings of comfort and trust. If these needs are not consistently met, the infant may develop a sense of mistrust. Premature infants requiring long hospitalization or those who are irritable or difficult to feed may have a disruption in their development of trust. Parents may

TABLE 2–4. Physiologic Postural Reflex Responses*

Postural Reflex	Stimulus	Response	Age of Emergence	Clinical Significance
Head righting	Visual and vestibular	Align face/head vertical, mouth horizontal	*Prone*—2 months *Supine*—3–4 months	Delays or absent in CNS immaturity or damage
Head and body righting	Tactile, vestibular proprioceptive	Align body parts in anatomic position relative to each other and gravity	4–6 months	As above
Protective extension or parachute reactions	Displacement of center of gravity outside supporting base in sitting, standing	Extension/abduction of lateral extremity toward displacement to prevent falling	*Sitting anterior*— 5–7 months *Lateral*—6–8 months *Posterior*—7–8 months *Standing*—12–14 months	As above
Equilibrium or tilting reactions	Displacement of center of gravity	Adjustment of tone and posture of trunk to maintain balance	*Sitting*—6–8 months *Standing*—12–14 months	As above

* Emerge with CNS maturation, present through life, modulated by volition, used in gross motor activities.
CNS, Central nervous system.
Data from references 44, 45, 63–67, 77, 78.

feel inadequate to meet the infant's needs. Professional assistance may be needed to guide the parents with basic information regarding their infant's special needs and to facilitate positive activities for the parent and the infant. During the toddler stage, children master autonomy versus shame and doubt. With the achievement of walking, they exercise some self-direction and control. The all-too-common phrase "Me do it" is proclaimed. With increased control, children learn mastery over their bodies, and toilet training may be initiated. For those with physical disabilities, the issue of autonomy is critical, and they need to be given opportunities for control and mobility. Professionals working with the child and family should assist with the promotion of independence rather than inadvertently encourage assuming a passive role by the child. During the third stage, at 3–5 years, children master initiative versus guilt. They demonstrate an increased understanding of task and plan strategies for play. During this period, the child becomes aware of his or her own sex and experiences a sexual attraction to the parent of the opposite sex. With resolution of this crisis, the child identifies with the same-sex parent.

In the next stage, children enter school and seek their place among their peers. For the parents of children with special needs, this time may be an increased awareness of their child's limitations intellectually or physically, arousing concerns about school entry. For children with limitations in their ability to learn or to compete in recreational activities, stress may occur from finding adjustment with school peers.[72,73] Professional guidance may assist the family in understanding the child's specific strengths and weaknesses while offering opportunities for choice and continued encouragement of independence.[73]

Out-of-school opportunities with community or church organizations may give the child a sense of identity and an opportunity to participate with peers on a noncompetitive basis. The adolescent years bring an increase in the sense of identity. Adolescents are concerned about how they appear in the eyes of others, as compared with how they perceive themselves. They need to evaluate and formulate their roles and ways of behavior.[72] Those with chronic disability may have to confront the reality of permanent disability and conflicts with the fantasy of sudden cure. The opportunities for more mobility in relationship to driving and dating may not be easily attainable for them. Finally, the transition from high school to independent living, college, or vocational training may present a time for reevaluation and new adaptation for the adolescent or young adult with a chronic physical or cognitive disability. Counseling should be offered for the family and adolescent, but the focus should shift primarily to the adolescent to assist with social, sexual, marital, and vocational attitudes; coping; and adaptation to the future.[73]

The *learning theory* is another framework for personality development. The premise is that behavior is based on learning, and, as such, it is dependent on experienced events. Perception and interpretation of social experiences generate rules and patterns of behavior. A criticism of the learning theory is that it does not take into account biologic preparedness and emotional development. Nevertheless, the learning theory provides a basis for useful behavior therapy techniques. Techniques may be applicable to youngsters with physical or cognitive disabilities. The term *learned helplessness* is a behavior described in this group of individuals implying a learned perception that situational outcomes are not dependent on their behavior.[74] In such cases, therapeutic intervention may be useful whereby these individuals learn that their actions can influence subsequent events and interactions.

Developmental Milestones

The key milestones are listed in four descriptive areas of development, along with cognitive and emotional milestones, in Table 2–5.

Newborn

In the newborn, muscle tone is predominantly with semiflexion of the extremities.[75] When positioned in prone, there is head turning from side to side with neck hyperextension, sweeping the mouth against the surface. If held in sitting, full support is required, the back is rounded, and the head falls forward. Hands are loosely fisted, and grasp reflex can be elicited. With bright, bold objects, the newborn can visually fix and follow to limited extent. When held in supported standing and tilted forward, automatic reflex stepping may be seen for approximately 3–4 weeks. The infant's crying at first consists of vowel-like sounds. In quiet states, the head turns toward the sound of a rattle or voice. Many primitive reflexes can be seen or elicited but should not be obligatory in nature. Reflex sucking and swallowing is present. The state of alertness has a significant influence on all behaviors. A characteristic behavior of newborns included in the Brazelton scale is cuddliness.[76,77] Temperamental characteristics are discernible during the first few months and contribute to parent–child interaction.[78] In cognitive development, this is the reflex stage of the sensorimotor period.[70] Emotionally, this age is considered a symbiotic phase in which a sense of basic trust develops while the infant's needs are satisfied.[72]

4 Months

With progressive central nervous system maturation, the young infant displays increasing motor control with more balanced flexion and extension tone. Most primitive reflexes become integrated; some of the righting responses are emerging.[79] When placed supine, the head is generally in midline. When pulled to sitting from supine, the infant tucks the chin holding the head in midline; some abdominal muscle activity and flexing of the upper and lower extremities may be noted on this maneuver.[80] In supported sitting, the thoracic spine is straight. In prone, the infant raises the head to 90 degrees and may even lift the chest slightly. Gross motor achievements include rolling from prone to supine. The hands are now generally open and brought to the midline for hand play. A crude palmar prehension may be present. The infant recognizes his or her bottle and turns to a voice or the sound of a bell consistently. Social interaction blossoms with responsive vocalization, laughing, squealing, blowing bubbles, and *raspberries*. The infant is developing a sense of basic trust, which is important for later life relationships.[72] For the premature infant or those at risk of developmental delay, early intervention programs may assist the parents with handling and positioning techniques to facilitate the child's opportunity for motor development and to accept and adjust to their child's special needs.

7 Months

Primitive infantile reflexes, such as asymmetric and symmetric tonic neck reflexes, are becoming integrated at this age and allow the infant an increased freedom of movement and higher transitional skills.[77,79] Gross motor accomplishments include rolling both prone and supine and moving from prone to quadruped on hands and knees.[19,81] Although the legs are still abducted and externally rotated and the abdomen is sagging, there may be an ability to rock in quadruped position. The infant can maintain sitting if placed and can also attain it from a quadruped position. While sitting, there is active rotation of the upper trunk and reaching with hands in a limited range. Pulling to stand and starting to cruise sideways with lateral leg abduction movements is generally obtained at this age. A well-directed accurate reaching and inferior radial grasp with the thumb as stabilizer is achieved. Objects are banged together and transferred from hand to hand. If an object is dropped, the infant looks for it. The infant can hold a bottle. Oral motor skills are improving with more accurate and stronger lip closure for spoon-feeding although drooling may continue. Increased vocalization is noted with single-consonant and double-consonant and vowel combinations. Stranger anxiety begins to develop because the infant can now differentiate between familiar persons and strangers.

Late acquisition of sitting or rolling and the lack of suppression of primitive reflexes may indicate a neuromuscular disease.[79] Delay in oral motor skills may affect transition from breast-feeding or bottle-feeding to solid foods. It may be a cause for parental anxiety and failure to thrive with inadequate caloric intake.

TABLE 2–5. Milestones in Child Development

Age	Gross Motor	Fine Motor Adaptive	Personal/Social	Speech and Language	Cognitive	Emotional
Newborn	Flexor tone predominates In prone, turns head to side Automatic reflex walking Rounded spine when held sitting	Hands fisted Grasp reflex State-dependent ability to fix and follow bright object	Habituation and some control of state	Cry State-dependent quieting and head turning to rattle or voice	Sensorimotor 0–24 months Reflex stage	Basic trust vs. basic mistrust (first year) Normal symbiotic phase—does not differentiate between self and mother
4 months	Head midline Head held when pulled to sit In prone, lifts head to 90° and lifts chest slightly Turns to supine	Hands mostly open Midline hand play Crude palmar grasp	Recognizes bottle	Turns of voice and bell consistently Laughs, squeals Responsive vocalization Blows bubbles, raspberries	*Circular reaction*, the interesting result of an action moti- vates its repetition	*Lap baby*, developing a sense of basic trust
7 months	Maintains sitting, may lean on arms Rolls to prone Bears all weight; bounces when held erect Cervical lordosis	Intermediate grasp Transfers cube from hand to hand Bangs objects	Differentiates between familiar person and stranger Holds bottle Looks for dropped object "Talks" to mirror image	Uses single-words and double- consonant– vowel combinations		At 5 months began to differentiate be- tween mother and self, i.e., beginning of separation– individuation Has a sense of be- longing to a central person
10 months	Creeps on all fours Pivots in sitting Stands momentarily Cruises Slight bow leg Increased lumbar lordosis; acute lumbosacral angulation	Pincer grasp, mature thumb to index grasp Bangs two cubes held in hands	Plays peek-a-boo Finger feeds Chews with rotary movement	Shouts for attention Imitates speech sounds Waves bye-bye Uses "mama" and "dada" with meaning Inhibits behavior to "no"	Can retrieve an object hidden from view	Practicing phase of separation–individ- uation, practices initiating separations
14 months	Walks alone, arms in high guard or midguard Wide base, ex- cessive knee and hip flexion Foot contact on entire sole Slight valgus of knees and feet Pelvic tilt and rotation	Piles two cubes Scribbles spon- taneously Holds crayon full length in palm Casts objects	Uses spoon with overpronation and spilling Removes a garment	Uses single words Understands simple commands	Differentiates available be- havior patterns for new ends, i.e., pulls rug on which is a toy	Rapprochement phase of separation–indi- viduation; ambiva- lent behavior to mother *Stage of autonomy vs. shame and doubt* (1–3 years) Issue of holding on and letting go Pleasure in controlling muscles and sphincters
18 months	Arms at low guard Mature support- ing base and heel strike Seats self in chair Walks backward	Emerging hand dominance Crude release Holds crayon butt end in palm Dumps raisin from bottle spontaneously	Imitates housework Carries, hugs doll Drinks from cup neatly	Points to named body part Identifies one picture Says "no" Jargons	Capable of *insight*, i.e., solving a problem by mental combi- nations, not physical groping	
2 years	Begins running Walks up and down stairs alone Jumps on both feet in place	Hand dominance is usual Builds eight-cube tower Aligns cubes horizontally Imitates vertical line Places pencil shaft between thumb and fingers Draws with arm and wrist action	Pulls on garment Uses spoon well Opens door turning knob Feeds doll with bottle or spoon Toilet training usually begun	Two-word phrases are common Uses verbs Refers to self by name Uses "me," "mine" Follows simple directions	*Preoperational period* (2–7 years) Able to evoke an object or event not present Object permanence established Comprehends symbols	

(Table continued on following page.)

TABLE 2–5. Milestones in Child Development *(Continued)*

Age	Gross Motor	Fine Motor Adaptive	Personal/Social	Speech and Language	Cognitive	Emotional
3 years	Runs well Pedals tricycle Broad jumps Walks up stairs alternating feet	Imitates three-cube bridge Copies circle Uses overhand throw with anteroposterior arm and trunk motion Catches with extended arms hugging against body	Most children toilet trained day and night Pours from pitcher Unbuttons; washes and dries hands and face Parallel play Can take turns Can be reasoned with	Three-word sentences are usual Uses future tense Asks what, who, where Follows prepositional commands, i.e., put it under Gives full name May stutter in eagerness Identifies self as boy or girl Recognizes three colors	*Preoperational period* continues: Child is capable of: deferred imitation symbolic play drawing of graphic images mental images verbal evocation of events	*Stage of initiative vs. guilt* (3–5 years) Deals with issue of genital sexuality
4 years	Walks down stairs alternating feet Hops on one foot Plantar arches developing Sits up from supine position without rotating	Handles a pencil by finger and wrist action, like adults Copies a cross Draws a froglike person with head and extremities Throws underhand Cuts with scissors	Cooperative play—sharing and interacting Imaginative make-believe play Dresses and undresses with supervision distinguishing front and back of clothing and buttoning Does simple errands outside of home	Gives connected account of recent experiences Questions why, when, how Uses past tense, adjectives, adverbs Knows opposite analogies Repeats four digits		
5 years	Skips; tiptoes Balances 10 seconds on each foot	Hand dominance expected Draws man with head, body, and extremities Throws with diagonal arm and body rotation Catches with hands	Creative play Competitive team play Uses fork for stabbing food Brushes teeth Is self-sufficient in toileting Dresses without supervision except tying shoelaces	Fluent speech Misarticulations of some sounds may persist Gives name, address, age Defines concrete nouns by composition, classification, or use Follows three-part commands Has number concepts to 10		*Stage of industry vs. inferiority* (5 years–adolescence) Adjusts himself to the inorganic laws of the tool world
6 years	Rides bicycle Roller skates	Prints alphabet; letter reversals still acceptable Mature catch and throw of ball	Teacher is an important authority to child Uses fork appropriately Uses knife for spreading Plays table games	Shows mastery of grammar Uses proper articulation		*Stage of industry vs. inferiority* continues
7 years	Continuing refinement of skills		Eats with fork and knife Combs hair Is responsible for grooming		*Period of concrete operational thought* (7 years–adolescence) Child is capable of logical thinking	

Data from references 1, 5, 9, 20–22, 76, 77, 80–86.

10 Months

Mobility and exploration continue to expand rapidly.[80,81] Safety in the home should be reviewed, particularly stairs, patio, and other potential areas for falls and poison hazards. The infant can creep on hands and knees with reciprocal movements. Transition to standing continues to improve through half-kneeling. Momentary independent standing begins. While sitting, the infant can reach up to 10 inches forward without losing balance. Mature pincer grasp between thumb and index finger is present. The infant can finger-feed and bang blocks together.[19] Oral motor skills continue to advance with increasing lip closure and rotational jaw movements on chewing. Socially the infant waves bye-bye, shouts for attention, and imitates speech sound. The infant uses *mama* and *dada* and inhibits behavior when told no. Emotional maturation reflects the characteristic stage of separation and individuation.[72]

14 Months

The infant has now become independent and autonomous. Gait advances with independent walking are clearly descriptive of a *toddler*.[82] The arms are in high guard position, with wide base of support and excessive hip and knee flexion in swing phase. There is slight valgus of the knees and ankles, and on foot strike the entire sole contacts the floor. Soon the toddler may start to crawl upstairs. The toddler can stack two cubes and enjoys scribbling. The toddler holds the crayon or marker in full length of the palm.[80,81] The toddler can insert a pellet in a bottle. Feeding skills advance further with the ability to use a spoon.[19] The toddler holds the spoon with overpronation and frequent spilling. Comprehension of single commands is achieved. The toddler may indicate some desire or need by pulling things and hugs the parents.

18 Months

Gait pattern continues to mature with more narrow base of support, heel strike, and arms in low guard position.[83,84] The toddler can walk backward and sit in a low chair. Fine motor skills advance with emerging hand dominance, building a three-cube tower, and turning two to three pages in a book at a time. Socially the toddler imitates the parent's daily routines, such as sweeping and dusting, and carries and hugs a doll. The toddler can drink from a cup neatly.[80,81] Language development includes pointing to body parts, few words, saying no quite frequently, and speaking in jargon with inflection to convey mood or desires.[20] The toddler may seek help when in trouble and complain when wet or soiled. The toddler kisses the parents with a pucker.[85] The child's cognitive development expands with the capability of insight and finding new ways of doing something not by trial and error but by mental combination, for example, dumping a raisin from an inverted bottle. This is the final stage of the sensorimotor period.[70]

A physical handicap that limits an infant's mobility to explore his environment actively or manipulate objects may interfere with cognitive development. Early intervention programs offer guidance for the parents to alternative activities or opportunities to facilitate the child's cognitive development.

2 Years

The ability to run is added to the child's mobility as is jumping on both feet in place and walking up and down the steps without help but not with alternating feet. The child explores the environment by opening doors and climbing onto furniture.[80,81] Hand dominance is established. With improved coordination, the child helps with dressing by pulling on a garment. Self-feeding improves in efficiency with better use of a spoon. The child can build an eight-cube tower or align cubes horizontally.[70] Holding a pencil is advanced to securing its shaft between the thumb and fingers. The child can copy a vertical line and fold a paper imitatively. Language skills expand to two-word phrases and the use of verbs, often telling immediate experiences, referring to self by name, and using *me* and *mine*. The child can turn pages in a book one at a time and listens to stories with pictures. Following simple directions and parallel play with friends are expected behaviors.

3 Years

The 3-year-old can run well, pedal a tricycle, and broad jump. Stair mobility advances to alternating feet when ascending the stairs.[80,81] Fine motor adaptive skills include imitation of a three-cube bridge and copying a circle. A ball is tossed by overhand throw with anteroposterior arm and trunk motion. Catching it is with arms extended and hugging it against the body. The child parallel plays, but also starts to take turns. The child can be reasoned with. Most children at this age show improved self-help skills with achievement of toilet training day and night. They can wash and dry their hands and face and unbutton or unzip their clothing.[20] Questions are frequent—*what, who, where*—and three-word sentences are usual.[86] The child uses future tense and can follow prepositional commands, such as *put it under*. With excitement, the child may stutter. The child can give his or her full name, identify self as girl or boy, and recognize three colors. Cognitively the preoperational stage is achieved, making the child capable of symbolic, imaginative play and drawing graphic images.[70]

At this age, children with various types of cerebral dysfunction may show discrepancies in different areas of development. Language skills are often a modality of relative strength unless there is a central communication disorder or cognitive deficit. Visual motor integration may lag behind, suggesting the possibility of a learning disability at a later age. The diagnosis of motor dysfunction is well established by this age, and accurate prognostication is feasible in most cases of static encephalopathy. Individuals in the trainable range of moderate mental retardation function around this cognitive level in adulthood.

4 Years

A 4-year-old child is able to walk up and down the stairs using alternating feet and can hop on one foot. The plantar arches are developing, giving a more mature appearance to the feet. With adequate strength of the abdominal muscles, the child can sit up directly from supine without rolling to the side at first.[20,80,81] Mature manipulation of the pencil, moving it by finger and wrist movements, is present. Children can now copy a cross and draw a crude person with head and extremities. They can cut with scissors and throw a ball underhand. Playing with peers includes the concepts of sharing and is interactive rather than parallel. The child may also engage in make-believe play. Self-care skills improve to dressing and undressing with supervision and the ability to distinguish the front and the back of a garment. The child is able to assist with tasks at home and run simple errands outside nearby the home. Cognitive linguistic skills mature with the ability to give an account of recent experiences and tell a story using past tense, adjectives, and adverbs. Constant questions expand to include *why, when, how.* The child can repeat 4-digit series and knows opposite analogies.

5 Years

Entrance into kindergarten usually occurs at this age. Children at 5 years of age enjoy participating in team play.[20,80,81] Motor behavior is mature, and self-care skills have developed. The 5-year-old enjoys skipping and often does it. The child walks on tiptoes or heels and can balance on one foot for 10 seconds. Throwing a ball is with diagonal arm and body rotation movements, whereas catching is with the hands, rather than hugging the ball with full arms against the body. The child kicks with one foot. Limited adult supervision is necessary to dress. In grooming, the child may brush teeth and comb hair, but initially may still need some assistance to tie shoelaces. Speech is fluent at this age, and the child can

follow three-part commands; count to ten; and recite address, age, and phone number.[86] The child knows colors, can draw a triangle, and can draw a picture of a person that includes not only head and extremities, but also the body.

6 to 12 Years

As the child grows and matures, the transition from care-free play activities to structured learning occurs.[21] A 6-year-old enters full-day school and is expected to work on academic tasks while sitting quietly at a desk. Motor skills and eye-hand coordination continue to develop with skills such as riding a bicycle without training wheels, roller-skating, and mature catching and throwing a ball. Self-help skills include appropriate use of a fork, spreading with a knife, and in most cases tying shoelaces. By 7 years, most children have learned the days of the week, can tell time, and are beginning to reason in concrete terms. Handwriting is becoming better organized, although written letters may occasionally be reversed, but this error generally disappears by 8 years. Children with physical disabilities that impede the ability to write legibly may find success with computer use.

The ability to read with the mastery of decoding the written words and understanding the content of a passage occurs during the first grade. The child also learns basic addition and subtraction. With advancing grades, the child must apply reading comprehension and follow written directions and use mathematic principles. Cognitive development has reached the concrete operational stage.[70]

The 9-year-old child can demonstrate true sequencing such as day, month, and year. Simple multiplication and division concepts are performed by this age. Most 10-year-olds understand rules and comply with them. Lasting friendships are formed. Preadolescents can reason through problems and situations and begin to understand social and political issues.[87]

Developmental delay in language skills or cognitive maturation or shortened attention span may represent delay in maturity or a true learning disability. In either situation, close monitoring and appropriate evaluation should occur to maximize the child's potential and to minimize negative outcomes.

13 to 18 Years

The adolescent or teenage years are those of physical and sexual maturity and intellectual and social expansion.[87] Physical growth, along with sexual maturation, occurs at a faster pace.[22]

Intellectual functioning is in the stage of formal operational thought and expands to abstract thinking, planning from hypothetical ideas, mental problem solving, insight into motives, and a sense of morality and social judgment.[70] During the adolescent years, there is a transition from complete dependence on the family to the individual with an evolution of own identity. All teenagers, with or without disability, may experience anxiety and mood changes as they try to make sense of the adolescent world.[86]

For the adolescent with chronic disability, individual counseling may be beneficial to assist with transition to college or vocational training. Perpetuation of dependency and unresolved issues of identity may hinder development of a mature personality. Additional therapy of physical disabilities may be necessary at this age to adapt to changes in body size and dimensions that occur with the growth spurt during this age.[86] Also, direct therapy can assist with transition to independent living, in learning how to organize and plan for personal care assistance and manage daily living tasks such as meal preparation and homemaking activities.

Conclusion

Knowledge of normal growth patterns, functional milestones, and potential deviations is important to the comprehensive management of children with developmental or acquired disabilities. With this understanding, a detailed treatment plan can be derived and assist with facilitating the maximal developmental potential of the individual child.

References

1. Behrman RE, Kliegman RM, Arvin AM (eds): Nelson's Textbook of Pediatrics. Philadelphia, WB Saunders, 1992.
2. Palmer CD: Study of the center of gravity in the human body. Child Dev 1944;15:99.
3. Hay W, Groothuis J (eds): Current Pediatric Diagnosis and Treatment. Stamford, CT, Appleton & Lange, 1995.
4. Smith DW: Growth and its disorders: Basics and standards, approach and classifications, growth deficiency disorders, growth excess disorders, obesity. Major Problems in Pediatrics 1977;15:1.
5. Tachdjian M: Pediatric Orthopedics, 2nd ed. Philadelphia, WB Saunders, 1990.
6. Cooley WC, Graham JM: Down Syndrome: An update and review for the primary pediatrician. Clin Pediatr 1991;30:233.
7. Eng GD, Koch B, Smokvina MD: Brachial plexus palsy in neonates and children. Arch Phys Med Rehabil 1980;59:458.
8. Paryani S, Arvin A: Intrauterine infection with varicella-zoster virus after maternal varicella. N Engl J Med 1986;314:1542.
9. Lowrey GH: Growth and Development of Children. Chicago, Year Book Medical Publishers, 1986.
10. Barone M (ed): The Harriet Lane Handbook: A Manual for Pediatric House Officers. St. Louis, Mosby, 1996.
11. Ross Laboratories. Columbus, OH, 1989.
12. Nellhaus G: Head circumference from birth to eighteen years: Practical composite international and interracial graphs. Pediatrics 1968;41:106.
13. Swaiman KF (ed): Pediatric Neurology, 2nd ed. St. Louis, CV Mosby, 1994.
14. Volpe JJ, Hill A: Neurologic disorders. In Avery GB (ed): Neonatology: Pathophysiology and Management of the Newborn. Philadelphia, JB Lippincott, 1987.
15. Finkelstein JW: The endocrinology of adolescence. Pediatr Clin North Am 1980:27:53.
16. Scherzer A, Tscharnuter I: Early Diagnosis and Therapy in Cerebral Palsy: A Primer on Infant Developmental Problems. New York, Marcel Dekker, 1990.
17. Egan DF: Developmental examination of infants and preschool children. Clin Dev Med 1990;112.
18. Fiorentino M: A Basis for Sensorimotor Development Normal and Abnormal: The Influence of Primitive, Postural Reflexes on the Development and Distribution of Tone. Springfield, IL, Charles C Thomas, 1981.
19. Gesell AL, Amatruda CS: Developmental diagnosis. In Knobloch H, Pasamanick B (eds): The Infancy and Early Childhood. New York, Harper & Row, 1974.
20. Gesell A, Halverson HM, Ilg FL, et al: The First Five Years of Life. New York, Harper & Row, 1940.
21. Gesell A, Ilg FL: The Child from Five to Ten. New York, Harper & Row, 1946.
22. Gesell A, Ilg FL, Ames LB: Youth, The Years from Ten to Fifteen. New York, Harper & Row, 1956.
23. Frankenburg WK, Dodds JB: The Denver Developmental Screening Test. J Pediatr 1967;71:181.
24. Frankenburg WK, Dodds JB, Fandal AW: Denver Developmental Screening Test, Revised Manual. Denver, CO, University of Colorado Medical Center, 1970.
25. Gross Motor Function Measures: Gross Motor Measure Group Chedoke-McMaster Hospital. Hamilton, Ontario, 1990, revised September 1993.
26. Russell DJ, Rosenbaum PL, Cadman DT, et al: The Gross Motor Function Measure: A means to evaluate the effects of physical therapy. Dev Med Child Neurol 1989; 31:341.
27. Campbell S: Physical Therapy for Children. Philadelphia, WB Saunders, 1995.
28. Rosenbaum P, Russell D, Cadman D, et al: Issues in measuring change in motor function in children with cerebral palsy: A special communication. Phys Ther 1990;70:125.
29. Palisano R, Rosenbaum P, et al: Development and reliability of a system to classify gross motor function in children with cerebral palsy. Dev Med Child Neurol 1997; 39:214.
30. Granger C, Braun S, et al: Guide for Use of the Uniform Data Set for Medical Rehabilitation, Functional Independence Measure for Children (WEEFIM) Version 1.5. Research Foundation, State University of New York, 1991.
31. Haley S, Coster W, et al: Pediatric Evaluation of Disability Inventory (PEDI): Development, Standardization and Administration Manual: Version 1.0. Boston, New England Medical Center Hospital and PEDI Research Group, 1992.
32. Haley SM, Inacio C, Gans BM: Tufts Assessment of Motor Performance, Pediatric Clinical Version. Boston, New England Medical Center Hospital, 1991.
33. Sousa JC, Gordon LH, Shurtleff DB: Assessing the development of daily living skills in patients with spina bifida. Dev Med Child Neurol 1976;17(suppl 37):134.
34. Sousa JC, Telzrow RW, Holm RA, et al: Developmental guidelines for children with myelodysplasia. Phys Ther 1983;63:21.
35. Oi S, Matsumoto S: Purposed grading scoring system for spina bifida: SPINA BIFIDA, Neurologic scale (SBNS). Child Nerv Syst 1992;8:337.

36. Pruitt S, Varni J, Setogughi Y: Functional status of children with limb deficiency: Development and initial validation of an outcome measure. Arch Phys Med Rehabil 1996;77:1233.

37. Pruitt S, Varni JW: Functional status in limb deficiency: Development of outcome measure for preschool children. Arch Phys Med Rehabil 1998;79:405.

38. Huggins M, Wright S, et al: The Prosthetic Upper Extremity Functional Index (PUFI): Presentation of an approach to measurement of a child's use of an upper extremity prosthesis. Grand Rapids, MI, ACPOC, 1998.

39. Evans P, Alberman E: Recording motor defects of children with cerebral palsy. Dev Med Child Neurol 1985;27:404.

40. Evans P, John A, Mutch L, Alberman E: Report of the recording and reporting of cerebral palsy. Dev Med Child Neurol 1986;28:547.

41. Evans P, Johnson A, Mutch L, et al: Standardized recording of central motor deficit and associated sensory and intellectual deficits. Dev Med Child Neurol 1989;31:117.

42. Semans S: Specific tests and evaluation tools for the child with central nervous system deficit. J Am Phys Ther Assoc 1965;45:456.

43. Semans S, Phillips R, Romanoli M, et al: A cerebral palsy assessment chart: Instructions for administration of the test. J Am Phys Ther Assoc 1965;45:463.

44. Milani-Comparetti A, Gidoni EA: Routine developmental examination in normal and retarded children. Dev Med Child Neurol 1967;9:631.

45. Milani-Comparetti A, Gidoni EA: Pattern analysis of motor development and its disorders. Dev Med Child Neurol 1967;9:625.

46. Fiorentino MR: Reflex Testing Methods for Evaluation C.N.S. Development. Springfield, IL, Charles C Thomas, 1963.

47. Hoskins TA, Squires JE: Developmental assessment: A test for gross motor and reflex development. Phys Ther 1973;53:117.

48. Bayley N: Manual for the Bailey Scales of Infant Development. New York, Psychology Corp, 1969.

49. Folio R, Fewell RR: Peabody Developmental Motor Scales and Activity Cards. Hingham, MA, Teaching Resources Corporation, 1983.

50. Sparrow SA, Balla DA, Cicchetti DV: Vineland Adaptive Behavior Scales. Interview Edition. Survey Form Manual. Circle Pines, MN, American Guidance Services, 1984.

51. Bruininks RH: Bruininks-Oseretsky Test of Motor Proficiency. Examiner's Manual. Circle Pines, MN, American Guidance Services, 1978.

52. Steel KO, Glover J, Spasoff RA: The Motor Control Assessment: An instrument to measure motor control in physically disabled children. Arch Phys Med Rehabil 1991;72:549.

53. Chandler LS, Andrews MS, Swanson MW: Movement Assessment of Infants: A Manual. Seattle, WA, Child Development and Mental Retardation Center, University of Washington, 1980.

54. Rogers DS, D'Eugenio DB: Developmental Programming for Infants and Young Children. Vol 1. Assessment and Application. Ann Arbor, MI, University of Michigan Press, 1977.

55. Miller LJ: Miller Assessment of Preschoolers. Littleton, CO, Foundation for Knowledge in Development, 1982.

56. Ayres AJ: Sensory Integration and Praxis Tests. Los Angeles, Western Psychological Services, 1989.

57. Deaver FF, Brown ME: Physical Demands of Daily Life. Institute for the Crippled and Disabled, 1945.

58. Parks S, Furuno S, O'Reilly KA, et al: HELP ... at Home. Palo Alto, CA, VORT Corporation, 1988.

59. Coley IL: Pediatric Assessment of Self-Care Activities. St Louis, CV Mosby, 1978.

60. Jebsen RH, Taylor N, Trieschmann RB, et al: An objective and standardized test of hand function. Arch Phys Med Rehabil 1969;50:311.

61. Taylor N, Sand PL, Jebsen RH: Evaluation of hand function in children. Arch Phys Med Rehabil 1973;54:129.

62. Erhardt RP: Developmental Hand Dysfunction Theory Assessment Treatment. Baltimore, RAMSCO Publishing Company, 1982.

63. Bobath K: A neurophysiologic basis for the treatment of cerebral palsy. Clin Dev Med 1980;75.

64. Taft LT, Cohen HJ: Neonatal and infant reflexology. In Hellmuth J (ed): Exceptional Infant. Seattle, Special Child Publication, 1967.

65. Twitchell TE: Attitudinal reflexes. Phys Ther 1965;45:411.

66. Twitchell TE: Normal motor development. Phys Ther 1965;45:419.

67. Menkes JH: Textbook of Child Neurology, 5th ed. Baltimore, Williams & Wilkins, 1995.

68. Capute A, Accardo P: Developmental Disabilities in Infancy and Childhood. Baltimore, Paul H. Brookes, 1991.

69. Mussen PH, Conger JJ, Kagan J: Child Development and Personality. New York, Harper & Row, 1974.

70. Piaget J, Inhelder B: The Psychology of the Child. New York, Basic Books, 1969.

71. Newman B, Newman P: Development Through Life: A Psychosocial Approach. Brooks, Cole Publishing Company, 1991.

72. Hoffman L, Paris S, Hall E, Shell R: Developmental Psychology Today. New York, McGraw-Hill, 1988.

73. Harper D: Psychosocial aspects of physical differences in children and youth. Phys Med Rehabil Clin North Am 1991;2:765.

74. Seligman ME: Learned Helplessness. San Francisco, WH Freeman, 1975.

75. Dubowitz V, Dubowitz L: The neurologic assessment of the preterm and full-term infant. Clin Dev Med 1981;79.

76. Brazelton TB: Neonatal behavioral assessment scale. Clin Dev Med 1984;88.

77. Brazelton TB: Behavioral competence of the newborn infant. In Avery GB (ed): Neonatology: Pathophysiology and Management of the Newborn. Philadelphia, JB Lippincott, 1987.

78. Capute AJ, Accardo PJ, Vining EPG, et al: Primitive Reflex Profile. Baltimore, University Park Press, 1977.

79. Thomas A, Chess S: Temperament and follow-up to adulthood. In Porter R, Collins GM (eds): Temperamental Differences in Infants and Young Children. London, Pitman, 1982.

80. Paine SR, Brazelton TB, Donovan DE, et al: Evolution of postural reflexes in normal infants and the presence of chronic brain syndromes. Neurology 1964;14:1036.

81. Knobloch H, Stevens F, Malone AF: Manual of Developmental Diagnosis: The Administration and Interpretation of the Revised Gesell and Amatruda Developmental and Neurological Examination. Hagerstown, MD, Harper & Row, 1980.

82. Illingsworth RS: The Development of the Infant and Young Child: Normal and Abnormal. Edinburgh, Churchill Livingstone, 1987.

83. Statham L, Murray MP: Early walking pattern of normal children. Clin Orthop 1971;79:8.

84. Burnett CN, Johnson EW: Development of gait in childhood. Dev Med Child Neurol 1971;13:196.

85. Sutherland DH, Olshen R, Cooper L, Woo-Sam J: The development of mature gait. J Bone Joint Surg 1980;62A:336.

86. Stern DS: The Interpersonal World of the Infant. New York, Basic Books, 1985.

87. Bax M, Hart H, Jenkins S: Assessment of speech and language in the young child. Pediatrics 1988;66:350.

88. Miller F, Bachrach S: Cerebral Palsy: A Complete Guide for Caregiving. Baltimore, The John Hopkins University Press, 1995.

Chapter 3

Psychological Assessment in Pediatric Rehabilitation

Anne R. Robbins, PsyD
Jane Crowley, PsyD

Nature of the Population

Children's needs within rehabilitation involve perhaps some level of recovery of mastered skills, but in the case of a child, a return to baseline is not sufficient. Rehabilitation with children is more cogently a habilitation process. The goal in pediatric rehabilitation is not an end point but a process toward continued development of ever-changing abilities and emotional and cognitive structures. The goal is to allow the child to continue with the business of childhood—to grow. To ensure the progress of that development, psychological assessment may be appropriately sought across a much longer time line than adults and hence on a more frequent total basis in a given child.

The challenges of hospitalization, a disruption of familiar routine, absence of parents, and intrusive medical procedures are faced by a child with no armamentarium of coping. The procedures required to save a life or reduce the morbidity of injury or illness may have the potential for as much emotional harm as physiologic good. Complicating the picture is the fact that these experiences can form their own brand of trauma that affects a child's emotional development in its most basic form and spawn a legacy of anxious, hopeless responding to future events, with a level of stress out of proportion to the actual event. It is widely acknowledged that certain developmental periods, notably adolescence, can bring a profound reformulation of an individual's management of chronic illness, in that regimens formerly adhered to are now dropped, with dire potential results.[1]

For the children that clinicians see every day, their medical history can masquerade as merely a list of procedures and number of days in the hospital. In actuality, these events often represent direct challenges to the continuity or integrity of development. The task is to have them remain *challenges* to development and not become *barriers*. In a study by Cadman and colleagues,[2] it was demonstrated that children with a chronic physical disability had a significantly higher number of social problems. There was a further differentiation in that the children with a physical disability stood out, apart from those with chronic disease only. The study showed that those with chronic disease without physical disability were not distinguishable from the *healthy* children in regard to social activities, isolation, and peer problems. Incidence figures for children with chronic physical conditions found that 30% of these children would be expected to have *secondary psychosocial maladjustment*.[3] Other studies demonstrated that those with chronic health conditions or disabilities as a group have more behavior and social problems than children in the general norm sample.[4]

It is important to recognize the distinction between psychiatric disturbance and the increased risk for adjustment problems. Psychiatric disturbance is not common in children with chronic conditions, as their adjustment is reported as better than children in the mental health clinic population. Children in need of rehabilitation have a greater risk for adjustment problems.[1] Essentially, chronic health concerns are life stressors. Additionally, for children with physical disability, evidence shows that functional limitations and societal response (e.g., prejudice) represent an additional dramatic influence.

Another higher-risk group within that of children with chronic conditions are those whose illness or trauma involves the brain. They exhibit difficulties that are different in character, incidence, and chronicity from those whose condition has no brain involvement. First, such children have more behavioral and social difficulties.[5] Additionally, these difficulties last longer as compared with the fluctuating nature of psycho-social problems in those with a condition that did not involve the brain.[6] Cognitive impairment becomes a primary aspect of difficulties in these children.[7]

An additional distinguishing dimension of pediatric rehabilitation relates to the central feature of development in this population. First, in acknowledging that normal development assumes an intact sensory, motor, and overall neurologic system for interaction with the environments of family and the world, these children do not approach that task with the same equipment. For example, a child's physical status may intrinsically alter basic emotional developmental tasks. The protraction of physical dependence on another person that is a reality for a motor-impaired child greatly alters the psychological milestone of separation/individuation.[8] Clearly, standard developmental schema often do not apply.

Then there are the issues of the unique developmental milestones that exist in this population. Self-catheterization, independent dressing with one arm, and safe and independent mobility using a wheelchair are just a few of these milestones. These are unique skills that do not have to be mastered by children without disabilities, as they are for many of the children in rehabilitation.

Psychological assessment in rehabilitation is useful in determining the quality of an individual child's cognitive abilities and emotional survival when the physical counterpart is ensured or stabilized. Physical medicine and rehabilitation specialists have long been recognized for this broader approach to medical practice.

Nature of Measurement

Psychological assessment attempts to evaluate an individual in the context of his or her unique circumstances so that the information derived from the assessment can address the particular needs of that person. Tests and the scores represent one method of gathering data, which are used to generate hypotheses about the individual and his or her capacities. Physicians need to be aware of basic properties of *tests*. Their role as informed consumers is vital to evaluate the quality of work done and to serve the role generally taken as an ongoing consultant to parents and the growing child.

Normative Data

In choosing what instruments to use for psychological assessment, the examiner must be knowledgeable regarding the appropriateness of the standardization sample and the adequacy of its reliability and validity as it applies to the test in a general way. Norm-referenced tests are standardized on a clearly defined group, referred to as the *norm group*, and scaled so that each individual score reflects a rank within the norm group. The examinee's performance can thus be compared with that of a specific group. The comparison is done by converting the child's raw score into some form of relative measure, termed *derived scores*, which indicates the child's standing relative to the norm group. Examples of derived scores include standard scores, stanines, percentile ranks, and age-equivalent and grade-equivalent scores.

Standard Scores

Standard scores are raw scores that have been transformed to have a given mean and standard deviation and can therefore express how far a child's score lies from the mean of the distribution curve in standard deviation units or Z-scores (Fig. 3–1). A positive Z-score is above the average, whereas a negative Z-score is less than the mean. Often, transformations of Z-scores are used in reporting test results. Multiplying by 10 and adding a constant of 50 yields T-scores ranging from 20 to 80, with an average of 50. Another transformation occurs by multiplying the standard score by 15 and adding 100. This provides a range from 55 to 145, with a mean of 100. This method is used in reporting most intelligence quotient (IQ) tests. Scholastic Aptitude Test (SAT) scores use yet another calculation. By multiplying the standard score by 100 and adding 500, a range of scores from 200 to 800, with a mean of 500, is obtained. Finally, stanines provide a single-digit score expressed as whole numbers from 1 to 9, with a mean of 5 and a standard deviation of 2.

Norms provide a way to relate a child's test scores to a group who have previously taken the test and provide the normative reference. Critical factors in judging the appropriateness of norm groups include their size and degree of representativeness.

Percentile ranks are derived scores that indicate a child's position relative to the standardization sample or any other specified sample. The percentile rank reflects the point in a distribution at or below which the scores of a given percentage of individuals fall. This is often confused with the percentages, which are not referenced to a normative population—only to the number correct. For example, functioning at the 50th percentile is normal, whereas a grade of 50% on a test is considered poor performance.

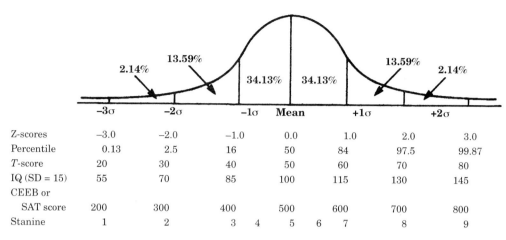

	−3σ	−2σ		−1σ	Mean	+1σ		+2σ	
Z-scores	−3.0	−2.0		−1.0	0.0	1.0	2.0		3.0
Percentile	0.13	2.5		16	50	84	97.5		99.87
T-score	20	30		40	50	60	70		80
IQ (SD = 15)	55	70		85	100	115	130		145
CEEB or									
SAT score	200	300		400	500	600	700		800
Stanine	1	2		3	4	5	6	7	8	9

FIGURE 3–1.   Normal curve and relationships among scales.

Often, test scores are reported as age-equivalent and grade-equivalent scores. Reporting in this manner can be helpful in that it places performances in a developmental context and provides information with a frame of reference that is easily understood by parents and the public. Equivalency scores of this nature are psychometrically impure, however, and should be interpreted with caution.

Reliability

In addition to issues of standardization, factors of reliability and validity are integral to the selection of appropriate measures for psychological assessment. Reliability refers to the consistency and stability of test scores and the extent to which nonsystematic variation affects what is being measured. In a behavioral sense, reliability can be defined as the ability of a test to elicit stable performance from the subject in the absence of outside influences.[9] Reliability indices range from 0.00, indicating no reliability, to 1.00, indicating perfect reliability. High reliabilities are considered particularly important for tests used for individual assessment, 0.80 or higher for most tests of cognitive and special abilities. Variations within the test situation may influence reliability. The fewer variations there are, the higher the reliability of the test procedure. In the context of psychological assessment of the pediatric population in a rehabilitation setting, factors such as misleading or misunderstood instructions, illness, and inattention may pose significant sources of error.

Validity

Validity is the extent to which a test actually measures what it intends to measure. The extent to which this is the case affects the appropriateness with which inferences can be made on the basis of the test results. Validity of a given test is expressed as the degree of correlation with external criteria generally accepted as an indication of the trait or characteristic.

Validity is discussed primarily in terms of *content*—whether test items represent the domain being measured—or *criterion*—the relationship between test scores and a particular criterion or outcome. The criterion may be concurrent, such as comparison of performance on neuropsychological test measures with neurophysiologic measures (e.g., computed tomography, electroencephalography). Alternatively the criterion may be predictive—the extent to which test measures relate in a predictive fashion to a future criterion (e.g., school achievement). In the rehabilitation context, various events and contingencies may affect predictive validity. Acute disruption in physical or emotional functioning could certainly interfere with intellectual efficiency, leading to nonrepresentative test results. In contrast, chronic conditions would be less likely to invalidate the child's performance from a predictive standpoint because significant change in performance as a function of illness or impairment would not be expected over time. An appropriate determinant of predictive validity may be the likelihood that the individual's test performance reasonably reflects performance weeks after the test administration. Finally, construct validity refers to the extent to which the test relates to relevant factors and not to irrelevant factors.

Many factors inherent in the population under discussion may affect validity of test measures because they affect performance. Some of these factors are test-taking skills, anxiety, motivation, speed, understanding of instructions, degree of item or format novelty, rapport, physical and sensory handicaps, bilingualism, deficiencies in educational opportunities, and unfamiliarity with the test material.[10] For an inpatient population, the effects of acute medical conditions (e.g., pain, the stress of hospitalization or medical interventions [fatigue] would, in some cases, affect the validity of test measures. Wendlend and colleagues[11] acknowledged the potential variance caused by factors other than impairment when they noted that an apparent decrease in the intellectual functioning of individuals after poliomyelitis might be a function of hospitalization rather than the disease. In this regard, consistency of performance several weeks after initial testing reflects the validity of results. Lezak[12] reviews considerations in testing individuals with severe disabilities. Lezak notes the importance of establishing that the individual engaged in test taking, in fact, has adequate verbal comprehension and a reliable response modality. In addition, Lezak[17] distinguishes between *optimal* and *standard* testing conditions in brain injury because of the strong possibility that many of these individuals may not have the capacity to "perform well within the confines of the standard instruction."[12]

Issues of standardization, reliability, and validity present specific dilemmas in the context of assessment of a pediatric population. Most instruments of assessment were developed for and normed on unimpaired or nondisabled individuals. As such, most measures of assessment presume the presence of intact physical, sensory, and cognitive functioning. The validity of testing of individuals with sensory deficits has been questioned. For example, most instruments standardized on hearing subjects are likely not valid for a child who is deaf "because of violation of the assumption of a normative range of experience and level of language comprehension."[13] The author notes a possible discrepancy between those with and without hearing impairment as it may affect performance on items included in common instruments.

Application of traditional measures of assessment to the population of children in rehabilitation therefore poses unique challenges. Questions raised in the context of psychological assessment with this population include the selection of appropriate instruments, consideration for administration and interpretation of performance in a particular disability, and type of modifications that may be appropriate in accommodating specific impairments. A critical consideration is to gain an understanding of the possible differences experienced by the child with a disability on interaction with the environment. Similarly

the clinician must consider in what ways the child's behavior and development are affected by a specific impairment. Furthermore, the challenge of the entire process is to promote and enhance the goal of development and expectation for *any* child to grow.

Uses of Assessment

The use of psychological assessment in all its forms is to further the function and adjustment of children with disabilities or chronic illness. Interpretation of results must take into account not only the individual child's medical status, but also the context for which the information is sought. This context may mean the family, school, or hospital or may turn on the developmental challenge to be met. There could be many decision points and different critical issues that must be addressed. Assessment is one tool to promote the ultimate goal of reducing the *gap* between normal and disabled children. In this way, the spirit of normal development (i.e., growing independence) can be presented in a manner in which that individual child can achieve it. It is a diagnostic process with the information gained to be used in treatment and promotion of coping behavior.

Intellectual function has a primary influence on overall functioning and psychological adjustment.[14] School is children's work. The interface with this system is critical because it provides the arena in which many of the psychological and key identity issues of middle and late childhood and adolescence are played out. Furthermore, it is the mechanism by which children acquire the basic academic skills to function in society, skills such as reading and mathematics. Psychological assessment performed by the schools typically includes intellectual and achievement testing as its prime components. This serves for the classification of the largest populations needing special services within the educational system—children with learning disabilities and mental retardation. Diagnoses that predominate in a pediatric rehabilitation population also include children with spina bifida, cerebral palsy, or traumatic brain injury. A broader notion of evaluation is often required to explore fully the nature of these young people's abilities.

This broader notion entails the assessment of *cognitive* abilities, not merely *intellectual* as represented by tests that yield an IQ score. A demonstration of this need is that in the intellectual assessment of children with spina bifida or brain injury, often the component portions of the full-scale IQ score are so divergent that it does not represent a true summary score. Schools often find it difficult to classify children with such profiles. The delineation of primary abilities seen as critical to these children's success in school is not addressed by an assessment limited to IQ and achievement testing only. Pertinent abilities are attention, concentration, memory, and executive functions. Fuller evaluation is appropriate to ascertain the status of these factors known to be affected by the central nervous system abnormalities of such disorders. In the past, a triennial schedule of reevaluation within the schools was the standard for special education students. This is often not the case now, so it may be incumbent on the rehabilitation clinician to request an evaluation, either in the schools or through referral to psychologists within the hospital or community. To advise parents as to the appropriateness of the special education plan, known as the *individualized educational plan* (IEP), requires current pertinent data.

Accommodations sought under Section 504 of the Rehabilitation Act do not require classification within the special education system. Instead, these can be accessed within a mainstream curriculum, but evidence of need is still required. Results of psychological evaluations can be useful in demonstrating such need related to cognitive issues. For example, deficits in information processing speed can have quite specific and global effects on functioning within the group instructional environment of school. Accommodations such as reduction in homework, extended time for tests, or receiving copies of another student's lecture notes can all be sought with the documentation provided by evaluation results. The issue of how long the accommodations are required can be answered by repeated testing as in the case of brain injury; where recovery occurs, problems may no longer be present. These are rare issues to a school but are frequent in a rehabilitation medicine practice, where traumatic brain injury is a common patient group.

Effective September 1992, the concept of *transition services* was inaugurated in federal regulations relevant to the Individuals with Disabilities Education Act. This pertains to students aged 16–21 or younger if they are thought to be at risk, whether receiving special education services or not. This new concept in service delivery to students with disabilities is discussed further in Chapter 6. Psychological assessment can be useful not only in determining needs across the broad service categories available (e.g., using public transit), but also for families and students in the determination of

postponing traditional graduation time frames to access these enhanced services because eligibility lasts until the twenty-first birthday.

Cognitive functioning is of primary importance in children whose conditions have known brain involvement, but an argument can be made for its utility beyond school functioning. As mentioned in the preceding section, unique learning demands exist for this population inherent in the rehabilitation process itself. In the authors' practice within a comprehensive hospital-based physical medicine and rehabilitation service, difficulties in therapeutic progress or compliance are not an infrequent consultation request. Individual characteristics such as learning styles and attention may be primary considerations in this *extra learning* that children with physical disabilities or chronic medical conditions often must undertake. Children with physical disability are often required to do consciously what other children do naturally and without effort once mastered.

An example of this in children is ambulation training. A discrete *picture* of a child's predilections for one modality over another could add efficacy to physical therapy efforts in any child—even one without accompanying cognitive deficit. In a related vein, the treatment of children with pain, whether acute or chronic, can benefit from input as to how best to approach the amelioration of discomfort in situations in which medication is inappropriate or not completely effective. Decisions about a specific child's capacity to benefit from biofeedback, relaxation training, distraction, or operant conditioning can save valuable treatment time and conserve treatment resources. There is a dearth, if not outright absence, of research in this regard. It can nonetheless become an arena where the results of an assessment pertinent to learning would seem to have considerable import.

Understanding the individual experience of the child represents a major realm for assessment. Increased vulnerability of this population to adjustment difficulties and behavioral problems was addressed in the previous section. A full treatment of psychosocial issues is found in Chapter 6. Whether this assessment is approached in terms of personality functioning or the experience of one's body—as sought in a pain questionnaire—the degree and quantification of deviation from the normative experience is vital diagnostically. Posttraumatic stress disorders are also possible in children who have been injured or as a result of the experience of treatment involving invasive medical procedures. The differentiation of posttraumatic stress disorder versus other more characterologic components, such as avoidant or conduct disorders, is important.

Determination of treatment effectiveness also serves as a primary reason to secure assessment for a child. Although perhaps not the primary outcome of formalized assessment, changes in functioning compared before and after treatment are possible. Often, this means using other instruments or techniques because individual instruments have practice effects that can obscure a primary change as a result of intervention. With the extension of entitlement for evaluation and intervention to the delayed or disabled infant, toddler, and preschooler, the number of young children presenting to practitioners has increased. Their developmental status covers a broader and more dynamic spectrum than seen in practice previously. Additionally the issue of treatment efficacy acquires a much longer spectrum. Assessing the appropriateness of interventions (e.g., group versus individual) has a wholly different character than in older children because the nature of the intervention is open to question: What methods work in these ages? What about frequency, timing, or duration of treatment in the form of rehabilitation therapies? Children at such young ages are in a pivotal stage of unique rapid development, so the role of assessment is primary not only as a research tool, but also to the clinician in day-to-day practice.

Types of Assessment

A variety of assessment tools are available, and the format is often tied to the domain to be assessed. Although the most readily identifiable with psychological assessment are probably the individually administered tests, various other ways exist to perform a psychological assessment depending on the area of functioning. In the individually administered test, such as the IQ test, a single examiner sits with a child and poses questions or challenges in verbal and nonverbal outplays. The other dominant association to the individually administered test is the projective test; the best known is the Rorschach Inkblot Test. Scrupulous accounting of responses to a set of 10 inkblots is given and later assessed for normative content and the perceptual integrity of the response.

Individually administered tests are only one type of many tools that are used in a well-reasoned and balanced assessment strategy. In preschoolers, for instance, some of the normative behaviors of limit testing render an individually administered test a truncated and highly

inaccurate view of the child's global capacities. It does let the clinician know about the child's reaction to novelty and an unfamiliar environment. This reaction is only one aspect of the relevant domain of their abilities: What is known is only what the child felt comfortable or happy about showing on that day to that examiner.

Another major type of evaluation device is the *structured interview*. Such a format is often used to explore adaptive behavior in children and can be done with several informants. Respondents are asked about the demonstration of a given skill or behavior in the setting in which they function in a child's life. The most useful of these interviews covers both home and school environment so that parents and familiar but nonfamily members are included in the informant pool. This variety in informants, however, can introduce some reporting bias. People bring certain preconceived notions and, in fact, can interpret a situation differently than another person also present. The frame of reference could vary as well as a result of the child's status as one with a disability. Abnormal behaviors or interpretation of intent and capacity may be skewed. Multiple informants are useful so that the interobserver consistency of responses can be determined. Acknowledgment of possible bias and distortion in the use of these instruments still allows a valuable place in competent assessment.

Behavioral checklists ask for frequency ratings of specific behaviors by informants and are another frequently used tool. They typically include a *pull* toward identification of unusual behavior resulting from many different factors. With these devices, scale summary scores can lead to misinterpretation, particularly when a disability makes the acquisition of regular behavior in a standard time frame impossible. As was mentioned in the section on psychometric properties, when using these instruments in rehabilitation populations, it is incumbent on the evaluator to recheck each significant response to ensure that it is not due to sensory or physical impairment. As a consumer, the referring rehabilitation clinician needs to be aware of limitation in such checklists because they are not standardized on populations of children with disabilities.

Again the perspective of several informants across different settings allows for the fullest understanding of a child's activities. The same issues of reliability and informant bias apply, perhaps more so, to behavioral questionnaires. Such questions can elicit a more personalized interpretation not only of the behavior itself, but also by the motivation ascribed to it by the informant. Variables operant on the informants can have an effect on the mindset invoked in answering. The best demonstration of this is that nondistressed families have been shown to have higher levels of agreement than distressed families.[15] Finally, the form of a question can itself lead to more potential disagreement among informants. Specific information is sought as to frequency and time ratings: for example, "How often has the child violated rules in the last month?" compared with a general query, "Would you judge this child as happy?" Teachers bring a wide range of normative experiences with a given age group to the process and are able to observe the child in the most instrumental environment in which he or she functions. In addition to the bias introduced by informants, the type of problem can influence the level of agreement across raters or even temperament that the child displays (i.e., internalizing versus externalizing as a prime example).

The other major form of assessment of behavior is by observational methods. It is not appropriate for those behaviors that occur infrequently, such as incontinence. These are best used when the object of interest is global, such as shyness or one of high frequency, or to assess progress after an intervention. In any form, observational methods are based on the assumption that a valid sample of behavior is being observed that is representational of standard activity in the area of focus.

As Sattler[15] has elucidated, behavioral observation serves the following valuable functions in the assessment process:

1. It provides a picture of the child's spontaneous behavior in everyday life settings, such as the classroom, playground, home, or hospital ward, or in specially designed settings, such as a clinic playroom.

2. It provides information about the child's interpersonal behavior and learning style.

3. It provides a systematic record of both the child's behaviors and the behaviors of others that can be used for evaluation and intervention planning.

4. It allows for verification of the accuracy of parental and teacher reports regarding the child's behavior.

5. It allows for comparisons between behavior in the test situation and in more naturalistic settings.

6. It is especially useful in the study of young children or disabled children who may not be easily evaluated by other procedures.

The process can be a structured one, with actual counts of observed behavior and carefully noted time intervals. Detailed coding systems exist, some aimed at specific behaviors, such as the one by Roberts and colleagues[16] that evaluates hyperactivity in a structured playroom situation using a seven-category system.

When targeted at a particular behavior, factors that precede, follow, and coexist with a disordered behavior are the prime targets of the encounter.[17] External factors such as the setting as well as the internal dialogue inside a child as internal factors are sought to be quantified. The specific behavior under study is also dissected to discern possible entire points for intervention, including those obtained from analysis of the preceding and maintaining factors cited previously. The concept of disordered behavior here encompasses both excess (e.g., screaming during physical therapy) and lack (a behavioral deficit), and the aim of intervention is to increase the behavior or just to produce it by a variety of approaches, such as operant conditioning.

Often the interest is in the description and evaluation of the child's functioning in a more global way. Issues such as interactions with peers, relationship to adult authority figures, play style, preferences, and spontaneous language are the variables of interest. In these situations, there is reference to the normative levels of behavior observed, either provided by a specific system, as in the Transdisciplinary Play Based Assessment,[18] or through general developmental references. Observation of play is particularly revealing in preschoolers and can be done in a free play situation or a more staged analogue to a natural situation. The latter approach of an analogue is more effective with older children because it acts to inhibit the fantasy and imaginative play in younger children. The most ecologically sound approach is natural or free and can offer substantial input to the assessment of a preschool child particularly.[19] At a basic level in a naturalistic observation, the nature of play can be observed—within the categories of unoccupied, solitary, onlooker, parallel, associative, and cooperative play.[20]

Within a general ecologic perspective, some new approaches have been suggested that seem particularly applicable to a population of children with disabilities. The concept is mastery motivation and its expression in infants, toddlers, and preschoolers. An assessment of this nature attempts to garner where a child is focusing her or his energies in terms of a developmental domain and the effectiveness and perseverance seen in this focus. One form of this assessment looks at the *structured mastery-task situation*, in which the objective is "to elicit and to observe systematically the child's attempts to master challenging tasks."[21] Mastery pleasure and persistence are specifically observed in task simulation. Information is also gathered about the parent's perceptions of the child's motivation. A global rating is available from a scale that can be used in conjunction with the Bayley Scales of Infant Development, probably the most widely used test of individual ability in infants and young children, although this scale has not been updated as the Bayley has been with a revision.

The idea of this specific type of assessment is presented to highlight the role of nontraditional assessment in the unique circumstance of children seen in rehabilitation. This includes attention to a vital concept in a population of patients in which there may be substantial physical or cognitive barriers to normal experience of mastery. The realistic expenditure of intervention, both for the child and the larger system in terms of financial resources, argues for "picking one's battles." Directed efforts at producing a feeling of effectiveness and training in persistence would seem a valuable intervention and one with far-reaching effect for many children in this population.

Traditional personality assessment devices are of several types: *objective* and *projective* measures. The objective measures have undergone the most dramatic changes over time in their format and approach. In this population, they represent the most useful of the individual approaches in the authors' view because they can best address the normative issues and the realm of psychological functioning in terms of assessing adjustment and coping. Although literature is sparse compared with other groups of exceptional children, there are studies that employ these measures in a rehabilitation population, so a context exists. Depending on the instrument, the projective tests can encompass the agenda of understanding broader issues in personality in addition to deviation type. The administration and interpretation of projective testing, however, demand much more sophistication and experience on the part of the professional. There is no literature that looks specifically at these results in children with chronic illness or disability, so application carries significant potential liabilities and is more dependent on the individual professional's clinical judgment.

The use of computers for administration, scoring, and interpretation of many psychological assessments has exploded in this decade. Studies have shown that the administration of tests by computers does not reduce reliability or validity.[22] It is often useful in the rehabilitation population because it can circumvent some visual and fine motor difficulties. With the advent of voice input technology, it can provide the privacy that is a primary aspect of some tests. Voice is the only response modality but registered in written format with the computer.

The use of computer-generated interpretative reports is one of considerable debate. Depending on such output as the only data on which to base important clinical determinations is a misuse of this primarily technical device—used best when it is only one part of evidence to consider.

Specific Instruments

Cognitive and Intellectual Measures

A central component of all psychological assessment has been measurement of intellectual or cognitive ability. As this pertains to children, the purpose is typically to provide prediction and planning around academic capacity and appropriate educational programming. Tests of this nature have also allowed clinicians and educators to detect students who may be at risk for learning problems and benefit from special services.

The Wechsler scales are considered excellent instruments for measuring general intelligence in relatively normal individuals. Limitations exist in the fact that the standardization samples do not incorporate individuals with various impairments (e.g., sensory, physical, or language). As a result, it may be difficult to generate meaningful or valid scores based on these scales.

The *Wechsler scales* include the Wechsler Intelligence Scale for Children–Third Edition (WISC-III, 1991),[23] the Wechsler Adult Intelligence Scale–Revised (WAIS-R, 1981),[24] and the Wechsler Preschool and Primary Scale of Intelligence–Revised (WPPSI-R, 1989).[25] Each of these three tests follows a basic format of verbal and performance subtests that yield summary scores referred to as *verbal IQ* and *performance IQ* as well as a composite score of general intellectual ability referred to as the *full-scale IQ*. The WISC-III is designed for use with children aged 6.0–16.11 years. Twelve subtests are grouped into two summary scales—verbal and performance scales. Factor analytic studies yield four factors with potential significance—verbal comprehension, perceptual organization, freedom from distractibility, and processing speed factors. The WAIS-R is used with individuals 16 years and older. The WPPSI-R is designed for children aged 3.0–7.0 years. Across the Wechsler tests and virtually all tests of intellectual ability, subtests should not be viewed as a means of describing specific cognitive skills with precision. Subtest scores should be used to generate hypotheses about a child's abilities.

The *Stanford-Binet Intelligence Scale–Fourth Edition (SB4)*[26] was released in 1986 as a revision of the Stanford-Binet Intelligence Scale–Form LM (SB-LM) edition. This test assesses cognitive ability of individuals from age 2 years to adult. In addition to providing a global index of cognitive functioning, the 15 subtests yield standard scores in four theoretically derived areas: verbal reasoning, abstract and visual reasoning, quantitative reasoning, and short-term memory. Certain subtests may accommodate nonverbal administration for children with limited proficiency in English or language impairments. Also, modifications can be made for children with physical impairments. In addition, guidelines are provided for meeting the specific testing needs of children with hearing, visual, or motor handicaps.

Instruments for Young Children

Tests of infant ability have been developed in an attempt to measure developmental status of infants and young children. Such tests are primarily useful in describing *current* developmental status, with minimal relationship of these early childhood competencies to skills considered crucial during later developmental phases.[27] Predictive validity is considered viable only with infants who are significantly developmentally delayed in the first year of life.[28,29] Rather than providing direct measurement of cognitive skills, tests of infant abilities emphasize motor skills and cooperative behavior, representing areas compromised in a child with chronic or acquired disability, which provides additional complications for achieving test validity in this population.

Research generally indicates that the younger the child, the less predictive intelligence tests are of later school-age and adolescent test scores and academic performance.[30] Stabilization of IQ does not occur until 4 years of age.[31] The assessment of young children typically requires adaptation and expansion of existing tests to obtain relevant and valid information. Factors to be considered are that the young child cannot be expected to perform on request; exceptional efforts may be necessary to elicit the degree of responsiveness and cooperation necessary to obtain sufficient and meaningful information. According to Stevenson and Lamb,[32] an infant's response to a strange adult influenced test performance and "sociably friendly" infants scored higher on measures of cognitive competence. Ulrey and Schnell[27] noted that preschool children have had minimal experience with test situations, show minimal concern for responding correctly, and have limited experience with the feedback process that is

contingent on being *right*. Usually the process of merely asking young children to complete a task may not yield an accurate indication of their capabilities. It is therefore incumbent on the examiner to make a judgment about the extent to which the child's performance represents optimal functioning. The likelihood of obtaining ecologically valid information can be enhanced by incorporating observations and analyses of infants' or young children's interactions with the environment (e.g., parents, siblings, or caregivers) during spontaneous play.

The *McCarthy Scales of Children's Abilities*[33] measures the cognitive abilities of children from ages 2.5–8.5 years. In addition to providing a general measure of cognitive functioning, it also provides a profile of a wide variety of functions, including verbal ability, nonverbal reasoning, quantitative knowledge and skills, short-term memory, and gross and fine motor coordination. Hand dominance is also assessed. The McCarthy Scales incorporate some unique features useful for assessing young children with learning problems or other neuropsychological deficits. Studies have suggested that this test can serve as a useful psychoeducational assessment tool for English-speaking Mexican-American children.[34] One disadvantage is the fact that it cannot be used for serial evaluation beyond the 8-year-old age limit.

The *Kaufman Assessment Battery for Children (K-ABC)*[35] is the most recently developed test of intelligence. It is designed for use with children aged 2.6–12.5 years. The K-ABC is constructed from a different theoretical model—specifically Das and coworkers'[36] notion of a sequential and simultaneous processing dichotomy, which, in turn, is purported to be related to Luria's theoretical framework. In addition to three mental processing scales—sequential, simultaneous, and mental—the K-ABC also provides independent achievement scores. The number of items in the achievement subtests are limited to the extent that they may be primarily useful for screening purposes. Measures of verbal cognitive processes are not incorporated into the composite score; instead a nonverbal scale is used for the benefit of assessing children with linguistic differences or impairments. Directions in Spanish are provided in the manual. In its application, the teaching of tasks is both encouraged and standardized. Materials are highly visual, which may limit the appropriateness for visually impaired children. The validity of the neuropsychological model on which the sequential-simultaneous distinction is based has not been well substantiated.[37] In general, the K-ABC may not be optimal for use as the primary instrument to delineate intellectual ability.

The *Bayley Scales of Infant Development–Second Edition (BSID-II)*[38] is based on normative maturational developmental data. It is designed for young children between 1 and 42 months of age. Depending on which items are administered, scores may be generated in three domains—mental, motor, and behavioral. The mental scale measures sensory perception, object constancy, and early verbal ability. The motor scale measures body control, coordination, and dexterity. The infant behavior record assesses qualitative aspects of the child's test-taking behavior, including rating for attention and arousal; orientation and engagement toward tasks, the examiner, and caregiver; emotional regulation; and quality of movement. The indices report current intellectual status and deviation from age norms. The test has a strong standardization sample and is the most psychometrically sound instrument for assessing young children. Infants who score 2 standard deviations below the mean on this test have a high probability of testing in the retarded range later in life.[39]

The *Cattell Infant Intelligence Scale (CIIS)*[40] is a downward extension of the Stanford-Binet designed to assess children between 2 and 30 months of age. It is also based on normative developmental data. As compared with the Bayley test, the standardization sample is much smaller and not representative of the general population. Administration time is shorter, but it yields more limited results.

The *Gesell Developmental Schedules (GDS)*[41] considers the developmental status of children from 2.5–6 years of age. The scale is based on normative data from a longitudinal study of early developmental milestones. The schedules yield developmental quotients (DQs) obtained by dividing the child's maturity age by chronologic age. This measure provides a standard format for observing behavior in young children but relies on an inadequate standardization sample and does not meet acceptable psychometric standards.

The *Brazelton Neonatal Assessment Scale (BNAS)*[42] is administered to infants between 3 days and 4 weeks of age to generate an index of a newborn's competence. This scale includes 27 behavioral items and 20 elicited responses to assess reflexes, responses to stress, startle reactions, cuddliness, motor maturity, ability to habituate to sensory stimuli, and hand-mouth coordination. No norms are available with which to compare, rank, or interpret performance.

The *Infant Psychological Development Scales*[43] assesses cognitive-intellectual development in children from the age of 2 weeks to 2 years. Research has shown that these scales are valid for children with developmental delays through age 4 years.[44] Eight subscales are presented in ordinal sequence based on Piagetian theory. Subscales include visual pursuit and object permanence, means for obtaining desired environmental events, vocal and gesture imitations, imitation of gestures, understanding causality, conception of object relations in space, and schemes for relating to objects. The scales are based on Piaget's assumption that development in infancy is multifaceted; therefore, assessment should span several domains. This is in contrast with the single-factor view of intelligence on which most standardized tests are based.

Developments in testing infant intelligence are emerging from the cognitive sciences, with a focus on evaluating skills such as memory and abstraction rather than sensorimotor development.[45] It has been demonstrated that visual recognition memory at 3 months of age was predictive of later IQ, in contrast with Bayley scale scores, which were not predictive.[46]

Alternative Tests of Cognitive Function

Alternative tests of ability have been generated to allow for more appropriate assessment of children with various impaired abilities (Table 3–1). This, in part, reflects the fact that standard measures of intelligence are heavily mediated by both expressive and receptive language. In contrast, some of the alternative measures rely less on verbal responding or reading ability. The child may be required to point or indicate *yes* or *no* rather than generate a response. Some measures simplify the demands for complex integration of visual and motor skills or mitigate the impact of speed on performance. In a pediatric rehabilitation population, it is often necessary to use alternative assessment measures to accommodate a range of conditions that may interfere with the child's ability to meet requirements of standardized test administration. Given that many of these alternative measures were designed for particular populations, scores generated are not interchangeable with scores of the major intelligence scales. Instead, these instruments may be most useful as screening or supplemental tools in the assessment or interpretation processes.

Achievement Tests

The assessment of academic achievement represents an integral component of the evaluation

TABLE 3–1. Alternate Tests of Cognitive Ability

Instrument	Description	Comments
Peabody Picture Vocabulary Test–Revised (PPVT-R)[47]	Nonverbal, multiple-choice test that measures receptive vocabulary. For individuals aged 2.6–40 years. Items span very low and above-average ranges of mental ability. Offers two equivalent alternate forms and a Spanish version	Useful as a screening device for measuring range of vocabulary, particularly for children with expressive and/or motor difficulties
Pictorial Test of Intelligence (PTI)[48]	Can be administered to normal and impaired children aged 3–8 years. Includes six subtests: Picture Vocabulary, Form Discrimination, Information and Comprehension, Similarities, Size and Number, and Immediate Recall. No time limits are applied	Eye movements can be used to indicate responses for children unable to use pointing for response selection. A viable nonverbal measure of learning functions for young children with motor and speech impairment. Norms are outdated, and reliability has been implicated.
Leiter International Performance Scale (LIPS)[49]	Nonverbal test developed for use with hearing- or language-impaired subjects. Measures perceptual organization and discrimination ability. Does not impose time limits. Originally developed for ages 2 years to adult; subsequent adaptations[50] address ages 2–12 years	May be less culturally loaded than other more verbally mediated measures. Items allow the examiner to observe the examinee's ability to learn new tasks. Test norms are outdated, and standardization sample is not adequately described. Can provide clinically useful information but should not be used as a measure of general intellectual ability
Raven's Progressive Matrices[51–53]	Measures nonverbal reasoning ability using figures. Three different forms are available: Coloured Progressive Matrices, for children aged 5–11 years; Standard Progressive Matrices, ages 6–17 years; and Advanced Progressive Matrices, older adolescents and adults, particularly those considered to have above-average intelligence. No time limits are applied. Raw scores are converted into percentile ranks	Stratified random sampling procedures were not used; however, large samples were obtained from a variety of school districts, yielding norms that are likely representative of the school-aged population. Easy to administer. Involves minimal sensory demands, making it useful for individuals with auditory, linguistic, or physical disabilities and non–English-speaking individuals. Absence of language mediation may reduce the effect of cultural bias in the test results
Test of Nonverbal Intelligence, 2nd Edition (TONI-2)[54]	Provides a language-free assessment of general intelligence consisting of abstract/figural problem-solving items. Instructions provided by gesture. Subject responds by pointing to correct response option. Scores are presented in percentile ranks and deviation quotients	Culture-reduced test. No time limit. Norms are based on large and representative sample. Useful for individuals with poor or impaired linguistic and/or motor skills. Does not replace broad-based intelligence measures

of children and adolescents. Several academic achievement measures have been devised that address reading, spelling, and mathematical ability. Some measures also attempt to assess written expression (structure, content, or both). In the context of psychoeducational assessment, it is common to use results of achievement measures that are discrepant from intellectual functioning indices to target children with learning difficulties. The more comprehensive achievement measures can provide valuable information about learning style, function, and application of skills.

Some of the more frequently used, individually administered, norm-referenced, and wide-range screening instruments for measuring academic achievement spanning kindergarten through twelfth grade include the *Kaufman Test of Educational Achievement (K-TEA)*[55] and the *Wechsler Individual Achievement Test (WIAT)*.[56] The *Woodcock Johnson Psycho-Educational Battery–Revised (WJ-R)*[57] also includes a college-age

sample. The *Wide Range Achievement Test–Third Edition (WRAT-3)*,[58] although frequently used, represents a brief measure, yielding limited information regarding the individual's achievement in the areas of reading, spelling, and arithmetic. The *Peabody Individual Achievement Test–Revised*[59] addresses generally similar content areas as the other major assessment tools but minimizes the verbal response requirement by using a recognition format (e.g., point to correct response based on four choices). Although this format may allow assessment of children presenting with certain impairments, language or motor, the results may not provide the best indication of expectations for student performance in the classroom, where recall and more integrated answers are required. See Table 3–2 for additional information regarding these specific achievement measures.

In conjunction with the information obtained from these wide-range screening instruments, it can be beneficial to incorporate supplemental

TABLE 3–2. Measures of Achievement

Instrument	Description	Comments
Kaufman Test of Educational Achievement (K-TEA)[55]	For ages 5.0–18.0 or grades K–12. Subtests include Math Applications, Math Computation, Reading Decoding, Reading Comprehension, and Spelling. Provides fall and spring age and grade equivalent scores	Spring and fall standardization samples acknowledge qualitative differences in performance over course of an academic year. Includes an error analysis summary, which organizes the errors and helps pinpoint specific areas of strength and weakness to aid in planning and intervention
Wechsler Individual Achievement Test (WIAT)[56]	For ages 5.0–19.11 or grades K–12 differentiating fall from spring expectancies. Includes eight subtests: Basic Reading, Mathematics Reasoning, Spelling, Reasoning Comprehension, Numerical Operations, Listening Comprehension, Oral Expression, Written Expression. Requires approximately 50 minutes for younger children and 1 hour for children grade 3 and above	Yields composite scores for Reading, Math, Language, and Writing. Linked to the Wechsler scales, which facilitate estimates of ability-achievement discrepancies. Covers all areas of learning disability specified in the Public Law 94-142, 1975
Woodcock Johnson Psycho-Educational Battery–Revised (WJR)[57]	Comprehensive battery of tests organized into Tests of Cognitive Ability and Tests of Achievement. For ages 3 to adult. Provides alternate forms. Contains 27 subtests. Battery may be administered in its entirety, or single subtests may be administered to meet specific evaluative needs	Extensive standardization and reliability data. Includes both younger and college-age individuals in normative sample. Yields information about more advanced skills, e.g., math and writing samples. Yields a variety of scores, some of which are not easily calculated
Wide Range Achievement Test, 3rd Edition (WRAT-3)[58]	Brief screening measure. Two alternative test forms cover three subtests—Reading, Spelling, and Math. Uses a single-level format for individuals 5–75 years old	Reading measure involves strictly word recognition, not reading comprehension, thus restricting the value of information provided
Peabody Individual Achievement Test–Revised (PIAT-R)[59]	For ages 5–18.11 or grades K–12. Includes subtests for General Information, Reading Recognition, Reading Comprehension, Mathematics, Spelling, and Written Expression	Uses a recognition format that accommodates individuals with language and possibly motor impairments

measures of academic functioning. For example, it can be helpful to obtain a sample of the child's comprehension for multiple-paragraph text because this is more representative of what is required in the actual school situation. Also, the *Test of Written Language (TOWL-2)*[60] provides a test of thematic maturity that can be informative regarding the individual's capacity to write spontaneously in a logical, organized fashion. Criteria used by the examiner to evaluate the story include the use of paragraphs, dialogue, humor, specificity of characters, whether the story integrates the themes depicted, and ending.

Neuropsychological Evaluation

Originally, neuropsychological assessment was directed at diagnosing the presence, nature, and sites of brain dysfunction. The focus has shifted from diagnosis to assessment of a child's function to identify and implement effective management, rehabilitation, or remediation services. Over the past 20 years, neuropsychological assessment has developed as an integrated and comprehensive approach for evaluating behavioral

aspects of brain function.[61] Neuropsychological evaluation incorporates multiple standardized measures assessing several functional areas: (1) motor, including strength, dexterity, integrative control, and visuopraxic and graphomotor abilities; (2) sensory, including basic and complex aspects of visual, auditory, and tactile perception; (3) attention, concentration, and information processing; (4) language, both expressive and receptive abilities; (5) psychoeducational aspects of reading, spelling, writing, and mathematics; (6) memory, both verbal and nonverbal and short-term and long-term memory; and (7) metacognition or executive functions, including measures of reasoning, problem solving, and judgment and standardized intellectual tests.

In a neuropsychological evaluation, measures that allow a sampling of various complex cognitive functions are incorporated to reveal the child's performance as a reflection of brain function. Selection of test measures in a comprehensive neuropsychological assessment requires not only an appreciation of the relationship between the brain and behavior, but also the developmental process that unfolds over the course of growth and development.[62]

Neuropsychological Batteries

The three most widely used standardized neuropsychological test batteries for children represent downward extensions of those initially developed and validated on adult clinical populations. As a result, the type of stimuli used in tasks to assess brain function also reflect downward extensions of the stimulus items presented to adults. As noted by Lyon and colleagues,[63] neuropsychological assessment of children should consider the fact that (1) the tasks employed and their content are based primarily on models of adult brain function and dysfunction that occur after a period of normal development; (2) many tasks are designed to assess the effects of focal neuropathology typically seen in adults (e.g., tumors, cerebrovascular accidents, penetrating head wounds), rather than the generalized neural disorders usually observed in children (e.g., closed head injury, anoxia, epilepsy, perinatal trauma); and (3) the neuropsychological task content may bear minimal relationship to the ecologic demands that the child is facing in home and school environments.

The *Luria-Nebraska Neuropsychological Battery–Children's Revision (LNNB-CR)*[64] was developed by Golden as a downward extension of this test and based on Luria's conceptualization of the brain as composed of functional units. The battery is composed of 11 clinical scales and 3 supplemental scales that assess sensorimotor, perceptual, and cognitive abilities and is normed on children aged 8–12 years. Interpretation is based on the level and pattern of scale elevations. Analysis of performance on the individual items included in the battery can be informative. The reliability of this level of analysis is questionable, however, in that the assessment of specific component skills generally relies on a minimal number of items. No specific items measure attention or learning, and the sample of visual-spatial processes is minimal. The battery requires approximately 2.5 hours administration time.

Reitan and Wolfson[65] developed two neuropsychological test batteries for children. The *Halstead-Reitan Neuropsychological Test Battery for Older Children*[65] is used for children aged 9–14 years and takes approximately 4–6 hours to administer. The *Reitan-Indiana Neuropsychological Test Battery*[65] is designed for children between 5 and 8 years of age and requires a similar time interval for administration. Both batteries include many tests from the adult Halstead-Reitan Neuropsychological Battery,

with some modifications. The Reitan tests have been used extensively and as such have a substantial research database. Research efforts have shown adequate validity for discriminating brain-damaged, learning-disabled, and normal children.[66] Limitations include the fact that the composition does not lend itself to analysis of a child's functional capabilities. Certain tests require a complex interplay of abilities that make it difficult to distinguish the precise components of deficient performance. Assessment of memory and language functions is minimal, and there are no direct measures of attention.

An option for comprehensive neuropsychological evaluation with children has become available in the NEPSY.[67] The NEPSY also reflects a measure based on the theoretical framework of brain function developed by Luria. The authors state several purposes for developing the NEPSY, including the intent to provide a reliable and valid instrument that could contribute to the study of normal and atypical neuropsychological development with sensitivity to subtle deficiencies and that could enhance the understanding of the effects of brain damage in young children with congenital or acquired dysfunction and could be used for long-term follow-up. It is designed for children aged 3–12 years and includes several options for test and battery selection, including (1) a core assessment for an overview of the child's neuropsychological status, (2) an expanded or selective assessment for a more thorough analysis of specific cognitive disorders, and (3) a full assessment for a comprehensive neuropsychological evaluation. Five functional domains are assessed, including (1) attention and executive functions, (2) sensorimotor functions, (3) language, (4) visuospatial processing, and (5) memory and learning functions. The manual indicates that the core assessment requires approximately 45 minutes for preschool-aged children and 1 hour for school-aged children. The full NEPSY would be expected to take 1 hour for preschool-aged children and 2 hours for school-aged children. Customized selection of the most appropriate elements for the individual child is allowed. The NEPSY was standardized on 1000 children and validated for use with various clinical populations.

Flexible Battery Approach

The *flexible* and *eclectic* approach to child neuropsychological assessment emphasizes the use of standardized test procedures to quantify aspects of cognitive and behavioral functions. This approach incorporates a variety of test options based on the more specific needs and deficits presented by the individual and the particular referral question. When using this approach, a core battery of measures is used to obtain information regarding an array of cognitive functions. Additional tests are then selected to supplement a description of the individual's cognitive strengths and weaknesses. Examples of tests spanning the various domains to be considered in evaluating a child's neuropsychological functioning are described or mentioned in the following sections and tables.

Attention, Concentration, and Information Processing

Assessment of attentional functioning can be a particularly difficult cognitive construct to differentiate and measure but is nevertheless central to the neuropsychological evaluation. Attentional deficits may appear as distractibility or impaired ability for focused behavior, regardless of the patient's intention.[61] Concentration problems may be due to a simple attentional disturbance and be a function of the individual's inability to maintain a purposeful attentional focus. To clarify the nature of an attention problem, it is important to observe behavior as well as performance on tests involving attention, concentration, and information processing to differentiate the possible areas of disruption.

Reaction time tests assess the examinee's vigilance or attention span by his or her response to a signal. The primary dependent measure is the speed with which the subject presses a button after the signal appears. Tests of this nature require the maintenance of vigilance to

simple stimuli or the inhibition of responses to competing stimuli over prolonged periods of time. Deficits in sensory perception, motor programming and execution, language comprehension, and rule-governed behavior may impair reaction time.

Continuous performance tests are used to assess vigilance and impulsivity in children. These tasks are similar to reaction time tasks but differ in that they require the examinee to respond only to one type of stimulus while inhibiting responses to others. Continuous performance tasks yield measures of total correct responses and errors of commission and omission. Commission errors are viewed as reflection of impulsivity, whereas omission errors reflect inattention. Gordon[68] has provided the first commercially marketed continuous performance test for use in the assessment and diagnosis of children. The electronic device relies on visual stimuli; however, the manual indicates that an unstandardized version may be presented through auditory modality. Some specific tests of attention and information processing are described in Table 3–3.

Tests of Problem Solving and Executive Function

Executive function or metacognition, as applied to neuropsychological evaluation of children, refers to the capacity for planning and flexible use of strategies and the ability to generate, maintain, and shift cognitive set; to use organized search strategies; and to use self-monitoring and self-correction as well as the

TABLE 3–3.   Tests of Attention and Speed of Mental Processing

Instrument	Description	Comments
Gordon Diagnostic System (GDS)[68]	Normed for ages 6–16 years. Includes three tasks: Delay, Vigilance, Distractibiity. Has preschool version for children aged 4–5 years	Free-standing and portable, electronic device used for administration and calculation of summary data. Has parallel versions for Vigilance Task. Relies solely on visual stimuli
Paced Auditory Serial Addition Test (PASAT)[113]	Requires one to add pairs of digits presented at four rates of speed, controlled by the audiotape presentation. Norms exist for ages 16 years and above	Sensitive to deficits in information processing after mild concussion. Often perceived as stressful owing to perception of poor performance even when performing within normal limits. Performance correlates with educational level
Stroop Tests[114]	Requires timed reading of words and colored ink. Interference effect is then measured by timed reading of colored words printed in nonmatching colored inks	Measure of cognitive flexibility. Reflects deficits in response inhibition, selective attention, and concentration. Age and intellectual level may contribute to performance. Visual competence is important
Trail Making Tests[65]	Test of speed for visual search, attention, mental flexibility, and motor function. Subject draws lines to connect consecutively numbered (Part A) and alternating numbers and letters in order (Part B). Has children's form for ages 9–14 years	Part B is most sensitive. Motor speed contributes to task performance

capacity for working memory. The last-mentioned refers to the ability to maintain awareness of information relevant to the task while engaged in it and to manipulate such information mentally.[69] Tests designed to address these aspects of cognitive processes require the use of multiple component skills, including motor, visuospatial, attention, memory, and language functions. Abnormal performance does not lend itself easily to interpretation of the underlying deficit in component skills. Assessment of problem-solving abilities is relevant to understanding the functional capacities of the child.

A frequently used measure in standard neuropsychological practice is the *Wisconsin Card Sorting Test (WCST)*.[70] This test requires the inference of correct sorting strategies and their flexible implementation. Perseverative or inflexible responding has been described as symptomatic of prefrontal damage in adults.[71] A similar response style has been described in early treated phenylketonuric children.[72] Individuals with diffuse cerebral dysfunction also perform poorly on this test.[73] Other measures derived from the test include perseverative response tendencies and *learning to learn*. The revised manual includes normative data on a large sample with children as young as 6.5 years old. By approximately age 10 years, children's performances are reported to be comparable to those of young adults.[74]

The *Halstead Category Test*,[75] one part of the Reitan test battery, is designed to measure conceptualization and abstraction abilities. Sets are organized by principals, and subjects must use feedback provided by the examiner for their responses to infer the correct subtest rule. An intermediate version is available for children aged 9–15.6 years. A children's version also exists for subjects younger than 9 years old. Impairment on this test does not reflect a specific site of brain damage. The perceptual abstraction abilities required for the Halstead Category Test are considered more difficult than those required by the Wisconsin Card Sorting Test.[76]

Tower of Hanoi (TOH)[77] is a two disc-transfer task and is presumed to measure executive functions such as planning, working memory, and flexible, strategic thinking. The task evaluates the child's ability to plan an organized sequence of moves to transform the initial state into the goal state (i.e., duplicate the experimenter's disc configuration).

Tests of Visual Perception, Visuospatial Processing, and Visuomotor Integration

Tests of visual perception, visuospatial processing, and visuomotor integration are generally included in neuropsychological testing because of their sensitivity to various forms of brain dysfunction.[61] Tests of this domain of neuropsychological functioning include the ability to discriminate between objects, distinguish between left and right, judge spatial orientation and the relationship among objects in space, copy a model, understand symbolic representations of maps and routes, and solve nonverbal problems.

The *Bender Visual Motor Gestalt Test*[78] requires the child to copy nine geometric designs. The Developmental Bender Scoring System is designed for use with children aged 5.0–11.11 years. By 9 years, children of normal intelligence are not expected to make more than one or two errors. The *Developmental Test of Visual-Motor Integration–Third Revision (VMI-3R)*[79] consists of 24 geometric designs for the child to copy. Although similar to other visuographic measures, the VMI presents the geometric design stimuli in individual squares of space that match the original. Also the 24 designs follow a developmental gradient of difficulty starting with a vertical line for 2-year-olds and progressing to three-dimensional designs. The VMI-3R is designed for children 4–18 years old. This version provides weighted scoring to increase the sensitivity to individual differences. The scoring system provides percentile, age equivalents, and standard scores.

The *Rey Osterrieth Complex Figure*[80,81] permits assessment of a variety of cognitive processes, including planning and organizational skills; problem-solving strategies; and perceptual, motor, and memory functions. A copy score reflects the accuracy of the original copy and therefore provides a measure of visual-constructional ability. In addition, recall scores, 30-minute delay, and an optional immediate recall condition assess the amount of information retained over time. Various scoring procedures are available. Normative data are available for children as young as 6 years old. Copy scores increase with age, and adult levels are reached at about 13 years. Qualitative aspects of performance are useful in interpretation.

Tests of Language Functioning

Within the language domain, neuropsychological evaluation considers expressive and receptive aspects as well as the practical applications of language for academic functioning. Components of language function in children may include phonological processing; naming; receptive language comprehension, oral and written; and understanding the syntactic structure of language as well as the productive aspects of language. A variety of measures may be

TABLE 3–4.   Measures of Language Function

Instrument	Description	Comments
Token Test for Children[115]	Provides auditory commands to child to manipulate tokens varying along three dimensions—color, shape, and size. Provides standard scores for children aged 3–12.5 years. Involves immediate memory span for verbal sequences and capacity to use syntax	Sensitive to disrupted receptive language processes in aphasic conditions. 25% of children and adolescents with closed head injury showed impaired scores on the Token Test[82]
Peabody Picture Vocabulary Test–Revised (PPVT-R)[47]	A nonverbal, multiple-choice test that measures receptive vocabulary. For ages 2.6–18 years. Wide range of applicable age groups and absence of reading and motor requirements are useful in assessment of children with limited intellectual and physical abilities. Two equivalent alternate forms are available	Useful as a screening device for measuring range of vocabulary, particularly for children with expressive difficulties and/or motor difficulties. Items span both low age ranges and levels of mental ability and levels considerably above average adult ability. Not appropriate as measure of intelligence
Controlled Oral Word Association (Word Fluency)[83]	Elicits spontaneous production of words beginning with a given letter or of a given class within a limited amount of time. F, A, and S are the most commonly used letters for this test. Animal (or food) names have been used with younger children	Word fluency skills implicate frontal lobe damage[83] and may reflect later developing prefrontal skills[74]
Boston Naming Test (BNT)[84]	Assesses the ability to name pictured objects. Sixty line drawings ranging from simple high-frequency vocabulary to rare words are presented. Two prompting cues (semantic and phonemic) are provided if word is not spontaneously produced	Norms accompanying the test are based on small groups of adults aged 18–59 years and small groups of children grades K–5. Manual provides means for individuals with aphasia. Visual-perceptual integrity should be verified. Norms for small groups of children grades K–5 accompany the test. More recent norms are available for children aged 6–12 years[84]
Test of Written Language (TOWL)–Thematic Maturity Subtest[60]	Assesses capacity to formulate and express thoughts and ideas in writing in a structured fashion	Yields standard scores and percentile ranks from age 8–17 years
Woodcock Johnson–Revised Test of Achievement–Writing Samples Subtest[57]	Measures skill in writing responses to a variety of demands. Sentences are evaluated by quality of expression	Scores minimally address spelling or punctuation

used to elicit relevant information about a child's language capabilities (Table 3–4).

Memory Tests

Memory involves cognitive mechanisms used to register, store, retain, and retrieve previous events, experience, or information.[12] Memory abilities exhibit a clear and reliable developmental progression over a wide age span.[85] Developmental changes that mark the progression toward mnemonic competence are attributable to the child's growing proficiency in the use of strategies to aid encoding and retrieval of information. As summarized by Kail and Hagen,[86] the attainment of mnemonic competence follows an invariant developmental pattern: (1) infrequent use of strategies in children aged 6 years and younger; (2) a transitional phase from 7–10 years of age, when strategies begin to emerge, implemented with increasing consistency and become gradually refined; and (3) the beginning of mature strategy use with further gradual

refinement in the effectiveness and flexibility with which they are implemented. An understanding of memory and related learning processes represents a critical component in the evaluation of a child's neuropsychological functioning. These cognitive processes are particularly important in light of the fact that children are faced with the ongoing task of acquiring information and skills through the educational system. Various tests of memory and learning are listed in Table 3–5.

Psychosocial Evaluation

The assessment of psychosocial status has different conceptual bases depending largely on the age of the child. Furthermore, a variety of forms should be used, including structured interview, observational methods, performance evaluation, and careful analysis of both medical data and psychosocial variables. In the interpretation of any method, the biologic realities that

TABLE 3–5. Measures of Memory Function

Instrument	Description	Comments
Test of Memory and Learning (TOMAL)[116]	Includes four core indices. Verbal Memory, Nonverbal Memory, Composite Memory, and Delayed Recall. Supplementary Indexes include Learning, Attention and Concentration, Sequential Memory, Free Recall, and Associative Recall	Has clinically relevant features, e.g., the option to compare the examinee's own personal learning curve with a standardized learning curve
Wide Range Assessment of Memory and Learning (WRAML)[117]	For ages 5–17 years. Designed to evaluate the ability of children's learning and memory for verbal and visual information. Includes three verbal, three visual, and three learning subtests, yielding a subtest for each domain. Standard scores and percentiles can be derived. Has immediate, delayed, and recognition formats	Provides normative data from a large group of children. Recognition format for delayed retention of the narrative information facilitates consideration of storage versus retrieval abilities. A screening form is available, requiring 10–15 minutes. Children with special needs were included, but those unable to respond to items were excluded
Benton Visual Retention Test (BVRT)[118]	Assesses visual memory, visual perception, and visuoconstructive abilities for ages 7 years–adult. Includes three alternate forms composed of 10 designs. Has three administration options consisting of copy and recall. For children aged 7–13 years, exact number correct and error scores with standard deviations are given.	Sensitive to visual inattention problems. Spatial organization problems may emerge in errors of size and placement. Scoring allows both quantitative and qualitative analysis. Can note right- and left-sided errors. Requires relatively intact visual motor skills. German edition has recognition format to use with individuals with motor disabilities
Rivermead Behavioral Memory Test (RBMT)[119]	Designed to detect impairment of everyday memory functioning and to monitor change after treatment. Kit is designed for adults but supplementary children's materials are available. Adult version is for ages 11–95 years. Children's version is for children aged 5–10 years. Four parallel versions are provided. Includes a Screening score and Profile scores. Items involve remembering to carry out everyday tasks or retaining the type of information needed for adequate everyday functioning	Relates to practical effects of impaired memory. Complements more traditional memory assessment techniques. Is ecologically valid in that it relates to subjective ratings of everyday memory problems. Addresses prospective memory. Tables are provided in the RBMT manual for evaluating individuals with expressive language deficits or perceptual problems

impinge on functioning, and therefore development, must be taken into account. No real measures have been developed and substantially normed on populations of children with disabilities or chronic illness regarding global concepts of personality or emotional functioning. Confounding emotional factors such as depression exist in children who have somatic distress, such as pain. Thus, interpretation usually requires an awareness of the specific items that can elicit medical as opposed to psychological distress.[87] Essentially what must be appreciated is that a wide range of adjustment levels exists. As mentioned earlier, this population has adjustment issues at higher levels than the nondisabled population as opposed to outright psychiatric disability. For this group, more than others, grouping of children by nature of disability has limited merit aside from identifying possible risk factors. Assumptions based on group membership by disability or medical condition can be inaccurate. For example, intuitive reasoning would indicate that individuals with disfigurements, such as amputations or burns, would be particularly affected. Such is not the

case, however, as demonstrated in research of these groups.[88]

Unique to the arena of personality or psychosocial functioning is the *empirically based* or *criterion-group* strategy to assessment. This approach grew in response to the serious liabilities presented by self-report tests, which used items that had face validity. For example, an item that asks about arguing with others was a direct question, just as could be asked in a live interview. There are great liabilities to that approach; it assumes that subjects can evaluate their own behavior objectively and that they understand the item in the way it was intended. In a radical departure, the developers of what came to be known as the Minnesota Multiphasic Personality Inventory (MMPI) formulated the test with the main premise that *nothing* can be assumed about the meaning of a subject's response to a test item. The meaning can be discerned only through empiric research. Items are presented to criterion groups, for example, depressed, schizophrenic, or passive-aggressive personality disorders, and control groups. By their answers as a diagnostic group, the items become indicative of a given disorder or personality outplay. This indication is regardless of what the content of the items was or an intuitive judgment of what it *should* indicate. This approach also allows for the determination of respondent's bias—whether an adolescent self-reporting as in the case of the MMPI-A (Minnesota Multiphasic Personality Inventory–Adolescent) or parents filling out a behavioral checklist such as the Personality Inventory for Children.

In young children, temperament is a more cogent concept than that of personality. The dynamics of psychosocial functioning is the effect of this on interaction with parents and other caregivers within the basic sensorimotor exploratory nature of infancy and early childhood. If school is children's work, play is the work of this youngest group. What an interview or a self-report measure yields in older children, the observation of play provides in the preschooler. To quote Knoff,[19] "This information reflects the preschooler's unique perceptions of his or her world, perceptions that are important in any comprehensive assessment of a referred child's problems." Projective techniques such as the Rorschach are not recommended in this population because of the need to interpret ambiguous visual stimuli. The active developmental maturation of visual perceptual systems and the attendant normative variability mitigate against the appropriateness in preschoolers.

In older children, self-report measures can begin to play an important role. Whether specific dimensions of psychosocial functioning (as in the Revised Manifest Anxiety Scale) or more comprehensive devices (such as the MMPI-A), they can be an important source of information with considered interpretation. A more behavioral medicine approach is seen in measures specifically oriented to the physical experience, such as the Pediatric Pain Questionnaire.[89]

Additionally, behavioral functioning in the more natural settings of play, home, and school must be explored. A number of instruments afford such an opportunity with parents or other caregivers and teachers as the informants (Table 3–6).

Transdisciplinary Play Based Assessment (TPBA)[18] is a standardized observation of play. It provides an exhaustive listing of developmentally cogent play behaviors under four domains: cognitive, language and communications, sensorimotor, and social-emotional development. It allows the child to engage in the most natural of activities and is limited in that there may not be an expression of a specific behavior of interest but rather a global picture of the child in interaction with the environment. Because of the

limitations of individually administered tests in the young child, this acts as cross-validation of parental report and is less influenced by the demand characteristics of traditional testing. The advantage of hearing spontaneous language production is particularly useful, for this is often the primary *shutdown* of younger children in an evaluation setting.[90] There are other systems for play observation. Some are designed for the more evocative structure of play designed to tap certain themes (e.g., abuse) used in children. In the rehabilitation population, nonpathologic issues such as adjustment and developmental integrity predominate, so Linder's system offers an excellent choice.

With the *Infant Behavior Record / Behavior Rating Scales of Bayley Scales of Infant Development / Bayley Scales of Infant Development–Second Edition (IBR) (BSR)*,[38] as part of the evaluation of developmental status for infants aged 2 months to 2.5 years, a systematic record is provided for observing a child's behavior. There are 11 areas covered in the IBR and 6 in the BRS. These include motivational variables, interest in specific sensory modalities, emotional regulation, and interpersonal behaviors. Normative data are in the form of characteristic behavioral descriptions by age, which are provided in the manual of the Bayley. Sattler[15] notes that the behaviors oriented toward cognitive tasks, such as attention span and goal directedness in the IBR form, relate to mental scores, in which social behaviors have not shown predictive power.

Personality Inventory for Children–Revised (PIC-R)[91] consists of 280 true/false items answered by one or both parents. It is a revision of the original PIC. Different normative data checks are used to evaluate the nature of the different parent responses. Extensive validity data have been published for this test and its predecessor. There are 20 scales, three of which are designed to detect informant response style because it may affect the validity of a given parent's statement. Other scales measure cognitive status, behavioral adjustment, and family status. Four factors have been detected: undisciplined or poor self-control, social incompetence, internalization and somatic symptoms, and cognitive development. Cautions have been voiced about its use in some specific rehabilitation populations—notably those with brain injury.

The *MMPI-A*[92] is based on the criterion group strategy described in the introductory comments to this section. It is the first revision of the original MMPI specifically for use with adolescents. For the original test (MMPI), adolescent norms were developed in the 1970s, but it

TABLE 3–6. Measures of Psychosocial Functioning

Instrument	Description	Comments
Transdisciplinary Play Based Assessment (TPBA)[18]	Normed for 6 months–6 years. Administered in home or clinic. Structured play observation	Designed with intervention development as primary goal. Taps a naturalistic activity, more engaging
Infant Behavior Record/Behavior Rating Scales of Bayley Scales of Infant Development[38]	For newborns to age 4 years. Structured observation done during standardized administration	Not normed, but typical behaviors are listed in manual. Important adjunct to most widely used test in youngest children
Personality Inventory for Children–Revised (PIC-R)[91]	Parental report on children aged 3–5 and 6–16 years. Separate norms for mother and father as respondents	Well normed for clinical population, but less research in rehabilitation population. Not descriptive with traumatic brain injury population and can be misleading in that respect. Can assess respondent bias
Minnesota Multiphasic Personality Inventory–Adolescent (MPPI-A)[92]	Objective self-report for adolescents aged 14–18 years. Revision of most widely used personality test for this age. Detailed assessment of test-taking attitude	Excellent standardization and psychometric properties. Alternative formats available that can assist in valid administrations to those with disabilities affecting response or stimulus. Likelihood of continued widespread use facilitates comparison across different groups. Length can be problematic in terms of engagement by subjects
Child Behavior Checklist (CBCL)[96]	Parental report for children aged 2–3 and 4–18 years in separate forms. Basic personality typologies are yielded as well	Good psychometric properties. Most widely used instrument in children with chronic illness and disability, so potential for literature comparisons. No way to assess respondent bias
Teacher's Report Form (TRF)[98]	Behavior checklist for teacher for children aged 6–16 years. Survey of problem behaviors and personality style. By same authors as CBCL	Includes items about use of academic skills in functional ways, so broader focus than most school measures. No means to detect respondent bias
Youth Self-Report (YSR)[99]	Self-report inventory for ages 11–18 years. Requires 30 minutes to take	Ease for subject as is short, but not widely used. Validity questionable. Also no alternative format
Millon Adolescent Clinical Inventory (MACI)[100]	Self-report inventory for adolescents in true-false format. Test-taking attitude is assessed. Administration requires 20 minutes and uses adolescent language	One of a group of tests by this author based on a theory of personality. No studies in rehabilitation population. May be well received by adolescents
Rorschach Inkblot Technique[101]	Projective personality test using 10 inkblots as ambiguous stimuli. Norms for ages 2 years and up, but generally only given to ages 5 years and up	Requires considerable expertise by examiner. No literature on use with rehabilitation population. Great caution should be exercised in its use
Thematic Apperception Test (TAT); Children's Apperception Test (CAT)[102]	Ambiguous pictures for which subjects produce a story with some structured questioning. No normative sample	Can assess themes useful in this population but requires careful interpretation

was only a downward extension at best. Now new items tap specific adolescent developmental or psychopathologic issues. There are new supplemental scales that give feedback relative to alcohol and drug problems and immaturity. There are 15 new content scales in addition to the original 10 clinical scales. Development of the validity and response bias of the subject was expanded by devising response inconsistency scales. The original MMPI interpreted with adolescent norms had been used extensively with adolescent medical populations, including those with physical disability.[93] In fact, it was the most widely used objective assessment measure overall for adolescents.[92] For the development of the MMPI-A, extensive rewriting and some

revision of test items were done. A national representative adolescent sample was used for normative data (not the case in the original MMPI). The new length is 478 test items presented in a booklet form, with true/false response. Reading level required is best considered to be seventh grade, although it had been designed with the goal of fifth-grade comprehension. In actuality, the range is from fifth to eighth grade. It is available in an audiotape format as well, which takes about 1.5 hours. Each item is read twice. This aspect was designed for access by the visually impaired but doubles for individuals who have reading comprehension problems. Language comprehension level required for the audiotape formate is fifth grade. A computer administration is also available that presents items singly and with responses entered on the keyboard.

There is no published evidence to date of use of the MMPI-A or MMPI-2 in a rehabilitation population.[94] It could be used, however, with much the same caution as applied to its prior version. For example, there was a correction factor to be applied in its use with spinal cord–injured individuals.[95] This was to obviate responses to items that reflected the reality of the medical condition, as opposed to the criterion value assigned to the item. A new version has been developed for the MMPI-2 and awaits replication of the original study findings.

Child Behavior Checklist (CBCL)[96] is a group of behavioral checklists to be filled out by parents, caregivers, teachers, and the child. These checklists comprise the six different behavior rating scales that have been developed in the years since the first scale's introduction 15 years ago. Specifically, they are parent reports on children aged 2–3 years and then another form for ages 4–16 years. Concurrent teacher and caregiver forms exist, the latter being most recently added for ages 2–6 years. The scales are written for a fifth-grade reading level and can be completed in 20 minutes.

The items for the CBCL–ages 2–3 years (CBCL/2–3) are distinctly different from the form that parents fill out for older children (CBCL/4–16), and this differential speaks, in part, to the usefulness of these inventories. The two scales share only 59 items each. The scale for 4–16-year-olds has 112 problem statements and 1 open-ended item. The checklist for 2–3-year-olds consists of 99 items and 1 open-ended item. Between the two forms, no group differences between genders were found for the children aged 2–3 years. In the scale for older children and adolescents, however, normative work yielded different factor structure and scale score norms for gender in three separate bands for age, in the predictable demarcation of preschooler, latency age, and adolescence.

A three-point scale is used to indicate whether the behavior listed is considered to be 2—very true or often true; 1—somewhat true or sometimes true; or 0—not true at the present time or within the last several months. These scales yield scores on broader personality dimensions, such as internalizing versus externalizing, and more narrow band scales, such as withdrawal and depression. Knoff[19] notes the need to look at individual items because some scales register as clinically significant for an entire factor with only two or three two-point responses. In terms of validity, the CBCL forms are strong,

registering not only independence from developmental and intellectual assessment tests, but also from other behavior checklists. Reliability is also considered good.

Wallander and Thompson[1] consider the CBCL to be the *gold standard* for use with children with chronic physical conditions. They cite Perrin and colleagues,[97] who caution about CBCL on the basis that validity considerations exist, as the instrument was not specifically designed for this population. The CBCL's limited sensitivity to less serious adjustment problems and the special nature of the assessment of social competence in this population require further consideration in its use. Because a number of studies have used this instrument, however, there is a possibility for comparison of results that does not exist to the same degree in any other instrument. The general caution about using multiple methods and the perspective of multiple informants remains important. Again, garnering the child's own perspective is helpful with self-report.

Teacher's Report Form (TRF)[98] assesses the presence of problem behavior syndromes as well as adaptive behavior in the school arena. It is probably the best form for school-based behavior information. It describes behavioral areas such as social abilities but also yields scores on personality styles, such as obsessive-compulsive. It is considered to be well standardized with good psychometric properties.

Youth Self-Report (YSR)[99] is a self-report measure for adolescents, repeating many of the items on the CBCL. Although reliability and normative statistics are adequate, validity is thought to need further research even on a broad clinical sample. It takes about 30 minutes to complete.

Millon Adolescent Clinical Inventory (MACI)[100] is a self-report inventory for adolescents. Reading level is sixth grade, and most teens can complete the inventory in less than 20 minutes. Attention was paid to adolescent vocabulary and language to maintain interest in completion and use in a wide variety of settings. It has 12 personality scales that parallel DSM-IV disorders, this convergence being a major goal of its principal author in line with the personality theory on which it is based.

Rorschach Inkblot Technique[101] remains a widely used test in children and adolescents. It is the classic technique of 10 inkblots presented with the instruction to say what it looks like to the examinee. An alteration in administration with younger people is to follow up with the *inquiry*, asking why it looked like whatever the response was, whereas this is done only after all blots are viewed when given to adults. Normative data on this technique for these age groups began appearing in the 1970s; however, these are not representative of the general population, being overrepresentative of children with above-average intelligence with incomplete attention to race and socioeconomic status.[101] Despite the fact that some norms exist down to age 2 years, most authors agree that the Rorschach should not be used with children below the age of 5 years. There is little experience with this type of test in assessing the type of adjustment issues common to the rehabilitation population. It should be used guardedly.

Children's Apperception Test (CAT) and Thematic Apperception Test (TAT)[102] represent another type of projective test, but this time the stimuli are ambiguous pictures, and the subject is asked to make up a story concerning what is happening, what led up to the scene in the picture, and what will happen next. It requires considerable skill on the part of the examiner and should be given only by the professional, as is the case with all the projective techniques. There is usually follow-up questioning about the story given, and the recording is verbatim. There are no real normative data on the TAT, but some authors believe that it remains a powerful technique in discerning children's personalities.[103] Some believe it taps themes of confusion and conflict with the child's resolution being a central focus of interpretation. It is based on the author's personality theory as opposed to a pathologic model. The entire set of cards numbers 20, although a standard administration uses only selected pictures. Over the years, individual cards have been identified as particularly useful with certain age groups.

Adaptive Behavior

Adaptive behavior is defined as meeting the social, physical, and emotional demands of one's environment. There are two major issues as noted by Sattler:[15] the ability of individuals to function and maintain themselves independently and the ability of individuals to meet the social and personal responsibilities expected by society. These behaviors range widely from basic eating skills to raising a family. As a group of devices, the criticism has been the norms based in impaired population. Yet these can add considerably to the evaluation of children in whom scattered or idiosyncratic developmental schemas are the norm, as opposed to the exception. The ability to predict future functioning from current scores is limited.

In determining a diagnosis of mental retardation, there is a central place for the assessment of adaptive behavior. Along with significantly below-average intellectual abilities, there must also be a commensurate poor level of adaptive behavior.[104] Deficits are evaluated according to chronologic age milestones. Across different ages, different behaviors are required. In early childhood, for instance, deficits relate to communication skills, self-help, and socialization. Later the demand is of competence in using basic academic skills in daily life, showing judgment both in the community and in one's social interactions. Lastly, vocational issues and more complex social relations are examined.

These tests are structured interviews that can be independently completed with ratings gained from informants such as parents and teachers (Table 3–7). Consequently, they are open to the response bias that can exist from such sources. They can, however, provide direct programming assistance in terms of feedback and development. Basic dimensions of competence as shown in these instruments are often disparate with intellectual testing scores in a traumatic brain injury population because they represent more procedural learning and are

TABLE 3–7. Measures of Adaptive Functioning

Instrument	Description	Comments
AAMD Adaptive Behavior Scale (ABS)[105]	Covers ages 3–69 years, designed for institutional populations. Two parts—first along developmental lines; second part looks at maladaptive behavior. Done by interview or independently. Takes 15–30 minutes	Sound instrument with a rational focus on actual observation, as opposed to self-report or a rating scale. More predictive than standard IQ tests in terms of ultimate delay
Vineland Adaptive Behavior Scales (VABS)[106]	Birth–age 19 years covered. 20–90 minutes to complete, depending on form used. Has norms for several groups with disabilities. Assesses ADL and maladaptive social behavior	Questions about validity. Based on family-systems theory. Designed to facilitate intervention. Only instrument that has a Spanish version, with norms. Limited ability for longitudinal tracking owing to reliability. Studies suggest this instrument more useful than behavior rating scales in describing functioning in the TBI population specifically

ADL, Activities of daily living; IQ, intelligence quotient; TBI, traumatic brain injury.

often less affected directly after injury. The failure to gain subsequent abilities can be a source of substantial disability as time goes on because of impairments in sensory or cognitive abilities.

AAMD Adaptive Behavior Scale (ABS)[105] has 21 domains divided into two parts. The first 9 domains assess the presence of independence or dependence on a variety of issues, including dressing, toileting, personal hygiene, communication skills, and socialization. The next 12 domains are about social behavior, including disruptive and aggressive behaviors. The test can be used with caretakers or teachers and independently completed. With parents, structured interview is the preferred mode of assessment. It was designed for institutional populations and in that sense is limited when assessing children in a family setting. Psychometric properties are considered sufficient to make this a reasonable choice but with the caution that substantial limitations, such as blindness or use of nonverbal form of communication, require an item analysis. The normative group did control for degree of mental retardation, however.

Psychometric properties of the AAMD show limited reliability and validity for part II. In that arena of maladaptive behavior, the construction of the scale is such that major behaviors receive the same scoring weight as minor ones, and the limited range of items makes change in an individual difficult to detect. Most valid are the two general scores from each section, as opposed to individual subdomain scores.

Vineland Adaptive Behavior Scales (VABS)[106] are probably the most widely used adaptive behavior surveys. As with the ABS, these are administered in the structured interview format to a parent or caregiver. A teacher independently completes the classroom form. There are three versions of the Vineland: Interview Edition, Survey Form; Interview Edition, Expanded Form; and Classroom Edition. The informant answers on a three-point scale as to whether a given behavior usually occurs, sometimes or partially occurs, or never occurs. Each measures behavior in four domains. The communication domain covers receptive, expressive, and written forms. The daily living skills domain includes personal, domestic, and community areas. The socialization domain includes interpersonal relationships, play and leisure time, and coping skills. Finally, the motor skills domain includes gross and fine motor skills for children 5 years old and younger. Four domain scores result in a composite index as well. A maladaptive behavior domain surveys inappropriate social or behavioral displays. There is a composite score yielded as well as a maladaptive behavior domain for both interview editions.

The Expanded Form takes between 60 and 90 minutes to administer and the survey form between 20 and 60 minutes. The former edition has almost twice as many items as the latter. The Classroom Edition is completed independently by a teacher for ages 3–12 years and takes about 20 minutes. It has items from both the Survey and Expanded editions as well as ones pertinent to academics. Many consider the Vineland the most open format for discussion, making it feel less intrusive and less testlike for the caretaker.

Single Construct Measures

In these days of cost-efficiency considerations, more specialized and specific scales have been developed. The choice of a specific construct is often suggested by the results of other examinations or by knowledge of the presenting problem. The measurement of anxiety and pain seems particularly cogent in this regard, and to that end, the instruments presented here demonstrate typical ones for these constructs (Table 3–8). These devices are self-report measures and suffer from the limitation that a child may not always respond honestly or candidly. They should not be the only instrument used.

TABLE 3–8. Measures of Single Dimensions

Instrument	Description	Comments
Revised Children's Manifest Anxiety Scale for Children (RCMAS)[107]	For school-aged children 10 years and up. Self-report on anxious feelings. At third-grade reading level	The scale's brevity limits the use of the subscales generated; does include one that looks at respondent test-taking attitude. Reading level of third grade makes it accessible to wide variety of patients
Pediatric Pain Questionnaire (PPQ)[89]	Available from authors, this is a comprehensive assessment of pain in children and adolescents filled out as a self-report. It is specifically geared to their language and descriptive mentality, with a body outline and grading system to indicate location and quality of pain. Also a parent form	Expresses a clinical perspective on how to measure the dimension of pain in children. Cross-validated with good psychometrics for this type of instrument

Revised Children's Manifest Anxiety Scale for Children (RCMAS)[107] has 37 short statements to which the child responds *yes* or *no*. There is a Total Anxiety score as well as a Lie subscale that examines the candidness and honesty of the response set. The brevity of the instrument results in the three anxiety subscales that can be generated but are of limited use. The standardization sample was large and representative of socioeconomic status, demographics, race, and gender. Validity and reliability are extensively reported in the manual and are helpful in informed interpretation. Reading level is third grade, so a wide variety of children and adolescents can use this device. Again a caution is that in its brevity and specificity, it should be only one part of a battery.

Pediatric Pain Questionnaire (PPQ)[89] is modeled after the well-respected adult measures (McGill Pain Questionnaire) but conceptualized with the cognitive developmental status of children in mind. Three forms are used—for children, adolescents, and parents. The first two are self-report, with the last one added for cross-validation purposes. Both cover the intensity of pain and the emotional and perceptual experience. The adolescent form also covers the social and environmental influences on the experience. It reportedly covers acute, chronic, and recurrent pain. An integral part of the process is history taking, including extensive history of treatments, child and family pain history as well as conversant environmental aspects. The PPQ uses a body outline and a visual analogue scale to determine the specific physiologic aspects. The analogue scale provides no numbers or markings but instead elicits present and worst pain intensity of the past week. Different semantic anchors are used for children (*not hurting* versus *hurting a lot*) along with happy and sad faces. The adolescent and parent versions are anchored by *no pain* and *severe pain* and pain descriptors of *hurting* and *discomfort*. The body outlines are age-appropriate on the children and adolescent forms. Four levels of pain intensity can be indicated by the child by coloring in the body outline with a choice of eight crayons. The child chooses colors to demonstrate intensity gauged by four categories of pain descriptors. In this way, they can show multiple sites and register the appropriate range of intensity in each. Separately a list of pain descriptors is provided that assesses the evaluative, emotional, and sensory quality of the child's own experience. Words are provided for younger children or anyone who may have trouble generating labels.

The multidimensional aspect of the PPQ is appealing for anyone who has struggled to understand the experience of pain in children. It allows for engaging visual representations as well as standard language expression. Expecting parent reports to match the child's is erroneous. As in the adult literature, the subjectivity of pain experience mitigates against this being the case. It is useful more as a gauge of convergence in the relationship between parent and child, not as a validating measure. Despite the unusual venue of some of its components, reliability and validity have been shown for the PPQ, and it holds considerable promise.

Family Environment

The instruments noted here are part of the ever-growing recognition of the pivotal importance of family functioning in the face of a child's disability and adjustment. The most dramatic impetus has been because of the requirement of a Family Service Plan in all early-intervention services for children up to 3 years of age. Beyond the case to be made in the youngest age group, many studies show a strong relationship between family functioning and a child's psychological adjustment across a number of different medical conditions.[1] The importance of such considerations is clear. Following are synopses of two widely used instruments for populations

TABLE 3–9. Measures of Family Function

Instrument	Description	Comments
Home Observation for Measurement of the Environment Scale (HOME)[108]	Is a home-based observation of 1 hour of interaction between mother and child. For infants and toddlers, with good representative norms	Sound instrument with a rational focus on actual observation, as opposed to self-report or a rating scale. More predictive than standard IQ tests in terms of ultimate delay
Family Environment Scale (FES)[110]	Parent report on family's social climate. 90 items. Part of a tradition of environment assessment. Gives a sense of the family's personality and values	Recent questions about validity. Based on family-systems theory. Designed to facilitate intervention. Only instrument of its kind with any track record in rehabilitation populations, although to date all work has been with adults as patients

IQ, Intelligence quotient.

often within the scope of a rehabilitation practice (Table 3–9). They can offer an important adjunct to more child-focused assessment as they enlighten the status of the most important environment in any child or adolescent's life.

Home Observation for Measurement of the Environment Scale (HOME)[108] assesses the nature and quantity of support for a child in the home as well as the quality of child care. It has 45 items and includes observations and an interview administered in the home when the child and caretaker are present. This instrument was based on the early Head Start movement. Normal routine is observed for over 1 hour. Six subscales are scored and represented in the following areas: (1) emotional and verbal responsiveness of mother; (2) avoidance of restriction and punishment; (3) organization of physical and temporal environment; (4) provision of appropriate play material; (5) maternal involvement with child; and (6) opportunity for variety in daily stimulation. Each item is rated on a *yes* or *no* basis according to the interview and observation. The HOME can identify risk of developmental delay because of insufficient environmental support and can aid in intervention planning. Standardization data on 176 families were gathered and indicate that a wide range of scores can be registered regardless of socioeconomic status. Adequate reliability has been shown and, most impressively, predictive validity—to the extent that HOME scores are better predictors of developmental delay or normality than the Bayley Scales of Infant Development.[109]

Family Environment Scale (FES)[110] rates parental perception of the social climate of the family and is rooted in family systems theory. It contains 90 true-false items that break down into 10 subscales: cohesion, expressiveness, conflict, independence, achievement orientation, intellectual-cultural orientation, active-recreational orientation, moral-religious orientation, family organization, and family rules. Scores are plotted on a profile with two forms available—the actual state of the family as perceived by individual members and the ideal state. Profiles derived from each parent can be compared from which a Family Incongruence Score is calculated.

There has been controversy about the psychometric properties of the FES relative to the stability of its factor structure. It was suggested that the factor structure varies depending on which family member's perceptions were used. There is some caution expressed about its use as a clinical diagnostic tool in a rehabilitation setting with adults.[111] Others have used it successfully in studies of children with chronic medical conditions. In one such study by Wallander and colleagues,[4] family cohesion made a significant contribution to social functioning in children with spina bifida.

Nontraditional Methods

Presented here are two techniques that can provide important data to the rehabilitation professional that do not meet psychometric standards but rather provide information on conceptual issues central to work with children with challenged development (Table 3–10). They attempt to answer important questions, as in the second section here, where program effectiveness is measured. The first section addresses an area that is pertinent to the challenges of children with disabilities. These challenges often include the demand to exhibit mastery motivation in situations such as physical, occupational, and speech therapy. As alluded to earlier, children with disabilities have additional demands placed on them by virtue of their need for rehabilitation therapies. Because these therapies are necessary for the acquisition of adaptive behavior or physical integrity, they are vital but represent a unique demand compared with that on nondisabled peers.

TABLE 3–10.   Measures with Nontraditional Focus

Instrument	Description	Comments
Mastery Motivation[21]	New approach in early child development given to children from infancy to 3 years. Is an observation in a fixed situation that is scored and compared with an established normative hierarchy. Parent's perceptions also can be gathered. Also has a structure to be used with the first edition of the Bayley Infant Scales	Although no research directly in a rehabilitation population, this instrument is used with many children with suspected developmental delay, so appropriate to the youngest children seen. Reactions to frustration and ability to persist are especially demanded in pediatric rehabilitation population
Treatment Gains[112]	Common-sense formulas to be used as another way to judge therapeutic progress. Can yield a ratio expressing child's rates of improvement against status before intervention	Useful to add some quantification to the clinical judgment necessary about therapy duration and timing

Mastery Motivation[21] is receiving growing attention in the early childhood assessment literature. To date, used primarily in research studies, the dimensions addressed here of persistence and effectiveness have high importance for the daily clinical issues facing the youngest rehabilitation patients. The *structured mastery task situation* involves tasks to determine a child's desire to master a given task. Task-directed behavior is that which relates to trying to complete part of the task with no assistance. Brockman and colleagues[21] present a developmental hierarchy against which to calibrate a child's efforts. It includes the expression of exploration and curiosity at 5 months and older. Persistence is observed at 9 months in practicing emerging skills (e.g., cause-and-effect toys, getting a toy from behind a barrier) and completing a multipart task at 15 months, such as placing shapes in a form board or sorter. Finally, a preference for challenging tasks at 3 years of age is seen in a choice between building the relatively hard task of a six-block tower versus building a two-block tower. The pleasure as seen in the affect displayed in working or completing a task is noted as well as persistence as expressed in the time worked to find a solution.

From the same authors has come a scale used with the Bayley scales, to be observed while working with a child. Scoring systems can be used in observing a toddler during free play. Finally, the parent's perception of the child's mastery behavior is assessed by the *Dimensions of Mastery Questionnaire (DMQ)*. IT rates these behaviors across five types of play: (1) gross motor, (2) combinatorial, (3) means-end, (4) symbolic, and (5) social.

Treatment gains can be measured in a variety of ways. There are important considerations for avoiding the use of repeat standardized testing because there can be practice effects or conversely no change shown when real change has occurred. The inaccuracies grow proportionally to the degree of impairment a child shows because standardized instruments can bring more distortion to the determination. Finally, that was not the purpose of *any tests* covered, and yet feedback about effectiveness should and must occur. In the simple techniques given here, each child can be his or her *N* = 1.

Severe limitations exist about these derived scores. First, whether change is seen or not could be due to nontreatment factors such as environmental change or a normal plateau. All of the methods discussed are referenced in Benner and Brockmann.[112]

Comparison to the norm uses developmental gain in months divided by time in intervention to yield an intervention efficiency rate. Rates below 1.00 show slower rates, and those above 1.00 show developmental progress in excess of the time spent in treatment.

Comparison with ideal rates of development is an alternative procedure that weighs the child's developmental status. The score obtained is an efficiency index calculated so that [actual gain/ideal gain] / [developmental status] = *efficiency index*. Actual gain is the gain in months seen before and after treatment observation, and ideal gain is the actual time in intervention. Developmental status is an index score yielded from testing divided by 100.

Comparison with previous rates of development compares a child's progress with the rate of development before intervention. The resulting *proportional change index* is calculated in this fashion: [developmental gain / time in intervention] / [pretest developmental age / pretest chronologic age]. Lower rates during intervention yield proportional change indices below 1.00 and increased rates show proportional change indices over 1.00.

Conclusion

This chapter has sought to serve the physician as a major referral source for psychological assessment. The broad area beyond IQ determination, the unique considerations in this population, and methods, particularly for the youngest children, have been covered. Both the pros and cons of standardized tests in this population were delineated as well as the benefits of considering less well-known instruments or nonstandard techniques. Despite the contributions of these evaluative tools to diagnosis and treatment planning, an awareness of their limitations is important if the clinician is to fulfill the role of driving the treatment process either directly through treatment orders or referrals or indirectly as a parental consultant. The clinician must be comfortable with the expenditures of both economic and emotional resources in the pursuit of improvement through therapy, medication, or surgery. This chapter is meant as an ongoing reference to aid in that decision making.

References

1. Wallander JL, Thompson RJ: Psychosocial adjustment of children with chronic physical conditions. In Roberts MC (ed): Handbook of Pediatric Psychology. New York, Guilford Press, 1995.
2. Cadman D, Boylem B, Szatmari P, Offord DR: Chronic illness, disability and mental and social well-being: Findings of the Ontario Child Health Study. Pediatrics 1987;79:505.

3. Pless IB, Roughman KJ: Chronic illness and its consequences: Observations based on three epidemiological studies. J Pediatr Psychol 1971;79:351.

4. Wallander JL, Varni JW, Babani L, et al: Disability parameters: Chronic strain and adaptation of physically handicapped children and their mothers. J Pediatr Psychol 1989;14:23.

5. Austin JK, Huberty TJ: Development of Child Attitude toward Illness Scale. J Pediatr Psychol 1993;18:467.

6. Breslau N, Marshall IA: Psychological disturbance in children with physical disabilities: Continuity and change in a 5-year follow-up. J Abnorm Child Psychol 1985;13:199.

7. Rutter M: Introduction: Concepts of brain dysfunction syndromes. In Rutter M (ed): Developmental Neuropsychiatry. New York, Guilford Press, 1983.

8. Erikson EH: Childhood and Society, 2nd ed. New York, WW Norton, 1963.

9. Franzen MD: Reliability and Validity in Neuropsychological Assessment. New York, Plenum Press, 1989.

10. Sattler JM: Assessment of Children, 3rd ed. San Diego, Jerome M. Sattler, 1988.

11. Wendland LV, Urmer A, Safford H: The intellectual functioning of postpoliomyelitic patients. J Clin Psychol 1960;16:179.

12. Lezak M: Neuropsychological Assessment, 3rd ed. New York, Oxford University Press, 1995.

13. Cushman LA: History and context. In Cushman LA, Scherer MJ (eds): Psychological Assessment in Medical Rehabilitation. Washington, DC, American Psychological Association, 1995.

14. DeMaso DR, Beardslee WR, Silbert AR, et al: Psychological functioning in children with cyanotic heart defects. J Dev Behav Pediatr 1990;11:289.

15. Sattler JM: Assessment of Children, Revised and Updated, 3rd ed. San Diego, Sattler, 1992.

16. Roberts MA, Milich R, Loney J: Structured Observation of Academic and Play Settings (SOAPS). Iowa City, IA, Unpublished manuscript, 1984.

17. Haynes SN: Behavioral assessment. In Hersen M, Kazdin A, Bellak A (eds): The Clinical Psychology Handbook. New York, Pergamon Press, 1991.

18. Linder TW: Transdisciplinary Play-Based Assessment. Baltimore, Paul H. Brookes, 1990.

19. Knoff HM: Assessment of social-emotional functioning and adaptive behavior. In Nuttall EV, Romero I, Kalesnik J (eds): Assessing and Screening Preschoolers. Boston, Allyn & Bacon, 1982.

20. Yussen SR, Santrock JW: Child Development: An Introduction. Dubuque, IA, WC Brown, 1982.

21. Brockman LM, Morgan GA, Harmon RJ: Mastery motivation and developmental delay. In Wachs TD, Sheehan R (eds): Assessment of Young Developmentally Disabled Children. New York, Plenum, 1988.

22. Lee JA, Moreno KE, Sympson JB: The effects of mode of test administration on test performance. Educational and Psychological Measurement 1986;46:467.

23. Wechsler D: Wechsler Intelligence Scale for Children, 3rd ed. New York, Psychological Corporation, 1991.

24. Wechsler D: Manual for the Wechsler Adult Intelligence Scales–Revised. New York, Psychological Corporation, 1981.

25. Wechsler D: Manual for the Wechsler Preschool and Primary Scale of Intelligence–Revised. New York, Psychological Corporation, 1989.

26. Thorndike RL, Hagen EP, Sattler JM: Stanford-Binet Intelligence Scale, 4th ed. Chicago, Riverside Publishing Company, 1986.

27. Ulrey G, Schnell R: Introduction to assessing young children. In Ulrey G, Rogers S (eds): Psychological Assessment of Handicapped Infants and Young Children. New York, Thieme Stratton, 1982.

28. Honzik M: Value and limitation of infant tests. In Lewis M (ed): Origins of Intelligence. New York, Plenum Publishing, 1976.

29. DuBose RF: Predictive value of infant intelligence scales with multiply handicapped children. Am J Ment Defic 1976;81:14.

30. McCall RB, Hogarty PS, Hurlburt N: Transition in infant sensorimotor development and the prediction of childhood IQ. Am Psychol 1972;27:728.

31. Bloom BS: Stability and Change in Human Characteristics. New York, John Wiley & Sons, 1964.

32. Stevenson MB, Lamb ME: Effects of infant sociability and the caretaking environment on infant cognitive performance. Child Dev 1979;50:340.

33. McCarthy DA: Manual for the McCarthy Scales of Children's Abilities. New York, Psychological Corporation, 1972.

34. Valencia RR: Stability of the McCarthy Scales of Children's Abilities over a one-year period for Mexican-American children. Psychology in the Schools 1983; 20:29.

35. Kaufman AS, Kaufman NL: Administration and Scoring Manual for the Kaufman Assessment Battery for Children. Circle Pines, MN, American Guidance Service, 1983.

36. Das J, Kirby JR, Jarman RF: Simultaneous and Successive Cognitive Processes. New York, Academic Press, 1979.

37. Goldstein DJ, Smith KB, Waldrep EE: Factor analytic study of the Kaufman Assessment Battery for Children. J Clin Psychol 1986;42:890.

38. Bayley N: Manual for the Bayley Scales of Infant Development, 2nd ed. New York, Psychological Corporation, 1993.

39. Ames LB: Predictive value of infant behavior examination. In Hellmuth J (ed): Exceptional Infant, The Normal Infant, vol 1. Seattle, Straub & Hellmuth, 1967.

40. Cattell P: Cattell Infant Intelligence Scale. New York, Psychological Corporation, 1970.

41. Gesell A: Gesell Developmental Schedules. New York, Psychological Corporation, 1949.

42. Brazelton TB: Neonatal Behavioral Assessment Scale. Philadelphia, JB Lippincott, 1976.

43. Uzgiris I, Hunt J: Assessment in Infancy: Ordinal Scales of Psychological Development. Urbana, IL, University of Illinois Press, 1975.

44. Wachs TD, DeRemer P: Adaptive behavior and Uzgiris-Hunt Scale performance of young, developmentally disabled children. Am J Ment Defic 1978;83:2.

45. Fagan JF: A new look at infant intelligence. In Detterman DK (ed): Current Topics in Human Intelligence: Research Methodology, vol 1. Norwood, NJ, Ablex, 1985.

46. Bendell-Estroff D, Greenfield DB, Hogan AE, et al: Early assessment of sensorimotor and cognitive development in high-risk infants. J Pediatr Psychol 1989;4:549.

47. Dunn L, Dunn ES: Peabody Picture Vocabulary Test–Revised. Circle Pines, MN, American Guidance Service, 1981.

48. French JL: Manual: Pictorial Test of Intelligence. Chicago, Riverside Publishing, 1964.

49. Leiter RG: Leiter International Performance Scale. Chicago, Stoelting, 1948.

50. Arthur G: The Arthur Adaptation of the Leiter International Performance Scale. J Clin Psychol 1949;5:345.

51. Raven JC: Progressive Matrices. Lewis, 1938.

52. Raven JC: Guide to Using the Standard Progressive Matrices. London, Lewis, 1960.

53. Raven JC: The Coloured Progressive Matrices Test. London, Lewis, 1965.

54. Brown L, Sherbenou RJ, Johnson SK: Test on Nonverbal Intelligence, 2nd ed. A Language-Free Measure of Cognitive Ability. Austin, TX, Pro-Ed, 1990.

55. Kaufman A, Kaufman NL: Kaufman Test of Educational Achievement. Circle Pines, MN, American Guidance Service, 1985.

56. Wechsler Individual Achievement Test. San Antonio, TX, Psychological Corporation, 1992.

57. Woodcock RW, Mather N: Woodcock-Johnson Tests of Achievement. Allen, TX, DLM/Teaching Resources, 1989.

58. Wilkinson GS: WRAT3 Administration Manual. Wilmington, DE, 1993.

59. Dunn LM, Markwardt FC: Peabody Individual Achievement Test Manual. Circle Pines, MN, American Guidance Service, 1970.

60. Hammill DD, Larsen SC: Test of Written Language–2. Austin, TX, Pro-Ed, 1988.

61. Lezak MD: Neuropsychological Assessment, 2nd ed. New York, Oxford University Press, 1983.

62. Tramontana MG, Hooper SR (eds): Assessment Issues in Child Neuropsychology. New York, Plenum Press, 1988.

63. Lyon GR, Moats L, Flynn JM: In Tramontana MG, Hooper SR (eds): Assessment Issues in Child Neuropsychology. New York, Plenum Press, 1988.

64. Golden CJ: Luria-Nebraska Neuropsychological Battery: Children's Revision. Los Angeles, Western Psychological Services, 1987.

65. Reitan RM, Wolfson D: The Halstead-Reitan Neuropsychological Test Battery. Tucson, Neuropsychology Press, 1985.

66. Hynd GW: Neuropsychological Assessment in Clinical Child Psychology. Newbury Park, CA, Sage, 1988.

67. Korkman M, Kirk U, Kemp S: NEPSY. San Antonio, TX, Psychological Corporation, 1997.

68. Gordon M: The Gordon Diagnostic System. DeWitt, NY, Gordon Systems, 1983.

69. Goldman-Rakic PS: Working memory and the mind. Sci Am 1992;257:111.

70. Heaton RK, Chelune GJ, Talley JL, et al: Wisconsin Card Sorting Test (WCST) Manual Revised and Expanded. Odessa, FL, Psychological Assessment Resources, 1993.

71. Milner B: Effects of different brain lesions on card sorting. Arch Neurol 1963;9:90.

72. Pennington BF, Van Doorninck WJ, McCabe LL, et al: Neurological deficits in early-treated phenylketonurics. Am J Ment Defic 1985;89:467.

73. Robinson AL, Heaton RK, Lehman RAW, Stilson DW: The utility of the Wisconsin Card Sorting Test in detecting and localizing frontal lobe lesions. J Consult Clin Psychol 1980;48:605.

74. Welsh MC, Groisser D, Pennington BF: A normative-developmental study of measures hypothesized to tap prefrontal functioning. J Clin Exp Neuropsychol 1988;10:79.

75. Halstead WC: Brain and Intelligence. Chicago, University of Chicago Press, 1947.

76. Bond JA, Buchtel HA: Comparison of the Wisconsin Card Sorting Test and the Halstead Category Test. J Clin Psychol 1984;40:1251.

77. Simon HA: The functional equivalence of problem solving skills. Cognitive Psychology 1975;7:268.

78. Bender LA: Visual Motor Gestalt Test and Its Clinical Use. New York, American Orthopsychiatric Association Research Monograph, 1938.

79. Beery KE: The VMI Developmental Test of Visual-Motor Integration Administration, Scoring, and Teaching Manual, 3rd Revision. Cleveland, Modern Curriculum Press, 1989.

80. Rey A: L'examen psychologique dans les cas d'encephalopathie traumatique. Arch Psychol 1941;28:286.

81. Osterrieth PA: Le test de copie d'une figure complex: Contribution a l'etude de la perception et de la memoire. Arch Psychol 1944;30:286.

82. Ewing-Cobbs L, Levin HS, Eisenberg HM, Fletcher JM: Language functions following closed head injury in children and adolescents. J Clin Exp Neuropsychol 1987;9:575.

83. Benton AL, Hamsher K de S: Multilingual Aphasia Examination. Iowa City, IA, AJA Associates, 1989.

84. Kaplan EF, Goodglass H, Wintraub S: The Boston Naming Test, 2nd ed. Philadelphia, Lea & Febiger, 1983.

85. Hagen J, Jongward R, Kail R: Cognitive perspectives on the development of memory. In Reese HW (ed): Advances in Child Development and Behavior, vol 10. New York, Academic Press, 1975.

86. Kail RR, Hagen JW: Memory in childhood. In Wolman B, Stricker G, Ellman S, et al (eds): Handbook of Developmental Psychology. Englewood Cliffs, NJ, Prentice-Hall, 1982.

87. Kashani JH, Barbero G, Wilfley DE, Morris D: Psychological concomitants of cystic fibrosis in children and adolescents. Adolescence 1988;23:873.

88. Richard JS, Elliott TR, Cotliar R, Stevenson V: Pediatric medical rehabilitation. In Roberts MC (ed): Handbook of Pediatric Psychology. New York, Guilford Press, 1995.

89. Varni JW, Thompson KL: The Varni/Thompson Pediatric Pain Questionnaire. Unpublished manuscript, 1985.

90. Romero I: Individual assessment procedures with preschool children. In Nuttall EV, Romero I, Kalesnik J (eds): Assessing and Screening Preschoolers. Boston, Allyn & Bacon, 1992.

91. Wirt RD, Lachar D, Klinedinst JK, et al: Multidimensional Description of Child Personality: A Manual for the Personality Inventory for Children. Los Angeles, Western Psychological Service, 1990.

92. Butcher JN, Williams CL, Graham JR, et al: MMPI—A Minnesota Multiphasic Personality Inventory–Adolescent. Minneapolis, MN, University of Minnesota Press, 1992.

93. Harper DC: Personality correlates and degree of impairment in male adolescents with progressive and nonprogressive physical disorders. J Clin Psychol 1983;39:859.

94. Elliott TR, Umlauf RL: Measurement of personality and psychopathology following acquired physical disability. In Cushman LA, Scherer MJ (eds): Psychological Assessment in Medical Rehabilitation. Washington, DC, American Psychological Association, 1995.

95. Taylor GP: Moderator-variable effect on personality-test-item endorsements of physically disabled patients. J Consult Clin Psychol 1970;35:211.

96. Achenbach TM, Edelbrock C: Manual for the Child Behavior Checklist and Revised Child Behavior Profile. Burlington, University of Vermont, Department of Psychiatry, 1983.

97. Perrin JM, Stein RE, Drotar D: Cautions in using the Child Behavior Checklist: Observations based on research about children with chronic illness. J Pediatr Psychol 1991;14:411.

98. Achenbach TM, Edelbrock CS: Child Behavior Checklist and Youth Self-Report. Burlington, Author, 1986.

99. Achenbach TM, Edelbrock CS: Teacher's Report From. Burlington, Author, 1986.

100. Millon T, Green CJ, Meagher RB: Millon Adolescent Personality Inventory Manual. Minneapolis, National Computer Systems, 1982.

101. Aronow E, Reznikoff M, Moreland K: The Rorschach Technique. Boston, Allyn & Bacon, 1994.

102. Murray H: Explorations in Personality. New York, Oxford University Press, 1938.
103. Blau TH: The Psychological Examination of the Child. New York, Wiley & Sons, 1991.
104. Grossman HJ: Classification in Mental Retardation. Washington, DC, American Association on Mental Deficiency, 1983.
105. Lambert N, Nihira K, Leland H: AAMR Adaptive Behavior Scales–School, 2nd ed (ABS-S:2). Austin, TX, Pro-Ed, 1993.
106. Sparrow S, Balla D, Chicchetti D: Vineland Adaptive Behavior Scales. Circle Pines, MN, American Guidance Services, 1984.
107. Reynolds CR, Richmond BO: Revised Children's Manifest Anxiety Scale (RCMAS). Los Angeles, Western Psychological Services, 1985.
108. Caldwell BM, Bradley R: Home Observation for the Measurement of the Environment. Little Rock, University of Arkansas, 1984.
109. Nugent JK, Davidson CE: Newborn and infant assessment. In Nuptial EV, Romero I, Kalesnik J (eds): Assessing and Screening Preschoolers. Boston, Allyn & Bacon, 1992.
110. Moos RH, Moos VS: Family Environment Scale Manual. Palo Alto, CA, Consulting Psychologists Press, 1981.
111. Novack TA, Gage RJ: Assessment of family functioning and social support. In Cushman LA, Scherer MJ (eds): Psychological Assessment in Medical Rehabilitation. Washington, DC, American Psychological Association, 1995.
112. Benner SM, Brockmann BW: Is the child making expected progress? Measuring change in rate of development with young children. Early Education and Development 1990;1:424.
113. Gronwall D, Wrightson P: Memory and information processing after closed head injury. J Neurol Neurosurg Psychiatry 1981;44:889.
114. Colden JC: Stroop Color and Word Test. Chicago, Stoelting Co., 1978.
115. DiSimoni FG: The Token Test for Children. Hingham, MA, Teaching Resources Corp., 1978.
116. Reynolds CR, Bigler ED: Test of Memory and Learning. Austin, TX, Pro-Ed, 1994.
117. Adams W, Sheslow D: WRAML Manual. Wilmington, DE, Jastak Assoc., 1990.
118. Benton AL: Revised Visual Retention Test, 4th ed. New York, The Psychological Corporation, 1974.
119. Wilson BA: The Rivermead Behavioral Memory Test. Reading, England, Thames Valley Test Co.; Gaylord, MI, National Rehabilitation Services, 1985.

Chapter 4

Language Development and Disorders of Communication and Oral Motor Function

Cheryl Smith, PhD
Joy Hill, MA

When we consider the uniqueness of humans in the animal kingdom, we most certainly entertain the role of human language in social-communicative acts. Humans engage in social interaction using verbal symbols that are produced, for the most part, by the vocal tract. This tract has evolved in humans to provide us with the unique anatomy and physiology to produce a variety of speech sounds for the purpose of communicating ideas and feelings. Verbal symbols also can be produced and executed by the hand in the expression of written language or gestural/sign language. Thus, spoken, written, and gestural languages function to express and receive information from other humans using separate means and modes.

Language as a vehicle for the communication of ideas and feelings is distinguished from the execution or production of **speech**. Language denotes the structural and semantic properties of symbols and semiotic function, whereas speech conveys the idea of motor output or the production of speech sounds. Both speech and language are used in the act of **communication**. Each of these areas contains subparts, which can be recognized, viewed, and measured.

Language Components

Five aspects characterize language: phonology, morphology, syntax, semantics, and pragmatics. Each of these aspects can be assigned to one of three components of language: form, content, and use. The first three aspects—phonology, morphology, and syntax—are considered the **form** of language and provide the necessary rule-based structure for humans to form words, phrases, and sentences. The semantic component brings meaning and conceptual networks

for the coding of vocabulary and constructs and is considered the **content** of language. Finally, the pragmatic component governs the **use** of language in context. Humans use language to perform functions such as requesting, commenting, labeling, describing, questioning, and so forth. The interaction among form, content, and use is schematized in a Venn diagram (Fig. 4–1). Area D in the center of the diagram represents the integration and overlap of form, content, and use of language or language competence.

Phonology is concerned with the sounds or phonemes that comprise a language and the rules for determining how phonemes are used. The English language contains approximately 44 separate phonemes that are produced and recognized by native speakers as members of the sound system. Phonemes can be classified as either vowels or consonants, and such classification depends on how the air from the lungs passes through the oral cavity. Vowels are produced with little obstruction of the airflow; the variable position of the tongue and lips changes the size and shape of the oral cavity to form specific vowels. Consonants are produced by obstructing the airflow and, depending on the manner and degree of obstruction, provide the acoustic characteristics of different consonant sounds.

Morphology governs the rules for constructing words, deriving various word forms through the use of prefixes and suffixes, and using grammatical markers or inflections. Derived word forms include plurals, verb tenses, adverbs, and adjectives. For example, the word, *sleeping*, contains the root word *sleep* (made up of four phonemes: /s/, /l/, /i/, and /p/) and the suffix -*ing*, indicating a verb tense. The plural marker -*s* is used in English when we want to indicate the notion of

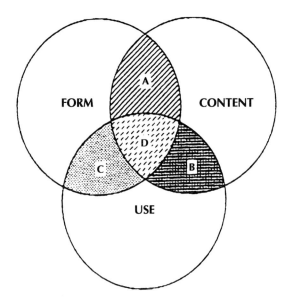

FIGURE 4–1.   The interaction of content, form, and use in language. (Adapted from Lahey M: Language Disorders and Language Development. New York, MacMillan Publishing Company, 1998.)

more than one, such as the distinction between the words *cat* and *cats*. Acquisition of morphemes and morphologic rules can be a source of difficulty when children are learning a language.

Syntax refers to the set of rules that governs how words are to be combined to form phrases and how phrases are to be combined to form a simple clause structure or sentence. English has a basic *s-v-o* construction, which means that we speak in a subject-verb-object word order. The sentence, *The young child carefully cradled the puppy in her lap*, contains the noun phrase *the young child*, the verb phrase *carefully cradled*, and the object noun phrase *the puppy in her lap* in the appropriate s-v-o order. Other languages may follow a different syntactic rule system, such as the Japanese syntactic frame s-o-v.

Semantics is the aspect of language that encompasses the meaning of words as they relate to objects, actions, events, and relationships among them. The semantic component, therefore, is conceptual and evident in what people talk about or the ideas that people express. The semantic component of language is related to culture, experience, and intellectual level.

Pragmatics is the use of language in context. It is a broad term that refers to the social functions of language or the reasons why we speak in terms of both personal and social goals. We use language to regulate others' behavior, to interact socially, and to fulfill personal functions that do not necessarily involve a social exchange with other persons.

Development of Language and Speech

The acquisition of speech and language ability in the function of communication has been the subject of intensive study for more than a century by linguists, scholars, philosophers, and biologists. How is it that children from a variety of cultures and human experiences arrive at a language? The question becomes more intriguing when one considers that more than 1,000 languages exist in the world. The answer lies in the biologic basis of human language and spoken communication.

Homo sapiens has unique central nervous, auditory, and vocal tract systems that function to support the acquisition of language and speech. The specialized function of the left hemisphere in the lateralization of language is well established. Important speech and language functions are localized in Broca's and Wernicke's areas, and damage to these areas results in deficits in the ability to comprehend and produce speech and language.

The vocal mechanism, including the structures of respiration and phonation, has evolved in humans to perform two functions. The primary function is to prevent the aspiration of food and liquid during deglutition. The secondary function is to provide a laryngeal valving mechanism necessary for phonation and production of speech sounds. Many children with congenital and acquired conditions interfering with sensory-motor neural control of the larynx and vocal tract present with dysphagia as well as aphonia or dysphonia.

In considering the roles of speech, language, and communication in children, one is faced with the dichotomy of both the development of symbolic and motor capacities and the effect of developmental arrests and acquired insults on speech communication. Developmental delays in speech, language, and communication are addressed by educational and health care professionals through the habilitative process. Maximizing function, learning, and acquiring are verbs that come to mind when one considers the concept of **habilitation** for children with a variety of congenitally based delays in speech communication. Habilitation is a process of developing a skill to be able to function within a given environment.[2] Rosen, Clark, and Kivitz[3] stated that habilitation is "a process by which various professional services are utilized to help a disabled individual make maximal use of his capacities in order that he might learn to function more effectively." In the realm of pediatric speech and language pathology, this concept involves establishing a functional mode of oral or nonoral communication and functional receptive language skills, spoken or written, for daily needs.

What then of acquired disorders of speech communication and oral motor function? Children who experience neurologic insults either from medical or accidental events frequently display dramatic deficits in speech, language, communication, and swallowing. The focus of intervention becomes **rehabilitation**, in which the educational and medical community attempt to reteach once automatic cognitive-linguistic and vegetative skills. Regain, recover, and restore are terms that come to mind when one considers the concept of rehabilitation for children with acquired disabilities such as traumatic brain injury or spinal cord injury and, in some cases, hearing loss or dysphagia. Nicolosi[2] defined rehabilitation as "restoration to normal, or to as satisfactory a status as possible, of impaired functions." Rosen et al.[3] refer to rehabilitation as a "process of 'restoring' the handicapped individual to the fullest physical, mental, social, vocational, and economic usefulness of which he is capable." In the pediatric population, the role of speech and language pathology translates into developing or restoring communication and oral motor function. Health care professionals must recognize the commonalities of habilitation and rehabilitation and essentially provide both, depending on the nature of the disorder (Fig. 4–2).

The Course of Language Development

The first year of life chronicles many cognitive and social achievements that relate to language development. The child's greatest achievements are the emergence of **intentional communication** and the beginnings of the **internal representation** of symbols. Researchers point to the onset of gestural communication in the performance of social intentions during the second half of the first year of life as evidence for the emergence of intentional communication. Two early gestural intentions appear. The first, called **protoimperative**, refers to the intention of using an adult agent as a tool in achieving some end. Protoimperative gestural intention is often expressed by 9–12 months of age and is characterized by the use of a pointing gesture toward an object in the act of request. The second gestural intention, called **protodeclarative**, refers to the preverbal effort to direct an adult's attention through the act of showing or gesture to some event or object in the world. These early gestural and vocal complexes culminate in the emergence of single words at age 10–14 months.

Children's first words are most likely for objects and people closely associated with the child. In studying the first 50 words of 18 children, Nelson[4] found that 65% were either general nominal words, such as *doggie*, or specific nominal words such as *Mama* or *Dada*. First words also included action terms (14%) such as *up* and *see*, modifiers (9%) such as *dirty*, personal-social terms such as *bye-bye* and *please* (8%), and general function words such as *on* (4%). The acquisition of at least 50 single words has been linked to the onset of two-word phrases and short sentences and is considered a critical milestone by 18–24 months. When combinatorial language

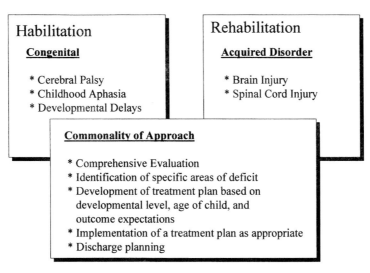

Habilitation & Rehabilitation

Habilitation	Rehabilitation
Congenital	**Acquired Disorder**
* Cerebral Palsy	* Brain Injury
* Childhood Aphasia	* Spinal Cord Injury
* Developmental Delays	

Commonality of Approach

* Comprehensive Evaluation
* Identification of specific areas of deficit
* Development of treatment plan based on developmental level, age of child, and outcome expectations
* Implementation of a treatment plan as appropriate
* Discharge planning

FIGURE 4–2.   The commonalities of habilitation and rehabilitation.

appears, the child is beginning to master the syntax, morphology, and phonology of the primary language. By 3 years of age, children usually have both simple and compound/complex sentences in their linguistic repertoire. From 3–6 years children refine the structural and conversational/discourse features of their language, including the use of narrative structure. Finally, at 6 years, the oral language competence provides the necessary but not sufficient grounds for the emergence and acquisition of written language competence. Children continue to refine their knowledge and use of spoken and written language through late adolescence.

Congenital Language Disorders

Congenital language disorders in children are characterized by late onset and slow development in the comprehension and/or use of language for any or all of the purposes of listening, speaking, reading, and writing. Historically, a number of approaches have been used to differentiate language disorders, which manifest in various forms. The traditional approach to congenital language disorders is to classify the disorders by the presumed etiology and to summarize clusters of language behaviors and variations in language acquisition for each group. One of the earliest classifications was made by Myklebust,[5] who included (1) etiologic categories of mental retardation, deafness and hearing impairment, emotional disturbance and autism, and childhood aphasia and (2) neurologically based disorders. Another approach is to classify language disorders not on the presumed etiology but by a descriptive, developmental approach.[1] This approach describes rather than classifies language disorders and uses data about normal language development as a point of comparison between language-delayed or language-disordered children and children acquiring language without difficulty. Language-disordered children demonstrate delays and differences in either the **form** of language (syntax, morphology, phonology), the **content** of language (semantics and cognitive ideation), or the functional **use** of language (pragmatic). Moreover, children may have a combination of some or all of the language components involved in their disorder, creating a number of possible variations and subtypes.

Finally, a number of researchers have attempted to define subtypes of language disorders based on statistical factor analysis of presenting behaviors and corresponding linguistic deficits. The nosologic subtypes of language disorders presented by Rapin and Allen[6] are among recent attempts to provide comprehensive profiles of

language-disordered children so that appropriate strategies for remediation can be applied. Rapin and Allen[6] described five subtypes of developmental language disorders: semantic-pragmatic syndrome, autism, phonosyntactic syndrome, verbal auditory agnosia, and severe expressive syndrome. Table 4–1 presents commonalities of classifications of language disorders based on etiology, description, or subtype. The following discussion of congenital language disorders focuses on the major etiologic categories along with descriptions of typical language behaviors and deficits as well as nosologic subtypes.

Mental Retardation

Children with mental retardation encompass a wide range of physical conditions, behaviors, and speech and language abilities. Generally, their speech and language abilities correspond to their overall cognitive abilities, including both intellectual functioning and adaptive behavior. The American Association of Mental Retardation (AAMR) defines mental retardation as "significantly subaverage general intellectual functioning existing concurrently with deficits in adaptive behavior and manifested during the developmental period."[7] All three components of the definition must be met to include an individual in the classification. An IQ of 70 or below is the standard benchmark of subaverage intellectual functioning, according the AAMR. A number of different tests are available to psychologists to measure intelligence, depending on the age and verbal ability of the child. For example, the Stanford-Binet Intelligence Scale[8] or the Wechsler Scales[9] are well normed instruments with excellent reliability and validity. The evaluation of adaptive behavior is more difficult because fewer well-standardized and reliable instruments are designed to measure an individual's ability to function socially with appropriate age and cultural expectations. Finally, the developmental period is regarded as the period between birth and 18 years. The AAMR recognizes four categories of mental retardation based on the level of intelligence and adaptive behavior. Table 4–2 contains the classification of mental retardation with corresponding IQ range, and speech/language ability.

Because speech, language, and communication are considered to be one aspect of intellectual functioning and adaptive behavior, it is reasonable to expect variations in ability and achievement in these areas according to level of severity. In general, an overall relationship has been found between language and IQ, including the relationship between mental age (MA), sentence

TABLE 4–1. Three Approaches to Understanding Congenital Language Disorders

Classification*	Description†	Subtype‡
Mental retardation	Content: children who exhibit difficulty in conceptualization and formation of ideas about objects, actions, events, and relationships among them Delay in development of content/form/use	Semantic-pragmatic syndrome: comprehension of discourse impaired; echolalia may be present; "cocktail party speech" Subcortical white matter; intrahemispherical disruption
Hearing impairment	Difficulty in auditory-vocal form	Excluded from nosology
Autism	Use: children who exhibit difficulty in language use; impaired in conveying range of communicative function Disruption in content/form/use interaction	Mute autistic syndrome: neurologic basis unknown Autistic syndrome with echolalia: may repeat well-formed utterances heard previously; may be hyperlexic; intact pathways between primary auditory cortex and primary motor cortex
Childhood aphasia	Form: children who exhibit difficulty with the phonologic, morphologic, and syntactic aspects of language	Phonosyntactic: deficits in auditory-verbal language primarily of phonologic and morphosyntactic systems; auditory comprehension may also be affected; oromotor dysfunction frequently noted; prefrontal pathology with encroaching motor cortex involvement; if comprehension affected, temporal or temporoparietal involvement Verbal auditory agnosia: severe deficit in language comprehension with overall appropriate social-cognitive skills (e.g., good eye contact) and adequate nonverbal cognition (e.g., average symbolic play skills), not attributable to sensory deficit Bilateral temporal lobe involvement Severe expressive syndrome with good comprehension: neurologic basis not known

* Mykelbust H: Auditory Disorders in Children: A Manual for Differential Diagnosis. New York, Grune & Stratton, 1954
† Lahey M: What is language? In Lahey M: Language Disorders and Language Development. New York, MacMillan Publishing Company, 1988.
‡ Rapin I, Allen DS: Developmental language disorders: Nosological considerations. In Kirk U (ed): Neuropsychology of Language, Reading and Spelling. New York, Academic Press, 1983.

length,[10] and vocabulary development.[11] The primary deficits appear to be in content and ideation of language[1] and application of meaning in functional communicative relationships, including social relationships.[6] The differences between the language of children with and without mental retardation have been an interest of several researchers during the 1960s and 1970s who were primarily concerned with investigating the nature of language itself.[12,13] The general consensus is that language and speech develop essentially in the same manner as in nonretarded individuals but at a slower rate. However, lifetime achievement in speech, language, and communication skills is affected by the extent of mental retardation.

Hearing Impairment

Developmental language disorder secondary to hearing impairment is frequently characterized by deficits in language comprehension, sentence structure, vocabulary development, and speech articulation. Studies of the syntax of hearing-impaired children have demonstrated significant delays in the onset and development of simple and complex sentence structure.[14] It is difficult to describe a single pattern of language development or delay because the speech and

TABLE 4–2. IQ Level, Classification, and Speech and Language Ability

IQ	Classification	Speech and Language Ability
69–55	Mild retardation	Usually develops social and communication skills, although language development is slower and linguistic difficulties may be subtle; vocabulary delay; conversational topic management poor
54–40	Moderate retardation	Able to learn functional communication, although often relies on earlier learned gestures to make a request or to gain attention, poor receptive language skills, concrete word meanings, articulation disorders
39–25	Severe retardation	Minimal speech, may have limited gestural repertoire to communicate functions, articulation disorders
< 25	Profound retardation	Frequently nonverbal, vocalizes, poor functional communication

TABLE 4–3.   Hearing Levels, Classification, and Speech and Language Ability

dB	Classification	Speech and Language Ability
15–30	Mild	Mild impact, voiceless consonants may be missed; may be inattentive, mild language and speech delay
30–50	Moderate	Need amplification to understand speech at conversational level although may miss unstressed words; difficulty with word meaning, limited vocabulary, confusion with grammar, speech has omitted and distorted sounds
50–70	Severe	Language and speech will not develop spontaneously without amplification and special intervention, severe speech, language, and learning problems
70+	Profound	Unable to hear sound without amplification, need intensive intervention, severe language retardation, speech problems, and learning difficulty

Adapted from Northern J, Downs M: Hearing in Children. Baltimore, Williams & Wilkins, 1984.

language abilities of hearing-impaired children vary in relationship to four significant factors:

1. Degree and scope of hearing loss
2. Age of onset
3. Congenital or acquired causative factors
4. Social-emotional factors, including intelligence and environment

Generally, the greater the hearing loss, the greater the difficulty in perceiving, understanding, and acquiring intelligible speech. Table 4–3 gives a generalized summary of hearing level, classification, and speech and language skills observed in children with congenital hearing losses. Difficulties with the content, form, and use of language are thought to be more of a delay in development rather than a disruption.[1] Children with severe hearing loss (50–70 dB) have delayed onset and slow development of the auditory-vocal form of language. They have significant difficulty in perceiving and understanding the morphosyntactic and phonologic properties of spoken language, which affects their comprehension and expressive language and speech development. Studies of severely hearing-impaired children learning sign language as their native language, however, do not show the same delay in development because sign language does not depend on the auditory modality for learning.

Early identification of hearing loss and appropriate intervention are critical factors in the habilitation of language and communication skills in children with hearing loss. Rehabilitation of children with hearing loss includes appropriate instrumentation, educational and intervention methods, and ongoing monitoring and follow-up. The philosophy of appropriate education and communication mode has changed dramatically over the past 30 years. Historically, children with moderate-to-profound hearing losses were educated in residential schools. Now children with congenital hearing impairment are mainstreamed into regular educational settings as a result of the mandate of the Education for All Handicapped Children Act (Public Law 94-142). Approaches to the education of children with hearing impairments usually focus on one of two methods. The **aural/oral method** incorporates speech and speech reading into the teaching method with auditory-vocal language as the primary goal. **Total communication** has as its goal the use of auditory-vocal language, speech reading, gestures, and sign language for communication. Choosing one method over the other for rehabilitation is a function of family beliefs and the philosophy of the educational setting available to the child and family. Moreover, the advances in **cochlear implants** for children with sensorineural hearing loss have affected the educational methods used for habilitation of hearing-impaired children.

Autism

One of the most devastating developmental disorders affecting communication and social relationships is autism. It is now accepted that autism is a serious developmental disorder and not an emotional or psychiatric disorder. Moreover, autism is present at birth and does not result from family stress and inadequate mothering or parenting.[16] What exactly is autism? How can it be differentiated from mental retardation or generalized developmental delay?

Autism refers to a clinical syndrome that is defined by a unique set of criteria. Diagnostic boundaries of autism have been identified by the American Psychiatric Association in the fourth edition of the Diagnostic and Statistical Manual of Mental Disorders (DSM-IV-R). Table 4–4 contains the diagnostic criteria for behavior and qualitative impairment that must be met for inclusion in the classification of autism.

A language disorder is an important part of the autism syndrome. Rapin and Allen[6] described two subtypes of autism based on the presence or absence of verbal communication (see Table 4–1). The **mute autistic syndrome** describes youngsters who demonstrate the most profound

TABLE 4–4. DSM-IV-R Diagnostic Criteria for Autistic Disorder*

Criteria for reciprocal social interaction (at least 2)	Example
1. Marked lack of awareness of the existence or feelings of others	Treats a person as if he or she were a piece of furniture
2. No or abnormal seeking of comfort at times of distress	Does not seek comfort even when ill, hurt, or tired
3. No or impaired imitation	Does not wave good-bye
4. No or abnormal play	Does not actively participate in simple games
5. Gross impairment in ability to make peer friendships	No interest in making peer friendships
Criteria for verbal and nonverbal communication (at least 1)	**Example**
1. No mode of communication, such as communicative babbling, facial expression, gesture, mime, or spoken language	No communicative babbling, facial expression, gesture, mime, or spoken language
2. Markedly abnormal nonverbal communication	Stiffens when held, does not make eye contact when making social approach, maintains fixed stare in social situations
3. Absence of imaginative activity	No playacting of adult roles, fantasy, characters, or animals
4. Abnormal speech production	Monotonous or questionlike intonation, high pitch
5. Abnormal language form or content	Immediate echolalia, use of "you" for "I," idiosyncratic language, irrelevant remarks
6. Inability to initiate or sustain conversation	Monologues are produced without allowing others opportunity to speak
Criteria for restricted repertoire of activities and interests (at least 1)	**Example**
1. Stereotyped body movements	Hand flicking or twisting, spinning, head banging, complex whole-body movements
2. Persistent preoccupation with parts of objects	Sniffs objects, repetitive feeling of texture of materials, attachment to unusual objects (e.g., carrying around a piece of string)
3. Distress over changes in trivial aspects of environment	Gets upset when a vase is moved from its usual position
4. Unreasonable insistence that routines be followed	Insists that the same route be followed when shopping
5. Restricted range of interests and preoccupation with one narrow interest	Interested only in lining up objects, amassing facts about meteorology, or pretending to be a fantasy character

* From American Psychiatric Association: Diagnostic and Statistical Manual of Mental Disorders, 4th ed. Washington, DC, American Psychiatric Association, 1994.

impairment in oral language, symbolic function, and social-communicative interaction. Children who present with this syndrome are nonverbal and display severe deficits in social-interaction and gestural communication. The **autistic syndrome** with echolalia includes autistic children who demonstrate the ability to repeat long sequences of well-formed utterances heard previously. Some demonstrate **hyperlexia**, or the ability to read in the absence of semantic comprehension. Lahey's[1] description of language behavior of autistic children (see Table 4–1) points to differences in the autistic child's use of language as the most prominent feature, including the lack of communicative gestures and limited communicative functions. In addition, the echolalic utterances and odd semantic properties of autistic children's language indicate disruptions in language content and form from language use.

Childhood Aphasia

Historically, the term developmental childhood aphasia has been used to describe children who show language impairment in the absence of hearing loss, mental retardation, or frank neurologic damage. In more recent clinical and research literature, **developmental language disorder** or **specific language impairment (SLI)** has replaced the term childhood aphasia. In contrast, the term **acquired childhood aphasia** is reserved for children who have experienced an accident or disease process that alters neurologic functioning, such as focal traumatic brain injury or stroke.

It is difficult to describe typical language behaviors in developmental language disorder or SLI. The label SLI does not predict which language behaviors to expect. However, the single most important characteristic of children with SLI is the delay and slow development in the form of language with better development in content and use[1] (see Table 4–1). Typically, children with childhood aphasia or SLI have a major deficiency in the acquisition and use of auditory-verbal language as it relates to the phonologic and morphosyntactic systems rather than in the conceptualization and formation of ideas related to the content of language.

Some children with SLI have difficulties with language expression only with normal or near-normal language comprehension. Others have a moderate-to-severe auditory-verbal language disorder that affects their comprehension and production. Rapin and Allen[6] describe three subtypes of language disorders that relate to the construct of SLI. The phonosyntactic syndrome is the most prevalent and is characterized by impairments in the phonologic and morphosyntactic (form) systems. Disturbances of form are noted in the restricted use of syntactic relations expressed within a single utterance as well as difficulty in learning the use of function words and inflections of nouns and verbs. Many such children have oromotor dysfunction that affects the onset and development of phonology and articulation skills, suggesting that the neurologic correlate is a prefrontal pathology that encroaches on the motor cortex. If language comprehension and/or reading is affected, the temporal or temporoparietal areas are suspected.

Severe deficits in language comprehension and expression with overall appropriate social-communicative skills and nonverbal cognitive skills are the hallmarks of **verbal auditory agnosia**. Children with this disorder have significant deficits in auditory comprehension but can be distinguished from autistic children by other than language behavior (i.e., good eye-contact, age-appropriate symbolic play skills). Researchers interested in childhood language disorders have recognized this syndrome as the one most often cited as childhood aphasia. Eisenson[17] defined developmental aphasia as follows:

> Congenital aphasia, dyslogia . . . refer(s) to the impairment for the child to acquire symbols for a language system. The impairment must be of a sufficient degree to interfere with the child's ability to communicate . . . . Use of the term implies that the child's perceptual abilities for auditory (speech) events underlies his impairment for the acquisition of auditory symbols . . . . Expressive disturbances are a manifestation of his intake or decoding impairment.

According to the classification nosology presented by Rapin and Allen[6] (see Table 4–1), the basis for this condition is bilateral temporal lobe pathology.

Assessment of Language Ability

Evaluating children's language performance in the domains of comprehension and oral expression requires the use of psychometrically valid instruments to compare their performance with that of a normal population. Such assessment determines whether the child is sufficiently delayed or different in language development and use to be called language-disordered. Procedures that are useful in gathering a sample of a child's language behavior can easily be implemented during a clinical evaluation. The first procedure is to observe **spontaneous language** and to gather a sizable corpus (between 50 and 100 utterances) to analyze the child's spontaneous use of phonology, morphology, syntax, semantics, and language pragmatics. Another procedure involves the use of **imitation**, in which the child repeats, word for word, the phrase or sentence produced by the clinician. Research has shown that children's imitative utterances are essentially the same in content and structure as their spontaneous language.[18] Finally, the use of an **elicited sample** of language performance is a useful clinical procedure to screen and assess oral language skills in children. Picture stimuli of either an object or an action scene are presented to the child, who then is asked to point to the picture describing an object or action (e.g., receptive tasks) or to name or describe a picture (e.g., expressive tasks).

Acquired Language Disorders

Acquired language disorders in children may be related to traumatic brain injury (TBI), cerebral vascular accident (CVA), brain tumor, or encephalopathy. Regardless of the etiology, the fact remains that the processing and use of language have been abruptly disrupted, not by congenital breakdown but by an acquired disorder. Language processing may be further compromised by concomitant impairments in critical cognitive or information-processing skills, such as memory, perception, attention, or organization, as well as behavioral impairment, such as disinhibition, poor self-monitoring, limited frustration tolerance, or poor judgment. Therefore, language and cognitive deficits must be critically assessed, identified, and addressed therapeutically in a manner appropriate to the patient's age and medical condition.

Assessment and Intervention

Ylvisaker[19] refers to three stages of recovery in discussing cognitive rehabilitation. **Early stages** of recovery refer to treatment programs of sensory and sensorimotor stimulation for medically stable patients emerging from coma as well as for patients who have begun to demonstrate stimulus-specific responses, functional use of common objects, following of simple commands, and attempts at verbal or nonverbal communication. **Middle stages** of recovery refer to treatment programs beginning to address cognitive/communicative functioning beyond a reflexive level. Such programs emphasize reduction of the patient's level of confusion, an increase in adaptive behaviors, appropriate environmental interactions, and reestablishment of organized thinking and structures of knowledge. **Later stages** of recovery refer to treatment programs focusing on residual or discrete deficits that compromise such skills as executive functions and pragmatics or altered behaviors that continue to affect the patient's successful return to an academic, family, or social setting. Many such patients fit the description "walking wounded," which often is used to describe traumatically brain-injured patients who may appear to be completely recovered but, when confronted with cognitively challenging tasks, continue to present significant deficits.

Specific assessment techniques and intervention strategies are discussed as they relate to each of the above stages of recovery for children and adolescents with acquired language deficits. The experiences of the family as a parallel process of recovery—not always synchronized with the patient—are also discussed. Because recovery from traumatic brain injury has not only immediate but also long-term repercussions for the family as well as the patient, family involvement, support, and education are critical elements of any comprehensive therapeutic program.

Early Stage of Recovery.   Because of the patient's limited responsiveness, assessment of language functioning in the early stage of recovery is typically completed through informal measures from which baseline responses may be documented and then tracked in the course of treatment. Sensory modalities in which the brain receives and interprets information are assessed by clinical questions such as those in Table 4–5; useful interventions are suggested below. Adamovich et al.[20,21] state that "early stimulation programs should include activities designed to excite patient activity. Next, attempts should be made to heighten or intensify that response." Receptive and expressive language functioning are initially marked by an absence of processing language input and verbal or gestural communication, respectively. As recovery continues, a progression in language functioning becomes apparent. The patient begins to follow commands, to demonstrate limited reading skills, to retain simple auditorily presented information, and to produce automatic verbal and gestural responses (i.e., names of family members, waving, head nods and shakes, or pointing) as well as simple verbal responses to external stimuli. Table 4–5 illustrates the skill

areas, clinical questions to be answered in the course of an assessment, and facilitation of treatment planning for the early stages of recovery. Family members initially experience shock, grief, and anger as family routines are drastically disrupted and feel a loss of control over their lives. As the patient begins to come out of the coma and responds to commands, the disruption in family routines persists, but families become more hopeful in their expectations.[22,23]

Middle and Late Stages of Recovery.   For children, language assessments and interventions in the middle and late stages of recovery focus on skills necessary for returning to home, school, and social settings. Assessments attempt to answer a series of clinical questions through a combination of standardized protocols as well as informal measures. Standardized protocols offer expectations and comparisons of specific language functions relative to noninjured peers, and informal measures allow the patient to be compared with him- or herself. Based on assessment findings, appropriate interventions are determined and implemented, with suggestions as listed below. Linguistic manifestations in the middle stages of recovery may include impairments in the rate of processing, retaining, categorizing, and associating information as well as verbalization of incoherent or bizarre utterances that are unrelated to the environment and reflect the patient's state of agitation and confusion. In the continuing process of recovery, improvements may be noted in auditory processing of phrases or brief sentences, but particular deficits persist in word finding, written expression, content of spoken connected utterances, and length of utterances. In the late stages of recovery, linguistic functioning is characterized by persistently delayed processing of auditorily or graphically presented material, difficulty in grasping new learning, difficulty in applying abstract reasoning and problem-solving skills, poor auditory retention for short paragraphs, inability to access taught compensatory strategies to facilitate language functioning, and anomia for confrontational naming. Table 4–6 illustrates the skill areas, clinical questions to be answered in the course of an assessment, and facilitation of treatment planning for the middle and late stages of recovery. Family experiences relative to the middle stages of recovery include fear of regression or embarrassment; agitation may begin to emerge, affecting the family's hopefulness. As agitation diminishes and early cognitive recovery begins, family members are confronted with the child's confusion, which often results in misinterpretations of the child's behavior. In some instances,

TABLE 4–5.   Facilitation of Treatment Planning for the Early Stages of Recovery

Clinical Questions	Sample Interventions
Arousal/alertness	
• Does the patient attend to his/her environment?	• Monitor the patient's attention to the presence or removal of auditory or visual stimuli in his/her room. Does behavior change when the radio or TV is turned on or off?
• Does the patient demonstrate any selective attending skills to a specific stimulus?	• Monitor the patient's ability to attend to family members, a favorite television program, or familiar photos. How long did the patient attend? Can this behavior be repeated or is it random?
Audition	
• Is there a reliable startle reflex?	• Abruptly present attention-getting auditory signals and watch for a reliable startle reflex (eye blink, head jerk, or generalized body movement).
• Does the patient exhibit search and localization behavior to nonsymbolic or symbolic auditory signals?	• Present nonsymbolic (noisemakers) and symbolic (speech) auditory signals in varying fields and observe for visual searching behaviors to the source of the signal as well as localization to the source of the signal. Monitor for rate of response.
• Are there any differential responses to familiar vs. unfamiliar voices?	• Observe for differential responses relative to facial expression, respiratory rate, or body posture in response to familiar vs. unfamiliar voices.
• Is the patient able to follow simple spoken commands?	• Present simple gross motor spoken commands for the patient to attempt to follow.
• Can the patient recognize common objects upon request?	• Present 3 common objects within the patient's visual field for him/her to point to upon request.
Vision	
• Is there a reliable blink in response to visual threat?	• Monitor reliability of the patient's ability to respond to a visual threat.
• Does the patient demonstrate visual regard/focus on faces or familiar objects at close proximity?	• Time the patient's ability to sustain visual regard/focus on faces or familiar objects at close proximity.
• Does the patient demonstrate differential responses to familiar or unfamiliar faces within his/her visual field?	• Monitor any overt changes in the patient's status as familiar persons enter his/her visual field as opposed to unfamiliar persons. Does the patient smile?
• Is there visual recognition of movement of persons within his/her visual field?	• Monitor the patient's ability to shift his/her visual gaze or visually track the movement of others as they move about the patient's room.
• Does the patient demonstrate horizontal and/or vertical visual tracking of common objects? If so, is this tracking for the full visual field?	• Monitor the patient's ability to visually track common objects horizontally or vertically for the full visual field.
• Is the patient able to use visual skills to match object pairs?	• Present an object to the patient to match to a corresponding object from a field of 3.
Expression	
• Does the patient demonstrate any alterations in oral postures or facial expression?	• Monitor for any smiles, grimaces, or changes in overall facial expression appropriate to a situation.
• Has the patient begun to demonstrate any spontaneous use of gestural responses?	• Encourage meaningful gestures to communicate such as waves, "thumbs up," head nods/shakes, or pointing to a desired item.
• Has there been any spontaneous vocalization attempts?	• Monitor and encourage any attempts to produce phonation, whether for vegetative functions such as yawns or sighs, or for single-word approximations.
• Have there been any productions of meaningful speech?	• Monitor and encourage any attempts to produce single words for desired items, automatic sequences such as counting, or expression of simple phrases.
Olfaction	
• Have there been any reliable response patterns to varied scents?	• Present pleasant as well as noxious scents for the patient to respond to. Observe for any generalized or localized responses and overall changes in behavior.
Sensation	
• Have there been any reliable response patterns to varied tactile stimuli?	• Present pleasant as well as noxious tactile experiences to the patient's extremities and observe for any generalized or localized responses and overall changes in behavior.
Oral motor function	
• What is the patient's general facial appearance?	• Address any alterations in facial tone or asymmetry as appropriate.
• What is the integrity of the oral structures?	• Document status of oral structures.
• What types of oral reflexes are present?	• Determine the presence of any protective, developmental, or pathologic oral reflexes, and treat as appropriate.
• What is the functional adequacy of the patient's oral mechanism?	• Pursue oral stimulation/facilitation or oral feeding attempts as deemed appropriate.

TABLE 4–6.   Facilitation of Treatment Planning for the Middle and Late Stages of Recovery

Clinical Questions	Sample Interventions
Behavior/orientation	
• What are the patient's attending skills?	• Increase the patient's attending skills for structured as well as unstructured tasks emphasizing sustained as well as focused attention.
• Is the patient oriented to person, place, and time?	• The patient may benefit from daily review of a calendar in his/her room or an orientation aid that may be kept in a pocket and easily accessed.
• Is the patient impulsive?	• Behavior modification programs may be beneficial in addressing behaviors such as disinhibition, impulsivity, distractibility, agitation, emotional ability, cognitive inflexibility, cognitive durability, and awareness of deficits.
• Is the patient verbally or physically disinhibited?	• Monitor improvement in cognitive durability and stamina as the patient continues to recover.
Auditory compensation	
Can the patient . . .	Ask the patient to . . .
• Recognize single words?	• Identify common objects or photos in varying fields as directed.
• Follow simple-complex oral directives?	• Follow simple as well as multi-step functional oral directives.
• Comprehend varied question types?	• Respond to a variety of question types in a meaningful and relevant manner using high-interest stories, games, or school texts.
• Comprehend simple-complex paragraphs?	• Respond to a variety of question types in a meaningful and relevant manner using high-interest stories, games, or school texts.
• Follow a conversational exchange?	• Follow structured and unstructured conversations.
• Comprehend figurative language?	• Define and demonstrate appropriate usage of varied idioms, proverbs, or metaphors.
Verbal expression	
Can the patient . . .	Ask the patient to . . .
• Adequately participate in a casual conversation?	• Discuss age-appropriate topical material (i.e., movies, TV, or sports), a funny story, or photos from a high-interest magazine. Critically listen to the patient's expressive language relative to content, form, and function.
• Express automatic speech sequences?	• Recite the numbers 1–21, days of the week, months of the year, and letters A-Z.
• Imitate words, phrases, or sentences?	• Imitate series of simple-complex words, phrases, and sentences, while listening for accuracy and style of expression.
• Retrieve targeted labels given descriptive, categorical, or functional cues?	• Retrieve targeted labels with varied cues such as an attribute of a common object, a category, a function of an object, or an initial letter. Imposing a time limit or specifying a desired number of responses may increase the complexity of this task.
• Verbally generate semantically and syntactically correct sentences and questions when given a visual or verbal cue?	• Verbally generate semantically and syntactically correct sentences or questions given a printed or picture cue.
• Appropriately respond to varied question types?	• Respond to varied question types such as yes/no, true/false, and multiple choice, WH-, or inferential, while attending to the patient's ability to determine the appropriate mode of response.
• Adequately participate in controlled narratives?	• Talk about a given topic for a designated amount of time, while attending to vocabulary, thought organization, topic maintenance, semantics, and syntax.
Oral and silent reading comprehension	
Can the patient . . .	Ask the patient to . . .
• Recognize letters and symbols?	• Identify letters and symbols in isolation or from a field of at least 3.
• Recognize simple-complex printed words?	• Identify simple-complex printed words in isolation or from a field of at least 3.
• Comprehend simple-complex printed words?	• Identify simple-complex printed words from a field of 3 given a definition.
• Comprehend simple-complex printed sentences?	• Match printed sentences to corresponding pictures.
• Comprehend simple-complex printed paragraph(s)?	• Match printed paragraph(s) to a corresponding picture.
Written expression	
Can the patient . . .	Ask the patient to . . .
• Write automatic/familiar information?	• Write full name, address, numbers, letters, or other personal data.
• Copy simple information?	• Copy letters, numbers, words, or sentences.
• Write symbols, words, or sentences to dictation?	• Write letters, numbers, words, or sentences to dictation.
• Write semantically and syntactically correct sentences?	• Write semantically and syntactically correct sentences given printed or picture cues.
• Write an organized and grammatically correct narrative?	• Write an organized and grammatically correct narrative given a specific topic or picture cue.

(Table continued on following page.)

TABLE 4–6. Facilitation of Treatment Planning for the Middle and Late Stages of Recovery *(Continued)*

Clinical Questions	Sample Interventions
Memory	
Can the patient . . .	Ask the patient to . . .
• Retrieve familiar background information?	• State full name, address, and names of family members, phone numbers, or other personally relevant information.
• Immediately recall targeted information?	• State series of 3–7 digits immediately following presentation, or series of simple words.
• Retrieve information from short-term memory?	• Retrieve targeted information following a brief delay.
• Retrieve information from long-term memory?	• Retrieve information from past events or old learning.
• Retrieve general factual information?	• State general factual information referring to basic academic subjects.
Executive functions	
Can the patient . . .	Ask the patient to . . .
• Identify concept similarities and differences?	• State similarities or differences for groups of 2–3 words.
• Complete interpolative thinking tasks?	• Determine what happened in the middle of a situation after given the beginning and the ending.
• Complete simple-complex analogies?	• Complete analogy phrases.
• Explain common idioms or proverbs?	• Explain or define common idioms or proverbs.
• Complete deductive reasoning tasks?	• Apply reasoning skills to draw conclusions in a step-by-step manner given a situation.
• Complete functional problem-solving tasks?	• Determine appropriate solutions to common day-to-day problems.
• Complete convergent and divergent thinking tasks?	• Apply convergent thinking skills to recognize relevant information and determine a main idea or central theme to silently read or orally presented age-appropriate material.
	• Apply divergent thinking skills to explain abstract concepts and demonstrate flexible thinking such as defining multiple meanings for a word or explaining visual or verbal absurdities.
• Sequence steps to complete functional tasks?	• List steps necessary to complete age-appropriate tasks such as making a sandwich or wrapping a birthday gift.

siblings may begin to experience more overt reactions to the changes in the family, ranging from anger over the personal effect of the changes to feelings of parental neglect. In other cases, however, siblings have offered additional support to their injured brother or sister and their parents. In the late stages of recovery, family members begin to increase their expectations for the injured child, and family life begins to return to pretrauma routines. However, the family is now confronted with the day to day issues of parenting a child recovering from a traumatic injury and understanding the effects of such an injury on home, school, and social settings.[22,23]

In addressing the speech and language deficits of children or adolescents following a traumatic brain injury, consideration must be given to age-appropriate understanding of formulating and producing communication. One must not lose sight of the fact that children and adolescents recovering from a traumatic brain injury experience a dynamic process with their own unique sets of strengths and weaknesses. Examples include variances in severity of injury, age, development at the time of injury, pretrauma personality traits, cognitive style, rate of recovery, and family background. However, some commonalities have been cited in the literature, including particular weaknesses in the areas of cognitive organization, psychosocial functioning, and potential for exaggeration of pretraumatic learning or personality styles. Effective treatment depends on recognition of these differences and similarities as well as family education and participation; the injury will have a long-term effect on both the patient and the family.[22,23]

Disorders of Speech and Voice Production

Congenital Speech and Voice Disorders

Congenital disorders of speech and voice production include disorders involving respiratory, phonatory, and articulatory structure and function. Any neuromuscular disease process that compromises any of these systems results in disordered speech.

Respiration. The biomechanics of breathing for quiet, vegetative function are significantly different from breathing for vocalization and speech. During quiet breathing, the inspiratory and expiratory phases are equal, but during speech production the inspiratory phase is brief compared with the longer exhalatory phase in which speech is produced. Moreover, during quiet vegetative breathing the respiratory tract is wide open with little resistance, whereas during speech breathing the respiratory tract undergoes pressure changes and alterations when vocal folds approximate within the larynx or placement of articulators constricts airflow through the vocal tract. Children experiencing significant medical problems that affect the lower respiratory function frequently have difficulty in maintaining the appropriate amount of pressurized air needed for speech production. Phonation may be brief with little perceptible loudness, and articulation targets during conversational speech may be shallow.

Phonation. Phonation occurs in the larynx when moving air within the vocal tract is transformed into acoustic energy by the reflexive approximation and vibration of the vocal folds. Phonation is a broad term referring to any sound produced in the larynx, including voice and whisper. The sound source for voicing is the rapid interruption of the air movement through the glottis. The opening and closing of the vocal folds involve a relatively rapid back-and-forth movement in the form of a complex vibration. Vocal fold vibration results from a dynamic alteration of forces that open and close the glottis. The laryngeal voice source can produce sounds with a large range of intensities, frequencies, and qualities. Whispering is the result of opening the glottis enough to create a narrow slit and the resulting turbulence produced from the rapid airflow.

Articulation. Speech articulation is the verbal means of communicating a message and results from specific motor behaviors and precise neuromuscular coordination. Speech sounds are produced in the oral cavity by changes in tongue height and shape and lingual placement against articulators such as the soft palate, alveolar ridge, and lips. In English, speech sounds are classified as either vowels or consonants; vowels are produced with relatively unrestricted airflow in the vocal tract, whereas consonants require a closed or narrowly constricted passage to create friction and air turbulence. It is generally accepted that children do not learn speech sounds as isolated phonemes; instead, they learn phonemes in relationship to other sounds within the context of a word.[24] Table 4–7 summarizes the sequence of sound acquisition.

Cerebral Palsy

Children with cerebral palsy frequently present with speech and voice disorders as a result of impaired respiration, phonation, and articulation. Variations in silent, vegetative breathing and speech breathing have been found for different types and severity of cerebral palsy. Solomon and Charron[25] provide a recent comprehensive review of the literature about speech breathing in children with cerebral palsy. Children with spastic cerebral palsy are more likely to have shallow inspirations and forced, uncontrolled expirations due to weak, spastic muscles of the chest wall. Children with athetoid cerebral palsy, on the other hand, demonstrate irregular and uncontrolled breath patterns, presumably related to abnormal involuntary movements of the chest wall and structures of the upper airway. These sudden changes in resting tone and involuntary chest wall movement result in sudden bursts of air during inspiration and expirations. Children with ataxic cerebral palsy demonstrate irregular rate, rhythm, and depth of tidal breathing.[26] The effects of compromised breathing on speech production are noted in Table 4–8.

Laryngeal and pharyngeal disorders are also characteristic of children with cerebral palsy. Tension in the laryngeal musculature during speech attempts contributes to laryngeal spasms, such as adductor spasms that cause difficulty with voice onset or abductor spasms that produce a breathy vocal quality.[27] Varying tension in laryngeal musculature causes corresponding variations in pitch, loudness, and vocal quality.[27]

TABLE 4–7. Phonemic Acquisition—Age at Which 75% of Children Tested Correctly Articulated Consonant Sounds

Age (yr)	Sounds
2	m, n, h, p, n (rING)
2.4	f, j, k, d
2.8	w, b, t
3	g, s
3.4	r, l
3.8	ʃ (shy), tʃ (chin)
4	δ (father), Z (measure)
4+	dz (jar), θ (thin), v, z

From Soifer LH: Development and disorders of communication. In Molnar GE (ed): Pediatric Rehabilitation, 2nd ed. Baltimore, Williams & Wilkins, 1985.

TABLE 4–8. Respiration and Speech Production in Cerebral Palsy

Respiration	Speech Production
Rapid breathing	Lack of vocalization in infancy
Shallow inspiratory breaths	Limited number of syllables per utterance
Reduced prolonged exhalation	Difficulty initiating voice onset for vocalization
	Difficulty with sustained vocalization
Involuntary movements in respiratory musculature	Speech breaks
	Difficulty modulating loudness

Adapted from McDonald E, Chance B: Cerebral Palsy. Englewood Cliffs, NJ, Prentice-Hall, 1964.

Articulation disorders are frequent in children with cerebral palsy and have been the subject of many investigations. The child with cerebral palsy often presents as nonverbal or with significantly delayed development of speech and language. The most distinctive speech characteristics are markedly reduced articulation targets generated at a slow rate with low pitch and a harsh vocal quality.[28] Speech may be slurred and labored and characterized as "spastic dysarthria" with indistinct articulation and breaks in velopharyngeal closure resulting in hypernasality. Speech often is accompanied by facial grimacing. Table 4–9 summarizes the evaluation of respiration, phonation, and articulation processes in children with cerebral palsy.

Acquired Speech and Voice Disorders

Children and adolescents recovering from a traumatic injury, such as brain or spinal cord injury, often present with acquired speech and/or voice disorders that result in altered speech intelligibility. Medical conditions may range from the persistence of a mildly breathy voice secondary to prolonged intubation to severe apraxia of speech, which requires the use of an augmentative communication system to express basic wants and needs.

Motor speech disorders include dysarthria and apraxia of speech. Dysarthria has been defined as "imperfect articulation of speech due to disturbances of muscular control which result from damage to the central or peripheral nervous system."[29] In the practice of speech and language pathology, this definition may be expanded to include effects, in any combination, on all five motor subsystems of speech production: respiration, phonation, resonation, articulation, and prosody. Furthermore, nonspeech actions, such as chewing, swallowing, jaw movements, or tongue movements, also may be impaired. Apraxia has been defined as "loss of ability to carry out familiar, purposeful movements in the absence of paralysis or other motor or sensory impairment."[29] In terms of speech, apraxia refers to the loss of purposeful acts to execute oral movements and initiate voice.

In the early stages of recovery after brain injury, the distinction between dysarthria and apraxia of speech is difficult because of the patient's limited communicative effort, level of confusion, and impaired language; furthermore, these disorders may coexist. Taking these factors into consideration, effective treatment programs may not be implemented until the patient is further along in the recovery process. In addition to careful assessment of oral motor functioning, Ylvisaker[19] suggests the following trends that may further facilitate the differential diagnosis:

1. Dysarthrias are more common than apraxia of speech in patients with severe physical involvement.

TABLE 4–9. Evaluating Respiration, Phonation, and Articulation

Respiration	Phonation	Articulation
• Does the child inhale upon request?	• Does the child have adductor spasms resulting in difficulty initiating phonation or an abrupt cessation of phonation?	• Does the child have proper oral movements necessary for facilitation of lip closure at rest, during sucking, swallowing, chewing, and speech?
• Does the child retain air?	• Does the child have abductor spasms resulting in a breathy voice pattern?	• Does the child have any involuntary movements of the lips, tongue, and mandible?
• Does the child whisper?	• Does the child have pitch, loudness, and quality changes in his or her voice due to changes in tension?	• Does the child have any dysarthric pattern in the lips, tongue, and mandible? • Lips: close on command • Tongue: lateralize right/left • Elevate, protrude, point • Dissociate from jaw movement • Mandible: open mouth, drooling • Hyperextension of mandible
• Does the child alternate retention and phonation on a single exhalation (i.e., a-a-a-a)?	• Does the child have increased bodily tension during phonation?	• Does the child have the ability to make rapid, alternating movements, i.e., diadochokinesis?
• Does the child exhibit reversed breathing or involuntary movement (at rest, during speech)?		
• Does the rate of inhalation/exhalation exceed 20 bpm?		

Adapted from Soifer LH: Development and disorders of communication. In Molnar GE (ed): Pediatric Rehabilitation, 2nd ed. Baltimore, Williams & Wilkins, 1985.

2. There is a greater incidence of persistent dysarthria among adolescents than among younger children.

3. Apraxia of speech appears more frequently among younger children.

Table 4–10, adapted from Ylvisaker,[19] illustrates diagnosis and treatment approaches for motor speech disorders.

For some children and adolescents, speech and voice production may be altered by the necessity of a tracheostomy, performed in an emergency situation to provide a patent airway and sustain life. Phonation is altered because the upper airway is bypassed; air enters and exits the lungs below the level of the vocal cords. The patient may become aphonic and unable to communicate orally or, at best, able to communicate

orally by breathy voice production using residual airflow around the tracheostomy tube. The quality of voice production depends on the following factors:

1. The type of tracheostomy tube (cuffed vs. uncuffed, fenestrated vs. unfenestrated)

2. The amount of airflow around the tracheostomy tube

3. The patient's ability to produce adequate diaphragmatic support to accomplish airflow beyond the level of the tracheostomy and through the vocal tract for oral communication.

The aim of speech/language intervention is to establish an effective means of restoring communication and to ensure that the patient has access to an appropriate communication system at all times (e.g., communication board, augmentative

TABLE 4–10. Diagnosis and Treatment Approaches for Motor Speech Disorders

Clinical questions	1. What is the integrity of the oral structures? 2. What is the status of isolated oral movements? 3. What is the status of sequential oral movements? 4. Is the patient verbal or nonverbal? 5. Can the patient execute diadochokinetic tasks? 6. Is respiration sufficient to support speech production? 7. What is the status of articulatory functioning? 8. What is the status of vocal quality and resonance? 9. Is the patient a fluent speaker? 10. Is the patient demonstrating appropriate intonation and prosody?
Potential charac- teristics of impairment	Mild dysarthria: imprecise articulation present; mild hypernasality; soft volume; slightly monotonal and breathy vocal quality; reduced rate of speaking; reduced length of utterance per breath Mild apraxia: mildly impaired articulatory searching and motor planning Moderate dysarthria: patient is fairly intelligible; soft and breathy voice produced; inaccurate articulation; hypernasality present (sometimes with nasal emissions); monopitch; reduced rate of speaking; muscle groups are involved rather than single muscles; reduced range of oral musculature present Moderate apraxia: improvement in speech intelligibility accomplished when using a reduced rate and pausing between words to allow for motor planning Severe dysarthria: not directly related to the degree of cognitive recovery; significantly impaired motor subsystems of speech resulting in production that may sound breathy, hyper/hyponasal, slurred, and/or executed at a reduced rate; patient may be nonverbal Severe apraxia: patient may only mouth or whisper words without phonation; vocalizations may occur spontaneously but are very difficult to produce upon command; patient may be nonverbal
Sample interventions	Mild dysarthria: refining of impaired speech parameters; instruction in compensatory strategies to maximize overall speech intelligibility; consideration of a voice amplification device Mild apraxia: refining of compensatory strategies to maximize overall speech intelligibility Moderate dysarthria: exaggerated articulation to compensate for slurring; use of incentive spirometry to improve respiratory support for speech; systematic drill and practice of targeted functional vocabulary and phrases; pool therapy may improve vocal volume and quality; use of phrasing techniques to maximize overall speech intelligibility Moderate apraxia: refining of word and phrase approximations in the context of age-appropriate activities; phrasing techniques; contrastive stress drills; gestural reorganization to augment oral communication Severe dysarthria: oral stimulation/facilitation; gross and fine motor treatment addressing muscle tone, coordination, posture, and strength; encourage any attempts at vegetative vocalizations such as yawns or sighs; shaping of vocalizations to achieve a core vocabulary for functional communication; consideration of a palatal lift or surgical intervention to achieve appropriate resonation; investigate augmentative communication options Severe apraxia: encourage, reward, and make the patient aware when vocalization occurs in varied settings; children may enjoy attempting to imitate animal or environmental sounds; gestures may facilitate phonation when attempting to orally communicate; develop a corpus of targeted vocabulary for the patient to master using progressive word approximations; pursue automatic speech sequences for the patient to master as well as singing or rhyming; investigate the patient's ability to use written language to facilitate communication; gestural reorganization to augment oral communication; establish a reliable yes/no system for basic communication; investigate augmentative communication options

Adapted from Ylvisaker MA (ed): Head Injury Rehabilitation: Children and Adolescents. San Diego, College-Hill Press, 1985.

system, call bell).[30] The Passey-Muir Ventilator Speaking Valve is often used in attempts to restore oral communication. This one-way valve fits over the outer cannula, allowing the patient to inhale. However, when exhalation occurs, the valve closes, forcing airflow through the vocal cords and upper airway, thus allowing phonation and oral communication. Not all patients, however, are considered appropriate candidates for this valve. Thought must be given to the degree of physical effort required for respiration when the valve is on as well as the risk of clogging when copious secretions are present. In addition, the patient must be able to tolerate a deflated tracheostomy cuff or have a cuffless tracheostomy. Many children need to acquire and build their tolerance gradually for wearing the valve to maximize its benefits.

Speech and voice production may be further compromised for tracheostomy patients when assisted ventilation is required. The patient must learn to initiate speech production on the inhalatory phase of the ventilator rather than the exhalatory phase, as in normal speech. By producing speech on the inhalatory phase of the ventilator, the patient takes advantage of the greatest amount of airflow provided to allow residual air leak around the tracheostomy tube, which, in turn, allows airflow upward through the vocal tract for oral communication. Some children and adolescents grasp this concept easily and quickly, whereas others may require specific instruction and practice. The resulting voice may have a breathy quality with reduced volume because the airflow through the vocal tract is reduced, but functional oral communication can be accomplished. In the early stages of the patient's adjustment to assisted ventilation and attempts to communicate orally, alternative means of communication, such as simple gestures, call bells, clinician-made communication boards, or augmentative systems appropriate for the patient's cognitive level, need to be investigated to ensure a functional mode of communication.[30]

Children and adolescents recovering from traumatic injury also may present with acquired laryngeal pathology. Such voice disorders may range from vocal cord irritation secondary to intubation to vocal cord weakness related to the patient's general physical weakness or to vocal cord paralysis related to nerve damage. Examination by an otolaryngologist ensures an accurate diagnosis beyond the clinical presentation. The speech/language pathologist may then use these findings to plan and implement an appropriate, individualized therapy program.

Disorders of Feeding and Swallowing

Feeding and swallowing impairments of varying levels of severity frequently occur in the pediatric population and may be temporary or long-term. The loss or impairment of the ability to meet nutritional needs through the oral mechanism is a debilitating experience for children and their families. In infants and young children, the inability to be fed orally interferes significantly with parent-child interaction and bonding. For older children and adolescents, a disruption in oral feeding and swallowing may deny the social experience of sharing a meal with friends and family.

Feeding and swallowing are separate yet integrally related functions of the eating experience. Feeding has been defined as (1) placement of food in the mouth, (2) manipulation in the mouth, and (3) posterior movement of the bolus by the tongue into the pharynx.[19] Swallowing includes these aspects of feeding as well as triggering of the swallowing reflex and movement of the bolus through the pharynx and esophagus into the stomach.[19] The role of the larynx in swallowing is critical: it provides airway protection by movement of the epiglottis as well as the true and false vocal folds to close the glottis and prevent aspiration. Anterior displacement and elevation of the larynx during the act of swallowing also provides protection by displacing the alignment of the trachea upward and away from the hypopharynx.

Phases of Swallow

Discussions of the pattern of normal oral feeding present differing opinions about the number of phases that comprise the feeding process as well as the labels given to each phase. However, a general consensus has been achieved about the sequence of these phases.[31] The following discussion addresses three discrete phases of swallowing and their synchronous relationship to accomplish oral feeding. Figure 4–3[32] illustrates the three phases and their integral relationship with each other.

Feeding begins with the **oral phase**, in which oral placement of food or drink is anticipated by orienting the mouth to the substance, responding to olfactory and other sensory input, depositing the food into the mouth, and maintaining a bilabial seal to prevent oral leakage. Lingual action varies depending on the consistency or temperature of the food or drink. Lingual movement patterns to formulate, manipulate, and/or masticate the bolus begin. Anterior-to-posterior lingual movement occurs

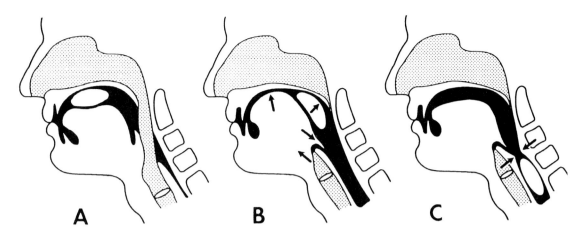

FIGURE 4-3. Three phases of normal deglutition. *A,* Oral. *B,* Pharyngeal. *C,* Esophageal. (From Braddom RL: Physical Medicine and Rehabilitation. Philadelphia, W.B. Saunders, 1996, with permission.)

along with lingual elevation to the hard palate to squeeze and propel the bolus toward the pharynx. Simultaneously, the soft palate elevates to contact the posterior pharyngeal wall and thus prevent nasal regurgitation. The oral phase concludes when the bolus has passed the anterior faucial arches and the swallow reflex is triggered.[31,33] This phase of swallowing becomes a voluntary action involving cranial nerves V, VII, and XII after the age of 6–9 months when the suck-swallow-breathe sequence is differentiated and individually controlled by the child.[34] During this phase, the airway remains open, nasal breathing continues, and the larynx and pharynx are at rest.

The second phase is the **pharyngeal phase**, which begins with the triggering of the swallow reflex. Numerous physiologic processes simultaneously occur to control bolus propulsion and airway protection. Specifically, the tongue prevents reentry of food into the mouth, the velopharyngeal port is completely sealed, and the upper pharynx is narrowed to prevent nasal regurgitation. Pharyngeal peristalsis begins to carry the bolus through the pharynx, the larynx is elevated and displaced to provide airway protection, and, finally, the bolus passes from the pharynx into the esophagus. This phase of swallowing is completely reflexive, involving cranial nerves IX, X, and XII. No pharyngeal activity may occur until the swallowing reflex is triggered.[31] Respiration ceases briefly during this phase.

The final phase is the **esophageal phase**, which begins with the descent of the larynx and the contraction of the cricopharyngeus muscle to prohibit regurgitation of food and gastric juices into the respiratory tract. A combination of gravity and synchronized peristaltic waves carries the bolus through the esophagus and into the stomach.[31] Respiration resumes during this phase.

Development of Feeding and Swallowing in Infants and Children

Swallowing is an extremely complex sensorimotor skill involving the coordination of a number of muscles in the mouth, pharynx, larynx, and esophagus. As early as 26 weeks' gestation, the swallowing and respiratory functions have separated and continue to develop independently.[35] The early onset of swallowing in fetal development appears to play a role in the regulation of amniotic fluid in a normal pregnancy.[36] Sucking, as a primary means for receiving nutrition, has been observed in utero as early as 15–18 weeks' gestation, but it is not fully functional for effective oral feeding until 34–35 weeks' gestation. Thus, infants born earlier than 34 weeks' gestation are significantly at risk for oral feeding dysfunction that may continue throughout life. There are important anatomic differences in the upper aerodigestive tracts of infants and adults. Figure 4–4[37] is a schematic lateral view of the infant and adult oropharyngeal structures. At birth, the infant's tongue fills the oral cavity and is in loose approximation with the cheeks, hard palate, and soft palate. The infant's tongue is considerably more anterior in the oral cavity than the adult tongue because the infant's larynx is positioned high in the neck, approximately at the level of the second or third vertebra. The epiglottis touches or nearly touches the soft palate. The mandible is small, and densely compacted sucking pads in the cheeks of infants help to stabilize the lips and mouth during sucking. Because of

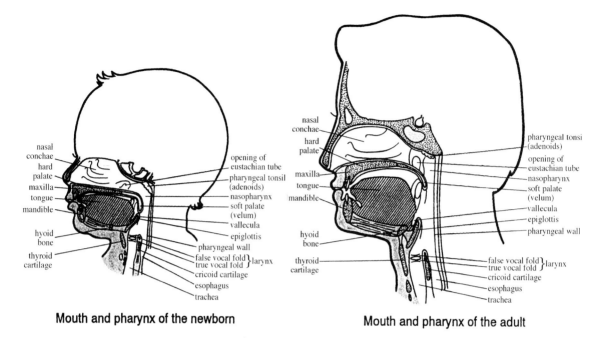

Mouth and pharynx of the newborn   **Mouth and pharynx of the adult**

FIGURE 4–4.   Infant vs. adult pharynx. Anatomy of the head and neck as it relates to feeding in the infant and the adult. (From Klein MD, Morris SE: Pre-Feeding Skills. Tucson, AZ, Therapy Skill Builders, 1987, with permission.)

the large tongue and the close proximity of the tongue, soft palate, and pharynx with the larynx, the term infant is an obligate nose breather. Oral breathing is not observed until 3 or 4 months of life after the cephalocaudal elongation of the pharynx and the subsequent descent of the hyoid, epiglottis, and larynx.

The oral motor and feeding skills of children progress gradually throughout the first 2 years of life from suckling liquids and accepting soft food from a spoon to increasing graded oral movements for chewing and the manipulation of various food textures. Finally, the child competently manages table food around 2 years of age. Table 4–11 illustrates this developmental progression.

Assessment of Feeding and Swallowing in Children

The assessment of oral feeding and swallowing disorders begins with a thorough case history

TABLE 4–11.   Stages of Oral Motor Activity Used in Feeding Progression

Age (mo)	Food Type	Oral Motor Activity	Method of Food Presentation
Birth–6	Milk, liquids	Suckling—progression to suck on bottle/breast	Bottle/breast
4–6	Cereals, pureed foods	Maturation sucking/swallowing	Spoon
5–7	Liquid, purees, teething biscuits	Diminishing bite/suck reflexes Cleaning spoon with lips Emergence munch/chew	Spoon
8–12	Ground, junior, mashed, finger foods, introduction of chopped fine	Active upper lip in spoon-feeding Lateralization of tongue begins with movement of food to teeth Biting on objects	Cup introduced
12–15	Chopped fine	Refinement of tongue lateralization Emergence of munching with rotary chewing Licking food off lips	Bottle/breast weaning Cup Spoon
15–24	Table food	Decreased drooling Increased maturity of rotary chew Internal jaw stability in cup drinking Tongue tip elevation for swallowing	Cup Spoon Fork

From Walter RS: Issues surrounding the development of feeding and swallowing. In Tuckman DN, Walter RS (eds): Disorders of Feeding and Swallowing in Infants and Children. San Diego, Singular Publishing, 1994.

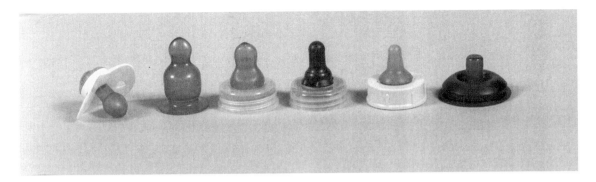

FIGURE 4–5.   Varieties of adaptive nipples.

and a clinical evaluation of oromotor structure and function. The case history should include information about general development as well as issues pertinent to feeding history in infancy, feeding behavior and milestones, feeding concerns, and current means of nutrition. A thorough clinical evaluation consist of two stages. The first stage focuses on general presentation, oral structure, and nonnutritive oral function. Critical components of this first stage are as follows:

1. Level of arousal/alertness
2. Sensitivity to the environment
3. General physical presentation
4. Positioning for optimal feeding
5. Facial appearance including tone, mouth posture at rest, and symmetry
6. Oromotor structure and function
7. Presence or absence of defensive, developmental, and/or pathologic oral reflexes

The second stage of the evaluation of feeding and swallowing focuses on the clinical observation of oral and pharyngeal phase management of varied food consistencies, including solids and liquids. Critical components of this stage are as follows:

1. Food consistencies clinically evaluated
2. Adaptive equipment used to facilitate feeding, including nipples, bottles, spoons, cups, or seating systems
3. Clinical evaluation of oral phase management according to food consistency
4. Clinical evaluation of pharyngeal phase management according to food consistency

Based on the findings of the clinical evaluation, decisions are made about the need for instrumental evaluation of oropharyngeal swallow competence, appropriate method of feeding (oral vs. enteral), appropriate equipment and positioning for feeding, and special feeding techniques to

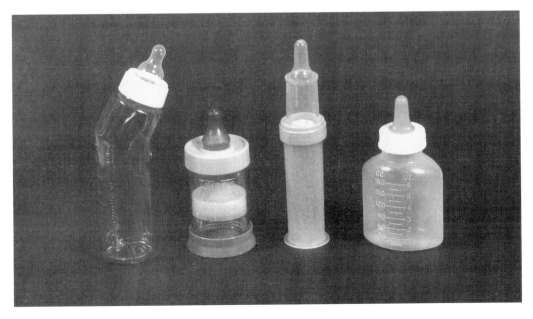

FIGURE 4–6.   Varieties of adaptive bottles.

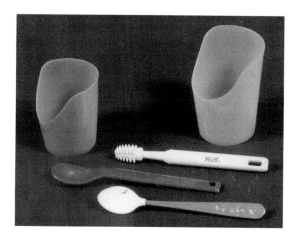

FIGURE 4–7. Cups and feeding aids.

maximize function and maintain safety. Figures 4–5, 4–6, and 4–7 illustrate adaptive feeding equipment commonly used in children. Table 4–12 contains additional information about adaptive feeding products, characteristics, and purchasing sources for review.

Videofluoroscopic Evaluation of Swallow

The modified barium swallow (MBS) study is considered the gold standard for assessing the anatomy and physiology of the oral and pharyngeal stages of swallow. The technique differs from a traditional upper GI or barium swallow in that the MBS focuses on the oral and pharyngeal stages of swallow for various food consistencies. It is one method for directly assessing the risk of aspiration as well as instances of frank aspiration.

During videofluoroscopy or MBS, the integrity of the oral and pharyngeal stages of swallow is assessed and the cervical esophageal region is observed. Typically, children are seated in a specialized chair (Fig. 4–8) and infants in a Tumbleform, both of which support the child's head, trunk, and neck in appropriate feeding alignment. These seating systems are designed

TABLE 4–12. Adaptive Feeding Products

Product	Characteristics	Source
1. Nipples		
Playtex Cherubs pacifier	Stimulates nonnutritive suck Calms infant by satisfying the natural sucking desire	Playtex Products, Inc. P. O. Box 1400 Dover, DE 19901
Nuk® orthodontic nipple	Similar to the nursing mother's breast Encourages oral exercise Allows for slow liquid intake	Gerber Products Co. P. O. Box 120 Reedsburg, WI 53959-0120
Newborn orthodontic nipple	Shape is similar to Nuk® orthodontic nipple, but shorter to allow for the oral cavity of a newborn	Ross Laboratories Columbus, Ohio 43216
Premature nipple	Longer length of nipple to facilitate posterior placement of liquid and reduce oral or nasal leakage Narrow nipple to allow for baby's smaller oral structures	Ross Laboratories Columbus, Ohio 43216
Neonatal nipple	Small, short nipple used with premature infants having small oral cavities	Mead Johnson Nutritionals Mead Johnson & Co. Evansville, IN 47721
Playtex nipple	Size and shape of nipple resembles mother's breast	Playtex Products, Inc. P. O. Box 1400 Dover, DE 19901
2. Bottles and nursers		
Angled bottle	Allows for more upright positioning of infant without disrupting the flow of the liquid Angle of the bottle helps to keep the nipple filled with liquid rather than air during feeding	Johnson & Johnson Consumer Products, Inc. Skillman, NJ 08558-9418
Baby food feeder	Allows for infant to have thickened liquids from a nipple when spoon-feeding may not be an option Eases the infant into foods and cereals	Kiddie Products, Inc. Avon, MA 02322-1171
Haberman feeder	Allows clinician to regulate the flow of liquid for infants with severe feeding problems via a one-way valve Recommended for infants with cleft lip and/or palate	Imaginart 307 Arizona Street Bisbee, AZ 85603
Cleft palate nurser	Cleft palate nipple and feeding system having a long, narrow nipple for posterior placement within the oral cavity Soft, squeezable bottle to permit adjustment of flow of liquid by the feeder Can also be used with other infant populations as appropriate	Mead Johnson Nutritionals Mead Johnson & Co. Evansville, IN 47721

(Table continued on following page.)

TABLE 4–12. Adaptive Feeding Products (*Continued*)

Product	Characteristics	Source
3. Cups, spoons, and brush		
Flexi-cut cups	Available in three sizes Soft plastic and easy for a child to hold The cut-out portion allows the feeder to better control the amount of liquid presented as this may be visualized without interference from the nose Bilabial approximation on the rim of the cup may be visualized	Imaginart 307 Arizona Street Bisbee, AZ 85603
Nuk® brush	Soft rubber nubbed tip may be used to provide intraoral stimulation	Imaginart 307 Arizona Street Bisbee, AZ 85603
Maroon spoon	Sturdy plastic spoon having a narrow, shallow bowl to allow food to slide off easily Useful for children having difficulty with lip closure, oral defensiveness, or tongue thrust	AliMed Inc. 297 High Street Dedham, MA 02026-9135
Coated baby spoon	Reduces sensory input from taste and temperature Safer for child who has a bite reflex	Gerber Products Co. Fremont, MI 49413

to fit between the upright fluoroscopic table and the filming surface.

A lateral view of the oropharynx during the dynamics of swallow is observed and videotaped for later review. The clinician is able to observe the duration and completeness of bolus transfer through the oral and pharyngeal stages and the movement patterns of the lips, tongue, mandible, velum, and larynx. Problems noted with bolus management during the oral and/or pharyngeal stages can be assessed for various food textures, consistencies, and temperatures, and appropriate recommendations can be made about the safety and appropriateness of oral feeding. Table 4–13[39] provides a summary of signs and symptoms that suggest a referral for a videofluoroscopic swallow study.

Considerations in Treatment of Children with Oral Pharyngeal Dysphagia

When any child is chronically ill or has experienced a traumatic injury, establishing realistic expectations for oral feeding is often difficult. Frequently it involves balancing the medical and nutritional needs of the infant or child with the need to develop or maintain oral function. Moreover, the expectations and desires of the families for feeding the child need to be considered. Management plans must be based on the development of coordinated oral-motor movements of the mouth and the relationship among the oral, respiratory, and neurologic systems of the child.[40] Therefore, treatment is based on an individualized oral motor and feeding plan, not simply on isolated techniques or discrete medical diagnosis.

Basic elements used in designing a treatment program have been discussed by Arvedson:[40]

(1) the feeding environment of the child, including the child's oral-motor, respiratory, and neurologic status; (2) tone and movement patterns in the body that affect oral motor movement

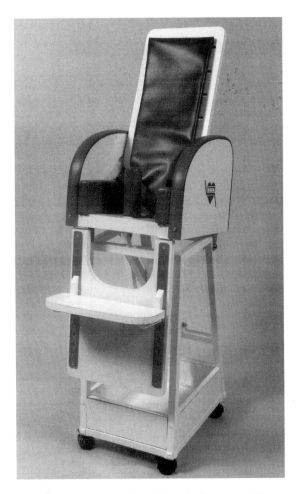

FIGURE 4–8. Specialized chair for barium swallow.

TABLE 4–13. Symptoms and Signs for Referral for Videofluoroscopic Swallow Study

Category	Symptoms/Signs
During feeding	Coughing, gagging, excessive drooling Increased congestion Gurgly voice quality Irritability Food refusal Lack of alertness or lethargy Mealtimes lasting more than 30 minutes
Pulmonary status	Frequent or recurrent pneumonia Recurrent upper respiratory infections Chronic lung changes Infiltrates on a chest x-ray
General health and gastro-intestinal status	Frequent or recurrent low-grade fevers Poor weight gain or weight loss Emesis Reflux (possible hoarseness)
Neurologic status	Oral-motor incoordination or weakness Reduced oral sensation
Structural status	Suspected tracheoesophageal fistula Vocal fold paralysis or paresis

From Arvedson JC: Management of swallowing problems. In Arvedson JC, Brodsky L (eds): Pediatric Swallowing and Feeding: Assessment and Management. San Diego, Singular Publishing, 1993.

during feeding and swallowing; (3) retention of primitive oral reflexes that may interfere with skill acquisition; and (4) facilitation of normal patterns of oral motor movement.

Frequently, adaptive equipment is recommended by the feeding clinician to facilitate accomplishment of treatment goals while maintaining adequate nutritional intake. For example, a specific type of nipple may be recommended to help the infant compensate for weak oral motor function during sucking. A coated spoon may be beneficial for the adolescent who is recovering from traumatic brain injury and demonstrates oral hypersensitivity and defensiveness. Table 4–14[41] outlines special considerations in treating dysphagia in brain-impaired patients.

Conclusion

This chapter provides a general overview of speech and language development and disorders of communication and oral motor function. The functional, practical approach provides easy reference tables and summaries for interested physiatrists. The habilitation or rehabilitation of oral communication and oropharyngeal skills for feeding and swallowing are skills that parents and caregivers frequently evaluate as critical to

TABLE 4–14. Considerations When Treating Dysphagia after Traumatic Brain Injury

Consideration	Rationale: The clinician will need to address the patient's . . .
Impaired cognitive abilities	Cognitive capacity to adequately comprehend and respond to visual, verbal, and/or tactile cues to maximize success with oral feeding/swallowing Ability to follow oral directives necessary for appropriately responding to verbal cues and maintaining safe oral feeding Understanding of specific precautionary measures and the rationale of such measures
Inability to self-initiate or inhibit	Dependency on external cues for safe feeding and potential for independent feeding Ability to inhibit inappropriate behaviors that may compromise successful oral feeding, such as impulsivity, distractibility, or use of a rapid rate of feeding
Impaired focused and/or sustained attention	Risk for choking or aspirating food due to environmental distractions, inability to maintain adequate attention to the feeding process and adequately sustain attention to complete a meal in a timely manner
Impaired cognitive/communi-cative abilities	Ability to effectively communicate orally or nonorally if a problem should occur during feeding Produce voice to allow for monitoring of maintenance of a clear vocal quality when feeding
Impaired oral motor functioning	Ability to functionally execute isolated and sequential oral motor movements necessary to achieve oral management (i.e., bolus formulation and manipulation) as well as timely posterior transit to trigger the swallow reflex at the juncture of the pharyngeal phase Awareness of and risk for premature entry of food or liquid into the hypopharynx Gag reflex integrity for airway protection
Severity of injury	Ability to successfully participate and progress through an oral feeding/swallowing treatment program to achieve that individual's optimal level of functioning Individualized pace for progressing through an oral feeding/swallowing treatment program
Developmental concerns	Oral feeding abilities before injury, taking developmental age into consideration as appropriate
Other physical and perceptual impairments	Ability to maintain an appropriate posture for oral feeding/swallowing Necessity of an occupational or physical therapy consultation to identify appropriate external supports or adaptive equipment to facilitate successful oral feeding/swallowing

Adapted from Blosser JL, DePompei R: Making communication work for the child/adolescent. In Blosser JL, DePompei R (eds): Pediatric Traumatic Brain Injury: Proactive Intervention. San Diego, Singular Publishing, 1994.

the child's success in the home and community. The goal is to facilitate normal functioning whenever possible and to maximize the child's potential in these areas.

References

1. Lahey M: What is language? In Lahey M: Language Disorders and Language Development. New York, MacMillan Publishing Company, 1988.
2. Nicolosi L, Harryman E, Kresheck J (eds): Terminology of Communication Disorders. Baltimore, Williams & Wilkins, 1978.
3. Rosen M, Clark GR, Kivitz MS: The concept of habilitation: Historical perspective. In Rosen M, Clark GR, Kivitz MS (eds): Habilitation of the Handicapped. Baltimore, University Park Press, 1977.
4. Nelson K: Structure and Strategy in Learning to Talk. Monograph of the Society for Research in Child Development, 1973.
5. Mykelbust H: Auditory Disorders in Children: A Manual for Differential Diagnosis. New York, Grune & Stratton, 1954.
6. Rapin I, Allen DS: Developmental language disorders: Nosological considerations. In Kirk U (ed): Neuropsychology of Language, Reading and Spelling. New York, Academic Press, 1983.
7. Grossman HJ (ed): Classification in Mental Retardation. Washington, DC, American Association on Mental Deficiency, 1983.
8. Terman L, Merrill M: Stanford-Binet Intelligence Scale. Boston, Houghton Mifflin, 1960.
9. Wechsler D: Wechsler Intelligence Scale for Children—III. San Antonio, Psychological Corporation, 1991.
10. Graham JT, Graham LW: Language behavior of the mentally retarded: Syntactic characteristics. Am J Ment Defic 1971;75:623.
11. Mein R, O'Connor N: A study of the oral vocabularies of severely sub-normal patients. J Ment Defic Res 1960; 4:130.
12. Lackner J: A developmental study of language behavior in retarded children. Neuropsychologia 1968;6:301.
13. Ryan J: Mental subnormality and language development. In Lenneberg F, Lenneberg E (eds): Foundations of Language Development, vol. 2. New York, Academic Press, 1975.
14. Quigley S, Power D, Steinkamp M: The language structure of deaf children. Volta Rev 1977;79:73.
15. Northern J, Downs M: Hearing in Children. Baltimore, Williams & Wilkins, 1984.
16. American Psychiatric Association: Diagnostic and Statistical Manual of Mental Disorders, 4th ed. Washington, DC, American Psychiatric Association, 1994.
17. Eisenson J: Developmental aphasia. In Eisenson J: Aphasia in Children. New York, Harper & Rowe, 1972.
18. Slobin D, Welsh C: Elicited imitation as a research tool in developmental psycholinguistics. In Ferguson C, Slobin D (eds): Studies of Child Language Development. New York, Holt, Reinhart, & Winston, 1973.
19. Ylvisaker MA (ed): Head Injury Rehabilitation: Children and Adolescents. San Diego, College-Hill Press, 1985.
20. Adamovich BB, Henderson JA, Auerbach S: Cognitive rehabilitation techniques. In Adamovich BB, Henderson JA, Auerbach S: Closed Head Injured Patients: A Dynamic Approach. San Diego, College-Hill Press, 1985.
21. Adamovich BB, Henderson JA, Auerbach S: Assessment of cognitive abilities. In Adamovich BB, Henderson JA, Auerbach S: Closed Head Injured Patients: A Dynamic Approach. San Diego, College-Hill Press, 1985.
22. Singer GHS, Glang A, Williams JM (eds): Children with Acquired Brain Injury: Educating and Supporting Families. Baltimore, Paul H Brooks, 1996.
23. Hughes BK: The impact of TBI on a child. In Hughes BK: Parenting a Child with Traumatic Brain Injury. Springfield, Charles C Thomas, 1990.
24. Soifer LH: Development and disorders of communication. In Molnar GE (ed): Pediatric Rehabilitation, 2nd ed. Baltimore, Williams & Wilkins, 1985.
25. Soloman NP, Charron S: Speech breathing in able-bodied children and children with cerebral palsy: A review of the literature and implications for clinical intervention. Am J Speech Lang Pathol 1998;7:2.
26. Hardy J: Intraoral breath pressure in cerebral palsy. J Speech Hear Disord 1961;26:309.
27. McDonald E, Chance B: Cerebral Palsy. Englewood Cliffs, NJ, Prentice-Hall, 1964.
28. Darley F, Aronson A, Brown J: Spastic dysarthria. In Darley F, Aronson A, Brown J (eds): Motor Speech Disorders. Philadelphia, WB Saunders, 1975.
29. Dorland WAN: Dorland's Illustrated Medical Dictionary, 28th ed. Philadelphia, WB Saunders, 1994.
30. Mason MF (ed): Speech Pathology for Tracheostomized and Ventilator Dependent Patients. Newport Beach, Voicing!, 1993.
31. Cherney LR, Cantieri C, Jones Pannell J: Overview. In Reiff Cherney L, Addy Cantieri C, Jones Pannell J (eds): Clinical Evaluation of Dysphagia. Rockville, MD, Aspen, 1986.
32. Grower M: The neurology of swallowing. In Grower ME: Dysphagia Diagnosis and Management, 2nd ed. Boston, Butterworth-Heinemann, 1992.
33. Bleile KM (ed): The Care of Children with Long-Term Tracheostomies. San Diego, Singular Publishing, 1993.
34. Morris S: Developmental implications for the management of feeding problems in neurologically impaired infants. Semin Speech Lang Disord 1985;6:293.
35. Tucker J: Perspective of the development of the air and food passages. Am Rev Respir Dis 1985;131:S7.
36. Pritchard J: Fetal swallowing and amniotic fluid volume. Obstet Gynecol 1966;28:606.
37. Dunn Klein M, Evans Morris S: Anatomy of the head and neck as it relates to feeding in the infant and adult. In Wolf LS, Glass RP (eds): Feed and Swallowing Disorders in Infancy: Assessment and Management. Tucson, AZ, Communication Skill Builders, 1992.
38. Tuchman DN, Walter RS (eds): Disorders of Feeding and Swallowing in Infants and Children. San Diego, Singular Publishing, 1994.
39. Arvedson JC, Christensen S: Instrumental evaluation. In Arvedson JC, Brodsky L: Pediatric Swallowing and Feeding: Assessment and Management. San Diego, Singular Publishing, 1993.
40. Arvedson JC: Management of swallowing problems. In Arvedson JC, Brodsky L (eds): Pediatric Swallowing and Feeding: Assessment and Management. San Diego, Singular Publishing, 1993.
41. Blosser JL, DePompei R: Making communication work for the child/adolescent. In Blosser JL, DePompei R (eds): Pediatric Traumatic Brain Injury: Proactive Intervention. San Diego, Singular Publishing, 1994.

Chapter **5**

Electrodiagnosis in Pediatrics

Craig M. McDonald, MD

Electromyography (EMG), nerve conduction studies (NCSs), and evoked potentials, including somatosensory evoked potentials (SSEPs), provide useful information to assist the clinician in the localization of pathology within the lower motor neuron and selected areas of the central nervous system. In acquired or hereditary disorders of the *lower motor neuron*—anterior horn cell, peripheral nerve, neuromuscular junction (presynaptic or postsynaptic region), or muscle—electrodiagnostic studies are a powerful diagnostic tool to be used as an extension of the physical examination. The information gained from electrodiagnostic studies may be invaluable in planning subsequent, more invasive diagnostic studies (e.g., muscle and nerve biopsy, CSF examination, and MR imaging, which at times require general anesthesia), or it may aid in the surgical management of peripheral nerve trauma, compressive lesions, or nerve entrapments. In immune-mediated disorders such as myasthenia gravis or Guillain-Barré syndrome, electrodiagnostic studies may allow prompt treatment.

Pediatric electrodiagnosis must be approached with knowledge of peripheral neuromuscular development and thoughtful planning of the study with regard to the most likely diagnostic possibilities, developmental status of the child, and likelihood that electrodiagnosis will be able to provide clinicians and family with useful diagnostic information. The physical examination and the developmental level of the infant or child direct the study. The examination requires patience and technical competence of an electrodiagnostic clinician experienced and skilled in the evaluation of children. This chapter will focus on considerations specific to infants and children with an emphasis on practical suggestions that may facilitate the completion of an accurate pediatric electrodiagnostic examination with minimal discomfort and distress to the child and parents.

Maturational Factors in Pediatric Electrodiagnosis

The normative neurophysiologic data relating to the maturation of peripheral nerves and muscle have greatly expanded over the past decade.[1,2] The reader is referred to the volume by Jones, Bolton, and Harper[2] for an excellent review of neurophysiologic norms in pediatric populations. Peripheral nerve myelination begins at about the 15th week of gestation and continues throughout the first 3–5 years after birth.[3] Conduction velocities are determined by myelination, diameter of the fiber, and internodal distances. Myelination occurs at the same rate, whether intrauterine or extrauterine. Conduction velocities are directly related to gestational and postconceptual age and are unrelated to birth weight.[4,5] Conduction velocities increase in direct proportion to the increase in diameter of fibers during growth. A direct relationship exists between the diameter of the axon and the thickness of the myelin sheath. The diameter of the fibers at birth has been shown to be one-half of that in adulthood. No unusual acceleration of myelination occurs subsequent to birth.[6] Peripheral fibers reach their maximum diameter at 2–5 years of age.[6,7] The nodes of Ranvier continue to remodel, with peak internodal distances being reached at 5 years of age.

Nerve Conduction

In general, normal standard adult values for conduction velocities are reached by age 3–5 years. Upper and lower extremity conduction velocities are similar for all infants under the age of 1 year. Subsequently, faster conductions are maintained in the upper extremities and comparatively slower conductions in the lower extremities, as in adults. Unique values for expected conduction velocities are observed for specific peripheral nerves.

TABLE 5–1. Normal Motor Conduction Velocities in Children (m/s)

	Median[12]	Ulnar[6a,16]	Peroneal[12]	Tibial[10,11]
7 days–1 month	25.43 ± 3.84	20.0–36.1	22.43 ± 1.22	25.3 ± 1.96
1–6 months	34.35 ± 6.61	33.3–50.0	35.18 ± 3.96	27.8 ± 3.89*
				36.3 ± 4.98[†]
6–12 months	43.57 ± 4.78	35.0–58.2	43.55 ± 3.77	39.9 ± 3.89
1–2 years	48.23 ± 4.58	41.3–63.5	51.42 ± 3.02	42.6 ± 3.80
2–4 years	53.59 ± 5.29		55.73 ± 4.45	49.8 ± 5.78
4–6 years	56.26 ± 4.61		56.14 ± 4.96	50.0 ± 4.26
6–14 years	57.32 ± 3.35	58.2 ± 9.7[‡]	57.05 ± 4.54	52.4 ± 4.19[§]

Data are presented as means ± SD or as normative ranges.
* 1–3 months
[†] 3–6 months
[‡] 4–16 years
[§] 6–11 years

Motor Nerve Conduction

Motor conduction velocities (MCVs) in infants are found to be one-half of those in adults. In infants, conduction studies should be at least greater than 20 m/s. At birth, mean MCVs for the median, ulnar, and peroneal nerves are 27 m/s. The median nerve may lag in maturation of MCV relative to the ulnar and peroneal nerves. Ulnar MCV values reach the lower adult range by the age of 3 years.[6] The slight difference between ulnar and median MCV values in the first three years of life disappears in children by 4–5 years of age. Careful and consistent measurements are necessary to achieve reliable and valid data. Normative values for selected motor nerve conduction velocities are shown in Table 5–1.

Distal latencies show maturational changes between infancy and 3–5 years of age, similar to motor conduction velocities. Normative data for distal latencies are generally more incomplete, with ranges of distances provided for stimulation point to active electrode. While the stimulation distance should always be recorded in the electrodiagnostic report, the specific distal latency is rarely of critical importance in determining a diagnosis in pediatric cases because distal peripheral entrapments are relatively uncommon. Rather, reported distal latencies that are either unusually fast or unusually slow in the setting of otherwise normal motor conduction velocities should raise a suspicion regarding technical problems and identification of appropriate wave forms. Compound muscle action potential (CMAP) amplitudes are important to consider in the evaluation of axonal loss, conduction block, and muscle fiber atrophy. In infants, CMAP amplitudes of lower extremity nerves are one-half to one-third those of adult values, and upper extremity CMAPs may be one-third to one-fourth those of adult values. As with motor conduction velocities, CMAP amplitudes increase in size with age, but adult values are generally not reached until the end of the first decade of life. Normal values for CMAP amplitudes are shown in Table 5–2.

Sensory Nerve Conduction

Modern EMG equipment, which includes amplifiers and signal-averaging capability, allows sensory nerve action potentials to be routinely recorded in the absence of peripheral nerve pathology. Maturational changes for orthodromic and antidromic sensory conduction are similar to those for motor fibers.[8–12] In infants and young children, two distinct peaks are often observed in the SNAP with proximal stimulation.

TABLE 5–2. Normal CMAP Amplitudes in Children (mV)

	Median[12]	Ulnar[6a,16]	Peroneal[12]	Tibial[10,11]
7 days–1 month	3.00 ± 0.31	1.6–7.0	3.0 ± 1.26	5.0–8.0
1–6 months	7.37 ± 3.24	2.5–7.4	5.23 ± 2.37	
6–12 months	7.67 ± 4.45	3.2–10.0	5.41 ± 2.01	
1–2 years	8.90 ± 3.61	2.6–9.7	5.80 ± 2.48	
2–4 years	9.55 ± 4.34		6.10 ± 2.99	
4–6 years	10.37 ± 3.66		7.10 ± 4.76	
6–14 years	12.37 ± 4.79		8.15 ± 4.19	4.0–20.0

Data are presented as means ± SD or as normative ranges.

TABLE 5–3. Normal Sensory Conduction Velocities in Children (m/s)

	Median[12]*	Ulnar[9]†	Sural[12]‡
7 days–1 month	22.31 ± 2.16	18.4 ± 3.97	20.26 ± 1.55
1–6 months	35.52 ± 6.59	27.7 ± 6.37 (1–3 mo)	34.63 ± 5.43
		37.1 ± 5.25 (3–6 mo)	
6–12 months	40.31 ± 5.23	40.0 ± 5.13	38.18 ± 5.00
1–2 years	46.93 ± 5.03	44.2 ± 7.79	49.73 ± 5.53
2–4 years	49.51 ± 3.34	48.8 ± 3.01	52.63 ± 2.96
4–6 years	51.71 ± 5.16	47.7 ± 6.75	53.83 ± 4.34
6–14 years	53.84 ± 3.26	46.6 ± 5.6	53.85 ± 4.19

Data are presented as means ± SD.
* Index finger to wrist using ring electrodes for stimulation.
† Fifth digit to wrist segment using ring electrodes for stimulation.
‡ Stimulation is below and distal to lateral malleolus; recording electrodes are over sural nerve 4–10 cm above ankle.

This two-peak potential has been attributed to differences in maturation between two groups of sensory fibers and often persists until 4–6 years of age.[13] Sensory nerve conduction velocities may be calculated from single distal antidromic or orthodromic stimulations by measuring the distance from stimulation point to active electrode and the distal latency. Normative values for sensory nerve conduction velocities in selected nerves using orthodromic stimulation and proximal recording are shown in Table 5–3. Normal values for orthodromic SNAP amplitudes are shown in Table 5–4.

F-waves

The F-wave is a late response that appears with supramaximal motor nerve stimulation and arises from the discharge of a small number of motor neurons in response to antidromic stimulation of the motor axon. The F-wave latency is measured from hand and foot intrinsic muscles and is useful for evaluating the motor nerve conduction velocity of proximal nerve segments. With the F-wave, the speed of motor nerve conduction is measured over a long distance; hence, F-wave latencies and velocities are less subject to errors inherent in the calculation of motor conduction velocities over short distances (10 cm or less). F-waves can be recorded from most limb nerves in newborns and young infants. The minimum F-wave latencies recorded from hand muscles with median or ulnar nerve stimulation at the wrist are generally less than 20 ms in normal children younger than 6 years.[12–14] In the lower extremities, the F-wave latencies recorded from intrinsic foot muscles with peroneal or posterior tibial nerve stimulation at the ankle are generally less than 30 ms in children younger than 6 years.[12,16]

Neuromuscular Transmission

The neuromuscular junction shows less stability and reserve in normal newborns. At low rates of stimulation (1–2 Hz), no significant incremental or decremental changes in CMAP amplitude are observed.[17] At higher rates of stimulation (5–10 Hz), normal infants may show slight facilitation. Decremental responses averaging 24% have been reported at high rates of stimulation (20 Hz) in normal newborns. At 50-Hz stimulation, normal newborns may show

TABLE 5–4. Normal SNAP Amplitudes in Children (μV)

	Median[12]*	Ulnar[9]†	Sural[12]‡
7 days–1 month	6.22 ± 1.30	5.5 ± 3.1	9.12 ± 3.02
1–6 months	15.86 ± 5.18	9.4 ± 3.2	11.66 ± 3.57
		13.2 ± 3.23	
6–12 months	16.00 ± 5.18	13.0 ± 5.6	15.10 ± 8.22
1–2 years	24.00 ± 7.36	16.3 ± 2.44	15.41 ± 9.98
2–4 years	24.28 ± 5.49	16.0 ± 3.6	23.27 ± 6.84
4–6 years	25.12 ± 5.22	14.2 ± 2.72	22.66 ± 5.42
6–14 years	26.72 ± 9.43	13.4 ± 4.2	26.75 ± 6.59

Data are presented as means ± SD.
* Index finger to wrist using ring electrodes for stimulation.
† Fifth digit to wrist segment using ring electrodes for stimulation.
‡ Stimulation is below and distal to lateral malleolus; recording electrodes are over sural nerve 4–10 cm above ankle.

decrements in the order of 50%.[17] In general, decremental changes greater than 10% at low rates of stimulation (2–5 Hz) and facilitatory changes greater than 23% at high rates of stimulation (20–50 Hz) are thought to be significant in the post-term infant.[18] Some authors have used high rates of stimulation in the order of 50 Hz for ten seconds to document facilitation greater than 20–23% in infantile botulism (at times over 100% increments are observed).[19,20]

Electromyography

Motor Unit Configuration and Amplitude

Amplitudes of motor unit action potentials (MUAPs) are lower in infants, ranging from 150 to approximately 2,000 µV. Generally, motor unit action potentials greater than 1,000 µV in 0–3-year-old children are rare.[21,22] In infants, motor unit action potentials are usually biphasic or triphasic.

Motor Unit Duration

Infantile motor unit action potentials are often shorter in duration. DeCarmo[21] found newborns to exhibit durations 17–26% shorter than those seen in adults. Durations of motor unit action potentials are often shorter than 5 ms in infants.

Motor Unit Recruitment

In infants and very young children, it is difficult to assess strength of voluntary contraction and determine when the interference pattern is full. In general, as strength of voluntary contraction increases, there is an increase in motor unit action potentials recruited. However, the recruitment pattern in infants may be disordered

and chaotic. As with adults, the recruitment frequency, defined as the firing rate of a motor unit action potential (MUAP) when a different MUAP first appears with gradually increasing strength of voluntary contraction, is helpful in differentiating a myopathic process (lower recruitment frequency values) from a neuropathic process (higher recruitment frequencies often greater than 20–25 Hz). An example of neuropathic recruitment is shown in Figure 5–1.

Technical Factors with Infantile Nerve Conduction Studies

Temperature

The maintenance of appropriate subject temperature is essential during nerve conduction studies. Neonates generally have difficulty with temperature homeostasis and low subject temperature may have profound effects on conduction velocities. A skin temperature of 36–37° C produces near-nerve temperatures of 37–38° C and avoids spurious reductions in nerve conduction velocities and prolongation of distal latencies. It is assumed that a 1° C drop in temperature produces a slowing of conduction in the order of 2–3 m/s. Every attempt should be made to maintain extremity temperature by using infant warmers, heating lamps, or warm blankets.

Volume Conduction

Volume conduction is defined as the current transmission from a potential source through a conducting medium, such as the body tissues. This may produce depolarization of peripheral nerves in proximity to the specific nerve being

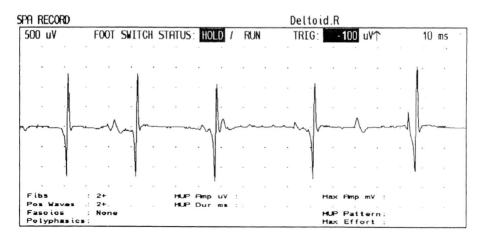

FIGURE 5–1.   Neuropathic recruitment of the deltoid in a 12-month-old child with a brachial plexus injury sustained at birth. The initial recruited MUAP is 2,500 µV, and it is firing at 25 Hz.

studied and is particularly problematic in smaller children with less soft tissue separating the nerves. For example, volume conduction can produce simultaneous stimulation of both the median and ulnar nerves at the wrist or elbow. Such volume conduction should always be suspected when higher stimulation intensities or durations are used and when CMAP configurations show an initial positive deflection or a multiple-peak configuration.

Shock Artifact

Shock artifact is a common problem with smaller subjects because of short distances between the stimulator and recording electrodes. Such artifact may be particularly problematic with distal stimulation. Whenever possible, the ground electrode should be placed between the stimulating and recording electrodes, and, in infants, often a standard 6-mm silver disc or ring electrode can be placed around the wrist or ankle. Alternatively, the ground disc may be taped to the dorsal surface of the hand. Other approaches to minimize shock artifact in young children include the use of pumice paste to reduce skin impedance and permit suprathreshold stimulation with lower electrical currents, use of a minimal amount of conduction gel or cream, and rotation of the proximal anode in relation to the distal cathode.

Measurement of Distances/Measurement Error

Distance measurements must be extremely meticulous in pediatric electrodiagnostic evaluations. Segment distances are often in the order of 6–10 cm. Thus, a measurement discrepancy of only 1 cm may produce as much as a 10–15% conduction velocity error.

Stimulating Electrodes

For neonates and young infants, small stimulators with short interelectrode distances are commercially available and simplify the testing of short nerve segments over small extremities (Fig. 5–2). The stimulation intensity may be reduced by the use of a small monopolar needle electrode as the stimulating cathode with a more proximal surface anode in close proximity. For example, for ulnar orthodromic sensory studies, the author has used ring electrodes on the fifth digit and recording electrodes over the ulnar nerve at the elbow. Generally, a standard bipolar stimulator may be used for children six months of age and older.

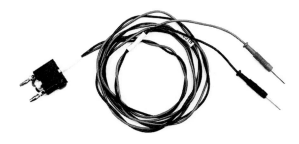

FIGURE 5–2.   Pediatric nerve stimulator. The interelectrode distance between cathode and anode is less than 2 cm.

Recording Electrodes
Sensory Conduction

Generally, sensory nerve action potentials (SNAPs) are easily recorded in newborns. The standard ring electrodes, needle recording electrodes, and/or pediatric-sized finger-clip electrodes may be used. While a 4-cm interelectrode distance is optimal for adults, this distance is not possible in small children. Hence, the pediatric electrodiagnostic clinician should attempt to obtain as much distance as possible between active and reference electrodes. Every attempt should be made to obtain at least a 2-cm interelectrode distance. Stimulation of the digits, palm, or wrist with recording electrodes located more proximally at the elbow for median and ulnar sensory studies provides longer distance and less measurement error. In general, normative data for sensory nerve conduction velocities are more readily available than normative data for distal latencies at specific distances.

Motor Conduction

Generally, standard 6-mm silver disc surface electrodes are used as active and reference electrodes for motor conduction studies. Some electrodiagnosticians prefer the use of ring electrodes on digits as the reference electrode and a standard surface electrode over the motor point of the muscle as the active electrode (Fig. 5–3). Often 4–6-cm distances are used from the stimulator to active electrode in small children. Conduction velocities and CMAP amplitudes are generally more important parameters in infants than motor distal latencies because distal nerve entrapments are rare. Thus, the distances used from distal stimulation to active electrode are less critical in children but should be reported.

Special Considerations for Nerve Conduction Studies

The best normative data for pediatric nerve conduction studies are available for the median,

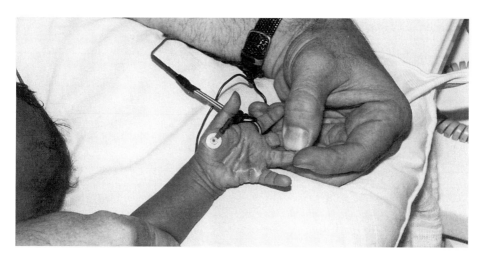

FIGURE 5–3. Recording electrodes for a median motor nerve conduction study in a small child. The active electrode is placed over the abductor pollicis brevis on the thenar eminence. The recording electrode is a ring electrode placed on the index finger. The ground electrode is a 6-mm silver disc surface electrode placed on the back of the hand.

ulnar, peroneal, tibial, facial, and phrenic nerves and the median, ulnar, and sural sensory nerves. Stimulation of the posterior tibial nerve (recording abductor hallucis brevis) produces a discrete CMAP more commonly than stimulating the peroneal nerve and recording over extensor digitorum brevis. The extensor digitorum brevis may be difficult to visualize or palpate in infants. Its CMAP configuration frequently has either an initial positivity or a low broad configuration. In addition, the CMAP amplitude may change substantially with slight changes in position for the active electrode over the extensor digitorum brevis.

The axillary and musculocutaneous motor nerve conduction studies may be helpful in the setting of infantile brachial plexopathy. Care should be taken to minimize volume conduction. Often, the intact side is studied for CMAP amplitude comparisons.

Evaluations of proximal nerves such as the axillary, spinal accessory, musculocutaneous, and femoral are often useful in the evaluation of severe demyelinating neuropathies (Fig. 5–4). The distal latencies of these nerves may be severely prolonged in the clinical setting with severe reductions in the CMAP amplitudes of more distal nerves because of conduction block or axon loss.

Percutaneous stimulation of the phrenic nerve is performed with techniques similar to those

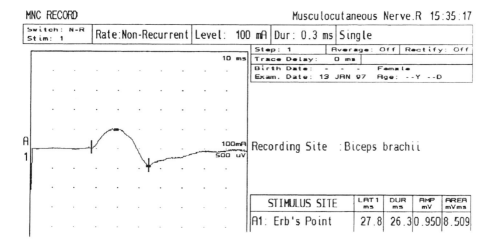

FIGURE 5–4. Nerve conduction study of the musculocutaneous nerve in hereditary motor sensory neuropathy type III. The nerve is stimulated at Erb's point, and recording electrode is over the biceps brachii. Distal latency is severely prolonged at 27.8 ms. Note the reduced CMAP amplitude presumably due to conduction block and the relative lack of temporal dispersion frequently seen in HMSN.

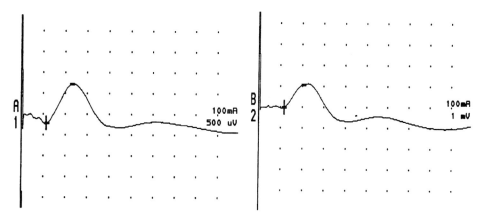

FIGURE 5–5.   Phrenic nerve conduction study in a 13-year-old child with C2 traumatic spinal cord injury. A1 is the CMAP obtained on the right side and B2 is the CMAP obtained on the left side. Latencies are approximately 5 ms and amplitudes from baseline to peak 1 mV. The viability of the phrenic nerves allowed placement of a phrenic nerve-diaphragm pacer for ventilation.

used in adults. The stimulus is applied to the posterior border of the sternocleidomastoid muscle at the level of the thyroid cartilage or, alternatively, with the cathode just medially, or occasionally laterally, to the sternal head of the sternocleidomastoid and the anode placed medially. Recording electrodes may be placed in the fifth to sixth intercostal space, 2 cm apart at the anterior axillary line. Alternatively, an active electrode may be applied immediately below the costal margin at the level of the nipple with recording electrode at the xiphoid. The active electrode may need to be moved to adjacent positions to obtain an optimal M-wave (Fig. 5–5). Normative values for phrenic latencies have been reported in children.[23] The author prefers to use ultrasound visualization of the diaphragm simultaneously with phrenic nerve stimulation to confirm downward deflection of the diaphragm. Volume conduction to the long thoracic nerve may produce a CMAP from the serratus anterior rather than the diaphragm. The downward deflection of the diaphragm, both spontaneously and with electrical stimulation, may be confirmed, and distance of diaphragmatic excursion can be quantitatively measured by ultrasound M-mode.

Repetitive Nerve Stimulation Studies

Every attempt should be made to stabilize the extremity of a child undergoing repetitive nerve stimulation studies with an infant- or pediatric-sized arm board. The author prefers to use a block electrode or 6-mm surface electrodes as cathode and anode taped over the nerve, as opposed to a hand-held stimulator. This placement helps to standardize the position of the stimulator for each stimulus during a train of 4–5 stimuli at low or high rates of stimulation. In newborns, the author prefers to stimulate the median or ulnar nerve at the elbow for repetitive stimulation studies to minimize shock artifact. Care should be taken to obtain a stable baseline between each stimulation in a train. Decrements or increments in amplitude should be accompanied by similar decrements or increments in area. If no concomitant area chances occur, then technical factors, i.e., changing baseline or changing temporal dispersion, may explain a decrement or increment in amplitude.

Technical Factors of Needle Electromyography

Electrodes

Generally, 26–28-gauge Teflon-coated monopolar electrodes, usually 25 mm in length, are used. Some laboratories routinely use disposable concentric facial needle electrodes. These electrodes have smaller calibrated recording areas and hence provide more stability of motor unit action potential (MUAP) configuration. In addition, concentric needle electrodes are more sensitive to changes in duration and amplitude than monopolar needle electrodes. Use of smaller electrodes, either small monopolar needles or small-diameter concentric needle electrodes originally designed for the examination of adult facial muscles, provides considerable psychological advantages in children of sufficient developmental age to associate needles with pain. The instrumentation used for needle EMG in children is essentially the same as that used in adults. In the intensive care unit (ICU), electrical interference may necessitate the use of either a facial concentric needle or a needle reference electrode. In addition, long electrode leads can create problems with ambient electrical interference.

Optimal Muscles to Study for Rest Activity

When evaluating an infant or young child for a generalized disorder, specific muscles are chosen for evaluation of insertional and spontaneous activity. The distal hand (first dorsal interosseous) and foot muscles of infants usually have minimal voluntary activity because of immature motor control at this developmental age, making them good sites to assess spontaneous activity. In addition, extensor muscles such as the vastus lateralis and gastrocnemius in the lower extremities and the triceps in the upper extremities are useful sites for the evaluation of insertional and spontaneous activity.

In the neonate and young infant, foot and hand intrinsic muscles exhibit high levels of end-plate noise because of the relatively larger end-plate area in the immature muscle. This end-plate activity may be confused with fibrillation potentials. Fibrillation potentials and positive sharp waves are not typically observed in the full-term normal newborn.

Optimal Muscles for Evaluation of Recruitment, Motor Unit Configuration, and Interference Data

In general, flexor muscles such as the tibialis anterior and the iliopsoas are useful for the evaluation of MUAPs and recruitment in the lower extremity. These muscles can be activated by tickling or pinching the bottom of the foot, producing a withdrawal response. In the upper extremity, the flexor digitorum sublimis and biceps muscles are frequently reflexively activated by newborns or young infants. More proximal muscles can be activated by moving the extremity or positioning it so as to produce antigravity stabilization of the limb by the firing of proximal musculature. Alternatively, reflex posturing techniques, such as the Moro reflex, can be used to activate the shoulder abductors but are usually not necessary.

Sedation

Physiatrists and neurologists performing pediatric electrodiagnostic evaluations have noted that extreme behavioral distress most frequently occurs among 2–6-year-olds.[24] Pain medication is occasionally or always prescribed by 50% of pediatric electromyographers.[24] General anesthesia is occasionally used by 25% of electrodiagnostic practitioners.[24] One study demonstrated that children exhibiting more behavior distress during electrodiagnostic evaluations were younger, had been uncooperative with previous painful procedures, were likely to have had more negative medical/dental experiences, and had mothers who themselves reported greater fear and anxiety about undergoing EMG/nerve conduction studies.[25]

Although some electromyographers never use sedation, there has been more interest in the use of sedation, analgesia, and, more recently, general anesthesia. Traditional sedative choices include chloral hydrate (50–100 mg/kg), DPT (meperidine hydrochloride, phenylephrine hydrochloride, and chlorpromazine hydrochloride), and midazolam hydrochloride nasal spray. EMLA cream (lidocaine 2.5% and prilocaine 2.5%) has been used during electromyographic evaluations as a topical anesthetic.[26] Mean duration of topical application in infants or older children was 45–145 minutes. Greater pain relief was obtained with use of EMLA over the extensor forearm muscles as compared with the thenar eminence muscles.

While general anesthesia is usually not necessary, the author has increasingly involved critical care and anesthesia colleagues who have used propofol (2,6-diisopropylphenol), an intravenous sedative-hypnotic agent for the electrodiagnostic evaluation of 18-month- to 6-year-old children who exhibit substantial behavioral distress during an initial attempt at an electrodiagnostic evaluation without sedation. This agent produces rapid onset of anesthesia (in 1–3 minutes) and sedation is maintained by either a continuous infusion or multiple boluses. Subjects usually awaken in less than 10 minutes after discontinuation of infusion. Sedation, analgesia, and particularly general anesthesia have inherent risks and require appropriate monitoring. Propofol should be administered by an anesthesiologist or pediatric intensive care specialist prepared to bag-mask ventilate or intubate the child if necessary. Adequate monitoring generally requires a sedation suite, pediatric ICU, recovery room, or operating room. The author usually obtains all nerve conduction studies and a thorough examination of multiple muscle sites for abnormal spontaneous rest activity while the subject is deeply sedated or anesthetized with propofol. The level of sedation is then titrated to a point at which appendicular movement is elicited with needle insertion or stimulation of the extremity. At this point, under lighter sedation, recruitment pattern and motor unit configuration are assessed. As the child awakens, interference pattern is evaluated with more vigorous motor activity. Children are usually amnestic to the EMG examination subsequent to propofol anesthesia. The costs and risks of general anesthesia must be weighed against the importance of the acquisition of a thorough, technically precise, and accurate electrodiagnostic evaluation.

The key to successful data acquisition in most pediatric electrodiagnostic evaluations remains a well organized, well planned approach with distinct diagnostic questions prospectively considered. If the examination is planned to answer a specific question, it is usually possible to proceed expeditiously, completing the examination within a reasonable time (30 minutes). As children approach six years of age, it becomes easier to talk them through an evaluation and elicit their participation and cooperation.

Nerve conduction studies are usually better tolerated than needle EMG and many pediatric electromyographers perform the nerve conduction studies first. Increased behavioral distress, subsequent to a needle examination, makes the motor nerve conductions, and particularly the sensory nerve conduction studies, technically difficult due to excessive EMG background noise.

Limitations of Single-fiber EMG in Pediatric Populations

While normative data for fiber density, mean consecutive difference, and jitter have been reported for different muscles among different pediatric age groups,[27] this procedure is difficult to use in younger children with limited ability to cooperate.

Specific Clinical Problems in Pediatric Electrodiagnosis

Electrodiagnostic Evaluation of the Floppy Infant

The most common referral for an electrodiagnostic examination in the infant is generalized hypotonia. The most frequent cause for infantile hypotonia is *central*, accounting for approximately 80% of cases. A differential diagnosis of infantile hypotonia is shown in Table 5–5. Electrodiagnostic abnormalities in selected conditions producing infantile hypotonia are shown in Table 5–6.[28]

Neurogenic causes of generalized weakness in infants are diagnosed more accurately with electrodiagnostic studies than myogenic causes.[29,30]

A study of the predictive value of the electrodiagnostic examination in the hypotonic infant showed that electrodiagnostic studies accurately predicted the diagnosis in 65% of infants with spinal muscular atrophy and only 10% of infants with myopathy. Seventy-five percent of the electrodiagnostic studies performed on infants with documented myopathies were considered normal.[31]

In the evaluation of hypotonia, a complete electrodiagnostic evaluation is critical, including motor and sensory nerve conduction studies, appropriate needle EMG examination with the highest-yield muscles examined initially, and, if necessary, repetitive nerve stimulation. It should be emphasized that nerve conduction studies and electromyography are an extension of the physical examination. Electrodiagnostic findings need to be interpreted in light of clinical examination. Care should be taken not to overinterpret subtle findings on needle EMG. Low-amplitude, short-duration, polyphasic MUAPs that would be considered myopathic in adults may be normal in young children. Motor unit amplitudes and durations may be reduced in the normal young child and mistaken for myopathic MUAPs. End-plate noise, abundant in the small intrinsic muscles of the hand and foot, may be difficult to distinguish from fibrillation potentials. Thus, borderline findings on needle EMG should not be overinterpreted in infants and young children.

Before an electrodiagnostic evaluation, parents should be cautioned that definitive diagnostic information is often not obtained, but that in many instances the results may help to guide further diagnostic studies. For example, EMG results may help to guide further studies, such as muscle biopsy, by providing information about the most appropriate muscle site for the biopsy. With spinal muscular atrophy (SMA), an electrodiagnostic evaluation may allow the clinician to defer a muscle biopsy and proceed with molecular genetic studies of the survival motor neuron gene. Electrodiagnostic studies in patients with hereditary motor sensory neuropathy help to categorize the neuropathy as either primarily demyelinating or axonal, and such information may help to focus subsequent molecular genetic analyses. In general, nerve conduction studies and electromyography provide powerful tools for the localization of lesions within the lower motor neuron.

Differential Diagnosis for Early Respiratory Distress in Infancy

The differential diagnosis of lower motor neuron disorders with perinatal respiratory

TABLE 5–5.   Differential Diagnosis of Infantile Hypotonia

Cerebral Hypotonia
  Chromosome disorders
    Trisomy
    Prader-Willi syndrome
  Static encephalopathy
    Cerebral malformation
    Perinatal CNS insult
    Postnatal CNS insult
  Peroxisomal disorders
    Cerebrohepatorenal syndrome (Zellweger syndrome)
    Neonatal adrenoleukodystrophy
  Inborn errors of metabolism
    Glycogen storage disease type II (Pompe's disease)
    Infantile GM1 gangliosidosis
    Tay-Sachs disease (infantile GM2 gangliosidosis)
    Vitamin dependency disorders
  Amino acid and organic acid disorders
    Maple syrup disease
    Hyperlysinemia
    Nonketotic hyperglycinemia
    Propionyl-CoA carboxylase deficiency
  Other genetic disorders
    Familial dysautonomia
    Cohen syndrome
    Oculocerebrorenal syndrome (Lowe's syndrome)
  Benign congenital hypotonia
 	
Spinal Cord Pathology
  Trauma (obstetric, postnatal)
    Hypotonia early with acute paraplegia
    Hypertonia
  Tumor or AVM
    Hypertonia may occur later or with slow-growing tumor
  Anterior horn cell
    Spinal muscular atrophy type I (Werdnig-Hoffman disease)
    Spinal muscular atrophy type II
    Poliomyelitis
    Neurogenic arthrogryposis
 	
Polyneuropathies
  Congenital hypomyelinating neuropathy
  Chronic inflammatory demyelinating polyneuropathy
  Acute inflammatory demyelinating polyradiculoneuropathy
    (Guillain-Barré syndrome)
  Hereditary motor sensory neuropathies
	Polyneuropathies *(cont.)*
	  Toxic polyneuropathy
	  Leukodystrophies (Krabbe's disease, Niemann-Pick disease)
	  Leigh's disease
	  Giant axonal neuropathy
	  Dysmaturation neuropathy
	Neuromuscular Junction
	  Presynaptic
	    Infantile botulism
	    Hypermagnesemia—eclampsia
	    Aminoglycoside antibiotics
	    Congenital myasthenia
	    Acetylcholine vesicle paucity
	    Decreased quantal release
	  Postsynaptic
	    Neonatal (autoimmune) disorders
	    Congenital myasthenia
	    Acetylcholinesterase deficiency
	    Slow changes
	    Acetylcholine receptor deficiency
	Myopathies
	  Congenital myopathies
	    Nemaline rod disease
	    Central core disease
	    Myotubular (centronuclear)
	    Congenital fiber-type disproportion
	  Congenital myotonic dystrophy
	  Congenital muscular dystrophy
	    Fukuyama-type (CNS involvement)
	    Merosin deficiency (with or without CNS involvement)
	    Atonic-sclerotic type (Ulrich's disease)
	    Undifferentiated
	  Inflammatory myopathies
	    Infantile polymyositis
	  Metabolic myopathies
	    Acid maltase deficiency (type II)
	    Muscle phosphorylase deficiency (type V)
	    Phosphofructokinase deficiency (type VII)
	    Cytochrome C oxidase
	    Carnitine deficiency
	  Endocrine myopathies
	    Hypothyroidism
	    Hypoparathyroidism

distress is fairly limited. Generally, respiratory distress within the first few days of life can be seen in spinal muscular atrophy type I, congenital hypomyelinating neuropathy, congenital myasthenia, transient neonatal myasthenia, congenital myotonic muscular dystrophy, neurogenic arthrogryposis, and X-linked myotubular myopathy. These disorders are easily differentiated with electrodiagnostic studies and, in some instances, molecular genetic findings. For example, congenital myotonic muscular dystrophy may be definitively diagnosed with molecular genetic studies of the chromosome 19q13.3 locus. In congenital hypomyelinating neuropathy, sensory conduction abnormalities are unrecordable and motor nerve conduction velocities are markedly slowed (2–5 m/s) with temporal dispersion and low-amplitude evoked potentials (Fig. 5–6). Patients with SMA type I show normal sensory

conductions, decreased CMAP amplitudes, occasional fibrillations, and decreased numbers of MUAPs. Patients with congenital myasthenia show normal sensory conductions, normal motor nerve conduction velocities, but often show abnormalities on repetitive nerve stimulation studies. X-linked myotubular myopathy patients may show profuse fibrillations and myopathic MUAPs on EMG, and diagnosis is confirmed by muscle biopsy.

Acute-onset Infantile Hypotonia

Acute-onset hypotonia in a previously normal infant warrants an evaluation to rule out acute inflammatory demyelinating polyneuropathy (AIDP), infantile botulism, infantile polymyositis, an infantile form of myasthenia, a toxic process, or acute-onset myelopathy. Repetitive motor

TABLE 5–6. Infant Hypotonia: Electrodiagnostic Abnormalities

Diagnosis	Motor Conduction	Sensory Conduction	Spontaneous Activity	Motor Units
SMA	Decreased amplitude; may show decreased velocity	Normal	Fibrillation ±; spontaneous rhythmic motor unit firing	Decreased number; may show mild increase in amplitude, duration
HMSN III	Markedly prolonged	Prolonged or absent	0	Reported normal
Hypomyelinating neuropathy	Markedly prolonged; markedly decreased amplitude	Prolonged or absent	0	Reported normal or increased in amplitude
Inflammatory polyneuropathy	Decreased amplitude; possibly decreased velocity; conduction block	±	Fibrillation may be present	Decreased number
Botulism	Decreased amplitude; normal velocity; decremental response to MNCV; facilitation > 20 Hz	Normal	Fibrillation	Decreased amplitude, duration
Spinal cord injury	Normal velocity and amplitude if nerves tested are not originating at area of injury; F-wave and H-reflex may be prolonged or absent	Normal	Fibrillations may be present in muscles innervated at level of injury	Decreased number at involved muscles; poor motor control below level of injury
Congenital myopathy	Normal velocity; amplitude may be decreased	Normal	Fibrillations may be present	Normal to decreased amplitude, duration; increased polyphasicity
Congenital myotonic dystrophy	Normal	Normal	Absent or few fibrillations; frequency-varying trains of positive waves	Poor activation; likely normal
Glycogen storage disease	Normal	Normal	Fibrillations (in types II, V, VII); frequency varying; trains of positive waves	Decreased amplitude duration
Metachromic leukodystrophy	Decreased velocity; decreased amplitude	Slowed		

From Turk MA: Pediatric electrodiagnostic medicine. In Dumitru D (ed): Electrodiagnostic Medicine. Philadelphia, Hanley & Belfus, 1995, pp 1133–1142, with permission.

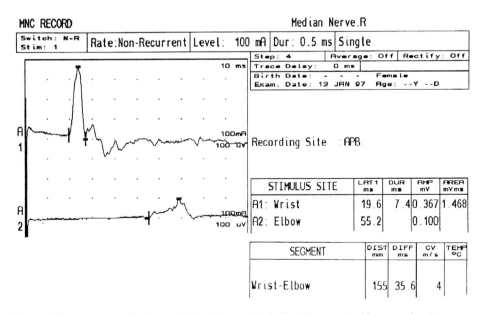

FIGURE 5–6. Median nerve conduction study in a 5-year-old child with congenital hypomyelinating neuropathy documented by sural nerve biopsy and molecular genetic studies of the EGRF 2 gene. Distal latency is markedly prolonged at 19.6 ms; there is reduced CMAP amplitude of 0.367 mV, conduction block (note the drop in amplitude from distal to proximal); and conduction velocity is 4 m/s.

nerve stimulation studies should be performed under the following circumstances: (1) there is constipation, bulbar involvement, and/or respiratory distress; (2) an infant presents with ptosis or extraocular muscle weakness; (3) CMAP amplitudes are severely reduced; (4) "myopathic" MUAPs are present; or (5) repetitive CMAP is observed after single supramaximal stimulation on routine nerve conduction study, suggestive of a diagnosis of congenital myasthenia with congenital acetylcholinesterase (AChE) deficiency or classic slow channel syndrome.

Motor Neuron Disorders

Spinal muscular atrophy (SMA) is perhaps the most common lower motor neuron disorder causing infantile hypotonia. The predictive value of needle EMG in the diagnosis of SMA has been established.[29–31] The findings in this motor neuron disorder have largely been consistent with motor axonal loss, denervation, and, among persons less severely affected, reinnervation. Traditional electrodiagnostic criteria for motor neuron disease are not suitable for patients with childhood SMA. For example, Buchthal[32] found that many infants with SMA did not meet strict criteria for motor neuron disease. If clinical findings suggest SMA, study of at least two muscles innervated by different nerve roots and peripheral nerves in at least three extremities is indicated.[33] In infants, spontaneous activity may be determined more readily with study of muscles that are not as commonly recruited, such as the vastus lateralis, gastrocnemius, triceps, and first dorsal interosseous. Recruitment and motor unit characteristics can be assessed in muscles that are readily activated, such as the anterior tibialis, iliopsoas, biceps, and flexor digitorum sublimis.[33] The paraspinal muscles usually are not studied because of poor relaxation, and the experienced pediatric electrodiagnostic medicine consultant usually defers needle evaluation of the tongue in the hypotonic infant.

Although some authors[62] have described high-density fibrillation potentials in infants with poorer outlook, most studies have not demonstrated abundant fibrillation potentials in the infantile form.[34–36] In SMA III, the incidence of fibrillation potentials ranged from 20–40% in one series[37] to 64% in another.[38] The incidence of fibrillation potentials in SMA III does not approach the level seen in SMA I. Additionally, spontaneous activity has been observed more frequently in the lower extremities than in the upper extremities, and proximal more than distal muscles in SMA III.[37] The degree of spontaneous activity has not been found to be independently associated with a worse prognosis in SMA.[31] Fasciculations are uncommonly observed in SMA I and appear more commonly in SMA II and III.[34,36,39] In younger patients, fasciculations are difficult to distinguish from spontaneously firing MUAPs. In relaxed muscles, some motor units exhibit a spontaneous rhythmic firing.[35,36,39]

Voluntary MUAPs often fire with an increased frequency, although recruitment frequency may be difficult to determine consistently in infants. Compared with age-matched norms, MUAPs show longer duration, particularly in older subjects, and higher amplitude; however, a bimodal distribution may be seen with some concomitant low-amplitude, short-duration potentials.[35] Large-amplitude, long-duration MUAPs may be absent in many infants with SMA I but more commonly observed in SMA II and III.[34] The percentage of large-amplitude MUAPs increases with the duration of the disease.[37] Other signs of reinnervation, such as polyphasic MUAPs, may be observed in more chronic and mild SMA. These polyphasic MUAPs may include late components, such as satellites or linked potentials. There also may be temporal instability of the waveform observed in individual MUAPs. Reduced recruitment (an incomplete interference pattern) with maximal effort is perhaps the most consistent finding in all SMA types (Fig. 5–7). In one series,[31] the amplitude of MUAPs and degree of decrement in recruitment pattern were not individually associated with worse prognosis.

Motor nerve conduction velocities and CMAP amplitude have been shown to be reduced in many patients with infantile SMA. The degree of motor conduction slowing (if present) tends to be mild and greater than 70% of the lower limit of normal.[36,38,40–42] Reduction of motor conduction to less than 70% of the lower limit of normal is described as an exclusion criterion for SMA.[43] The mild slowing of motor conduction is present to the same degree over distal and proximal segments as determined by M- and F-wave responses.[40] The slowing of conduction is generally seen in patients with correspondingly low-amplitude CMAPs and is thought to be due to selective loss of the fastest conducting fibers from large motor units. Alternatively, arrested myelination in utero has been proposed to explain this slowing in motor conduction noted in some SMA cases at birth.[31] Survival has been found to be longer for infants with normal motor conduction velocities over a distal segment.[31] Significant reductions in CMAP amplitudes have been reported frequently in SMA I–III.[31,34,38] Kuntz[38] reported a tendency toward greater reductions

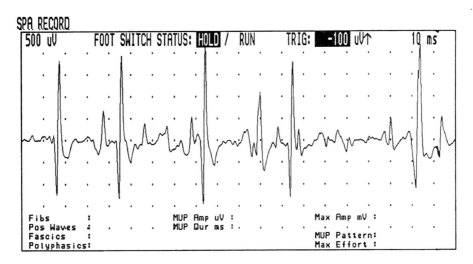

SPA RECORD

| 500 uV | FOOT SWITCH STATUS: HOLD / RUN | TRIG: -100 uV↑ | 10 ms |

Fibs :
Pos Waves :
Fascics :
Polyphasics:

MUP Amp uV :
MUP Dur ms :

Max Amp mV :

MUP Pattern:
Max Effort :

FIGURE 5–7. Incomplete or reduced interference pattern in SMA II. Note the large amplitude MUAP (3,000 μV) firing rapidly at 25 Hz.

in CMAP amplitude among patients with earlier age of onset and shorter survival.

Sensory nerve conduction studies in SMA show essentially normal sensory conduction velocities and sensory nerve action potential (SNAP) amplitudes. Significant abnormalities in sensory studies exclude a diagnosis of SMA,[43] whereas minor abnormalities in sensory conduction velocities have been noted infrequently in SMA.[41,44,45] Such rare sensory abnormalities have been reported in SMA patients with diagnostic confirmation by molecular genetic studies.

Spinal Cord Injury

Neonatal spinal cord injury may occur as an obstetrical complication or as a result of a vascular insult to the spinal cord. Typical clinical presentation may include findings of diffuse hypotonia, possible respiratory distress, hyporeflexia, and urinary retention. An anterolateral spinal cord injury due to a vascular insult will produce EMG findings of florid denervation in diffuse myotomes. Typically, 2–3 weeks may lapse before fibrillations and positive sharp waves are elicited. Anterior horn cell and axonal degeneration will result in decreased CMAP amplitudes in multiple peripheral nerves, whereas SNAP amplitudes are spared. Somatosensory evoked potentials may be spared if posterior columns are preserved.

Traumatic spinal cord injury often results in loss of anterior horn cells at a specific "zone of injury." For example, a child with C5 tetraplegia may have denervation present at the bilateral C6 and C7 myotomes. This zone of partial or complete denervation becomes particularly

relevant in the evaluation of a patient for possible placement of an implanted functional electrical stimulation system for provision of voluntary grasp and release (e.g., the Freehand System Neuro-Control, Inc.). Presence of denervation necessitates concomitant tendon transfers with electrical stimulation of the transferred muscle group.

Somatosensory evoked potentials may help to establish a sensory level in an infant or young child with spinal cord injury and is also useful in the evaluation of the comatose or obtunded child at risk for spinal cord injury without radiographic abnormality (SCIWORA).[46] Somatosensory evoked potentials are discussed below.

Brachial Plexus and Cervical Nerve Root Lesions

Traumatic obstetric brachial plexopathy usually results from traction on the brachial plexus (predominantly upper trunk) and its associated spinal roots. This traction can lead to stretching or rupture of the trunks of the plexus and/or partial axonotmesis or avulsion of the spinal roots. The most common cause is a dystocia of the anteriorly presenting shoulder causing excessive lateral neck traction. Injury to the upper trunk of the brachial plexus and/or C5–6 cervical roots is the more common injury known as Duchenne-Erb palsy. Damage to the lower trunk and/or C8–T1 cervical roots is referred to as Klumpke's palsy. Severe brachial plexus injuries may involve the entire plexus and C5-T1 nerve roots diffusely. Horner's syndrome, associated with injury of the C8 and T1 roots, results from injury to the superior cervical sympathetic

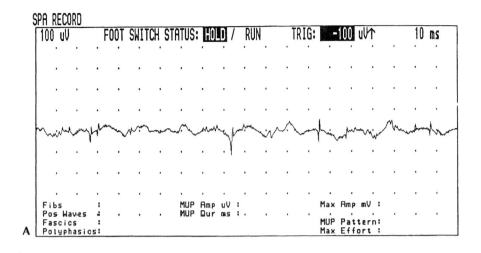

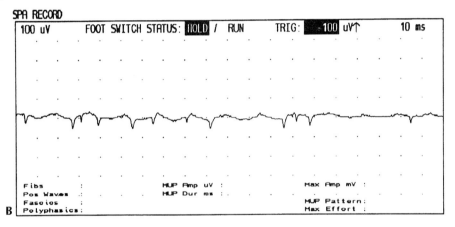

FIGURE 5–8. Fibrillation potentials (*A*) and positive sharp waves (*B*) indicative of acute denervation and axon loss.

ganglion. Isolated Klumpke's palsy is rare in the setting of traumatic birth palsy and usually results from a fall onto a hyperabducted shoulder, penetrating trauma, or tumor.

Electrodiagnostic studies help to determine the location (root and/or plexus), extent, and severity of the brachial plexus injury. Examination should be deferred until at least 3–4 weeks after the injury to allow for abnormal spontaneous rest activity (fibrillations and positive sharp waves) to develop in the setting of denervation and axon loss (Fig. 5–8). Complete injuries are characterized electromyographically by absent MUAPs and absent CMAP amplitudes in peripheral nerves supplied by the transected axons. In the setting of total motor paralysis, motor nerve conduction studies with measurement of the amplitude of the CMAPs in distal and proximal muscles provide useful prognostic information. For example, the preservation of the CMAP amplitude 10 days or more after the injury resulting in complete clinical paralysis suggests that the damage is, in

part, a neurapraxic injury with better prognosis. In this setting, F-waves are absent because of a conduction block. If motor function is absent and no MUAPs are observed, examination of the SNAP amplitude in the dermatomal distribution of the axons traveling through the affected brachial plexus trunks may help to distinguish plexus injuries from severe cervical root injuries or avulsions. The sensory dorsal root ganglion lies in the intervertebral foramen distal to the damaged segment with a root injury, leaving the sensory axon projection from the dorsal root ganglion to the limb intact. Thus, the sensory nerve action potential is obtainable in the setting of a root avulsion with absent clinical sensation.

In the setting of Erb's palsy, assessment of a superficial radial or median sensory response to the index finger is useful in making a distinction between a C6 root avulsion and a more distal lesion involving the trunk of the brachial plexus. The median SNAP to the middle finger provides information about the integrity of C7 axon projections distal to the dorsal root ganglion. The presence or absence of an ulnar sensory nerve action potential from the fifth digit can help to distinguish a lower trunk injury from a C8 nerve root injury.

In perinatal traumatic brachial plexopathy, positive sharp waves and fibrillations, indicative of true denervation, can be found by 14–21 days after injury.[34] Absence of fibrillations or positive sharp waves after this time frame suggests a neurapraxic lesion with intact axons. In this setting, the prognosis for recovery is favorable. Early in the course of recovery, before reinnervation, the interference pattern usually is reduced or discrete and recruitment frequencies increased into the neuropathic range (often > 20 Hz). A follow-up needle EMG evaluation 3–6 months after the injury is useful to determine subclinical evidence of reinnervation. Such reinnervation is characterized initially by "nascent" polyphasic MUAPs (Fig. 5–9). With reinnervation, the numbers of positive sharp waves and fibrillations decrease over time, amplitude of MUAPs increases as collateral spouting occurs, the MUAPs become less polyphasic (as shown in Fig. 5–1), and evaluation of interference pattern shows an increasing number of voluntary MUAPs present with greater contraction force.

For the electrodiagnostic work-up of an infant with a brachial plexus injury, the author prefers initially to perform sensory nerve conduction studies, occasionally with sedation, consisting of a median sensory nerve recording from the index finger (C6 dermatome), a median sensory nerve recording from the middle finger (C7 dermatome), and an ulnar sensory nerve recording from the fifth digit (C8 dermatome). Median and ulnar motor nerve conduction studies are useful to evaluate the integrity of axons traveling through the lower trunk. Axillary and musculocutaneous motor nerve conduction studies with assessment of CMAP amplitudes are useful if an upper trunk injury is suspected. These CMAP amplitudes may be compared with those on the intact side, depending on patient tolerance of the study. During the EMG study of the deltoid, the examiner should assess the clinical sensation of the C5 dermatome. The use of dermatomal and mixed nerve SSEPs in brachial plexus injuries are discussed below.

In addition to a complete needle EMG screen of paretic upper extremity muscles clinically affected, electromyographic examination of the infraspinatus or supraspinatus helps to localize an upper trunk injury proximal or distal to the takeoff of the suprascapular nerve. Although the examination of the rhomboid can be difficult in the infant, a finding of fibrillations or positive sharp waves supports the presence of a C5 root injury. Whereas in adults electromyographic evaluation of the cervical paraspinal muscles may help to determine the extent and severity of cervical root injuries, in infants such evaluation is extremely difficult because of poor relaxation. In young children, adequate relaxation of the cervical paraspinal muscles may be obtained with general anesthesia, but such measures usually are not necessary because the additional information does not usually influence management. In addition, study of the serratus anterior and rhomboids, usually performed to assess involvement of C5–C7 and C5 roots, respectively, may be technically difficult in infants because of intact sensation, the presence of trapezius overlying the rhomboids, depth of the rhomboids and serratus anterior, and the risk

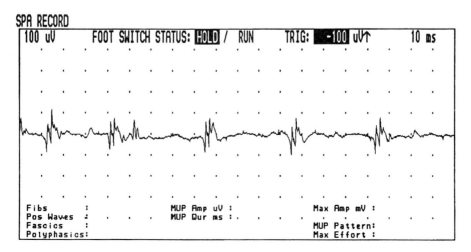

FIGURE 5–9.   Polyphasic MUAPs with a neuropathic firing frequency of 25 Hz. These polyphasic MUAPs obtained 4 months after brachial plexus injury are indicative of reinnervation.

that sudden movement may cause penetration of the needle into the pleural space. Usually a combination of needle EMG evaluation of affected muscles, sensory and motor conduction studies, and F-wave studies allows the electromyographer to determine the location and severity of the injury.

The natural history of conservatively managed brachial plexus birth palsy has recently been reported.[47] Seventy-two percent of those referred for rehabilitation evaluation showed stable functional status at follow-up. There has been a resurgence of interest in surgical exploration of obstetric brachial plexus palsy with external and internal neurolysis, neurotization, and, in selected cases, nerve grafting.[48–53] Upon reaching plateau of recovery (between 4 and 9 months after injury), an EMG evaluation may support the possible utility of a surgical exploration for neurolysis, neurotization, and/or nerve grafting if there is limited electrophysiologic evidence of reinnervation. Preoperative electrodiagnostic studies, intraoperative nerve conduction studies, and somatosensory evoked potentials are helpful in the surgical decision making. Preoperative and/or intraoperative somatosensory evoked potentials may provide evidence of upper cervical root avulsion as opposed to partial trunk and nerve root integrity, as discussed below.

Facial Paralysis in the Neonate

Facial paralysis or an asymmetric facies is a common finding in the neonate. Either condition may result from acquired traumatic facial palsy, a common iatrogenic problem with forceps deliveries; central nervous system conditions; congenital facial palsy; or congenital hypoplasia of the depressor anguli oris muscle. Facial nerve conduction studies may be helpful in the diagnosis of facial paralysis. Side-to-side comparisons of amplitudes and latencies are essential for evaluation. CMAP amplitude reduction and prolonged latency on the involved side indicate facial nerve involvement. Brain stem auditory evoked potentials and blink reflexes may be helpful in determining central nervous system involvement. Axonal integrity can be determined by electromyographic evaluation for abnormal spontaneous rest activity and motor unit recruitment. Improvement on serial testing provides favorable prognostic information, particularly when it occurs over 1–2 weeks. Normal facial nerve distal latencies in the newborn are ≤ 12.0 ms; in children from 1–12 months of age, ≤ 10.0 ms; from 1–2 years of age, ≤ 6.3 ms; from 2–3 years of age, ≤ 4.5 ms; from 3–4 years of age, ≤ 4.0 ms; and in children older than 4 years of age, ≤ 5.0 ms.[54]

Common Polyneuropathies
Hereditary Neuropathies (HMSN Subtypes)

Clinical findings associated with hereditary neuropathies and the current classification of these disorders are described in Chapter 15. The demyelinating form (HMSN type I) typically has onset in early childhood. Marked slowing of motor conduction velocities, usually to less than 50% of normal, is present in early childhood.[55,56] Generally, marked slowing of motor nerve conduction velocities is present by 3–4 years of age.[57] Distal latencies are usually severely prolonged. In HMSN there is usually less temporal dispersion than that observed in acute inflammatory demyelinating neuropathy (Guillain-Barré syndrome) because of fairly uniform demyelination of all axons. Needle EMG abnormalities include fibrillation with positive sharp waves, decreased interference pattern, and large amplitude polyphasic MUAPs resulting from reinnervation by collateral axonal sprouting.

HMSN type II is the axonal form of neuropathy. CMAP and SNAP amplitudes may be reduced, but nerve conduction velocities are either low normal or mildly reduced.[32] Needle EMG shows evidence of chronic denervation and reinnervation. HMSN type III (previously referred to as Déjérine-Sottas disease) and congenital hypomyelinating neuropathy often present in infancy. CMAP amplitudes are reduced because of a combination of conduction block and axonal loss; motor nerve conduction velocities are typically less than 12 m/s; and latencies may be three times the normal value.[58]

Acute Inflammatory Demyelinating Polyradiculoneuropathy (Guillain-Barré Syndrome)

These children often present with an acute rapid ascending paralysis initially affecting the lower limbs. While pain is common, sensory symptoms are usually mild and objective sensory loss is fairly rare. Electrophysiologically, criteria for poor recovery in adults may not apply to children. One study documented good recovery in children with low median CMAPs and fibrillation potentials.[59] Classic electrophysiologic findings include prolonged or absent F-waves early in the course of the disorder; slowing of conduction velocities, both proximally and distally; prolonged distal latencies; reduced CMAP amplitudes with evidence of conduction block; and significant temporal dispersion (Fig. 5–10). Electrophysiologic findings may lag behind the clinical signs and symptoms. In addition, electrophysiologic recovery may lag behind clinical recovery.

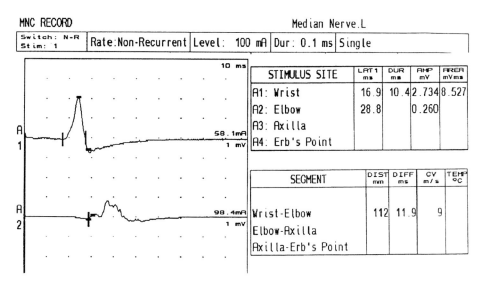

FIGURE 5–10. Median motor nerve conduction in a 4-year-old child with Guillain-Barré syndrome. Distal latency is prolonged at 16.9 ms, and conduction velocity slowed at 9 ms. Note the conduction block (amplitude drop from 2.734 to 0.260 mV) and temporal dispersion.

Chronic Inflammatory Demyelinating Polyradiculoneuropathy

This disorder has many features in common with acute inflammatory demyelinating polyradiculoneuropathy. These patients typically show a subacute or chronic onset lasting more than 4 weeks, and the disorder continues with either a chronic or relapsing course. Electrophysiologic findings generally show more marked slowing of conduction velocity, often below 10 m/s) and elevated stimulation thresholds. As in AIDP, there is evidence of focal conduction block, temporal dispersion, prolongation of distal motor latencies, and prolonged or absent H-wave and F-wave responses. These late responses may be absent because of proximal conduction block. Needle EMG may show a paucity of abnormal spontaneous rest activity and normal or slightly enlarged MUAPs that exhibit a neuropathic firing pattern.

Axonal Acute Inflammatory Demyelinating Polyneuropathy

In this disorder, children present with rapid onset, quadriparesis, bulbar dysfunction, and respiratory insufficiency.[60,61] The author has observed a case of axonal AIDP with clinical findings mimicking cerebral death.[62] The child had combined demyelinating and axonal findings and eventually achieved a near-complete recovery over 18 months. In general, children with the axonal form of AIDP are more likely to require assisted ventilation, develop severe quadriparesis, and require a much longer period of time to become ambulatory. *Campylobacter*

jejuni has been implicated as a precipitating agent in AIDP.[63]

Neuropathies Associated with Central Nervous System Disorders

Various metabolic disorders produce abnormalities of both the central and peripheral nervous system. Abnormalities of lipid metabolism, such as metachromatic leukodystrophy, may produce a severe demyelinating peripheral neuropathy with electrophysiologic findings of high stimulation threshold and low conduction velocities. Somatosensory evoked potentials may show both central and peripheral delay, and visual evoked potentials show central delay. Other disorders showing both central and peripheral nervous system involvement include Krabbe's disease, Refsum's disease (phytanic acid storage disease), Tangier disease (hereditary high-density lipoprotein deficiency), abetalipoproteinemia (vitamin E deficiency syndrome), Fabry's disease (α-galactosidase A deficiency), Niemann-Pick disease (a variant of sphingomyelin lipidosis), and others. Other disorders with combined central and peripheral nervous system involvement include peroxisomal disorders such as adrenoleukodystrophy; porphyria, which produces axonal degeneration of predominantly motor fibers; and tyrosinemia, which produces primary axonal degeneration with secondary segmental demyelination.

In ataxia telangiectasia, there is a loss of large, predominantly sensory, myelinated fibers due to a primary axonal degeneration. Friedreich's ataxia, an autosomal recessive condition, produces a primary axonal degeneration of peripheral nerve fibers resulting in reduced or absent sensory compound action potential amplitudes.

Acquired Metabolic Neuropathies

Toxic polyneuropathies with predominantly axonal involvement include lead-, mercury-, and vincristine-induced neuropathy, among others. Predominantly demyelinating neuropathies may be caused by organophosphate poisoning and arsenic poisoning. Although arsenic poisoning may clinically mimic Guillain-Barré syndrome or CIDP,[64] electrophysiologic studies have shown evidence of both axonal degeneration and severe demyelination.

Neuromuscular Junction Disorders

Infantile Botulism

Infantile botulism primarily occurs in infants 2–6 months of age. Clinical findings include diffuse weakness, hypotonia, weak cry, poor feeding, constipation, and occasionally respiratory distress. The onset is fairly rapid. Electrophysiologic studies may show a reduced CMAP amplitude, preserved motor conduction velocities and SNAPs, and abnormal repetitive nerve stimulation findings at high rates of stimulation (Fig. 5–11). One study demonstrated an incremental response to repetitive nerve stimulation at rates of 20–50 Hz in 92% of infants with infantile botulism.[20] The mean increment was 73% with a range of 23–313%. With the lower-frequency stimulation (2–5 Hz), variable changes occurred, but the majority of infants showed decremental responses. A recent study demonstrated that the isolation of *Clostridium botulinum* from stool obtained by enema effluent was actually more sensitive for the diagnosis of infant botulism than electrodiagnostic studies.[65]

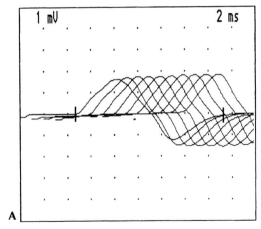

POT NO.	PEAK AMP mV	AMP. DECR %	AREA mVms	AREA DECR %	STIM. LEVEL
1	1.63	0	9.87	0	62.0mA
2	1.78	-9	10.00	-1	62.0mA
3	1.84	-13	9.95	-1	62.0mA
4	1.80	-10	9.91	0	62.0mA
5	1.79	-10	9.79	1	62.0mA
6	1.79	-10	9.85	0	62.0mA
7	1.84	-13	9.82	1	62.0mA
8	1.81	-11	9.83	0	62.0mA
9	1.80	-10	9.88	0	62.0mA
10	1.78	-9	9.81	1	62.0mA

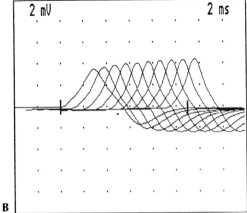

POT NO.	PEAK AMP mV	AMP. DECR %	AREA mVms	AREA DECR %	STIM. LEVEL
1	3.51	0	14.00	0	70.6mA
2	3.86	-10	14.80	-6	70.6mA
3	4.15	-18	15.80	-13	70.6mA
4	4.28	-22	16.20	-16	70.6mA
5	4.37	-25	16.30	-16	70.6mA
6	4.48	-28	16.40	-17	70.6mA
7	4.50	-28	16.70	-19	70.6mA
8	4.57	-30	16.90	-21	70.6mA
9	4.64	-32	16.90	-21	70.6mA
10	4.67	-33	16.80	-20	70.6mA

FIGURE 5–11. High-frequency repetitive nerve stimulation study in a 7-week-old infant with marked progressive weakness, respiratory failure, and botulism. *A*, Several days into the course, the repetitive stimulation study of the ulnar nerve at 50 Hz is normal; however, the CMAP amplitude is severely reduced (1.63 mV). *B*, Twelve days later, the infant is slightly improved clinically. A repeat study of the ulnar nerve at 50 Hz is diagnostic of infantile botulism with a 33% increment obtained between first and tenth stimuli. *Clostridium botulinum* was isolated from the stool.

EMG in infants with botulism demonstrates abnormal spontaneous rest activity with fibrillation potentials and positive sharp waves and short-duration low-amplitude MUAPs.[20]

Maternal Autoimmune Myasthenia Gravis

This disorder is caused by passage of antibodies from myasthenic mothers to their fetuses. Infants often present with hypotonia and respiratory distress. The diagnosis may be made by repetitive nerve stimulation studies. Given that normal infants exhibit less neuromuscular reserve than older children or adults, repetitive studies in this clinical setting use stimulation rates of 2–5 Hz almost exclusively. A decrement of greater than 8–10% between the first and fifth CMAP in the train is considered positive for myasthenia. The combination of repetitive motor nerve stimulation and administration of acetylcholinesterase inhibitors such as edrophonium

or neostigmine may improve the accuracy of the diagnosis.[66] If a decremental response is obtained utilizing a stimulation rate of 2–5 Hz, the repetitive nerve stimulation test may be repeated 30–120 seconds after administration of edrophonium, or 5–25 minutes after administration of the longer-acting neostigmine. Near-complete repair of the decremental response may be evident in the myasthenic infant (Fig. 5–12). Serologic antibody testing may be helpful if the mother has documented antibodies. Transient neonatal myasthenia gravis is self-limited with a reported duration of 5–47 days with a mean duration of 18 days.[67]

Toxic Neuromuscular Junction Disorders

Medications may interfere with neuromuscular transmission by inhibiting the release of acetylcholine, impairing the function of acetylcholinesterase (AChE), or binding directly to

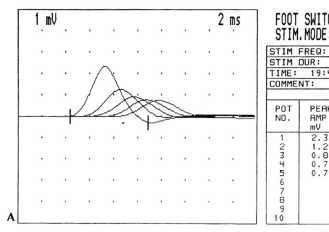

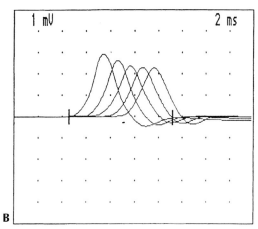

FIGURE 5–12. Low-frequency repetitive nerve stimulation study of the ulnar nerve in a 2-week-old infant with respiratory failure secondary to congenital myasthenia. *A*, At baseline, a 68% decrement in amplitude and 59% decrement in area is present between first and fifth stimuli with a stimulation frequency of 2 Hz. *B*, Twenty minutes after IV neostigmine is given, the initial CMAP has improved from 2.32 to 2.64 mV and the decrement has improved to 14%. The infant was treated with Mestinon and later extubated.

the acetylcholine receptor (AChR). Two drugs that may produce clinically significant weakness in normal children are magnesium and organophosphates.[68,69]

Congenital Myasthenic Syndromes

Numerous presynaptic and postsynaptic congenital myasthenic subtypes have been described by Engel.[70] These disorders often show decremental responses at low and high rates of stimulation. Typically, the decremental responses are greater at higher rates of stimulation. Although standard repetitive nerve stimulation studies do not adequately distinguish presynaptic from postsynaptic subtypes of congenital myasthenia, they do help diagnostically (Fig. 5–13). Based on clinical findings, repetitive nerve stimulation studies, and/or single-fiber EMG, a strong clinical suspicion of a neuromuscular junction (NMJ) disorder, such as a congenital myasthenic syndrome, may warrant further elucidation of the specific subtype of presynaptic or postsynaptic abnormality with application of a motor point biopsy. Ultrastructural evaluation of the neuromuscular junction with electron microscopy is usually performed on a biopsy of the deltoid or biceps, including the muscle region containing the NMJ (the "motor point"). For in vitro electrophysiologic and chemical studies of the neuromuscular junction, a short functionally nonrelevant muscle is usually removed from origin to insertion along with its entire motor branch and NMJ. Muscles obtained usually include the anconeus muscle near the elbow, the external intercostal muscle between the fifth or sixth intercostal space near the anterior axillary line, or the peroneus tertius muscle in the lower extremity. Often, patients undergo simultaneous motor point biopsy of the deltoid for EMG and anconeus or intercostal muscle for

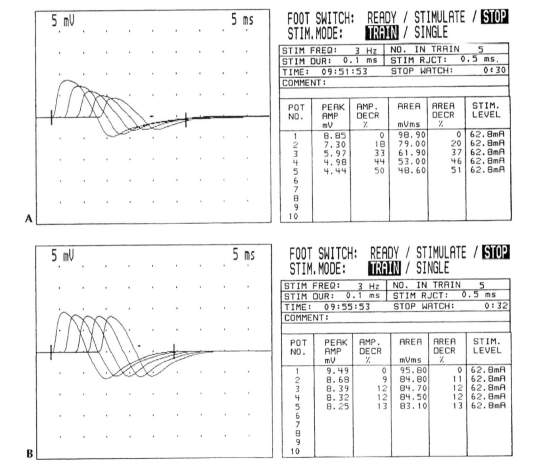

FIGURE 5–13. Low-frequency repetitive nerve stimulation study of the axillary nerve in a 12-year-old child with presynaptic congenital myasthenia. The active electrode is placed over the deltoid with stimulation at Erb's point using a block stimulator. A, A 50% amplitude decrement is obtained between first and fifth stimuli with 3-Hz stimulation frequency. B, After a 30-second isometric contraction of the deltoid, the amplitude decrement has improved to 13%. The child was later confirmed to have a presynaptic congenital myasthenia by motor point biopsy.

electrophysiologic studies. In vitro electrophysiologic studies often allow specific delineation of the congenital myasthenic syndrome into one of the numerous specific presynaptic or postsynaptic subtypes or may confirm a primary acetylcholinesterase deficiency.

Myasthenia Gravis

Myasthenia gravis presents in adolescents more frequently than in younger children. Muscle weakness typically increases with exertion but improves with rest and anticholinesterase medication. The disorder has an autoimmune cause due to circulating antibodies that bind to the postsynaptic membrane. Although elevated anti-AChR antibody levels may be diagnostic, a significant percentage of cases with autoimmune myasthenia gravis may have nondetectable circulating antibodies. Electrophysiologic studies demonstrate abnormal decremental responses at low stimulation rates (2–3 Hz). The limb should be well immobilized. A supramaximal train of 3–5 stimuli is applied. Typically, patients exhibit a smooth, reproducible decrement of the evoked synapse of greater than 8–10%. The defect in NMJ transmission can be partially repaired by exercise, which results in postactivation facilitation. Often, there is an increased decremental response to low stimulation rates (2–3 Hz) obtained 2–4 minutes after exercise, which results from postactivation exhaustion.[18] Proximal muscles may show increased sensitivity compared with distal muscles. Children with ocular myasthenia frequently exhibit normal responses with distal repetitive nerve stimulation studies, and sensitivity of the repetitive nerve stimulation is enhanced by use of a more proximal shoulder girdle muscle, e.g., axillary or spinal accessory nerve, or by study of the facial nerve.

Eaton-Lambert Syndrome

This presynaptic neuromuscular junction disorder usually found in adults with small cell carcinoma of the bronchus has been described in children.[71] The amplitude of the single evoked CMAP is low. With low rates of repetitive nerve stimulation, a decremental response is often obtained. After exercise or tetanic contractions, there is facilitation of the potentials by as much as 200%.

Myopathies

Polymyositis/Dermatomyositis

Polymyositis/dermatomyositis has been described in children of all ages ranging from infancy to adulthood. In children it may result in progressive proximal muscle weakness, dysphagia due to involvement of pharyngeal musculature, dyspnea, and muscle tenderness. A classic skin rash may or may not be present. Creatine kinase values are often markedly elevated. Classic EMG findings include (1) increased insertional activity with complex repetitive discharges; (2) fibrillations and positive sharp waves; and (3) low-amplitude, polyphasic, short-duration MUAPs recruited rapidly in relation to the strength of contraction. EMG of diffuse proximal and distal muscles in suspected inflammatory myopathy may be less subject to the risk of erroneous diagnostic information from sample error than muscle biopsy.

Congenital Myopathies

Congenital myopathies are a heterogeneous group of disorders usually presenting with infantile hypotonia, normal cognitive status, and primary structural abnormalities of the muscle fibers, which are elucidated on histologic and electron-microscopic evaluations of muscle biopsy specimens. Patients usually develop proximal greater than distal muscle weakness that is nonprogressive and static (these myopathies are described in Chapter 15). Nerve conduction studies are generally normal; however, there may be mild reductions in CMAP amplitudes. On needle EMG, findings are either normal or there may be mild, nonspecific changes, usually of a myopathic character, i.e., small-amplitude, short-duration polyphasic MUAPs. The only congenital myopathy consistently associated with abnormal spontaneous rest activity is myotubular (centronuclear) myopathy. In this disorder, the EMG reveals myopathic MUAPs with frequent complex repetitive discharges and diffuse fibrillation potentials.

Dystrophic Myopathies

The dystrophic myopathies are extensively described in Chapter 15. EMG is rarely used now for diagnostic evaluation of a suspected dystrophic myopathy because of the availability of molecular genetic testing and the importance of muscle biopsy in differentiating among Duchenne muscular dystrophy, Becker muscular dystrophy, and limb-girdle muscular dystrophies. EMG is characterized by low-amplitude, short-duration polyphasic MUAPs (Fig. 5–14). Recruitment is myopathic in nature, with increased recruitment or "early" recruitment demonstrated with slight effort. Interference pattern is usually full. Complex repetitive discharges (Fig. 5–15) and abnormal spontaneous rest activity may be present, reflecting muscle membrane instability.

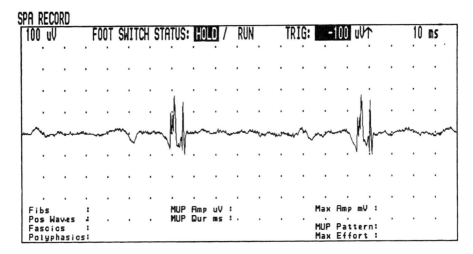

FIGURE 5–14.   Low-amplitude, short-duration, polyphasic MUAPs in a 14-year-old girl with limb-girdle muscular dystrophy.

Metabolic Myopathies

Nonspecific myopathic EMG findings may be demonstrated in metabolic myopathies. For example, absent maltase deficiency shows increased insertional activity, complex repetitive discharges, low-amplitude short-duration MUAPs, profuse fibrillations, and positive sharp waves. Carnitine deficiency, a disorder of lipid metabolism, demonstrates increased recruitment on effort, decreased MUAP amplitudes, and occasional fibrillations. EMG may be normal in many metabolic myopathies such as carnitine palmityltransferase deficiency.

Myotonic Disorders

Myotonic disorders such as myotonic muscular dystrophy (MMD) and Schwartz-Jampel syndrome may show myotonic discharges with either positive sharp wave or fibrillation configuration, and a waxing and waning firing frequency. The myotonic discharges are often described as exhibiting the sound of a "dive bomber." The changing frequency of the myotonic discharge differentiates it from a complex repetitive discharge. There may be profuse fibrillations and positive sharp waves in MMD. MUAPs often have low amplitude and short duration. There may be more involvement of distal musculature than proximal musculature in myotonic muscular dystrophy. Again, with a known family history of myotonic muscular dystrophy, confirmation of the diagnosis in an individual with classic clinical features can be provided expeditiously and cost effectively in the EMG laboratory rather than by costly molecular genetic studies.

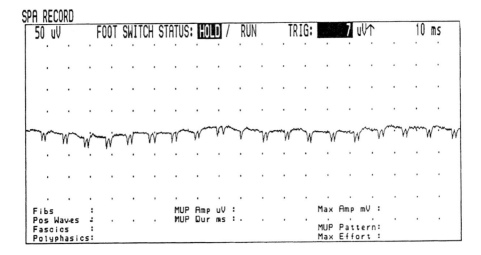

FIGURE 5–15.   Complex repetitive discharges in a dystrophic myopathy.

Somatosensory Evoked Potentials

General Principles

The somatosensory evoked potential (SSEP) is the sequence of voltage changes generated in the brain and the pathway from a peripheral sensory nerve following a transient electrical stimulus to the sensory cortex. Evidence suggests that these signals are related to large afferent fibers and peripheral nerves, which ascend through the dorsal column pathways of the spinal cord, proceed to the thalamus, and arrive at the somatosensory cortex. These are the same pathways that mediate light touch two-point discrimination, proprioception, and vibration. Sensitive amplification and averaging techniques enable discrimination between the evoked response and other larger and more random physiologic potentials with which the signal is mixed. As a general rule, SSEP studies may be considered whenever the disease process in question may involve the somatosensory system. SSEPs reflect neurophysiologic activity in the posterior column (medial lemniscus pathways). SSEPs do not reflect activity in the anterolateral column of the spinal cord and thus correlate better with clinical examinations of proprioception and vibration than pain or temperature sensation.

Individual components of the SSEP wave form are identified by their latency (i.e., the time at which they occur following a peripheral stimulus), polarity, position at which they are maximal, and to a lesser extent by the amplitude and shape of the wave form. Individual components are referred to by a letter and number. The letters (N for negative or P for positive) refer to the polarity of the wave and the number either to the latency (in milliseconds) of the signal from the time of the stimulus (e.g., N_{20}) or, alternatively, the order in which the component was observed (e.g., N_1, P_2), especially appropriate in pediatric SSEPs. Examples of median and tibial SSEPs are shown in Figures 5–16 and 5–17.

With mixed nerve stimulation, recording electrodes are placed over the peripheral nerve (more proximally), thoracolumbar or cervical spine, linked mastoids, and scalp. For upper extremity stimulation, the likely generator source for the cervical spine response is the incoming root, as well as postsynaptic excitatory potentials generated at the dorsal root entry zone.[72] For the lower extremity, the lumbar spine responses are similarly a reflection of the root or cauda equina activity and the postsynaptic activity of the cord. The linked mastoid response is generated at the brainstem level. The difference in the latency of scalp N_1 and the cervical spine response with median nerve stimulation gives a central conduction time. Similarly, the difference in latency between scalp P_1 for posterior tibial nerve stimulation and the spinal potential generated over T12 or L1 gives a central conduction time.

Filter settings vary from a low-frequency filter of 3–30 Hz to a high frequency filter of 1.5–3 kHz. The peripheral nerve is typically stimulated with a rate of 3.1 Hz. Our laboratory uses a stimulation intensity of 1.5 times motor threshold for mixed nerve stimulation and 2.5 times sensory threshold for dermatomal stimulation. Electrodes are positioned according to a modified international 10–20 electrode system.

SEP latencies decrease with age until well into childhood.[72–75] The maturation of SSEPs with growth is mainly associated with cell growth processes, such as myelination, cell differentiation, and synaptic development. Conduction velocity along the central pathways progressively increases until 3–8 years of age, remaining constant between 10 and 49 years of age, and slowing thereafter. The N_1 scalp latency of the median SSEP decreases until 2–3 years of age because of peripheral myelination and then increases with body growth until adulthood. The cervical spine latency is relatively stable during the first 2 years because of concomitant peripheral myelination and body growth, and then increases with age from 2–3 years until adulthood. The median SSEP central interpeak latency between cervical spine latency and scalp N_1, which reflects central conduction time, decreases from a mean of 11.6 ms at 4–8 months of age to a mean of 7 ms at 6–8 years of age, and remains constant between 6.9 and 7.0 ms until adulthood.[76,77]

In infants younger than 4 months of age, the study is best performed on the awake infant because sleep can affect the cortical components. With children older than 4 months of age, sleep or sedation usually has little effect on the SEP waveform during mixed nerve stimulation. Indeed, the author has had no difficulty obtaining median nerve scalp responses in the pediatric ICU in comatose children with head trauma or heavily sedated children. Dermatomal SSEPs, on the other hand, are state-dependent responses influenced by both sleep and sedation.

Clinical Applications of SSEPs in Children

SSEPs in Brain Injury

Abnormalities of median SSEPs can be predictive of poor prognosis in the situation of brain injury due to head trauma or hypoxia. A loss of bilateral SSEP scalp wave forms, as demonstrated in Figure 5–16B, portends a poor

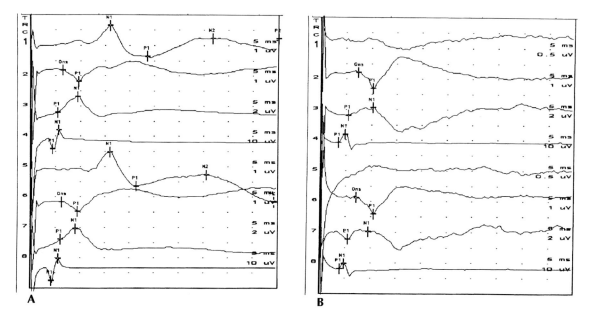

FIGURE 5–16. Median nerve SSEPs obtained in the pediatric intensive care unit. Channels 1 to 4 are responses with left median nerve stimulation, and channels 5 to 8 are responses with right median nerve stimulation. Channels 1 and 5 are scalp responses (C4' and C3' referenced to Fz); channels 2 and 6 are brain stem (C4' and C3' referenced to linked mastoids); channels 3 and 7 are lower cervical spine responses (C7 spine referenced to Fz); channels 4 and 8 are peripheral responses obtained at the axillae. *A,* Normal median SSEP responses obtained from a child with an epidural hematoma who was paralyzed with vecuronium for intracranial pressure control. There is no evidence of myelopathy. The child later recovered with minimal sequelae. *B,* Abnormal median SSEP responses in a comatose child with severe brain injury and C1–2 vertebral injuries. Note the bilaterally abnormal scalp responses. Brain stem, C7 spine, and peripheral responses show no evidence of a spinal cord injury affecting posterior column pathways.

prognosis in comatose children.[78,79] Asymmetric scalp responses in a comatose child may be associated with the development of motor abnormalities such as hemiparesis because of the proximity of the sensory cortex to the motor cortex (see Fig. 5–17B). Recently, posterior tibial nerve SSEPs performed on neonates at high risk for future neurodevelopmental impairment have demonstrated a highly significant relationship between bilaterally abnormal posterior tibial nerve SSEPs and the presence of cerebral palsy at 3 years of age.[80] Normal posterior tibial nerve SSEPs were associated with a normal outcome in 24 of 25 infants. In this study, posterior tibial nerve SSEPs were more predictive than cranial ultrasound. Another study of 43 children with hemiplegic cerebral palsy found a positive correlation between median nerve SSEPs and the affected side using the amplitude of the responses rather than the latency.[81] Other studies have confirmed the prognostic value of SSEPs in infants at risk for neurodevelopmental impairment.[82-85]

Traumatic Spinal Cord Injury

SSEP results combined with early American Spinal Injury Association (ASIA) motor scores

have been shown to predict ultimate ambulatory capacity in patients with acute spinal cord injury.[86] Other authors have shown that SSEP improvement over a 1-week interval during the first 3 weeks after spinal cord injury was associated with motor index score improvement over a 6-month period.[87] Dermatomal somatosensory evoked potentials also have been shown to be more sensitive for the detection of sacral sparing and of more prognostic value than mixed nerve somatosensory evoked potentials.[88]

The author has a great deal of experience in using somatosensory evoked potentials in the pediatric intensive care unit to evaluate head-injured children at risk for spinal cord injury without radiographic abnormality (SCIWORA), which is an entity commonly observed in pediatric spinal cord injuries.[46] The SSEPs are particularly helpful in situations in which children are comatose, too obtunded to cooperate with the examination, or of an age that precludes a detailed sensory examination. Figure 5–17A shows an example of a normal tibial SSEP, whereas Figure 5–17C demonstrates the impaired posterior column conduction between the lower cervical spinal cord and brain stem with

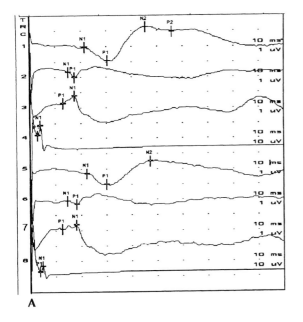

FIGURE 5–17. Tibial SSEPs obtained in the pediatric ICU. Channels 1 to 4 are responses with left tibial stimulation, and channels 5 to 8 are responses with right tibial stimulation. Channels 1 and 5 are scalp responses (C2′ to Fz); channels 2 and 7 are spine responses (L2 spine referenced to flank); and channels 4 and 8 are peripheral responses obtained at the popliteal fossae. A, Normal tibial SSEP study. B, Abnormal tibial SSEPs in a child with left hemispheric brain injury. Peripheral and lumbar spine (L2 and T12 level) responses are normal bilaterally. The scalp response is normal with left tibial nerve stimulation (channel 1) but absent with right tibial nerve stimulation (channel 5). C, Abnormal tibial SSEPs bilaterally in an awake 4-year-old child with low cervical SCIWORA. Peripheral (channels 4 and 8) and L2 spine (channels 2 and 7) responses are normal. Scalp responses (channels 2 and 5) are absent as a result of the low cervical spinal cord injury.

a SCIWORA injury sustained by a 4-year-old child.

Tethered Cord Syndrome

Posterior tibial somatosensory evoked potentials have been shown in some studies to be a sensitive indicator of declining neurophysiologic status and a more sensitive diagnostic tool than the clinical testing of sensation in patients with tethered spinal cord after myelomeningocele repair.[89–92] In addition, improvement of the evoked potentials after untethering has been documented.[89,90,92] In the author's experience, the spine response is often caudally displaced in

myelomeningocele. Absent or reduced-amplitude lumbar spine potentials or prolonged lumbar spine or scalp latencies with tibial nerve stimulation in the setting of normal median somatosensory evoked potentials (i.e., normal spine latencies and amplitudes with median nerve stimulation, normal cervical-to-brain central conduction time, and normal median scalp latencies) are suggestive of electrophysiologic impairment due to tethered cord syndrome.

Intraoperative Spinal Monitoring

There are many reports detailing efficacy of intraoperative SSEP monitoring during scoliosis surgery,[93–96] as well as during other surgical procedures of the spine. Continuous electromyographic monitoring is being used increasingly to detect nerve root injury during thoracolumbar scoliosis surgery.[97] In addition, the corticospinal tracts are being monitored by many investigators intraoperatively using transcranial electrical stimulation of the motor cortex,[98] with motor evoked potentials recorded from either peripheral motor axons or as a CMAP from innervated muscles.[96,98]

Brachial Plexus Injury

The dermatomal SSEPs can be a useful supplement to the assessment of the child with a brachial plexus injury.[99] The child needs to be awake during the study. In the author's experience, the C5 and C6 dermatomal SSEPs are generally most useful. The C5 dermatome is stimulated over the lateral proximal shoulder using a proximal disc as cathode and distal disc as anode. Intraoperative SSEPs with direct stimulation of exposed nerves may demonstrate incomplete injuries of upper cervical roots; a proximal stump of the ruptured C5 root with functional central continuity, thus potentially suitable for grafting; or complete root avulsion. Preoperative diagnostic SSEPs, although a useful adjunct to conventional electrodiagnosis, do not discriminate incomplete cervical root avulsion from intact roots.[100]

Demyelinating Diseases

Both SSEPs and brainstem auditory evoked potentials have been reported to be abnormal in children who have, or are carriers of, leukodystrophy. Peripheral and/or central abnormalities have been documented in metachromatic leukodystrophy, Pelizaeus-Merzbacher disease, Krabbe's disease, adrenoleukodystrophy, Canavan's disease, Alexander's disease, and multiple sulfatase deficiency.[101]

Pediatric multiple sclerosis (MS), while relatively rare, does occur in preadolescents and adolescents.[102] MRI has been shown to be slightly more sensitive than multimodal evoked potentials in confirming the clinical diagnosis of childhood MS. However, in suspected or probable MS, both SSEPs and visual evoked potentials may contribute to the determination of clinical diagnosis because of their capacity to demonstrate asymptomatic involvement in central somatosensory and central optic nerve pathways.[103,104]

Acute transverse myelitis often results in severe myelopathy because of inflammation and demyelination. SSEPs have been shown to be abnormal in this condition and may provide prognostic information regarding ultimate outcome.[105]

The extent and location of nerve involvement in demyelinating peripheral neuropathies have been evaluated with SSEPs; however, SSEPs do not usually provide necessary additional information to standard nerve conductions. Hereditary motor sensory neuropathy type I shows impaired peripheral conduction in both proximal and distal nerve segments with normal central conduction.[106] Acute inflammatory demyelinating polyradiculoneuropathy (AIDP) patients have been shown to exhibit prolonged posterior tibial peripheral SSEP latencies in addition to prolonged or absent median F-waves.[107] In contrast, posterior tibial F-wave latencies and median nerve SSEPs were less sensitive in detection of demyelination in AIDP.

Conclusion

Pediatric electrodiagnostic studies are a powerful diagnostic tool that aids in the localization of abnormalities within the lower motor neuron and often provides useful prognostic information. Practical suggestions concerning pediatric electrodiagnostic evaluation have been provided. Study results must be interpreted in light of developmental and maturational issues affecting both clinical findings and electrophysiologic processes. A skilled electrodiagnostic evaluation requires careful strategic planning to provide accurate diagnostic information in an expeditious manner, with the least distress possible for the child and parents. Continuing electrodiagnostic experience with the pediatric population provides increasing diagnostic acumen regarding pediatric lower motor neuron disease processes and sufficient technical skills to provide the referring physician with accurate diagnostic information.

References

1. Harmon RL, Eichman PL, Rodriguez AA: Laboratory Manual of Pediatric Electromyography. An Approach to Pediatric EMG. 1992;1–66.
2. Jones HR, Bolton CF, Harper CF (eds): Pediatric Clinical Electromyography. Philadelphia, Lippincott-Raven, 1996.
3. Gamble HJ, Breathnach AS: An electron-microscope study of human foetal peripheral nerves. J Anat 1965;99:573.
4. Miller G, Hekmatt JZ, Dubowitz LMS, Dubowitz V: Use of nerve conduction velocity to determine gestational age in infants at risk and in very-low-birth-weight infants. J Pediatr 1983;1103:109.
5. Schulte FJ, Michaelis R, Linke I, Nolte R: Motor nerve conduction velocity in term, preterm and small-for-dates newborn infants. Pediatrics 1968;42:17.
6. Thomas JE, Lamber EH: Ulnar nerve conduction velocity and H-reflex in infants and children. J Appl Physiol 1960;51:1.
6a. Baer RD, Johnson EW: Motor nerve conduction velocities in normal children. Arch Phys Med Rehabil 1965;46:698.

7. Cottrell L: Histologic variations with age in apparently normal peripheral nerve trunks. Arch Neurol 1940;43:1138.

8. Gamstorp I, Shelburne SA Jr: Peripheral sensory conduction in ulnar and median nerves in normal infants, children and adolescents. Acta Paediatr Scand 1965;54:309.

9. Cruz Martinez A, Perez Conde MC, del Campo F, et al: Sensory and mixed conduction velocity in infancy and childhood: I. Normal parameters in median, ulnar and sural nerves. Electromyogr Clin Neurophysiol 1978;18:487.

10. Cruz Martinez A, Perez Conde MC, Ferrer MT: Motor conduction velocity and H-reflex in infancy and childhood: II. Study in newborns, twins and small-for-dates. Electromyogr Clin Neurophysiol 1977;17:493.

11. Cruz Martinez A, Ferrer MT, Perez Conde MC, Bernacer M: Motor conduction velocity and H-reflex in infancy and childhood. II. Intra- and extrauterine maturation of the nerve fibers: Development of the peripheral nerve from 1 month to 11 years of age. Electromyogr Clin Neurophysiol 1978;18:11.

12. Parano E, Uncini A, De Vivo DC, Lovelace RE: Electrophysiologic correlates of peripheral nervous system maturation in infancy and childhood. J Child Neurol 1993;8:336.

13. Wagner AL, Buchthal F: Motor and sensory conduction in infancy and childhood: Reappraisal. Dev Med Child Neurol 1972;14:189.

14. Kwast O, Krajewska G, Kozlowski K: Analysis of F-wave parameters in median and ulnar nerves in healthy infants and children: Age-related changes. Electromyogr Clin Neurophysiol 1984;24:439.

15. Shahani BY, Young RR: Clinical significance of late response studies in infants and children [abstract]. Neurology 1981;31:66.

16. Miller RG, Kuntz NL: Nerve conduction studies in infants and children. J Child Neurol 1986;1:19.

17. Koenigsberger MR, Patten B, Lovelace RE: Studies of neuromuscular function in the newborn: 1. A comparison of myoneural function in the full term and premature infant. Neuropediatrics 1973;4:350.

18. Cornblath DR: Disorders of neuromuscular transmission in infants and children. Muscle Nerve 1986;9:606.

19. Pickett J, Berg B, Chaplin E, et al: Syndrome of botulism in infancy: Clinical and electrophysiological study. N Engl J Med 1976;295:770.

20. Cornblath DR, Sladky J, Sumner AJ: Clinical electrophysiology of infantile botulism. Muscle Nerve 1983;6:448.

21. De Carmo RJ: Motor unit action potential parameters in human newborn infants. Arch Neurol 1960;3:136.

22. Sacco G, Buchthal F, Rosenfalck P: Motor unit potentials at different ages. Arch Neurol 1962;6:366.

23. Moosa A: Phrenic nerve conduction in children. Dev Med Child Neurol 1981;23:434.

24. Hays RM, Hackworth SR, Speltz ML, Weinstein P: Physicians' practice patterns in pediatric electrodiagnosis. Arch Phys Med Rehabil 1993;74:494.

25. Hays RM, Hackworth SR, Speltz ML, Weinstein P: Explorations of variables related to children's behavioral distress during electrodiagnosis. Arch Phys Med Rehabil 1992;73:1160.

26. Lamarche Y, Lebel M, Martin R: EMLA partially relieves the pain of EMG needling. Can J Anaesth 1992;39:805.

27. Gilchrist JM: Ad hoc committee of the AAEM special interest group on single fiber EMG. Single fiber EMG reference values: A collaborative effort. Muscle Nerve 1992;15:151.

28. Turk MA: Pediatric electrodiagnostic medicine. In Dumitru D (ed): Electrodiagnostic Medicine. Philadelphia, Hanley & Belfus, 1995, pp 1133–1142.

29. Packer RJ, Brown MJ, Berman PH: The diagnostic value of electromyography in infantile hypotonia. Am J Dis Child 1982;136:1057.

30. David WS, Jones HR Jr: Electromyography and biopsy correlation with suggested protocol for evaluation of the floppy infant. Muscle Nerve 1994;17:424.

31. Russell JW, Afifi AK, Ross MA: Predictive value of electromyography in diagnosis and prognosis of the hypotonic infant. J Child Neurol 1992;7:387.

32. Buchthal F, Behse F: Peroneal muscular atrophy and related disorders. I. Clinical manifestations as related to biopsy findings, nerve conduction and electromyography. Brain 1977;100:41.

33. Jones HR: EMG evaluation of the floppy infant: Differential diagnosis and technical aspects. Muscle Nerve 1990;13:338.

34. Eng GD, Binder H, Koch B: Spinal muscular atrophy: Experience in diagnosis and rehabilitation in management of 60 patients. Arch Phys Med Rehabil 1984;65:549.

35. Hausmanowa-Petrusewicz I, Karwanska A: Electromyographic findings in different forms of infantile and juvenile proximal spinal muscular atrophy. Muscle Nerve 1986;9:37.

36. Parano E, Fiumara A, Falsperla R, Pavone L: A clinical study of childhood spinal muscular atrophy in Sicily: A review of 75 cases. Brain Dev 1994;16:104.

37. Hausmanowa-Petrusewicz I, Fidzianska A, Dobosz I, Strugalska MH: Is Kugelberg-Welander spinal muscular atrophy a fetal defect? Muscle Nerve 1980;3:389.

38. Kuntz NL, Daube JR: Electrophysiological profile of childhood spinal muscular atrophy. Muscle Nerve 1982;5:S106.

39. Buchthal F, Olsen PZ: Electromyography and muscle biopsy in infantile spinal muscular atrophy. Brain 1970;93:15.

40. Imai T, Minami R, Nagaoka M, et al: Proximal and distal motor nerve conduction velocities in Werdnig-Hoffmann disease. Pediatr Neurol 1990;6:82.

41. Moosa A, Dubowitz V: Motor nerve conduction velocity in spinal muscular atrophy of childhood. Arch Dis Child 1976;61:975.

42. Russman BS, Iannoccone ST, Buncher CR, et al: Spinal muscular atrophy: New thoughts on the pathogenesis and classification schema. J Child Neurol 1992;7:347.

43. Munsat TL, Davies KE: Meeting report: International SMA consortium meeting. Neuromuscul Disord 1992;2:423.

44. Raimbault J, Laget P: Electromyography in the diagnosis of infantile spinal amyotrophy of Werdnig-Hoffmann type. Pathobiology 1972;20:287.

45. Schwartz MS, Moosa A: Sensory nerve conduction in the spinal muscular atrophies. Dev Med Child Neurol 1977;19:50.

46. Pang D, Wilberger JE: Spinal cord injury without radiographic abnormalities in children. J Neurosurg 1982;57:114.

47. Eng GD, Binder H, Getson P, O'Donnell R: Obstetrical brachial plexus palsy (OBPP) with conservative management. Muscle Nerve 1996;19:884.

48. Laurent JP, Lee R, Shenaq S, et al: Neurosurgical correction of upper brachial plexus birth injuries. J Neurosurg 1993;79:197.

49. Ochiai N, Nagano A, Sugioka H, Hara T: Nerve grafting in brachial plexus injuries: Results of free grafts in 90 patients. J Bone Joint Surg Br 1996;78:754.

50. Clarke HM, Al-Qattan MM, Curtis CG, Zuker RM: Obstetrical brachial plexus palsy: Results following neurolysis of conducting neuromas-in-continuity. Plast Reconstr Surg 1996;97:974.

51. Tonkin MA, Eckersley JR, Gschwind CR: The surgical treatment of brachial plexus injuries. Aust N Z J Surg 1996;66:29.

52. Sherburn EW, Kaplan SS, Kaufman BA, et al: Outcome of surgically treated birth-related brachial plexus injuries in 20 cases. Pediatr Neurosurg 1997;27:19.
53. Kay SP: Obstetrical brachial palsy. Br J Plast Surg 1998;51:43.
54. Waylonis GW, Johnson EW: Facial nerve conduction delay. Arch Phys Med Rehabil 1964;45:539.
55. Berciano J, Combarros O, Calleja J, et al: The application of nerve conduction and clinical studies to genetic counseling in hereditary motor sensory neuropathy type I. Muscle Nerve 1989;12:302.
56. Feasby TE, Hahn AF, Bolton CF, et al: Detection of hereditary motor sensory neuropathy type I in childhood. J Neurol Neurosurg Psychiatry 1992;55:895.
57. Gutmann L, Fakadej A, Riggs JE: Evolution of nerve conduction abnormalities in children with dominant hypertrophic neuropathy of the Charcot-Marie-Tooth type. Muscle Nerve 1983;6:515.
58. Benstead TJ, Kuntz NL, Miller RG, Daube JR: The electrophysiologic profile of Dejerine-Sottas disease (HMSN III). Muscle Nerve 1990;13:586.
59. Bradshaw DY, Jones HR Jr: Guillain-Barré syndrome in children: Clinical course, electrodiagnosis and prognosis. Muscle Nerve 1992;15:500.
60. Triggs WJ, Cros D, Gominak SC, et al: Motor nerve inexcitability in Guillain-Barré syndrome: The spectrum of distal conduction block and axonal degeneration. Brain 1992;115:1291.
61. Reisin R, Cersosimo R, Alvarez MG, et al: Acute "axonal" Guillain-Barré syndrome in childhood. Muscle Nerve 1993;16:1310.
62. Bakshi N, Maselli R, Gosep S, et al: Fulminant demyelinating neuropathy mimicking cerebral death. Muscle Nerve 1997;20:1595.
63. Yuki N: Pathogenesis of axonal Guillain-Barré syndrome: Hypothesis. Muscle Nerve 1994;17:680.
64. Donofrio PD, Wilbourn AJ, Albers JW, et al: Acute arsenic intoxication presenting as Guillain-Barré–like syndrome. Muscle Nerve 1987;10:114.
65. Graf WD, Hays RM, Astley SJ, Mendelman PM: Electrodiagnosis reliability in the diagnosis of infant botulism. J Pediatr 1992;120:747.
66. Hays RM, Michaud LJ: Neonatal myasthenia gravis: Specific advantages of repetitive stimulation over edrophonium testing. Pediatr Neurol 1988;4:245.
67. Fenichel GM: Clinical syndromes of myasthenia in infancy and childhood. Arch Neurol 1978;35:97.
68. Besser R, Gutmann L, Dillman U, et al: End-plate dysfunction in acute organophosphate intoxication. Neurology 1989;39:561.
69. Lipsitz PJ: The clinical and biochemical effects of excess magnesium in the newborn. Pediatrics 1971;47: 501.
70. Engel AG: Myasthenic syndromes. In Engel AG, Franzini-Armstrong C (eds): Myology, 2nd ed. New York, McGraw-Hill, 1994, pp 1798–1835.
71. Chelmiska-Schorr E, Bernstein LP, Zurbrugg EB, Huttenlocher PR: Eaton-Lambert syndrome in a 9-year-old girl. Arch Neurol 1979;36:572.
72. Desmedt JE, Brunko E, Debecker J: Maturation of the somatosensory evoked potentials in normal infants and children, with special reference to the early N1 component. Electroencephalogr Clin Neurophysiol 1976;40:43.
73. Tomita Y, Nishimura S, Tanaka T: Short-latency SEPs in infants and children: Developmental changes and maturational index of SEPs. Electroencephalogr Clin Neurophysiol 1986;65:335.
74. Gilmore RL, Bass NH, Wright EA, et al: Developmental assessment of spinal cord and cortical evoked potentials after tibial nerve stimulation: Effects of age and stature on normative data during childhood. Electroencephalogr Clin Neurophysiol 1985;62:241.

75. Gilmore R, Brock J, Hermansen MC, Baumann R: Development of lumbar spinal cord and cortical evoked potentials after tibial nerve stimulation in the preterm newborn: Effects of gestational age and other factors. Electroencephalogr Clin Neurophysiol 1987;68:28.
76. Fagan ER, Taylor MJ, Logan WJ: Somatosensory evoked potentials. Part I. A review of neural generators and special considerations in paediatrics. Pediatr Neurol 1987;3:189.
77. Taylor MJ, Fagan ER: SEPs to median nerve stimulation: Normative data for paediatrics. Electroencephalogr Clin Neurophysiol 1988;71:323.
78. Lutschg J, Pfenninger J, Ludin H, Vassella F: Brainstem auditory evoked potentials and early somatosensory evoked potentials in neurointensively treated comatose children. Am J Dis Child 1983;137:421.
79. Emerson R, Pavlakis S, Carmel P, DeViro D: Use of spinal somatosensory evoked potentials in the diagnosis of tethered cord. Ann Neurol 1986;20:443.
80. White CP, Cooke RW: Somatosensory evoked potentials following posterior tibial nerve stimulation predict later motor outcome. Dev Med Child Neurol 1994;36:34.
81. Laget P, Salbreux R, Raimbault J, et al: Relationship between changes in somesthetic evoked responses and electroencephalographic findings in the child with hemiplegia. Dev Med Child Neurol 1986:28:633.
82. Gorke W: Somatosensory evoked potentials indicating impaired motor development in infancy. Dev Med Child Neurol 1986;28:633.
83. Klimach VJ, Cooke RW: maturation of the neonatal somatosensory evoked response in preterm infants. Dev Med Child Neurol 1988;30:208.
84. White CP, Cooke RWI: The use of somatosensory evoked potentials (SEPs) in the prediction of motor handicap in the preterm infant. In Gennser G, Marsal K, Svenningsen N, Lindstrom K (eds): Fetal and Neonatal Physiological Measurements, vol. III. Proceedings of the Third International Conference on Fetal and Neonatal Physiological Measurements. Malmo, Ronneby, 1989.
85. Willis J, Seales D, Frazier E, et al: Somatosensory evoked potentials predict neuromotor outcome after periventricular hemorrhage. Dev Med Child Neurol 1989;31:435.
86. Curt A, Dietz V: Ambulatory capacity in spinal cord injury: Significance of somatosensory evoked potentials and ASIA protocol in predicting outcome. Arch Phys Med Rehabil 1997;78:39.
87. Li C, Houlden DA, Rowed DW: Somatosensory evoked potentials and neurological grades as predictors of outcome in acute spinal cord injury. J Neurosurg 1990;72: 600.
88. Schrader SC, Sloan TB, Toleikis JR: Detection of sacral sparing in acute spinal cord injury. Spine 1987;12:533.
89. Roy MW, Gilmore R, Walsh JW: Evaluation of children and young adults with tethered spinal cord syndrome: Utility of spinal and scalp recorded somatosensory evoked potentials. Surg Neurol 1986;26:241.
90. Boor R, Schwarz M, Reitter B, Voth D: Tethered cord after spina bifida aperta: A longitudinal study of somatosensory evoked potentials. Childs Nerv Syst 1993; 9(6):328.
91. Polo A, Zanette G, Manganotti P, Bertolast, et al: Spinal somatosensory evoked potentials in patients with tethered cord syndrome. Can J Neurol Sci 1994;21:325.
92. Kale SS, Mahapatra AK: The role of somatosensory evoked potentials in spinal dysraphism—do they have a prognostic significance? Childs Nerv Syst 1998;4:328, discussion 332.
93. Helmers SL, Hall JE: Intraoperative somatosensory evoked potential monitoring in pediatrics. J Pediatr Orthop 1994;14:592.

94. Nuwer MR, Dawson EG, Carlson LG, et al: Somato-sensory evoked potential spinal cord monitoring reduces neurologic deficits after scoliosis surgery: Results of a large multicenter survey. Electroencephalogr Clin Neurophysiol 1995;96:6.

95. Fisher RS, Raudzens P, Nunemacher M: Efficacy of intraoperative neurophysiological monitoring. J Clin Neurophysiol 1995;12:97.

96. Owen JH, Sponseller PD, Szymanski J, Hurdle M: Efficacy of multimodality spinal cord monitoring during surgery for neuromuscular scoliosis. Spine 1995;20:1480.

97. Holland NR, Kostuik JP: Continuous electromyographic monitoring to detect nerve root injury during thoracolumbar scoliosis surgery. Spine 1997;22:2547.

98. Burke D, Hicks RG: Surgical monitoring of motor pathways. J Clin Neurophysiol 1998;15:194.

99. Date ES, Rappaport M, Ortega HR: Dermatomal somatosensory evoked potentials in brachial plexus injuries. Clin Electroencephalogr 1991;22:236.

100. Hashimoto T, Mitomo M, Hirabuki N, et al: Nerve root avulsion of birth palsy: Comparison of myelography with CT myelography and somatosensory evoked potential. Radiology 1991;178:841.

101. De Meirleir LJ, Taylor MJ, Logan WJ: Multimodal evoked potential studies in leukodystrophies of children. Can J Neurol Sci 1988;15:26.

102. Guilhoto LM, Osorio CA, Machado LR, et al: Pediatric multiple sclerosis report of 14 cases. Brain Dev 1995;17:9.

103. Scaioli V, Rumi V, Cimino C, Angelini L: Childhood multiple sclerosis (MS): Multimodal evoked potentials (EP) and magnetic resonance imaging (MRI) comparative study. Neuropediatrics 1991;22:15.

104. Riikonen R, Ketonen L, Sipponen J: Magnetic resonance imaging, evoked responses and cerebrospinal fluid findings in a followup study of children with optic neuritis. Acta Neurol Scand 1988;77:44.

105. al Deeb SM, Yaqub BA, Bruyn GW, Biary NM: Acute transverse myelitis: A localized form of postinfectious encephalomyelitis. Brain 1997;120:1115.

106. Scaioli V, Pareyson D, Avanzini G, Sghirlanzoni A: F-response and somatosensory and brainstem auditory evoked potential studies in HMSN type I and II. J Neurol Neurosurg Psychiatry 1992;55:1027.

107. Gilmore RL, Nelson KR: SSEP and F-wave studies in acute inflammatory demyelinating polyradiculoneuropathy. Muscle Nerve 1989;12:538.

Chapter 6

Psychosocial Aspects of Childhood Disabilities

Jessie K. M. Easton, MD, MPH
Bruce Rens, BA, EdS, NCSP
Michael A. Alexander, MD

There is no joy in easy sailing
When the skies are clear and blue
There is no joy in merely doing
Things which anyone can do
But there is some satisfaction
That is mighty sweet to take,
When you reach a destination
That you thought you'd never make.[1]

Disability in infants most often presents as a delay in physical development, such as feeding, head control, or independent sitting, or as an obvious physical abnormality, such as spina bifida or amelia. Parents and caregivers tend to concentrate on managing the physical problems and only later are able to attend to the child's cognitive, psychological, and emotional needs. It is important that these aspects be dealt with appropriately. Although physical ability may limit the child's mobility or communication, eventual success in life is more dependent on the ability to relate to people socially in an acceptable, comfortable, nonthreatening way. The eventual level of function appears to be primarily determined by a person's degree of physical involvement, cognition, and various cultural influences, as depicted in Figure 6–1.[2,3] Most of these factors can be assessed and influenced or manipulated as development progresses from infancy to adulthood. Internal motivation, more difficult to determine and perhaps impossible to change, can be the decisive factor in children having a successful and satisfying life.

Many adults are able to function in society despite physical, cognitive, or educational disabilities. Some of the factors influencing success are the nature and severity of the disability, accommodations available in society, attitudes toward the disabled, individual personality characteristics, the ability to learn age-appropriate social skills, and the person's ability to pursue inclusion in society's mainstream. Werner and Smith[4] have identified aspects of child and family that affect function as resilience, protective factors, and risk factors, which help to explain some of the differences in outcome in outwardly similar situations of deprivation or disability.[4]

Kokkonen and colleagues[5] compared social outcome in 52 young adults with cerebral palsy or spina bifida to a group of 209 controls. Of the study group, more had divorced parents, fewer completed high school or went on to further training, and fewer were living away from home or married. Social contacts were more likely to be primarily with family members, and fewer were employed. The level of social maturation was less in the study group, without relation to severity of disability.

Legislation has provided the opportunity for families and individuals to access materials, professionals, and facilities to gain personal independence. In 1976, the Education for All Handicapped Children Act (EHA) (PL 94-142) was passed.[6] This legislative act mandated a free and appropriate education to be provided in the least restrictive environment for children with handicapping conditions. PL 94-142 requires the development of an individualized educational plan for all children between the ages of 3 and 21 to address their needs and modifications required to ensure that the student will succeed in the educational environment. Public Law 99-457, the Education of the Handicapped Act Amendments of 1986, Part H, expanded this to include infants and toddlers in a comprehensive, coordinated, multidisciplinary, interagency program of early intervention services. An Individualized Family Services Plan is meant to facilitate families' goals by identifying and organizing formal and informal resources (Table 6–1).[7]

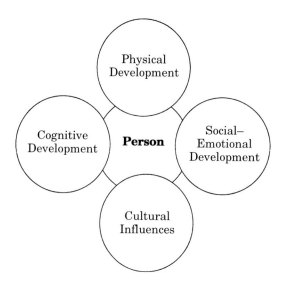

FIGURE 6–1. Interaction of societal factors.

Another major federal provision protecting students with handicaps is Section 504 of the Rehabilitation Act of 1973,which states that no "otherwise qualified" handicapped person can be discriminated against in any federally assisted program or activity "solely by reason of his handicap." Section 504 also applies to teachers, administrators, and others and requires that reasonable accommodation be made to the handicapping condition. This act has wide application to education, employment, and federally aided social service programs, such as housing and transportation. In 1986, when the Rehabilitation Act (PL 99-506) was reauthorized, the amendments added the provision of assistive technology services to clients who qualified for vocational rehabilitation services. Assistive technology services include the selection, fitting, maintaining, and replacing of equipment needed for access to the educational environment, such as power wheelchairs, voice output computers, or microswitches.

The Individuals with Disabilities Education Act Amendment of 1997 (IDEA) (PL 105-17) reiterated the right of a free and appropriate education for children with handicaps and expanded the definition of related services to special education.[8] Legislation has helped to improve the probability of independence by requiring appropriate education, access to and accommodation at the workplace, and assistance with communication where needed. Regardless of legislation and the terminology used, from *mainstreaming* to *inclusion*, people with physical disabilities still need to be accepted by individuals and organizations if they are to develop social competence.

Attitudes in society at large are not easily changed. The worker with a physical handicap may be seen as displacing a more able-bodied person; his or her work may not be valued even when production is equal to others. The ideal of inclusion is not achieved because the person is not perceived as equal or is seen as taking

TABLE 6–1. History of Federal Legislation of Benefit to the American Child with Disabilities

Year	Law	Title	Action	Provisions of Act
1968	90-480	*Architectural Barriers Act*	*Requires*	Federal building accessibility
1979	91-453	*Urban Mass Transportation Act*	*Requires*	Plan and design of accessible transportation
1973	90-87	*Federal Aid Highway Act*	*Requires*	Federal funds be used to make crosswalks accessible
1973	93-112	*Rehabilitation Act*	*Prohibits*	Discrimination against disabled when federal resources are used
			Establishes	Architectural and Transportation Barriers Board
1975	93-391	*Department of Transportation Appropriations Act*	*Requires*	Purchased or build mass transit facilities be accessible
1975	94-103	*Developmental*	*Establishes*	Protection and advocacy systems for developmentally disabled
1975	94-142	*Education for All Handicapped Children Act*	*Provides*	Free and appropriate education in least restrictive environment
1978	95-602	*Rehabilitation Comprehensive Services, and Developmental Disability Amendments*	*Establishes*	Independent living priorities funding
1980	96-265	*Social Security Disability Amendments*	*Removes*	Disincentives to work by making independent living expenses deductible
1990	101-336	*Americans with Disabilities Act*	*Establishes*	Clear comprehensive prohibition of discrimination on the basis of disability
1990	101-613	*National Advisory Board of Medical Rehabilitation Research*	*Establishes*	Board within the NICHD of the National Institutes of Health

resources from the normal person. Individuals with a physical handicap then must deal with society's lack of understanding and acceptance. They need to develop social skills and persevere to overcome the fears, ignorance, and prejudice of those around them, if they are to live the most normal life possible in society.

Although a child's physical disability cannot be eliminated, adults can influence the successful development of psychosocial skills. Early in a child's development, parental involvement is the strongest predictor of future success in home, school, and community activities. Siblings are also important in shaping the future for children with disabilities. Their contributions and their needs are part of the family's resources and stress.[9] When raising a child with physical disabilities, parents need both personal and professional resources available to them.[10,11] During adolescence, peers, relatives, teachers, and community members can help or hinder this process. For adults, professionals and family are the primary support system. It is critical for all persons involved at any developmental stage to remember that children's rate of learning or ability to comprehend varies significantly and depends on their level of cognition, functional communication skills, and learning style. Throughout the life span, physicians can play a critical role in providing needed information and emotional support and as a liaison to other agencies (school-, community-, and home-based).[12,13]

This chapter outlines the challenges encountered at different ages by persons with physical disabilities in developing and maintaining social skills or social competence. The roles of parents, relatives, peers, and support personnel are discussed as they assist the person with physical disabilities throughout life. Possible interventions and resources to help achieve optimal functioning are also discussed.

Birth to 2 Years

The developmental achievements for age group birth to 2 years are considered an essential base for further growth. Parents tend to focus on motor performance and to reinforce any behavior displayed by the child. Children's primary task is play because they learn through exploring their environment. During this time, parents or professionals can assess the child's motor, cognitive, and psychosocial abilities.

To facilitate an infant's socioemotional development, early in life parents can use slightly different strategies during different age spans as recommended by Wilson.[14] For the first 6 months, parents are encouraged to respond to their infant's vocalizations by holding, touching, stroking, and talking to facilitate bonding with their infant and to condition the infant to calm to their voice or touch.

One of the difficult tasks for parents at this young age is to determine when their infant learns cause and effect and, more importantly, when the infant can learn to comply. Research studies have shown that infants as young as 2.5 months can learn limited aspects of cause and effect, such as "I cry, then someone comes."[15] An appropriate way for parents to respond is trying to determine if there is a physiologic reason for the crying, such as being hungry, being cold, having a soiled diaper, or having discomfort from their current physical position. Parents then need to remember to provide attention for physiologically based discomfort and not to reinforce crying inadvertently. Instead of immediately picking up the infant, parents should check to determine whether the infant's physical needs are met and then offer a favorite toy or music to calm them. The goal is for infants to learn to comfort themselves and to learn self-regulation.[16]

Around 6 months of age, infants start to observe what other children are doing or playing. This is an opportunity to place them in closer physical proximity to peers to observe them and begin interaction. Around the age of 1 year, children start to initiate interaction with peers, gesturing to them, offering toys and taking toys away. During this age, it is critical that children are provided with toys they can play with independently, which may entail using a switch-activated toy. Around 2 years, children tend to be more cooperative in turn-taking, although they still frequently state "no," "mine," and "go." It is important that children with handicaps are not forced to give up their toys when they cannot physically prevent others from taking them; they need to have some sense of independence and what is theirs. Children should be taught to say "no" verbally when peers take toys away but also to share and to participate in interactive turn-taking.

Infants and toddlers begin to display unique personality characteristics. Despite physical impairments, emotional development tends to follow a typical pattern of development. Anger, fear, and happiness are experienced at the same stage of development unless cognitive functioning is significantly impaired (Table 6–2).[17] Parents have specific emotional milestones they can look for and encourage in the child. If there are significant cognitive impairments, the child may not be able to remember past events for extended periods of time, may not display prolonged anger or frustration when a desired object is denied, or

TABLE 6–2. Infant Psychosocial Development

Emotional Expression	Approximate Time of Development
Interest	Present at birth
Neonatal smile (a half-smile that appears spontaneously for no apparent reason)	
Startle response	
Distress	
Social smile	4–6 weeks
Anger	3–4 months
Surprise	
Sadness	
Fear	5–7 months
Shame/shyness	6–8 months
Guilt	2 years old

may be more easily distracted by other toys. Concurrently, at times, the child may be more difficult to calm because parents' voices or familiar objects may not serve as consolation, and the child may lack the capacity to calm him- or herself.

Definite temperament styles are evident shortly after birth. *Temperament* is defined as a child's behavioral response repertoire to situations. Chess and Thomas[18] have found that young children demonstrate one of three basic temperament responses: the easy child, who generally is positive in mood and adapts easily to new experiences; the difficult child, who tends to react negatively, to cry frequently, and to be slow to accept change in routines; and the slow-to-warm child, who has a low activity level, is slow to adapt, and displays low level of mood. Forty percent of the children studied fell within the easy category, 10% in the difficult category, and 15% in the slow-to-warm category, with the rest not in a specific category. Parents should be able to respond to their child's temperament by being sensitive to and respecting the individual style. Parents are more successful when they structure environments to suit their child's temperament (e.g., not bringing a difficult child into loud, crowded environments for long periods of time or forcing a slow-to-warm child to be held immediately by other people).

Behavioral concerns of parents need to be acknowledged and addressed. Parents should learn how to teach their children to make their wants and needs known appropriately. Maladaptive behaviors, such as temper tantrums, crying for long periods of time, and demanding large amounts of adult attention, may reflect limited ability to learn by trial and error or inappropriate parental response to a child's behavior. Careful analysis of the child's level of understanding and responses can help parents to plan realistic performance goals, appropriate

reinforcement, and teaching strategies that suit the child's learning style.[19] Children with disabilities may need to be specifically taught various basic social and coping skills because they do not necessarily learn through modeling or trial and error as their peers do, but rather require direct training. Various techniques may be helpful for the nonverbal or preverbal child, such as teaching simple sign language (yes, no, help, please, more, drink, eat), how to use gestures appropriately, or even how to use an augmentative communication system.[20] Children need to be able to communicate their wants and needs to feel some level of control and self-determination and to minimize frustration, without the need to display maladaptive behaviors. Parents may seek assistance with behavioral concerns from sources such as psychologists, nurses, relatives, and friends. The family physician or pediatrician who sees the child for well-baby visits can help, either directly or by referral to other resources.[21]

2 to 6 Years

A child's emotional development and personality emerge further between 2 and 6 years of age. During this stage, the child develops a much more secure sense of self or personality. The initial phase of development of self occurs around the age of 2 years when children recognize themselves in a mirror. Around the age of 3–5 years, children start to define themselves by physical and behavioral characteristics they believe are important or distinguishing about themselves. Therefore, it is not uncommon to hear children with a physical disability state what that disability is: "I have spina bifida," "I need to catheterize myself," or "I wear braces." Instead of discouraging this behavior, parents should encourage honest expression and acknowledgment of the physical disability to foster positive self-esteem and avoid a sense of shame or guilt.

As children become older, they do not view themselves just in terms of physical and behavioral characteristics but rather in terms of personality traits and disposition. Statements such as "I like to be bossy and tell others what to do" or "I'm shy and don't like to talk to strangers" need to be acknowledged, with parents encouraging a child's positive characteristics. Parents therefore should not force their shy child to tell the physician about the troubles he or she is having, but rather should start the conversation and prompt the child to supply short, concise, factual information to the physician—e.g., "Which leg brace is it that doesn't work right, this leg brace or that one?"—in order to respect their child's emerging personality. The physician should begin to include children in discussions, to prepare for the time when they take more control over their own lives as they get older.

Children between 2 and 6 years old want to be more independent and to attempt tasks by themselves. Because of their physical disability, however, they may become easily frustrated, give up, or make statements such as, "I'll never be able to do this." When this happens, parents need to provide verbal encouragement and break down tasks into easier, more manageable steps. Success in small tasks is the first stage to independence. Children need to assist as much as possible when doing activities of daily living, such as eating, drinking, dressing, and toileting. These activities need frequent, daily repetition. More difficult and time-consuming activities of daily living may need to be practiced during less structured times, such as on the weekends when longer periods of time are available to complete the task.

In general, parents of a child with a physical disability tend to protect their child and not push or encourage him or her to be as independent as possible. Parents frequently do not believe their child should be made to do activities of daily living because these tasks are harder for the child and it is difficult for parents to watch the child struggle with tasks that come naturally for their child's age peers. Often, time constraints limit families' ability to have children do activities themselves, particularly at the beginning of a busy day.

Preschool children start to display a wider array, level of intensity, and duration of emotions. Around age 2–3 years, children tend to mirror emotions of others around them. It is not uncommon for them to start crying or laughing in response to others' emotions and be unable to tell adults why they are crying or laughing. As they get older, around the age of 4 or 5 years, if they are distressed or hurt they seek out an adult for comfort. Children also display their anger and frustration more directly and outwardly at this age. A 2-year-old may express anger by crying or hitting. Between the ages of 4 and 6 years, children may show anger or frustration through physical aggression; telling an adult; leaving the area; or yelling, screaming, or crying. A child with a physical disability tends to become more frustrated or angry if unable to leave the area or physically manipulate the object being fought over. This child tends to be more prone to verbal aggression or relying on an adult to intervene or resolve the conflict. Parents must be careful not to foster an overreliance of

the child on adults to fix the problem. The child should be taught how to resolve conflict appropriately verbally and to request adult assistance only after unsuccessful attempts to settle the dispute.

Childhood fears begin to emerge during this phase of development. Warren and Minirth[22] state that fears are especially common during the preschool years, such as fear of the dark, being lost or abandoned, or being hurt by a monster or *bad people*. Children with physical disabilities may have more pronounced fears of abandonment or being left alone because of their limited motor ability. Parents may find their child needs reassurance, more structured bedtime routine, and security items such as blankets or teddy bears to calm or waylay these fears. Parents should not be overly concerned about the expression of these fears. They should actively seek methods that reassure the child while allowing more autonomy and independence.

For children, play is essential to the development of appropriate social and emotional competence. *Play* is defined as engaging in an activity for the enjoyment gained. Play facilitates interaction with peers of the same age, stimulates cognitive development, and increases the opportunity to learn appropriate social skills. During play, children also practice possible roles they may fulfill later in life. One study found that 4-year-olds engaged in pretend play more than 12 minutes out of every hour of play.[23] During these times of imaginary play, children may act out various themes or roles. Garvey[24] found three primary components of pretend play: props, plot, and roles. Children use various props, such as cups, dishes, or phone, to act out a story line, such as going to the store or the hospital, while assuming different roles, such as mother, father, doctor, or friend. It is important that parents and professionals take note of what themes or plots are being acted out because these may indicate children's anxieties or perception of their future role in society. Parents should encourage the use of imaginary play by participating in it and modeling possible positive outcomes of themes that they are acting out, for example, that the child with the physical disability could be a teacher, doctor, parent, or whatever other role seems to be indicated by the imaginary play. Physical assistance or adaptations may be needed to facilitate the imaginary play activities.

Interactive or social play is equally important. A child with a physical disability may not necessarily initiate play with age-appropriate peers but may be more content to be a passive onlooker.[25] As Parten[26] has found, children generally

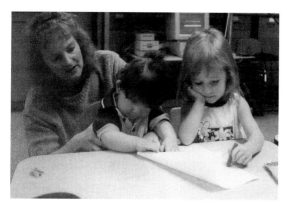

FIGURE 6–2. Parallel play. In a *reverse integration* preschool situation, the girl uses crayons as the teacher assists her playmate.

go through various stages of play: (1) unoccupied play, playing at random; (2) solitary activities, playing alone; (3) onlooker play, watching others; (4) parallel play, separate but copying others; (5) associative play, interactive, social, but not structured or organized; (6) cooperative play, with others in an organized manner. The child has numerous social skills to master during play, such as attending, turn-taking, and sharing. Parents and caregivers should assist the child's progress through these stages by providing situations in which the child with the physical disability and nondisabled peers can interact to reach a common goal, such as completing a puzzle, modeling clay, painting, coloring, or playing a game together. Children may not seek out these opportunities, but adults can

facilitate the process by setting up events where the children need to interact to achieve a shared success (Fig. 6–2).

6 to 12 Years

The stage spanning ages 6–12 years represents a significant time of transition in a child's life with progress from the home environment to a more structured, peer-oriented school environment. Before entering school, children have a number of social skills they need to master (Table 6–3). Children with physical disabilities experience the same apprehension as their peers, with the added concerns of needing more time to move from one classroom to another or assistance in personal self-care and having numerous people questioning them about the physical disability, braces, wheelchair, or other equipment. Parents can ease this transition by talking to school personnel before enrollment, explaining their child's physical condition, accommodations needed, and how classmates should be educated about the child's physical disability. Classmates should be told in an honest, question-and-answer format what the child's physical disability is, how all children have unique needs and strengths, and how to help the child feel part of the class. Classroom adaptations should be made as soon as possible so that the student can have access to the educational environment. Minor modifications, such as lowered coat hooks, slanted desk top, and nonskid desk surfaces, can significantly improve a student's ability to function independently. Physical

TABLE 6–3. Survival and Academic Skills Identified as Important for Children to Exhibit on Entry into Kindergartens*

Social Behaviors and Classroom Conduct	Task-related Behaviors
Separates from parents and accepts school personnel	Finds materials needed for task
Expresses emotions and feelings appropriately	Holds and manipulates materials
Understands role as part of a group	Does not disrupt peers during activities
Respects others and their property	Stays in *own space* for activity
Plays cooperatively	Works on activity for appropriate time frame
Shares and takes turns	Asks peers or teacher for information or assistance
Initiates and maintains peer interactions	Seeks teacher's attention appropriately (e.g., raises hand)
Interacts without aggression	Completes tasks on time
Plays independently	Completes tasks of ability level near criteria
Imitates peer actions	Replaces materials and cleans up work space
Lines up	Follows routine in transition
Waits appropriately	Complies quickly with teacher instructions
Willing to try something new	Generalizes skills across tasks and situations
Defends self appropriately	Recalls and follows directions for tasks previously described
Controls voice in classroom	Follows two- to three-part direction by teacher
Follows classroom rules	Follows group instructions
Responds to warning words (e.g., no, stop)	Attends to teacher in large group activity
Modifies behavior when given verbal feedback	Makes choices

* This list was developed from various research studies examining prerequisite kindergarten skills.

adaptations to buildings, bathrooms, or classrooms may also be needed. Playgrounds may need to be modified to maximize the child's level of independence, functioning, and ability to play with peers.[27] Any special equipment that the child will need should be available and its operation and maintenance understood. School personnel should be instructed in the equipment's use and contribution to the student's ability to function.

Social and psychological concerns may be overshadowed or exacerbated by physical problems. The child with incontinence who needs bladder catheterization deserves privacy and school personnel who can provide willing, tactful assistance. If odor is a problem, this issue should be addressed with the child and family and, if necessary, explained to staff. Whether this issue should be discussed with classmates may be a decision best made by the child.

Participation in school activities should be as normal as possible, with clear, appropriate behavioral expectations explained to the child. Academic assignments may need to be shorter because of physical fatigue or difficulty learning the task at the same rate as the rest of the class. Learning disabilities may become evident as tasks become more complex, especially by third grade. Accurate definition of problems and remediation of learning difficulties during the primary grades is important to ensure positive self-esteem and academic success in later years. The parents, occupational therapist, speech and language clinician, and regular and special education teachers need to work together with the child to find the best ways to compensate for deficits. When the child needs to be out of the regular classroom for special help or therapies, this time should be scheduled without interfering with critical academic subject areas.

As children with physical disabilities enter school, their sense of self or self-esteem is challenged. The primary influences on a child's self-esteem at this age are acceptance or support from significant others, parents, siblings, teachers, and extended family and the child's self-evaluation of academic, athletic, and social skills. Children with physical disabilities may have good skills and an excellent adult and peer support system but still consider their abilities as inadequate because of their physical limitations. Children can easily develop *learned helplessness*,[28] believing that their behavior has minimal effect on any outcome in their environment, with a feeling of having no control over what is happening to them. Parents, educational staff, and other support personnel need to point out situations in which the student has

success and to foster areas of interest. This is an ongoing and changing process as the child progresses through the educational system. Developing positive self-esteem is a long-term process that requires frequent verbal encouragement, awareness of accomplishments, and sharing accomplishments with others. When a child does appear to have poor self-esteem, parents and professionals need to break the pattern of negative thinking and failures by setting up situations in which the child can have several small successes throughout the day.

Friendships and peer groups become more important as the child becomes older. In the early elementary years, peer groups tend to be same sex. These groups typically have two to five members and demonstrate different styles of playing, communicating, and behaving. In a peer group, children develop basic social skills and gain a sense of belonging. Through peer interaction, they are able to form a basis for comparison or a realistic gauge of their own abilities and skills. Children with physical disabilities can appreciate their physical limitations more clearly as well as any unique skills they may possess compared to their peers.

Children frequently ask, "What can I do to make the kids at school like me?" and worry about not being popular. A study conducted by Kennedy[29] found that children rated as popular were able to communicate clearly with peers, appropriately gain their attention, and maintain conversations. Parents and professionals working with children who have a physical disability may find that to foster friendships, direct social skills teaching is needed, in a small group setting, focusing on how to initiate, maintain, and appropriately terminate conversations.

The development of friendships appears to go through five phases, as outlined by Selman:[30]

Stage 0—momentary playmateship occurs typically from ages 3–7 years. Children at this stage are egocentric and have difficulty seeing another person's perspective. Friends typically are defined in terms of proximity, as being next door, and value of material possessions, as having a computer.

Stage 1—one-way assistance typically occurs between ages 4–9 years, with children defining a good friend as someone who does what they want them to do. It is not uncommon to hear, "He isn't my friend any more because he won't play the games I want to play."

Stage 2—two-way fair weather cooperation can take place from the ages of 6–12 years. This type of friendship does involve give and take but still is self-serving and based on self-interest rather than common interests: "We are friends because he gives me the baseball cards he doesn't want."

Stage 3—intimate, mutually shared relationships can occur around the ages of 9–15 years. These friendships tend to be easygoing, committed to each other, and based on mutual interests. Friendships tend to be progressive and may demand exclusivity: "She is my best friend and no one else's."

Stage 4—autonomous interdependence can begin at age 12 years. Children at this stage respect the other's need for dependence and independence: "We went to his house to watch TV, which was boring, but we both like to go to baseball games."

Children may go through the stages at different rates; however, adults should be concerned if a child appears *stuck* at a certain friendship stage for an extended period of time and is not progressing. These situations may require intervention, such as formal counseling, peer tutors, or structured peer interaction activities.

Adults must remember that at early ages children tend to change friends frequently and for minor reasons. Parents should not be overly concerned about changes in friends. As children grow older, however, they change friends less often, demand more of them, find it more difficult to make new friends, and are more upset when a friendship ends. Children tend to choose friends who are similar to them not only in terms of interests, but also in gender, ethnicity, and socioeconomic status. Adults attempting to foster friendship may find that peers they view as appropriate because of personality, behavioral, or academic traits are not necessarily interesting to the child as friends. Adults are more likely to be successful if they determine ahead of time what qualities or traits their child desires in a friend and then attempt to make a match accordingly. Parents can foster friendships by inviting peers to their house for short, specific event-driven times, such as watching a

football game on television, planning a community outing with a peer invited, and even having children stay overnight. Activities may include clubs and special or regular camps. Activities including other children with a physical handicap can help with separation issues and provide a comparison group of peers for the child. During the development of friendships, parents of a child with a physical handicap may find it helpful to tell the friend's parents some of the basic information about their child's disability and special needs (Fig. 6–3).[31]

Adolescence—12–21 Years

Strax[32] states that unless there are successful relationships both in the family and within peer groups, the adolescent cannot establish a successful relationship later on in adult life. Tasks to be accomplished include consolidating identity, achieving independence from parents, establishing love objects outside of the family, and finding a vocation. The first issue to be resolved during adolescence is, "Who am I?" This process of definition entails self-evaluation of the adolescent's emotional status, cognition, and behavior as they relate to interactions with people and to situations he or she encounters daily. Adolescents typically try out multiple selves or personalities as they attempt to determine, "Who is the real me?" or "Who do I want to be?" It is not unusual for adolescents to change behaviors with different peer groups, alternating between being quiet, pensive, and withdrawn, and being rude, opinionated, or obnoxious. An adolescent's physical disability may limit ability to try different styles of behavior. Parents may also inhibit experimentation if the physically dependent child fears loss of needed help. To promote self-expression, parents should allow exploration of options, within reason and safety,

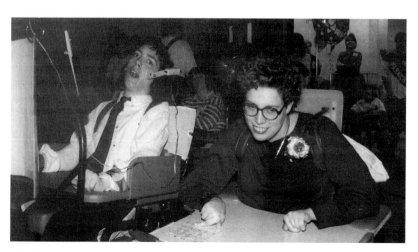

FIGURE 6–3. Teenagers with physical disabilities relate using augmentative communication at a school party.

such as different clothing, hairstyles, music, jewelry, or makeup. Parents may even need to assist in this process. Adolescents need to explore their own identity and not be expected to demonstrate the identity that parents believe they should possess.[33]

While adolescents attempt to develop a firmer identity and simultaneously seek more independence or freedom, conflict with parents is not unusual. Generally, early adolescence, as children begin to assert their independence, appears to be a time of greater conflict compared with later adolescence. At this age, parents should encourage some risk taking for new tasks, such as getting a drivers' license or a job or going on a date, that the adolescents may have some reservations about. Physical disability may interfere with opportunities for self-expression (for example, the need for leg braces limits clothing styles available) or for risk taking, as when assistance is needed with transportation. Similar to all young people, adolescents with a physical handicap should be allowed the opportunity to fail; to learn to accept limited physical abilities, and to succeed within those limitations. Support and realistic encouragement are essential during this developmental phase. To minimize conflict and foster independence, parents should be more willing to listen, negotiate, and exert less control. Parents of a child with a physical disability often find that they need to push or encourage their adolescent to be more independent. This can be difficult if their own identity is so firmly enmeshed in being the parent of a child with a physical disability that they as parents are apprehensive about allowing more independence. In either scenario, parents should encourage their child to develop needed skills to be independent and successful in life after graduating from high school. This includes learning daily tasks, doing laundry, budgeting for needed items, and even discerning what qualities to look for in a possible future spouse.

In the school environment, adolescents appear to have the most difficult adjustments to make at about 12–13 years old, when they make the transition to middle or junior high school. They move from small class size and frequent teacher interactions to larger classes, less teacher interaction, more responsibility to do assignments on their own, and higher academic standards. The school counselor or psychologist is an available resource to answer questions and advocate with school personnel who may not be willing to modify curriculum or assignments as needed.

During this time, adolescents typically experience the onset of puberty, when they are concerned over facial complexion, body size, vocal timbre, and perceived attractiveness. These changes tend to affect adolescents with physical disabilities to a greater degree because they feel that the already enhanced unwanted attention because of their physical disability increases with physical maturation.

Peer groups are an important part of an adolescent's social development. These are larger numbers of children who are not necessarily close friends but have mutual interests or friends. Peer groups serve as a source of information about new experiences or challenges, provide support in adjusting to changes such as new rules or different types of classes, and can serve as a sounding board for exploring values or aspirations. If possible, teenagers with physical disabilities need to be included in these peer groups to avoid the stigma of not being part of an accepted societal group. Adolescents may need to be encouraged and assisted to go to school activities, dances, and sporting events and to participate in extracurricular events, such as plays, debate club, or as student manager of the basketball team, because these activities are an essential part of learning, growing, and preparing for adulthood.[34] Some modifications within these events may be needed for the student to be successful. Activities independent from family members should be encouraged because these experiences can help teach adolescents responsibility and how to make arrangements for activities on their own.

Friendships take a more central role as friends many times have more influence than parents over adolescent choices. Adolescents tend to choose friends who share their parents' values and belief system, although this seldom is a conscious decision because choices are based on mutual interests and interactions.[35] Friendships tend to be more intimate, with the adolescents discussing thoughts and feelings on a multitude of subjects while taking into consideration the other's point of view. Although parents may not necessarily approve of the type of friend an adolescent makes, they need to understand that the friend obviously sees something positive and likable in their child and is able to provide much-needed social interaction or ties outside the family. The exception to this statement comes when adolescents with physical disabilities become involved with others who use drugs or break the law. The young person with a physical disability may be more susceptible to negative influence or exploitation because of the desire for friendship and acceptance within a peer group.

Young people with disabilities need to learn to become as independent as possible and to develop strategies for times when they do need assistance from others.[36] They need to have realistic expectations of what their peers, who are now physically able to provide assistance, can do to help them. Teenagers need to realize that friends and others in society are not obligated or willing to provide assistance as freely as family or school personnel have in the past. It is critical that adolescents be able to do tasks by themselves as much as possible or to ask for assistance. When needing assistance, they should ask appropriately and not demand help from others. They also need to know how any assistive technology or equipment, such as an electric wheelchair or communication device, works and be able to explain to others how it is used and maintained. Individuals also should have a phone number of someone to call who can help in time of emergency. A portable phone can be useful away from home because strangers are less apt to volunteer help. Medical concerns and cares should become the responsibility of these adolescents. They should be encouraged to direct their medical care, which would include knowing their medical history, taking their medication, learning how to voice concerns when they are ill, and making and keeping medical appointments. The physician and parent should expect adolescents to be interested, informed participants in any interaction involving their care.

Social interaction between males and females also changes during adolescence. Dunphy[37] has studied the development of opposite-sex relationships. Adolescents typically participate in isolated, unisex groups evolving into larger same-sex groups, which start to engage in some gender group-to-group interaction. During middle adolescence, there is more interaction between males and females at large group activities, such as dances or athletic events. During later adolescence, teens engage in more dating behavior and participate less and less frequently in large group activities. As they develop more intimacy and deeper relationships with the opposite sex, they tend to rely more heavily on one particular person for acceptance and affirmation than the large group peer setting. Dating relationships are viewed as serious, with breaking up or fights as significant stressors in their lives. Teenagers also need to learn to distinguish different types of relationships, recognizing that peers are not necessarily interested in a romantic relationship but may just want to be friends. They have to understand degrees of friendship can develop under different circumstances, ranging from an acquaintance to a close friend.

Sexuality becomes a major issue during adolescence.[38–40] Physical changes occurring at this time should be explained in understandable terminology by adults, preferably the adolescent's parents. The physiatrist or family physician should be prepared to assist with information, particularly relating to the effect of disability on sexual functioning. Teenagers should have the opportunity to ask questions about sexual development, individual sexuality, and appropriate expression of sexuality. Parents need to know that adolescents with a physical disability are more prone to sexual abuse and exploitation than their peers. Teenagers should know that sexuality is a natural aspect of becoming an adult that needs to follow personal, family, and cultural norms. They also have to know how to protect themselves. Individualized strategies for dealing with unwanted sexual advances should be developed and taught.

In high school, adolescents need to start investigating available postsecondary options.[41] These options may include college, vocational schools, sheltered employment or adjustment training center, or independent employment. School personnel; medical personnel, including physical and occupational therapists; parents; and, most importantly, the adolescents themselves should evaluate available skills and aptitudes.[42–44] All parties involved have to accept what the student truly can and cannot do. A teenager usually identifies jobs that appear ideal or are based on role models; however, adolescents with a disability have to be more reality based. Part-time employment during high school may not be an option because of limited energy level or transportation issues. In some areas of the United States, this may limit the student's social opportunities, as contacts at work tend to supplement or displace school- or community-based group interactions.

Family dynamics tend to change during this time, as siblings leave home, parents become older, and less physical assistance may be available. The young adult may need more assistance because of decreasing physical ability, growth, or weight gain. Grandparents may not be able to help as much. During adolescence, the relationship between siblings and the teenager with a physical handicap tends to be more congenial, cooperative, and mutually enjoyable, because adolescents feel less responsibility for their sibling with a physical disability.[45]

Adulthood

If not previously accomplished, the disabled adult has all the usual tasks of growing up with the added problems of obtaining needed help and access to the world (Fig. 6–4). Choice of occupation

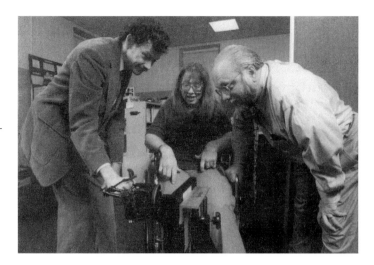

FIGURE 6–4. Adults with physical disabilities working on a research panel.

may be determined by the disability's ruling out some options. Finances may also dictate choices, although Vocational Rehabilitation Services can help. Societal and cultural factors also influence the vocational choices available. For some, competitive employment may not be feasible, and alternatives have to be explored, such as supported employment, enclaves, sheltered work, or activity training centers.[46] When performing activities of daily living uses a large part of the person's available physical energy, social activities may be more important than any benefit obtained from employment. The Americans with Disabilities Act does not excuse the disabled from being able to perform the duties required of specific employment. It does mandate no discrimination based solely on the presence of a disability. Accommodations usually are not costly. Worker's Compensation costs do not increase. The individual's abilities should be assessed for appropriate job placement. Safety measures can be adapted as necessary.[47]

At this stage of life, the adult's parents are aging, siblings and other family members have their own lives, and personal assistance is not within the scope of most friendships. If outside help is needed at home or work, funding must be arranged and managerial skills acquired. Independent living centers, vocational rehabilitation, or medically based rehabilitation centers can help with training for the assistant and the disabled person as employer. The person with a physical disability is still responsible for deciding use of the assistance, budgeting payment, and the personal relationship that is essential if the assistant is to be a stable part of the person's life. Obtaining medical care may be more difficult for the adult, who has to transfer from pediatric to adult providers. Special clinics may be an answer where population density permits.[48]

Considering quality of life for people with physical disabilities, life satisfaction was found to depend more on leisure satisfaction than on employment or other aspects of living.[49] Marriage is often not considered to be a viable option by people with disabilities, their parents, or society. This relates to the issues of sexuality and the possibility of children. It also relates to perceptions of personal worth as depending on the person's ability to work and support a family.[50] Sexual activity and child care can be accomplished with adaptations and sometimes assistance. Decisions regarding sexual activity, marriage, and parenthood are to be made by the persons involved rather than agencies or other people. These decisions do need to be informed ones, and the responsibility for providing that information is shared by caregivers, family, teachers, social workers, and physicians.

The pool of potential partners for people with disabilities is smaller because of fewer opportunities to meet people and difficulties in establishing friendships likely to lead to a committed relationship. The difficulties may influence or be affected by the choice of living situation. A group home or institution may be better than independent living if social contacts through work or organized activities are not feasible.[51]

Psychosocial issues for the older person with a physical disability relate to issues of change: physical change in ability to do self-care or to work requires adaptation to more care and less income or income not derived from work, with subsequent loss of self-esteem. Transportation needs may change, with more expense and less flexibility. The person must cope with a different level of independence.[52]

As abilities change, interests must too, and ways of interacting with others may need adjustment. Relationships centered on work activities, if no longer available, have to be replaced by more social interaction, such as clubs and games or just visiting. Interest in community activities helps, and even political activism may be possible if energy is no longer needed for work. Relationship skills gained in adolescence can be used again to renew old friendships and find new ones.

Depression is a risk at this stage because losses occur and change is forced on the person. Physical or medical reasons for decreased interest and endurance should be considered and dealt with, if present, to avoid unnecessary loss of function. Medical personnel should be aware of psychological as well as physical problems and provide appropriate treatment or referral to other resources, such as senior centers, counselors, geriatric-trained physicians, psychologists, social workers, vocational rehabilitation services to change work situations, or Social Security for help with pension and Medicare. Accessible wellness or senior centers or health clubs can provide less strenuous activities that help maintain physical health and contact with people. Physical and occupational therapists can help with adaptations to maintain abilities, using equipment and training or exercises.

Conclusion

Psychosocial issues for children with disabilities are similar to those of the nondisabled population. Dealing with them requires thought, consideration, and resources, both physical and personal. Psychosocial factors may be more important determinants of overall success in life than is severity of a disability. Physicians, especially physiatrists, need to include social abilities in their assessment of patients' function, and plan remedial action as needed, in the same way as assistive devices or exercises are prescribed for mobility.

Acknowledgments

The authors thank the Wegner Health Science Information Center staff and Children's Care Hospital and School, especially Peggy Schumacher, for support in preparing this chapter.

References

1. Cain H: Leadership is Common Sense. New York, International Thomson Publishing Company, 1997.
2. Brookins G: Culture, ethnicity, and bicultural competence: Implications for children with chronic illness and disability. Pediatrics 1993;91:1056.
3. Patterson J, Blum R: A conference on culture and chronic illness in childhood: Conference summary. Pediatrics 1993;91:1025.
4. Werner E, Smith R: Overcoming the Odds. Ithaca, NY, Cornell University Press, 1992.
5. Kokkonen J, et al: Social outcome of handicapped children as adults. Dev Med Child Neurol 1991;33:1095.
6. Fischer L, Sorenson GP (eds): School Law for Counselors, Psychologists and Social Workers. New York, Longman, 1985.
7. Public Law 99-457, the Education of the Handicapped Act Amendments of 1986, Part H.
8. OSERS IDEA '97 Home Page. *http://www.ed.gov/offices/OSERS/IDEA/index.html*. 1997.
9. Miller S: Living with a disabled sibling—A review. Pediatr Nurs 1996;8:21.
10. Beresford B: Resources and strategies: How parents cope with the care of a disabled child. J Child Psychol Psychiatry 1994;35:171.
11. Patterson J: Family resilience to the challenge of a child's disability. Pediatr Ann 1991;20:491.
12. Taylor EH: Understanding and helping families with neurodevelopmental and neuropsychiatric special needs. Pediatr Clin North Am 1995;42:143.
13. Marshall RM, et al: Physician/school teacher collaboration. Clin Pediatr 1987;26:524.
14. Wilson LC: Infants and Toddlers Curriculum and Teaching. Albany, NY, Delmar, 1990.
15. Ronee-Cullier C: Learning and memory in children. In Mussen PH (ed): Handbook of Child Psychology, vol. 4, 4th ed. New York, Wiley, 1987.
16. Brazelton TB, Cramer BG: The Earliest Relationship. Reading, MA, Addison-Wesley, 1990.
17. Santrock JW (ed): Children. Dubuque, IA, Brown & Benchmark Publishers, 1994.
18. Chess S, Thomas A: Temperamental individuality from childhood to adolescence. J Child Psychiatry 1977;16:218.
19. Carr EG, et al (eds): Communication-based Interventions for Problem Behavior. Baltimore, Paul H Brookes, 1994.
20. Reichle J, et al (eds): Implementing Augmentative and Alternative Communication Strategies for Learners with Severe Disabilities. Baltimore, Paul H Brookes, 1991.
21. Parette HP, et al: The family physician's role with parents of young children with developmental disabilities. J Fam Pract 1990;31:288.
22. Warren P, Minirth F: Things That Go Bump In The Night. Nashville, TN, Thomas Nelson, 1992.
23. Haight WL, Miller PJ: Pretending at Home. Albany, State University of New York Press, 1993.
24. Garvey C: Play. Cambridge, MA, Harvard University Press, 1977.
25. Missiuna C, Pollock N: Play deprivation in children with physical disabilities: The role of the occupational therapist in preventing secondary disability. Am J Occup Ther 1991;45:882.
26. Parten M: Social play among preschool children. J Abnorm Social Psychol 1932;27:243.
27. Stout J: Planning playgrounds for children with disabilities. Am J Occup Ther 1988;42:653.
28. Seligman ME: Learned Helplessness. San Francisco, WH Freeman, 1975.
29. Kennedy JH: Determinants of peer social status: Contributions of physical appearance, reputation and behavior. J Youth Adolesc 1990;19:233.
30. Selman RL: The Growth of Interpersonal Understanding. New York, Academic Press, 1980.
31. Mulderij KJ: Peer relations and friendships in physically disabled children. Child Care Health Dev 1997;23:379.
32. Strax TE: Psychological issues faced by adolescents and young adults with disabilities. Pediatr Ann 1991;20:507.
33. Marcia JE: The empirical study of ego identity. In Boxma HA, Graafsma TLG, Groterant, et al (eds): Identity and Development. Newbury Park, CA, Sage, 1994.

34. Ervin M: Dance an expression of the soul. Enable 1998; Jan/Feb:72.

35. Cowardin NW: Adolescent characteristics associated with acceptance of handicapped peers. Adolescence 1986; 21:931.

36. Blum RW: Adolescents with chronic conditions and their families: The transition to adult services. In Hostler SL (ed): Family-Centered Care: An Approach to Implementation. Charlottesville, University of Virginia, 1994.

37. Dunphy DC: The social structure of urban adolescent peer groups. Society 1963;26:230.

38. Modaras L: The What's Happening to My Body? Book for Girls. New York, Newmarket Press, 1988.

39. Modaras L: The What's Happening to My Body? Book for Boys. New York, Newmarket Press, 1988.

40. Alexander MA: Sexuality and the adolescent. In Leyson JF (ed): Sexual Rehabilitation of the Spinal-Cord Injured Patient. Totowa, NJ, Humana Press, 1990.

41. Rowley-Kelly FL, Reigel DH (eds): Teaching the Student with Spina Bifida. Baltimore, Paul H Brookes, 1993.

42. McDonnell J, Mathot-Buckner C, Ferguson B (eds): Transition Programs for Students with Moderate/Severe Disabilities. Pacific Grove, CA, Brooks/Cole Publishing Company, 1996.

43. Brollier C, et al: Transition from school to community living. Am J Occup Ther 1994;48:346.

44. White PH: Success on the road to adulthood: Issues and hurdles for adolescents with disabilities. Rheum Dis Clin North Am 1997;23:697.

45. Faux SA: Siblings of children with chronic physical and cognitive disabilities. J Pediatr Nurs 1993;8:305.

46. Will MC: Youth with disability: The transition years. J Adolesc Health Care 1985;6:79.

47. Seaver ME: Employing persons with disabilities. AAOHN J 1989;37:513.

48. Mann NR: Primary care for persons with disabilities: The Rehabilitation Institute of Michigan Model Program. Am J Phys Med Rehab 1997;76(3 suppl):547.

49. Kinney WB, Coyle CP: Predicting life satisfaction among adults with physical disabilities. Arch Phys Med Rehab 1992;73:863.

50. Haseltine FP et al (eds): Reproductive Issues for Persons with Physical Disabilities. Baltimore, Paul H Brookes, 1993.

51. Spencer JC: An ethnographic study of independent living alternatives. Am J Occup Ther 1991;45:243.

52. Breske S: Gearing up for the golden years. Advance for Directors in Rehabilitation 1997;6:22.

Appendix
Resources Available

Organizations

Easter Seals Organization

Special Olympics

NICHCY
PO Box 1492
Washington, DC 20013
(800) 999-5599

The National Information Center for Handicapped Children and Youth (NICHCY) is a national clearinghouse that provides personal responses to specific questions.

HEAT
Higher Education and Training for People with Disabilities (HEAT) provides services regarding postsecondary education for the handicapped.

ERIC
Counsel for Exceptional Children
1920 Association Drive
Reston, VA 22091
(703) 620-3660

Clearinghouse on the Handicapped and Gifted Children

International Shriners Hospitals
1-800-237-5055

Canadian Rehabilitation Council for the Disabled
One Yonge St., Suite 2110
Toronto, Ontario, Canada M5E 1E5
(416) 862-0340

American Academy for Cerebral Palsy and
    Development Medicine
P.O. Box 11086
Richmond, VA 23230-1086
(804) 282-0036

Magazines/Journals

Exceptional Parent: a magazine for families and professionals involved with disabled children

en·able: the official magazine of the American Association of People with Disabilities

Advance: for directors in rehabilitation

Exceptional Child: research journal for professionals

Developmental Medicine and Child Neurology: Services for Children with Disabilities in European Countries, Supplement No. 76, Vol. 39

Government

Refer to local:

Office of Vocational Rehabilitation

Office of Special Education

Office of Social Services for assistance in respite care, SSI

Maternal and Child Health Services—Title V Program for Children with Special Healthcare Needs

Individual states have parent training and information centers

Chapter 7

Therapeutic Exercise

Patricia Taggart, MBA, PT
Christine Aguilar, MD

Planning an effective rehabilitation program for a child with congenital or acquired motor dysfunction requires an understanding of the interaction of biologic, environmental, and developmental factors. The multisystemic nature of physical disability necessitates the use of a multidisciplinary team well versed in a variety of treatment techniques and methods. The pediatric physiatrist, working with the child, family, and rehabilitation team and using the knowledge of interaction between structure and experience, seeks to foster an optimal developmental course so that the functional potential allowed by the organic deficits can be fully realized.[1]

Realistic rehabilitation goals should be established based on the diagnosis, degree of motor dysfunction, and anticipated functional potential. Consideration should be given to the life-long nature of physical handicap with periodic reassessment and update dependent on the child's level of ability.

When developing a rehabilitation program for a child with physical disability, care should be taken to involve the child and family. The realization that families provide the context of life for children has opened up new ways of relating to families and of providing services to children.[2] Care should be given to respecting ethnic and cultural factors that may affect the course of rehabilitation. The ultimate prognosis for any disabled child is as much dependent on the functional effectiveness of the family in dealing with the problems as on the child's own capabilities.[3]

This chapter describes the general principles of therapeutic intervention for motor dysfunction. Therapeutic exercise for specific conditions related to childhood disability is discussed. Traditional and nontraditional theories of therapeutic exercise and their application to common neuromotor impairment are reviewed.

Children and Exercise

Physical fitness is generally viewed as having two facets—health-related fitness and more traditional motor fitness. Health-related fitness includes abilities related to daily function and health maintenance, and motor fitness generally includes physical abilities related to athletic performance.[4] When designing exercise programs for children with disabilities, it is important to understand childhood physical fitness. Assessing the patient's level of fitness helps in establishing appropriate goals related to specific disabilities.

Health-related fitness is generally divided into four categories: cardiorespiratory endurance, muscular strength and endurance, flexibility, and body composition.[5] The rationale for each component is presented in Table 7–1.

Development of strength depends on the development of force production and is influenced by numerous factors.[6] Muscle strength increases linearly with chronological age from childhood in both sexes until the age of 13–14 years. During this growth period increase in strength is closely related to increase in muscle mass. Boys have greater strength than girls at all ages (seen as early as age 3 years) and have larger absolute and relative amounts of muscle.[6,7] Deficits of muscular strength in children with disabilities should be a primary focus for the rehabilitation team in attempts to improve function.

Children with disabilities often demonstrate decreased or limited exercise capacity relative to their nondisabled peers. This decrease in capacity may result from their limited participation in exercise, which leads to deconditioning, or from the specific pathologic factors of their disability that limit exercise-related functions. Children with disabilities may enter a cycle of decreased activities demonstrated in Figure 7–1.

TABLE 7-1. Health-related Fitness Components and Their Importance in Health Promotion and Disease Prevention

Component	Importance
Cardiorespiratory endurance	Improved physical working capacity Reduced fatigue Reduced risk of coronary disease Optimal growth and development
Muscular strength and endurance	Improved functional capacity for lifting and carrying Reduced risk of low back pain Optimal posture Optimal growth and development
Flexibility	Enhanced functional capacity for bending and twisting Reduced risk of low back pain Optimal growth and development
Body composition	Reduced risk of hypertension, coronary disease, and diabetes Optimal growth and development

Principles of Therapeutic Exercise in Pediatrics

Developmental Considerations

There are numerous developmental considerations one must be aware of when designing an exercise program for an infant or child, including the child's age and mental capacity, home and family environment, level of mobility, and school placement.

Therapy to elicit active movement in infants is delivered in the form of handling and by inducing spontaneous interaction. Babies frequently cry during vigorous stretching or handling; parents need to be forewarned that the activities are not hurting the baby. Many therapists believe that infancy is a period when the quality of a child's motor performance is most important.

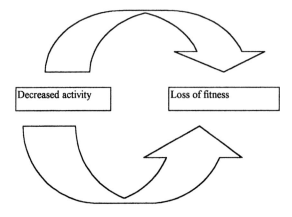

FIGURE 7–1. Cycle of decreased activity in children with disabilities.

Movement patterns are learned through repetition, and once a pattern is learned incorrectly, it is considered more difficult to break the "bad habit" than to facilitate a normal movement pattern.

Toddlers and preschoolers may exhibit stranger anxiety; therefore, children may need time to adjust to the therapeutic setting and to accept handling. A period of gradual weaning from parents may be necessary. Whenever possible, parental involvement in the therapeutic activity should be encouraged. Carry-over of the exercise program into the home is usually necessary to achieve goals.

Children may be motivated during therapy through the use of developmentally appropriate toys, songs, and games. Colorful equipment such as bolsters, balls, and benches may also encourage participation. Mirrors may help to provide visual feedback when a particular motor output is desired. Group settings may be useful in cases in which children are uncooperative, although some children may find the extra stimulus distracting and need quiet treatment rooms. Further incentives may be provided through behavioral modification techniques; however, incentives must be meaningful to the child and linked to the desired response.

As children enter preschool and school age, coordination of education and therapy is essential. There is often increased emphasis on the child's education and less on supportive therapies. In a school setting, therapists often function in a consulting role to enhance the child's educational experience and potential. Occupational therapists may work with the teacher in selecting appropriate adaptive devices, while physical therapists may assist with suggestions for mobility, seating posture, and body alignment.

Adolescence presents special challenges to children with disabilities. Accelerated growth predisposes the child to development of contractures and postural malalignment. Low self-esteem, poor body image, emotional problems, and obesity may further compound the motor disability. Therapeutic exercise in combination with psychological counseling may be necessary. Vocational rehabilitation offers disabled adolescents the opportunity to participate in advanced skills training. The number of students with disabilities attending college has increased over the past decade.

Sports, either as leisure activities or on a competitive basis, provide significant physiologic and emotional benefits to children with disabilities. Virtually all sports have been adapted for disabled participants.[8,9] Local, national, and international sports organizations assist children with disabilities in establishing healthy, active lifestyles.

Theories of Motor Learning, Development, and Intervention

Motor Learning

How is the task of motor learning accomplished? Many have attempted to understand and explain motor learning in a simple manner. Initially motor learning was proposed to be "a habit."[10] Sherrington stated that reflexes affect motor function. He proposed that reflex-chaining, the coordination of single reflexes, both excitatory and inhibitory, results in movement.[11] Some form of feedback is necessary for motor learning. The closed-loop theory of motor control[12] notes that sensory input and feedback influence motor learning. Take, for example, someone who wants to learn to play the banjo. He or she arrives at the first lesson and holds the banjo, getting to know its touch. Carefully, the student listens to and watches the teacher. The sensory map by which the fingers will navigate begins to take shape. Eventually, the listening, watching, and an increasing familiarity with the touch of the instrument in the hands brings the child a growing ability as a musician. This example includes learning through many aspects of sensory feedback: touch, hearing, and visualization. As motor learning progresses and becomes more proficient, the need for sensory feedback decreases.[13]

In contrast, there is the open-loop theory in which motor movements are primarily responsible for selection and execution of sequential movements.[14] This theory minimizes the need for sensory feedback and was first explained by those who studied fast-paced movements.[15] Examples include anticipatory postural changes and adjustments, such as in karate.

In the child, there are considerations not only of motor skill, but of developmental issues as well. Many have attempted to sort out the much-debated controversy about whether motor coordination problems are related to physiologic deficit or a developmental delay. The progression of development from infancy through childhood is well described. Schmidt brought to the forefront the importance of memory in the learning scheme. He recognized the importance of cognition in motor learning.[16] Researchers, using a movable platform, found that training can affect postural adjustments and accelerate the development of sitting posture in infants.[17] Most recently, motor-learning theorists have described a dynamic theory in motor learning.[18,19] According to this theory, motor learning results from previous experience, cortex changes, cerebellar coordination, and sensory input. To better understand motor skill, researchers have used imaging techniques such as single photon emission computed tomography (SPECT), positron emission tomography (PET), and functional magnetic resonance imaging (MRI).[20] Karni et al.[21] revealed that a few minutes of daily practice on a sequential finger opposition task produced large, incremental performance gains over a few weeks of training. These gains did not generalize to the contralateral side, suggesting that learning evolved through practice. This observation was supported by functional MRI.[21] The development of a therapeutic exercise program is dependent on the theories of motor learning adhered to by the practitioners.

Early Intervention Programs

Early intervention programs provide a range of educational and therapeutic options to families and their children with developmental delays.[22–24] These programs generally target children between the ages of 0 and 3 years; however, the age of onset varies depending on the type of disability, identification of developmental delay, or the risk for developmental delays. Predominant risk groups and the effect of early intervention in each group are described in Table 7–2. The

TABLE 7–2.   Pediatric Risk Groups and Effects of Early Intervention

Group	Description	Outcome of Early Intervention
Environmentally vulnerable children	Children deemed disadvantaged as a result of a deprived physical and social environment that may limit growth and development	Improved cognitive function, less need for special education
Children at biologic risk	Children deemed at risk due to presence of a condition that can result in developmental delay, i.e., fetal alcohol syndrome, maternal drug use, asphyxia, prematurity	Improved parenting skills, short-term gains in growth and development, more long-term follow-up is needed
Children with established risk	Children diagnosed with a medical condition known to adversely affect development, i.e., cerebral palsy, Down syndrome	Evidence conflicting, short-term gains in developmental achievement, especially in less severely disabled children, positive effects of family acceptance and caregiving abilities

primary objective of early intervention is to enhance the competence of participants in all developmental domains in order to prevent or minimize delays.[22] Intervention programs also assist families in managing and coping with daily challenges effectively at home and in the community.[25–27]

Early intervention programs have been available for some time but have evolved dramatically since the 1960s. Programs initially geared primarily for the socially disadvantaged, such as Head Start, have paved the way for important changes in legislation related to early intervention in the United States. Public Law 94–142, enacted in 1975, mandated that all children with disabilities were entitled to education in the least restrictive environment with the right to all related services needed within the school environment. The Education of the Handicapped Act Amendments of 1986 (Public Law 99-457) ensured federal incentives that were already available to children through PL 94-142. Public Law 99-457 was enacted to extend services provided in PL99-142 to children 0–6 years of age. The Individuals with Disabilities Education Act (IDEA) Amendments of 1991 (PL102–119) strengthened early intervention service provision through its emphasis on family-focused programming, prevention strategies, and better coordination of transition service.[22]

The risks and benefits of early intervention programs have been highlighted in numerous studies over the past decade. The authors of these reviews emphasize the following points:[22,28–37]

1. Identification of infants who will do poorly is complicated and must include assessment of the infant, the family, and the environment.

2. Early intervention programs are effective, particularly for children in whom biologic risk is compounded by environmental risk.

3. Structured programs that continue throughout childhood appear to have long-lasting effects, especially when they combine a child focus with a parent focus.

4. Initial gains in IQ scores may be transient, but other benefits, such as enhanced school performance, lower need for special education service, greater independence, and lower criminal activity, are evident in follow-up studies.

5. Earlier referral seems to be more effective than later intervention.

Early intervention programs for infants with developmental disabilities or those at high risk should be multi- or transdisciplinary in nature and include occupational and physical therapists, speech/language pathologists, and early-childhood specialists. These professionals provide therapeutic interventions to eliminate or minimize the diverse impairments that may be present across all developmental domains.[22,25,38] Programs that are most successful not only instruct and support parents in carrying out activities at home, but also help them to deal with irregularities of feeding, sleeping, crying, and other problems that lessen the chances of appropriate family functioning.[29]

Studying the effects of early intervention programs on children with established disabilities presents challenges, which include the following:

1. Unsuitability or lack of sensitivity of existing standardized measures

2. Ethical considerations, which limit the application of a control (no treatment), group

3. Heterogeneity of degree and type of disability in populations of interest

4. Small numbers of children available for study that meet selection criteria

5. Use of a structured, standardized curriculum, which is less likely to meet the individual treatment needs of disabled children.

There is, however, a general consensus that these programs help to improve the participants' functioning, particularly in terms of communication, socialization, and self-help skills, while providing considerable guidance and support to parents.

Therapeutic Treatment Approaches

The fundamental goals of therapeutic intervention for physical disabilities include prevention or correction of impairments that are secondary to the underlying pathologic condition or to normal physiologic adaptations superimposed on the pathologic condition.[39] Therapeutic intervention can take many forms, including traditional exercises, specific treatment approaches, and nontraditional treatment approaches.

Traditional Exercises

Traditional exercises aimed at increasing strength, improving joint range of motion, and building endurance have a place in the treatment of children. The applicability of traditional methods may be limited in infants and preschool-aged children because of the need for cooperation and participation in some forms of therapeutic exercise.[40] Strengthening activities may take the form of progressive resistive exercise, isometric, and/or isotonic training programs. Age-appropriate games, play, and toys may be used with younger children when working on strengthening activities.

It is important to assess strength accurately in children in order to identify deficits and document changes that occur as a result of intervention. Methods to assess strength include traditional procedures of manual muscle testing, use of hand-held dynamometers, and use of computerized isokinetic testing systems.[39] The reliability of strength assessments in children is questionable because they have difficulty understanding concepts about movement and position that are necessary for accurate testing of muscle strength.

Assessing strength in muscles with spasticity is controversial. In the past, spastic muscles were not tested because hypertonicity was believed to compromise the results.[39] Current practice usually combines a formal strength assessment if the child can assume the test position, combined with other measures of muscle performance, such as movement against gravity, reflex responses, and functional performance.

The normal movement of each body part maintains mobility of the joints and soft tissues. Limitation in range of motion is of greatest importance when it interferes with normal movements or activities. It is easier to prevent tightness by frequently repeating an activity or movement than to correct limitations after they have developed. It is important to perform range of motion exercises through the full arc of motion several times per day. It is equally important to use the available range of motion in functional activities throughout the course of a day. Parents should be instructed to include range of motion and functional activities in home exercise programs.

Assessment of range of motion is performed most commonly through the use of a universal goniometer. Numerous studies have reported on the reliability of goniometric measurement in adult populations.[41] Pediatric studies with normal children have indicated that range of motion measurement is valid, but studies of children with pathologic conditions have shown varied reliability.[42–47]

Passive stretching to increase range of motion should be slow and gentle with the child relaxed. Stretching should stop just short of the point that produces joint pain, with the exception of burn patients (refer to Chapter 17). Although the child may experience some discomfort from the stretch of soft tissue, there should be no residual pain when the stretching is discontinued. Steady, prolonged stretching is more effective than vigorous intermittent stretching. Stretching combined with heat is usually well tolerated and may enhance the effectiveness of therapy.

Children with motor disabilities have increased energy demands and must develop endurance and the ability to maintain static and dynamic muscle activity. Numerous activities, such as bicycling, stair climbing, rowing, and walking on a treadmill, may be added to a child's therapy program. Therapeutic interventions in the pediatric population must also include training in functional activities, use of adaptive equipment when necessary, and activities of daily living. Oral motor function is addressed later in this chapter.

Feeding, dressing, and personal hygiene are basic skills of concern. The child should be expected to perform skills or any part of a skill that he or she is capable of, not only during formal therapy sessions but also at home, in school, and in all other situations. Consistent practice enhances physical independence and self-reliance, and success will increase motivation for further development.

Therapeutic Treatment Approaches

Over the past 40 years many therapeutic treatment approaches (Table 7–3) have been developed. Most evolved empirically from clinical observations, and a theoretical framework was devised later to explain the possible neurophysiologic principles. To date, few controlled studies exist on the outcome of various treatment techniques despite proclamations by various proponents.[48,49] The variables discussed earlier regarding the study of early intervention programs for children with disabilities also come into play in attempts to study therapeutic methods.

There is little reliable scientific evidence or clinical observation to indicate superiority of one method over another. Basic assessment tools are lacking and, in many cases, may not be valid or reliable.[50] Assessment of developmental progress does not separate the effect of treatment from maturation in individual cases. For these reasons, long-term follow-up into adulthood would be necessary to establish the ultimate influence of different treatment methods in childhood.

Proprioceptive Neuromuscular Facilitation

Proprioceptive neuromuscular facilitation (PNF), developed by Kabat and further refined by Knott and Voss, is based on motor learning incorporating the patient's volitional control and aspects of movement that can be elicited without voluntary effort.[51–53] This method emphasizes the use of specific spiral and diagonal movement patterns observed in normal

TABLE 7–3. Therapeutic Treatment Approaches

Treatment Approach	Founder	Appropriate Age Group	Principal Diagnosis	Major Features	Points of Controversy
Proprioceptive neuromuscular facilitation (PNF)	Kabat, Knott, Voss	Older children, young adults	Any neurologic condition	Diagonal movement patterns facilitate proprioceptive system	
Rood method	Margaret Rood	Any age, any cognitive level	Any neurologic condition	Sensory and motor response, stimulation with brushing and ice, posture and movement linked	
Neurodevelopmental treatment (NDT) approach	Karl and Bertha Bobath	Children and adults with hemiplegia	Cerebral palsy or other neurologic conditions	Abnormal reflexes produce abnormal muscle tone; tone influenced by inhibition followed by facilitation of motor response	Some advocates believe only pure NDT should be practiced
Brunnstrom method	Brunnstrom	Any age	Any neurologic condition	Facilitation of muscle groups within synergy, progress toward development of voluntary control	Strengthening synergistic pattern questioned
Conductive education (CE)	Peto	Preschool–school age	Cerebral palsy or other neurologic conditions	Holistic experience combining educational and therapeutic approaches uses verbal reinforcement to facilitate motor response	Requires separate classroom setting; children not mainstreamed; less emphasis on attaining cognitive skills
Doman-Delacato method	Temple Fay, Doman, Delacato	Any age	Cerebral palsy or other neurologic conditions	Normal movement based on primitive patterns similar to amphibians, reptiles, etc.; moving children through patterns improves motor development	Relies on family members or volunteers to perform patterning, highly labor-intensive, cerebral oxygenation questioned
Vojta method	Vojta	Any age	Cerebral palsy	Common neurogenic pattern in subcortical area of brain is responsible for infant movement; provoking and activating reflex movement may lead to "postural ontogenesis" and locomotion	Basis of treatment theory considered by many to be questionable
Myofascial release					
Awareness through movement	Feldenkrais				

development. Many additional therapeutic modalities such as use of stretch, resistance, traction, and approximation are incorporated into the diagonal patterns to increase facilitation of the proprioceptive system.[54] The agonist–antagonist interplay is stressed in PNF through the use of inhibitory techniques such as contract–relax and hold–relax and facilitating techniques such as rhythmic stabilization and slow-reversal. The appropriate combinations of diagonal movement and the rate, specific range, and degree of volitional effort are determined by the therapist based on the needs and developmental level of the patient.[54] These techniques have been applied most often to older children or young adults.

Rood Method

Margaret Rood based her treatment concepts on normal development, differentiating four general stages: mobility, stability, mobility in weight-bearing pattern, and mobility in a non–weight-bearing pattern. Her approach places equal emphasis on both the sensory and motor aspects of movement.[55,56] Specific stimulation techniques, such as the use of stretch, resistance, vibration, vestibular stimulation, color, sound, brushing, and icing, are selected according to the response desired from the patient. Rood stresses the importance of "duality of motor function," emphasizing the link between posture and movement. Her treatment procedures are based on one or the other of the two systems. She recommends minimal conscious effort of the child and argues that her method works well with infants and children of low intelligence as well as those capable of full cooperation. Rood was among the first to speculate that a motor response is a sensory input or feedback for the next aspect of a motor output.

Neurodevelopmental Treatment

The neurodevelopmental treatment (NDT) approach, developed by Karl and Berta Bobath, is the most widely used method for pediatric patients, particularly for those with cerebral palsy. The NDT philosophy postulates that children need to experience and incorporate normal automatic movement in the proper developmental sequence before being asked to carry out a volitional activity.[54] Treatment is based on the premise that the chief obstacle to performance of the normal movement is an impairment of postural mechanisms. The NDT hypothesis states that abnormal reflex activity produces abnormal distribution of muscle tone; therefore, tone should be influenced by inhibiting the patterns of abnormal reflex activity.[57–60]

The aim of treatment in the NDT approach is to alter abnormal postures, reduce or increase tone, improve balance in antigravity postures, and develop fundamental movement patterns following the normal developmental sequence. Movements are controlled through proximal joints, head, shoulders, and pelvis and clearly stress the rotatory components. Aides such as large balls or bolsters are used to elicit righting and equilibrium reactions. Parents are strongly encouraged and trained to handle the child in the same manner at home during daily activities.[61]

Brunnstrom Method

Brunnstrom recommended facilitating a predictable synergistic pattern to produce purposeful motion by developing control of flexion and extension. This treatment approach suggests facilitating the predictable activation of muscle groups within the synergy, progressing to isolated motion independent of the reflex synergy, and finally moving to development of voluntary control.[62] Training is directed first toward control of the head and trunk and then toward proximal and distal movements.

Conductive Education

The method of conductive education (CE), pioneered in Hungary by Peto, is a system of education aimed at maximal integration of the child with disability. It attempts to provide a holistic developmental experience that involves integration of educational and therapeutic approaches.[63] Emphasis is placed on developing skills that allow both psychological and physical independence. Activities are carried out by a "conductor" trained in education and movement therapy. The conductors use equipment and methods, such as rhythmic intention, to verbally reinforce the intended motor behavior. The child is taught to perform motor skills through sequence and rhythm, which eventually lead to an unconscious control of sequencing the movement.[64]

In several studies recently conducted in Australia,[63,65] children participating in a program based on the principles of CE showed greater improvement in motor performance than the children in the control group. Significant improvement was noted in gross motor performance, fine motor performance, and activities of daily living. Caregiver ratings in both groups reported improvements in all categories over time. Caregivers in the CE group showed a more positive outlook with respect to parent and family problems. Children in both groups demonstrated significant improvement in all standardized and nonstandardized cognitive tests over time, with the control group showing a tendency for greater improvement. Both studies were limited by small sample size, the nature of the control group, and the lack of random assignment to CE and control groups.

Nontraditional Approaches

Doman-Delacato Method

Expanding on the ideas of Temple Fay,[66–68] Doman and his associates recommended a program using reflex behaviors to lead to normal processing in lower centers of the brain, which eventually lead to higher level of integration. This highly controversial[69–71] therapeutic method uses a series of patterns repeated many times throughout the day. Patterning refers to the emphasis placed on passively guiding the child's body through certain patterns. Continued performance is believed to result in improved function and strength of spastic muscles and in reduction of tone and postural disturbances. The Doman-Delacato system recommends periods of carbon dioxide rebreathing, ventilatory-assisted breathing to increase cerebral oxygenation, and fluid restrictions.

Vojta Method

Vojta described a method of treatment based on clinical experience that shows that movements that can be provoked and observed in the child with cerebral palsy also can be seen in healthy newborns. He theorized the existence of a common pattern in the subcortical area of the brain from which these originate. He postulated that a child with cerebral palsy may retain some movement patterns from the newborn period that may be provoked and activated.[72] One can apply these patterns to reflex locomotion to isolate different muscle functions in children with cerebral palsy. Using the system of reflex locomotion, the child can develop postural and locomotion ontogenesis.[72]

Nontraditional Pediatric Therapeutic Approaches

Several other techniques originally developed for treating adult movement disorders, such as craniosacral technique,[73] myofascial release,[74] and the Feldenkrais method,[75] are now being applied to children with neurologic disorders. Controlled efficacy studies are not available in any population.

Therapeutic Exercise in Specific Conditions Associated with Childhood Disabilities

Fundamental goals of therapeutic intervention for children with physical disabilities include preventing and/or correcting impairments. Another major goal of therapeutic exercise is normalizing the physiologic adaptations superimposed on the pathologic conditions. The impediments to function are secondary to the underlying pathologic condition. If impairments are prevented or corrected, then presumably function is enhanced and disability decreased. Accomplishing maximal range of motion by increasing the length of the muscle/tendon unit and achieving maximal strength are frequently two fundamental goals of therapeutic intervention. Accurate assessments of the range of motion, muscle strength, and the neurologic processes are vitally important. Once the assessments are formulated, those factors that are inhibiting the desired function are identified. Priorities are set to develop an improved functional level. Various movements are then broken down into simple motions that the

child can control or almost control during the session. The motions are then practiced repeatedly until control is precise and dependable. As performance improves, movements are combined and the complexity is increased. In general, therapeutic exercises are designed to meet the patient at his or her functioning level. The appropriate starting point for these exercises may be any of the general modes of intervention[40] listed below:

1. Training for improved motor function
2. Assisting function through human or specialized devices
3. Substituting for function by specialized devices
4. Limiting requirements by modifying the environment
5. Training for substitute functions to compensate for a deficit
6. Modifying anatomic or physiologic abnormalities through surgical procedures or medications.

There are number of specific disorders in which therapeutic exercises require special techniques and aids.

Therapeutic Exercise in Patients with Hypotonicity

Hypotonicity is decreased passive resistance to stretch by a muscle group upon external manipulation.[76] The decrease may result from a number of causes occurring in infancy and childhood, which include initial stages of stroke, traumatic brain injury, cerebral palsy, and many other neuromuscular diseases. When assessing muscle tone in infants, the examiner should observe spontaneous activity in various positions before starting to handle the child, because handling may suppress spontaneous activity. Movement often can be elicited through sounds, visual tracking, placing toys where the child must reach for them, tickling, placing limbs in antigravity positions to elicit holding responses, and moving limbs to end-range positions. Handling techniques to facilitate head and trunk control should not only be used during therapeutic sessions but also be taught to all caretakers. These techniques should include sitting opportunities for the patients in order to facilitate the development of head and trunk control. Paucity of movements typically results in the infant's remaining in one position, which leads to joint contractures. The contractures are frequently seen in hip abduction, knee flexion, and elbow flexion. There is also a risk of hip subluxation because of ligamentous laxity. Thus, a program of gentle range of motion (ROM), proper positioning, and facilitated movement is essential. Ideally, exercises should be planned to keep pace with the normal timing of development so that the child is provided with similar developmental experiences. A combination of neurodevelopmental treatment and proprioceptive neuromuscular facilitation techniques may be beneficial. Muscle tone requires reassessment at each visit because hypotonicity is often a precursor of hypertonicity.

Therapeutic Exercise in Patients with Hypertonicity

Hypertonicity is an increase in passive resistance to stretch by a muscle group upon external manipulation.[76] It can result in decreased joint ROM, which can improve with passive stretching.

In the older child excessive muscle tone is a significant factor impairing motor control. In this case, volitional inhibition of dystonia—relaxation—should be taught. Techniques for inducing relaxation as advocated by Jacobson,[77] Rood,[78] or Bobath[49] may be used to make the relaxation available during the learning process. Spasticity is velocity-dependent tone and a type of hypertonicity. It is seen in a number of childhood disorders, including spinal cord injury, cerebral palsy, traumatic brain injury, and myelodysplasia. When a noxious stimulus enters a spinal cord in which central inhibition is lacking, a spastic response is elicited. Proper positioning of the patient in the early part of the course tends to reduce the complications of spasticity. Proper positioning can be achieved in young patients with splints and appropriate seating equipment. Muscle stretching is particularly important in the therapeutic realm. Local therapy such as heat may be useful prior to stretching, but cold in various forms is not very effective because its benefits are transient and not well tolerated by children. The gastrocnemius muscle is often the first to develop contractures in the spastic/hypertonic patients. The use of nighttime ankle-foot orthoses (AFO) may bring great benefits to these children. For children who are ambulatory during daytime, AFO with a dynamic foot plate may be beneficial. Oral medications may be used in conjunction with stretching. Diazepam, dantrolene sodium, and baclofen are used with varying degrees of success in achieving the therapeutic goals. Injectable chemical blocking agents temporarily produce a reduction in spasticity and/or hypertonicity. The result is an increase in the range of motion. An example is purified botulinum toxin A that is injected into skeletal muscles to decrease spasticity temporarily. This delay often allows the patient to perform the desired exercises or positions. In severe spasticity, range of motion exercises as well as oral and even injectable agents are probably not of much benefit in preventing contractures. In such cases, more invasive surgical procedures are used. These include tenotomies, dorsal rhizotomies, or continuous intrathecal chemical blocks via an implantable catheter and pump. All of the procedures require postoperative therapeutic interventions for the child to gain and maintain functional goals.

Therapeutic Exercise in Patients with Neuromuscular Disease

Neuromuscular diseases include disorders of the lower motor neuron from the anterior horn cells to the neuromuscular junction and muscle. The basic clinical picture is one of weakness, reduction of muscle tone, decrease or absence of tendon reflexes, and eventually visible muscular atrophy. The most common neuromuscular disorders are Duchenne muscular dystrophy and spinal muscular atrophy. The extent of exercise in the management of muscular dystrophy is controversial, although it is well accepted that overexertion and immobilization are detrimental.[79,80] Low resistance and high repetition in a submaximal early exercise program have been shown to produce beneficial effects. Upper body strengthening to maintain activities of daily living as well as lower body strengthening for ambulation should be considered, but the effects on family dynamics need to be followed cautiously. A formal exercise program that is burdensome to the child and caretakers may be too disruptive,[81] and, in these cases, encouragement of swimming, cycling, or walking may be more appropriate.

Another important consideration in the therapeutic management of the young is the maintenance of lower extremity range of motion. Contractures of gastrocnemius-soleus and tensor faciae latae are seen early and may progress rapidly. A home program of stretching with emphasis on regular timing is important. Often stretching linked to a particular activity or time of day can be helpful, e.g., first thing in the morning and/or as part of the bedtime routine or after brushing teeth. Nighttime use of ankle-foot orthoses is useful in slowing down the progression of equinovarus contractures. Scott and associates[82] found that boys with Duchenne muscular dystrophy who followed a program of stretching and splinting maintained ambulation longer than those who did not.

Therapeutic Exercise in Patients with Joint Diseases

In evaluations of patients with joint impairments, a thorough evaluation of their joint range of motion, ligamentous laxity, muscle strength, postural deviations, and level of pain is necessary.

Juvenile rheumatoid arthritis (JRA) is the most common childhood joint disease. Immobility and pain are very challenging. Nighttime immobility may result in joint stiffness. Morning stiffness may last for up to 2 hours. A warm bath with slow active range of motion exercises often relieves this stiffness. Active ROM exercises are preferred to passive ROM. A patient should perform full ROM of all joints at least once a day. With the guidance of occupational and physical therapists, a combination of movements in play can be taught for efficiency and maximal cooperation. Abnormalities of the hip occur in about 35% of cases.[83] Coxa valga may occur in young children. Forces across the femoral epiphysis may cause a widening of the femoral neck, resulting in restricted motion.

Avascular necrosis also can occur, sometimes as a complication of corticosteroid use. The result is disabling hip pain and decreased function. Hip motion should be closely monitored because children with active hip disease often develop difficulty with ambulation. The most common cause of avascular necrosis of the femoral head in childhood is sickle cell disease.[84] This pathology produces restricted ROM and, often, hip flexion contractures. Typically, therapists use hydrotherapy, analgesic hot packs, and reciprocal relaxation techniques to accomplish effective range of motion and pain relief.

Oral Motor Dysfunction

Therapeutic exercise in pediatrics must also address any disability resulting from oral motor dysfunction. When a child or infant has difficulty with chewing and swallowing, feeding is not an enjoyable activity and frequently becomes a source of major parental concern or danger. Poor coordination of the suck-and-swallow pattern can prolong feeding time and lead to frustration of the child and family. Teaching the caretaker to reduce abnormal oral tone through adequate positioning and proper handling optimizes oral motor function. Reducing abnormal tone may be as easy as swaddling the infant with hips and knees flexed or quieting the feeding environment and minimizing distractions.[85] Then, oral motor stimuli can be used to encourage sucking and/or swallowing.

Impairment of speech production is a later manifestation of oral motor dysfunction; thus, a cooperative team effort from parents, the physiatrist, nurses, occupational therapist, speech-language pathologist, psychologist, and physical therapist is vital.

Use of Modalities

Biofeedback

Biofeedback therapy consists of monitoring physiologic information rapidly enough for a person to potentially self-regulate the physiologic process. Skin temperature, galvanic skin response (GSR), electrical conductance of the skin, and electromyography (EMG) of muscle activity are some of the more traditional ways to monitor patients. EMG feedback is used most commonly in children. Therapists use this technique to help educate patients with physical disabilities to improve their motor control. Examples of exercises in which neuromuscular teaching can be enhanced include isometric contractions, relaxation of tense muscles, reduction of antagonistic muscle contractions during attempts to passively stretch a painful joint, and muscle retraining. Muscle retraining is especially important in Guillain-Barré syndrome, brachial plexus injury, and spinal cord injury because it strengthens muscles without unwanted substitution by other muscles. The patient must cooperate with the therapist for these techniques to work. Adequate carry-over requires that the child practice the same movements in a functional activity.

Electrical Stimulation

Electrical stimulation (ES) is commonly used in physical therapy to treat neuromuscular conditions, enhance local circulation and tissue healing, decrease pain, and increase range of motion. Therapists also use ES to overcome spasticity. Traditionally, methods of electrical stimulation used to decrease spasticity include direct stimulation of the spastic muscles, stimulation of muscles antagonistic to the spastic muscles, or reciprocal stimulation of spastic muscles and their antagonists. Most studies have shown short time effects of treatment and lack of carry-over,[86–88] but more recently there have been reports of long-term functional gains. A pilot study using continuous nighttime low-intensity electrical stimulation, so low that the level of stimulation does not cause a fused muscle contraction, found functional improvements in children with mild cerebral palsy.[89] In addition, case reports indicate that there may be long-term functional gains in submaximal stimulation of muscles when actively working.[90,91]

Further research is needed to prove the long-term efficacy of this modality.

Muscle pain and spasm can be treated with either intermittent electrical stimulation or high-frequency stimulation. The intermittent electrical stimulation causes alternating muscle contraction and relaxation. Rhythmic activation of the muscles causes an increase in local circulation, helps to remove metabolic irritants, and provides a mechanical stimulation to muscle fibers. These intermittent contractions can act like the routine pumping action provided by walking and thus improve circulation to the area. High-frequency stimulation is used to elicit sustained and continuous muscle contractions. The goal is to induce fatigue in the muscle in spasm. The patient's tolerance and the predisposition of the muscle to local ischemia should be assessed carefully before this approach is used. Because sustained muscle contractions may impede normal blood flow to the area, lower stimulation frequencies should be used. This treatment is not well tolerated by young children.

However, transcutaneous electrical nerve stimulation (TENS) is well tolerated by adolescents. It consists of low-voltage pulses to the nervous system by skin electrodes and is particularly effective in traumatic peripheral nerve injury.[92] There have been many theories that have attempted to explain its efficacy; the best known is the gate-control theory,[93] which states that stimulation of non-nociceptors or their axons can interfere with the relay of sensation from nociceptors to higher centers in the brain where pain is perceived.[94]

Conclusion

Therapeutic interventions in the pediatric population must take into account the child's developmental stage, the interaction of experience and dysfunction, physiologic trends in growth, and realistic long-term expectations. Reasonable and well-timed application of treatment techniques and modalities used in the framework of normal development can lead to accomplishment of optimal functional skills and quality of life.

Pediatric physiatrists, working with physical and occupational therapists and speech pathologists, should continue to investigate treatment approaches in order to validate outcomes in the pediatric population.

References

1. Molnar GE, Taft LT: Pediatric Rehabilitation, part I: Cerebral palsy and spinal cord injury. Curr Probl Pediatr 1977;7:1.
2. Ratcliffe K: Clinical Pediatric Physical Therapy: A Guide for the Physical Therapy Team. St. Louis, Mosby, 1998.
3. Pearson PH, Williams CE: Physical Therapy Services in the Developmental Disabilities. Springfield, IL, Charles C Thomas, 1972.
4. Stout JL: Physical fitness during childhood and adolescence. In Campbell SK (ed): Physical Therapy for Children, Philadelphia, WB Saunders, 1994.
5. Pate RR, Shephard RJ: Characteristics of physical fitness in youth. In Gisolfi CV, Lamb DR (eds): Perspectives in Exercise Science and Sports Medicine, Vol. 2: Youth, Exercise, and Sports. New York, Plenum Press, 1989.
6. Malina RM: Growth of muscle and muscle mass. In Faulkner F, Tanner JM (eds): Human Growth: A Comprehensive Treatise, Vol. 2: Postnatal Growth. New York, Plenum Press, 1986.
7. Blimkie C: Age and associated variations in strength during childhood: Anthropometric, morphologic, neurologic, biomechanical, endocrinologic, genetic, and physical activity correlates. In Gisolfi CV, Lamb DR (eds): Perspectives in Exercise Science and Sports Medicine, Vol. 2: Youth, Exercise, and Sports. Indianapolis, Benchmark Press, 1989.
8. Molnar GE: A developmental perspective for the rehabilitation of children with physical disability. Pediatr Ann 1988;17:12.
9. Molnar GE: Rehabilitation benefits of sports for the handicapped. Conn Med 1981;45:574.
10. James W: The Principles of Psychology, Vol. 1. New York, Holt, 1890.
11. Sherrington CS: The Integrative Action of the Nervous System. New Haven, CT, Yale University Press, 1947. (Original work published 1906.)
12. Mott FW, Sherrington CS: Experiments on the influence of sensory nerves upon movement and nutrition of limbs: Preliminary communication. Proc R Soc Lond 1895;57:481.
13. DeLisa JA: Rehabilitation Medicine, 2nd ed. Philadelphia, JB Lippincott, 1993.
14. Marteniuk RG: Information Processing in Motor Skills. New York, Rinehart & Winston, 1976.
15. Sheridan MR: Planning and controlling simple movements. In Smyth MM, Wing AM (eds): The Psychology of Human Movement. London, Academic Press, 1984.
16. Schmidt RA: A schema theory of discrete motor skill learning. Psychol Rev 1975;82:225.
17. Hadders-Algra M, Brogren E, et al: Training affects the development of postural adjustments in sitting infants. J Physiol 1996;439:289.
18. Kelso JA: Anticipatory dynamical systems approach to motor development. Phys Ther 1990;70:763.
19. Kamm K, Thelen E, et al: A dynamical systems approach to motor development. Phys Ther 1990;70:763.
20. Doyon J: Skill learning. Int Rev Neurobiol 1997;41:273.
21. Karni A, Meyer G, et al: The acquisition of skilled motor performance: Fast and slow experience-driven changes in primary motor cortex. Proc Nat Acad Sci USA 1998;95:861.
22. Majnemer A: Benefits of early intervention for children with developmental disabilities. Semin Pediatr Neurol 1998;5:62.
23. Humphry R: Early intervention and the influence of the occupational therapist on the parent–child relationship. Am J Occup Ther 1989;43:738.
24. Lawlor MC, Henderson A: A descriptive study of clinical practice patterns of occupational therapists working with infants and young children. Am J Occup Ther 1989;43:755.
25. Bashir AS, Ferketic MM, et al: The roles of speech-language pathologists in service delivery to infants, toddlers, and their families (Position statement). Am Speech Hearing Assoc 1989;39:31.

26. Stephans LC, Tauber SK: Early intervention. In Case-Smith J, Allen AS, et al (eds): Occupational Therapy for Children. New York, Mosby, 1996.

27. Dunn W, Campbell PF, et al: Occupational therapy services in early intervention and preschool services (Position paper). Am J Occup Ther 1988;42:793.

28. Bauchner H, Brown E, et al: Premature graduates of the newborn intensive care unit: A guide to follow-up. Pediatr Clin North Am 1988;35:4.

29. Chamberlin RW: Developmental assessment and early intervention programs for young children: Lessons learned from longitudinal research. Pediatr Rev 1987;8:8.

30. Green M, Ferry P, et al: Early intervention programs: Where do pediatricians fit in? Contemp Pediatr 1987; March:92.

31. Palfrey J, Walker D, et al: Targeted early childhood programming. Am J Dis Child 1987;141:55.

32. Ross G: Home intervention for premature infants of low-income families. Am J Orthopsychiatry 1985;54:263.

33. Russman B: Early intervention for the biologically handicapped infant and young child: Is it of value? Pediatr Rev 1983;5:51.

34. Simeonson R, Cooper D, et al: A review and analysis of the effectiveness of early intervention programs. Pediatrics 1982;69:635.

35. Denhoff E: Current status of infant stimulation or enrichment programs for children with developmental disabilities. Pediatrics 1981;67:32.

36. Gomby D, Larner M, et al: Long-term outcomes of early childhood program: Analysis and recommendations. Future Child 1995;5:6.

37. Yoshikawa HL: Long-term effects of early childhood programs on social outcomes and delinquency. Future Child 1995;5:51.

38. Short-Degraff MA: Human Development for Occupational and Physical Therapists. Baltimore, Williams & Wilkins, 1988.

39. Gajdosik CG, Gajdosik RL: Musculoskeletal development and adaptation. In Campbell SK (ed): Physical Therapy for Children. Philadelphia, WB Saunders, 1994.

40. Kottke FJ, Lehmann JF (eds): Krusen's Handbook of Physical Medicine and Rehabilitation. Philadelphia, WB Saunders, 1990.

41. Gajdosik RL, Bohannon RW: Clinical measurements of range of motion: Review of goniometry emphasizing reliability and validity. Phys Ther 1987;67:1867.

42. Haley SM, Tada WL, et al: Spinal mobility in young children: A normative study. Phys Ther 1986;566:1697.

43. Pandya S, Florence JM, et al: Reliability of goniometric measurements in patients with Duchenne muscular dystrophy. Phys Ther 1985;65:1339.

44. Stuberg WA, Fuchs RH, et al: Reliability of goniometric measurements of hip motion in spastic cerebral palsy. Dev Med Child Neurol 1988;30:657.

45. Ashton BB, Pickles B, et al: Reliability of goniometric measurements of hip motion in spastic cerebral palsy. Dev Med Child Neurol 1978;20:87.

46. Bartlett MD, Wolf LS, et al: Hip flexion contractures: A comparison of measurement of procedures. Arch Phys Med Rehab 1985;66:620.

47. Harris SR, Smith LH, et al: Goniometric reliability for a child with spastic quadriplegia. J Pediatr Orthop 1985;5:348.

48. Palmer F, Shapiro B, et al: The effects of physical therapy on cerebral palsy. N Engl J Med 1988;188:13.

49. Wright T, Nicholson J: Physiotherapy for the spastic child: An evaluation. Dev Med Child Neurol 1973;15:146.

50. Evans PR, Dachs Pehm MA: Testing and Measurement in Occupational Therapy: A Review of Current Practice with Special Emphasis on Southern California Sensory Integration Test. Monograph No. 15, Institute for Research on Learning Disabilities. Minneapolis, University of Minnesota, 1981.

51. Kabat H: Proprioceptive facilitation in therapeutic exercise. In Licht S (ed): Physical Medicine Library III. New Haven, E. Licht Publications, 1961.

52. Knott M, Voss D: Proprioceptive Neuromuscular Facilitation. New York, Harper & Row, 1968.

53. Voss DE: Proprioceptive neuromuscular facilitation: The PNF method. In Pearson PH, Williams CE (eds): Physical Therapy Services in the Developmental Disabilities. Springfield, IL, Charles C Thomas, 1972.

54. Umphred D: An integrated approach to the treatment of pediatric neurologic patient. In Campbell S (ed): Pediatric Neurologic Physical Therapy. New York, Churchill Livingstone, 1984.

55. Gilette HE: Systems of Therapy in Cerebral Palsy. Springfield, IL, Charles C Thomas, 1974.

56. Rood MS: Neurophysiological mechanisms utilized in the treatment of neuromuscular dysfunction. Am J Occup Ther 1956;10:4.

57. Bobath B: Motor development: Its effect on general development and application to the treatment of cerebral palsy. Physiotherapy 1971;57:526.

58. Bobath B: The very early treatment of cerebral palsy. Dev Med Child Neurol 1967;9:373.

59. Bobath B, Bobath K: Motor Development in the Different Types of Cerebral Palsy. London, Heinemann, 1975.

60. Bobath K: The normal postural reflex mechanism and its derivation in children with cerebral palsy. Physiotherapy 1971;57:515.

61. Bobath K: A Neurophysiologic Basis for the Treatment of Cerebral Palsy. Philadelphia, JB Lippincott, 1980.

62. Brunnstrom S: Walking preparation for adult patients with hemiplegia. J Am Phys Ther Assoc 1965;45:17.

63. Catanese AA, Coleman GJ, et al: Evaluation of an early childhood programme based on principles of conductive education: The Yooralla project. J Paediatr Child Health 1995;31:418.

64. Hari M, Tillemans T: Conductive education. In Scrutton D (ed): Management of the Motor Disorders of Children with Cerebral Palsy. Philadelphia, JB Lippincott, 1984.

65. Coleman GJ, King JA, et al: A pilot evaluation of conductive education-based intervention for children with cerebral palsy: The Tongala project. J Paediatr Child Health 1995;31:412.

66. Fay T: Basic considerations regarding neuromuscular and reflex therapy. Spastic Aura 1954;29:327.

67. Fay T: Rehabilitation of patients with spastic paralysis. J Int Coll Surg 1954;22:200.

68. Fay T: Use of pathological and unlocking reflexes in the rehabilitation of spastics. Am J Phys Med 1954;33:347.

69. Cohen HJ, Birch HG, et al: Some considerations for evaluating the Doman-Delacato "patterning" method. Pediatrics 1970;45:302.

70. Freeman RS: Controversy over "patterning" as a treatment for brain-damaged children. JAMA 1967;202:385.

71. Sparrow S, Zigler E: Evaluation of a patterning treatment for retarded children. Pediatrics 1978;62:137.

72. Vojta V: The basic elements of treatment according to Vojta. In Scrutton D (ed): Management of the Motor Disorders of Children with Cerebral Palsy. Philadelphia, JB Lippincott, 1984.

73. Upledger J, Vrevevoogd J: Craniosacral Therapy. Seattle, Eastland Press, 1983.

74. Manheim C, Lavett D: The Myofascial Release Manual. Thorofare, NJ, Slack Inc., 1989.

75. Feldenkrais M: Awareness Trough Movement. New York, Harper & Row, 1977.

76. Gans BM, Glenn MB: Introduction. In Glenn MB, Whyte J (eds): The Practical Management of Spasticity in Children and Adults. Philadelphia, Lea & Febiger, 1990.

77. Jacobson E: Progressive Relaxation. Chicago, University of Chicago Press, 1931.

78. Stockmeyer SA: An interpretation of the approach of Rood to the treatment of neuromuscular dysfunction. Am J Phys Med 1967;46:900.

79. Dangain J, Vrobova G: Response of normal and dystrophic muscles to increased functional demand. Exp Neurol 1986;94:796.

80. Vignos PJ, Spencer GE, et al: Management of progressive muscular dystrophy. JAMA 1963:184:103.

81. Fowler WM: Rehabilitation management of muscular dystrophy and related disorders: I. The role of exercise. Arch Phys Med Rehabil 1982;63:208.

82. Scott OM, Hyde SA, et al: Prevention of deformity in Duchenne muscular dystrophy: A prospective study of passive stretching and splintage. Physiotherapy 1981;67:177.

83. Scull SA, Dow MB, et al: Physical and occupational therapy for children with rheumatic diseases. Pediatr Clin North Am 1986;33:1053.

84. Styles LA, Vichinsky EP: Core decompression in avascular necrosis of the hip in sickle-cell disease. Am J Hematol 1996;52:103.

85. Finnie N: Handling the Young Cerebral Palsied Child at Home. New York, EP Dutton, 1975.

86. Walker JB: Modulation of spasticity: A prolonged suppression of spinal reflex by electrical stimulation. Science 1982;216:203.

87. Bowman B, Bajd T: Influence of electrical stimulation on skeletal muscle spasticity. In Proceedings of the International Symposium on External Control of Human Extremities. Belgrade, Yugoslavia, Committee for Electronics and Automation, 1981;561.

88. Lee WJ, McGovern JP, et al: Continuous tetanizing currents for relief of spasm. Arch Phys Med 1950;31:766.

89. Pape KE, Kirsch SE, et al: Neuromuscular approach to the motor deficits of cerebral palsy: A pilot study. J Pediatr Orthop 1993;133:628.

90. Carmick J: Clinical use of neuromuscular electrical stimulation for children with cerebral palsy. Part 1: Lower extremity. Phys Ther 1993;73:505.

91. Carmick J: Clinical use of neuromuscular electrical stimulation for children with cerebral palsy. Part 2: Upper extremity. Phys Ther 1993;73:514.

92. Wall PD, Sweet WH: Temporary abolition of pain. Science 1967;155:108.

93. Melzack R, Wall PD: Pain mechanisms: A new theory. Science 1965;150:971.

94. Hecox B, Mehreteab TA, et al: Physical Agents. Stamford, CT, Appleton & Lange, 1994.

Chapter 8

Adapted Sports and Recreation

Ellen S. Kaitz, MD
Michelle A. Miller, MD

Adapted sports for the disabled were initiated in the midtwentieth century as a tool for the rehabilitation of injured war veterans. Adapted sports have blossomed to encompass all ages, abilities, and nearly all sport and recreational activities, from backyards to school grounds to national and Paralympic competitions. The trend has been away from the medical and rehabilitation roots to school-based and community-based programs focused on wellness and fitness, rather than illness and impairment. Rehabilitation professionals remain connected in a number of important ways. Sports and recreation remain vital parts of a rehabilitation program for individuals with new-onset disability. Furthermore, rehabilitation professionals may be resources for information and referral to community programs. They may be involved in the provision of medical care for participants or act as advisors for classification. As always, research to provide scientific inquiry in biomechanics, physiology, psychology, sociology, technology, sports medicine, and many related issues is a necessary component.

This chapter provides an introduction to adapted sports and recreation for physically disabled children and adolescents. It includes a history of sports for the disabled and a discussion of the benefits of sports. Because the field is so young, research in this area has been limited, both in quantity and in quality. The use of sports as therapy, highlighting equestrian and aquatic therapies, and the professionals who are most commonly associated with the field are presented, followed by principles and controversies in the classification of athletes. Finally, some *common* sports and recreation activities and their adaptations for disabled participants are summarized. The focus is on children with motor disabilities. Information regarding sports and recreation for those with sensory and mental or emotional disabilities is beyond the scope of this chapter. The reader is encouraged to use this chapter and the resources listed in the appendices as starting points for further exploration.

History

Sports and exercise have been practiced for millennia. Organized activities for adults with disabilities have more recent roots, going back to the 1888 founding of the first Sport Club for the Deaf in Berlin, Germany. The International Silent Games, held in 1924, was the first international competition for disabled athletes. Deaf sports were soon followed by the establishment of the British Society of One-Armed Golfers in 1932. Wheelchair sports are younger still, having parallel births in Britain and the United States in the mid-1940s. Guttman[1] at the Stoke Mandeville Hospital in Aylesbury, England, invented polo as the first organized wheelchair team sport: "It was the consideration of the overall training effect of sport on the neuromuscular system and because it seemed the most natural form of recreation to prevent boredom in hospital . . ." Within a year, basketball replaced polo as the principal wheelchair team sport. In 1948, the first Stoke Mandeville Games for the Paralyzed were held, with 16 athletes competing in wheelchair basketball, archery, and table tennis. This landmark event represented the birth of international sports competition for athletes with a variety of disabilities. The games have grown steadily, now comprising more than 24 different wheelchair sports. The competitions are held annually in non-Olympic years, under the oversight of the International Stoke Mandeville Wheelchair Sport Federation (ISMWSF).

While Guttman was organizing wheelchair sports in Britain, war veterans in California played basketball in the earliest recorded US wheelchair athletic event. Popularity of wheelchair sports flourished, and a decade later, the first national wheelchair games were held. These games included individual and relay track events. With the success of these games, the National Wheelchair Athletic Association (NWAA) was formed. Its role was to foster the guidance and growth of wheelchair sports. It continues in this role today under its new name, Wheelchair Sports USA.

The US teams made their international debut in 1960 at the first Paralympics in Rome. The term *paralympic* actually means *next to* or *parallel to* the Olympics. In the 40 years since, the number and scope of sport and recreational opportunities have blossomed. The National Handicapped Sports and Recreation Association (NHSRA) was formed in 1967 to address the needs of winter athletes. It has been reorganized as Disabled Sports USA (DSUSA). The 1970s saw the development of the US Cerebral Palsy Athletic Association (USCPAA) and US Association for Blind Athletes (USABA). In 1978, Public Law 95-606, the Amateur Sports Act, was passed. It recognized athletes with disabilities as part of the Olympic movement and paved the way for elite athletic achievement and recognition.

In the 1980s, a virtual population explosion of sport and recreation organizations occurred. Examples of these organizations include the US Amputee Athletic Association (USAAA), Dwarf Athletic Association of America (DAAA), and the US Les Autres Sports Association (USLASA), an association for those with impairments not grouped with any other sports organizations. Within these and many other organizations are sport-specific groups, which help to provide training, opportunity for competition, funding, and governance (Table 8–1). Examples include the American Wheelchair Bowling Association (AWBA), National Amputee Golf Association, US Quad Rugby Association (USQRA), and the Handicapped Scuba Association.

Although the history of sports for the disabled can be traced back a century, the development of junior-level activities and competition

TABLE 8–1. Governing Bodies and Sports Organizations for Some Common Sports for the Disabled in the United States

Sport	Able-Bodied National Governing Body	Disabled National Governing Body	DAAA	DSUSA	WSUSA	SOI	USCPAA	USLASA
Archery	National Archery Association	Wheelchair Archery USA		X	X		X	
Basketball	USA Basketball	National Wheelchair Basketball Association	X	X	X	X		
Bowling	American Bowling Congress, Women's International Bowling Congress	American Wheelchair Bowling Association				X	X	
Football	National College Athletic Association	N/A						
Hockey	N/A	SOI American Sled Hockey Association				X		
Quad rugby	N/A	US Quad Rugby Association			X			
Racquetball	American Amateur Racquetball Association	National Wheelchair Racquetball Association						
Road racing	USA Track & Field	Wheelchair Athletics of the USA			X	X		
Skiing	US Ski Association	DSUSA		X		X	X	
Soccer	US Soccer Federation	N/A				X	X	
Softball	Amateur Softball Association	National Wheelchair Softball Association	X			X		
Swimming	US Swimming	US Wheelchair Swimming	X	X	X	X	X	X
Table tennis	USA Table Tennis	American Wheelchair Table Tennis Association	X	X	X	X	X	X
Tennis	US Tennis Association	Wheelchair Tennis Players Association		X		X		
Track and field	USA Track & Field	Wheelchair Athletics of the USA	X	X	X	X	X	X
Volleyball	USA Volleyball	N/A	X	X		X		

DAAA, Dwarf Athletic Association of America; WSUSA, Wheelchair Sports USA; USCPAA, US Cerebral Palsy Athletic Association; DSUSA, Disabled Sports USA; SOI, Special Olympics International; USLASA, US Les Autres Sports Association.

can be measured only in a few short decades. The NWAA created a junior division in the early 1980s, which encompassed children and adolescents from 6–18 years of age. It has since established the annual Junior Wheelchair Nationals. Junior-level participation and programming have been adopted by many other organizations, including the National Wheelchair Basketball Association (NWBA), DSUSA, and American Athletic Association of the Deaf (AAAD). Sports for youth with disabilities are increasingly available in many communities through adapted physical education (APE) programs in schools, inclusion programs in scouting, Little League baseball, and other groups.

Benefits of Sports for the Disabled

The physical benefits of exercise in adults have been well documented. Adult paraplegic athletes have fewer medical complications, such as decubitus ulcers and urinary tract infections; less risk of myocardial infarction; and fewer physician office visits and hospitalizations.[2–5] Exercise has also been shown to improve strength, range of motion, and flexibility in persons with cerebral palsy.[6] Improved body self-image, socialization, and higher self-esteem have also been reported.[7] Adult disabled athletes are typically better educated, more satisfied with life, and happier than disabled nonathletes.[8]

Less information is available about the effect of sports and physical activity on disabled children. Children with disability generally have greater levels of dependency and more quiet leisure time pursuits, such as television watching, than their able-bodied peers.[9,10] A study of self-concepts in young disabled athletes showed scores similar to those of able-bodied peers, including subscores for appearance.[11] Others have shown differences between those with congenital and acquired disabilities, with the former showing more positive mood, higher self-esteem, and lower trait anxiety.[12] More studies are needed to explore the impact of sports on physical, psychological, and social health and function in children with disabilities.

Equestrian Therapy or Hippotherapy

Therapeutic horseback riding, or hippotherapy, has been popular in Europe since the 1950s and spread to the United States in the 1970s. It uses the rhythmic motions and warmth of the horse to work on the rider's tone, range of motion, strength, coordination, and balance. The movement of the horse actually produces a pattern of movements in the rider that is similar to

human ambulation.[13] The rider may sit or be placed in various positions on the horse's back or, alternatively, may perform active exercises while on horseback.

Children with any of a variety of disorders that affect muscle tone, strength, or motor skills may benefit from this form of therapy. These disorders include, but are not limited to, cerebral palsy, myelodysplasia, cerebrovascular accident, traumatic brain injury, spinal cord injury, amputations, neuromuscular disorders, and Down syndrome. A careful screen of individuals with spinal pathology should be performed to rule out instability before participation. This screening includes the Down syndrome population, in whom 15–20% have atlantoaxial instability.[14] In addition, cognitive or behavioral impairments should not be so severe that they place the rider or others at risk.

Many potential physical, cognitive, and emotional benefits of hippotherapy have been reported. These include improvements in tone, posture, balance, strength, gait, hygiene, attention, concentration, language skills, self-confidence, and peer relations.[13,15] Wingate,[16] working with seven children with cerebral palsy, reported subjective improvements in strength, balance, posture, range of motion at the knees and hips, and self-image. Bertoti,[17] also working with the cerebral palsy population, noted decreased spasticity and better balance as well as a statistically significant improvement in posture. Significant gains in both standing and quadruped balance have been demonstrated in children with Down syndrome.[18]

Aquatic Therapy

Water has been an important therapeutic medium for centuries. In pool therapy, the water's intrinsic buoyancy nearly eliminates the effects of gravity. Therefore, less effort is required for movement, and the weight borne on the extremities is minimized. As recovery progresses, activity in the water can be graded to provide varying amounts of resistance. The water temperature can also be therapeutic, with warmer water producing muscle relaxation. Finally, children often view the pool as fun rather than therapy and are often encouraged by the ability to perform movements in water that they are unable to do on land (Fig. 8–1).[19]

The most common indication for pool therapy is muscle weakness, although gains are also noted in range of motion, coordination, endurance, and normalization of tone. It has been recommended for children with cerebral palsy, neuromuscular disorders, spinal cord injuries, myelodysplasia,

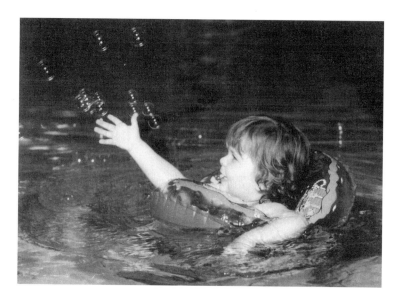

FIGURE 8–1. Aquatic therapy.

arthritis, brain injury, stroke, burns, fractures, and even asthma.[19] Children as young as neonates may benefit.[20] Aquatic therapy, however, is not indicated for everyone. Caution should be used in patients with hypertension or hypotension, open wounds, infective skin lesions, fever, or temperature instability.[19] It is contraindicated for children with uncontrolled seizures or excessive fear of the water, or whose cognitive status poses a safety risk for themselves or others.

There are a variety of approaches in aquatic therapy, including Bad Ragaz, Watsu, Halliwick method, Sequential Swim Techniques (SST), and task-specific approach.[21,22] Bad Ragaz is based on proprioceptive neuromuscular facilitation using active and passive techniques.[23] The Watsu approach is an energy-release technique in which a body segment is moved while the rest of the body is allowed to drag through the water, thus providing stretch.[24] The Halliwick method and SST work on distinct movement patterns with a specific goal such as swimming. The task-specific approach includes activities such as ambulation.[25]

Supportive literature for the benefits of aquatic therapy in the pediatric population is limited. Most studies report on aquatic therapy's effect on pulmonary function in the asthma, cystic fibrosis, and muscular dystrophy populations.[26,27] Endurance was increased and fewer exacerbations were noted in the asthma populations.[25] A significant increase in endurance but no objective change in pulmonary function tests was demonstrated in the cystic fibrosis population.[28] In children with muscular dystrophy, an increase in vital capacity was noted, although the study design was not optimal. Studies in the adult population have demonstrated relief of

pain, decreased spasticity, increased bone density, increased endurance, increased strength, improved range of motion, improved mood, and increased circulation.[25]

Adapted Sports and Recreation Professionals

Various fields provide training and expertise in adapted sports, recreation, and leisure. In pediatrics, they include APE teachers, child life specialists, and therapeutic recreation specialists. Physical and occupational therapists often incorporate sports and recreation into their treatment plans as well. Their involvement remains primarily within a medical framework, however, and is not discussed here.

APE developed in response to the Individuals with Disabilities Education Act, which states that children with disabling conditions have the right to free, appropriate public education in the least restrictive environment. Included in the law is *instruction in physical education*, which must be adapted and provided in accordance with the individualized education program. APE teachers receive training in identification of children with special needs, assessment of needs, curriculum theory and development, instructional design and planning as well as direct teaching.[29,30] The APE National Standards[31] were developed to outline and certify minimal competency for the field. The standards have been adopted by 15 states thus far. APE teachers provide some of the earliest exposure to sports and recreation for children with special needs and introduce the skills and equipment needed for future participation.

Therapeutic recreation had its roots in recreation and leisure. It provides recreation services to people with illness or disabling conditions. Stated in the American Therapeutic Recreation Association Code of Ethics, the primary purposes of treatment services are "to improve functioning and independence as well as reduce or eliminate the effects of illness or disability."[32] Clinical interventions used by therapeutic recreation specialists run the gamut from art, music, dance, and aquatic therapies to animal, poetry, humor, and play therapy. They may include yoga, tai chi, aerobic activity, and adventure training in their interventions. Although some training in pediatrics is standard in a therapeutic recreation training program, those who have minored in child life or who have done internships in pediatric settings are best suited for community program development. Therapeutic recreation specialists are often involved in community-based sports for the disabled, serving as referral sources, consultants, and support staff.

The child life specialty is quite different from therapeutic recreation. Its roots are in child development and in the study of the impact of hospitalization on children. Its focus remains primarily within the medical/hospital model, using health care play and teaching in the management of pain and anxiety and in support. Leisure and recreation activities are some of the tools used by child life specialists. In contrast to therapeutic recreation specialists, child life workers focus exclusively on the needs and interventions of children and adolescents. There is often overlap in the training programs of child life and therapeutic recreation specialists. The role of the child life specialist does not typically extend to community sports and recreation programs.

Classification Systems

Sport classification systems have been developed in an attempt to remove bias based on innate level of function. In theory, the systems would allow fair competition among individuals with a variety of disabilities. Early classifications were based on medical diagnostic groupings: one for athletes with spinal cord lesion, spina bifida, and polio (ISMWSF); one for ambulatory amputee athletes and a separate one for amputee athletes using wheelchairs; one for athletes with cerebral palsy (Table 8–2); one for les autres (International Sports Organized for the Disabled [ISOD]); and so forth. These early attempts reflected the birth of sports as a rehabilitative tool. This form of classification continues to be used in some disability-specific sports, such as beep ball for blind athletes and volleyball for amputee athletes (Table 8–3).

TABLE 8–2. Classification of Athletes with Cerebral Palsy (CP-ISRA)

Class	Description
C1	Quadriplegic, dependent on electric wheelchair or assistance for mobility
C2	Quadriplegic, poor functional strength in all extremities and trunk but able to propel a wheelchair
C3	Quadriplegic or severe hemiplegic, in a wheelchair with almost full upper extremity strength
C4	Good functional strength with minimal control problems in upper limbs and trunk
C5	May require the use of assistive devices in walking but not necessarily when standing or throwing
C6	All four limbs usually show functional involvement in sports movements, better functional control on dominant side
C7	Able to walk without assistive devices but may limp, good functional ability in dominant side of body
C8	Minimally affected, must have diagnosis of cerebral palsy or other nonprogressive brain damage with locomotor dysfunction

From US Olympic Committee, 1998.

With the growth of elite competitive sports came the need for more functionally based classification systems, which shifted the focus from disability to achievement. Functionally based classifications have the added advantage of reducing the number of classes for a given sport. This results in greater competition within classes and reduces the number of classes having only one or two competitors. Table 8–4 compares the older medically based classification with newer functional classifications of les autres.[33] Finally, classifications may be sport-specific, such as in basketball, quad rugby, and skiing (Table 8–5).

TABLE 8–3. Classification of Amputee Athletes

Class	Description
A1	Double AK—both legs amputated above the knee
A2	Single AK—one leg amputated above the knee
A3	Double BK—both legs amputated below the knee
A4	Single BK—one leg amputated below the knee
A5	Double AE—both arms amputated above or through the elbow joint
A6	Single AE—one arm amputated above or through the elbow joint
A7	Double BE—both arms amputated below the elbow, but through or above the wrist
A8	Single BE—one arm amputated below the elbow joint, but through or above the wrist
A9	Combinations of amputations of the upper and lower extremities

AK, above or through the knee joint; BK, below the knee, but through or above the talocrural joint; AE, above or through the elbow joint; BE, below the elbow, but through or above the wrist joint.
From US Olympic Committee, 1998.

TABLE 8–4. Comparison of Medical and Functional Classifications of Les Autres Athletes

	Medical Classification of Les Autres	
Level	**Athletes with**	**Examples**
L1	Severe involvement of all four limbs	Severe multiple sclerosis Muscular dystrophy Juvenile rheumatoid arthritis with contractures
L2	Severe involvement of three or all four limbs but less severe than L1	Severe hemiplegia Paralysis of one limb with deformation of two other limbs
L3	Limited functioning of at least two limbs	Hemiparesis Hip and knee stiffness with deformation of one arm
L4	Limited functioning in at least two limbs; limitations less than in L3	Contracture/ankylosis in joints of one limb with limited functioning in another
L5	Limited functioning in at least one limb or comparable disability	Contracture/ankylosis of hip or knee Paresis of one arm Kyphoscoliosis
L6	Slight limitations	Arthritis and osteoporosis Ankylosis of the knee

	Functional Classification of Les Autres (DSUSA, ISOD)
Level	**Description**
L1	Uses a wheelchair. Reduced function of muscle strength and/or spasticity in throwing arm. Poor sitting balance
L2	Uses a wheelchair. Good function in throwing arm and poor-to-moderate sitting balance or reduced function in throwing arm with good sitting balance
L3	Uses a wheelchair. Good arm function and sitting balance
L4	Ambulatory with or without crutches and braces or problems with balance together with reduced function in throwing arm
L5	Ambulatory with good arm function. Reduced function in lower extremities or difficulty in balancing
L6	Ambulatory with good upper extremity function in throwing arm and minimal trunk or lower extremity impairment

DSUSA, Disabled Sports USA; ISOD, International Sports Organized for the Disabled.
From US Olympic Committee, 1998.

The issue of inclusion in elite sports has been quite controversial. Debate exists not only within sports for the disabled, but also in the inclusion of disabled athletes in sports with able-bodied competitors. A few sports, such as archery, have now fully integrated able-bodied and disabled competitors. In sports such as marathon racing, the able-bodied athlete is at a distinct disadvantage, being unable to achieve the speeds or times of the wheelchair racer. Having classification systems and segregation in disabled sports allows for achievement based on ability rather than disability. Yet there continues to be a discrepancy between the recognition and reward for able-bodied and for disabled athletes. The issues of integration and classification have been identified as major research areas for the future.[34,35] Inclusion at the educational and recreational levels remains much more feasible through APE and community-based programs.

TABLE 8–5. Alpine Classes for Men and Women with Mobility-related Disabilities

Class	Description
Standing Classes	
L1	Disability of both legs, skiing with outriggers and using two skis or skiing on one ski using a prosthesis
L2	Disability of one leg, skiing with outriggers or poles and on one ski
L3	Disability of both legs, skiing on two skis with poles
L4	Disability of one leg, skiing on two skis with poles
L5	Disability of both arms or hands, skiing on two skis with no poles
L6	Disability of one arm or hand, skiing on two skis with one pole
L9	Disability of a combination of arm and leg, using equipment of choice
Mono-ski Classes	
L10	All athletes above T-10 inclusive with involvement of upper limbs and little or no sitting balance and all athletes with spinal cord level above T-10 with major disability of one arm
L11	Athletes with spinal cord level below T-10 through LS, double above-knee amputations, and other neurologic conditions

From Disabled Sports USA.

SPORTS

Archery

With the exception of the adaptive equipment, archery is essentially unmodified. It is a popular recreational and competitive activity in which individuals with virtually any disability can participate (Fig. 8–2).

Equipment

Trigger release or release cuff—designed for individuals with a poor grasp or weakness; assists in the smooth draw and release of the bowstring. Its use is permitted in sanctioned competition only by those with tetraplegia from cerebral palsy or a spinal cord injury.

Wrist and elbow supports—provide support and stability for the bow arm.

Standing supports—give the wheelchair user a choice between sitting and standing while shooting.

Bow supports—provide support and stability of the bow for individuals with weakness or a poor grasp. Its limited use is permitted only in USCPAA competition.

Crossbows and compound bows—for recreational use primarily, although compound bows are allowed in USCPAA competition.

Mouth pieces—allow archers with upper extremity impairments to draw the bowstring with the mouth.[36]

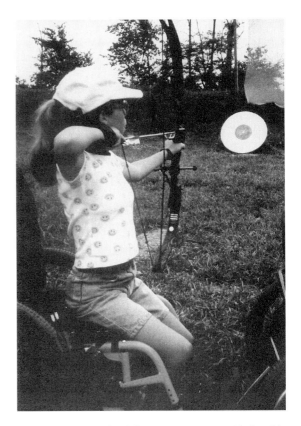

FIGURE 8–2. Wheelchair users compete side-by-side with able-bodied archers.

Basketball

Basketball may be played either as an ambulatory or a wheelchair sport. Teams of five play on a regulation basketball court following National Collegiate Athletic Association (NCAA) rules with only slight modifications to accommodate the wheelchairs. The NWBA uses a classification point system during competition. A junior program was developed by NWBA with four divisions each having different age requirements, ball sizes, court measurements, time restrictions, and basket heights. It is a popular sport spanning all disabilities. Adapted versions with no contact, no running, no dribbling, or lower baskets are useful for developing skills.[36]

Equipment

Sports wheelchair, basketball.

Super Sport—upper extremity prosthesis designed for ball sports.[37]

Bowling

Rules for competitive bowling may be divided into three divisions: AWBA, Special Olympics, and USCPAA. Lane measurements, rules, and bowling balls are the same as in the able-bodied population under the AWBA. Assistive devices, such as a handle ball, bowling stick, and bowling prosthesis, are allowed. Under the Special Olympics, target bowl and frame bowl are also allowed. Target bowl uses regulation pins, a 2-pound bowling ball, and a carpeted lane that is half regulation length. Frame bowl uses plastic pins and ball and a shortened lane. Under the USCPAA, there are four divisions, with a ramp or chute allowed in divisions A and B. Bowlers with a CP classification of 3–6 participate in division C. Division D is composed of classes 7 and 8. Other rules follow the AWBA recommendations.

Equipment

Handle ball—a bowling ball with a spring-loaded retractable handle for individuals with poor finger control.

Bowling stick—a two-pronged stick similar in appearance to a shuffleboard stick.

Bowling ramp/chute—a wooden or metal ramp down which bowlers can push the ball using their hands, feet, or a head stick.

Bowling prosthesis—attaches to a standard prosthetic wrist and fits into one of the holes of the bowling ball. It has a release mechanism activated by stretch on the expansion sleeve.[36]

Football

Rules for wheelchair football vary from league to league. There is one national competition, the Blister Bowl, which is held in California. There are six players per team, one of whom must be female or quadriplegic. The asphalt field measures 60×25 yards and is divided into 15-yard segments. Play follows NCAA rules and is similar to touch football with players advancing the ball by running or passing. All players are eligible receivers. Four 15-minute quarters are played. Participants primarily include individuals with amputations, cerebral palsy, spinal cord injury, and les autres.

Equipment

Sports wheelchair, regulation football[36]

Hockey

Floor hockey is in some respects similar to ice hockey. It is played in a gymnasium with a minimal playing area of 12×24 m and a goal at each end. Teams are composed of six players who play three 9-minute periods. The puck is a felt disc, and hockey sticks are wood or fiberglass rods. Games may be either ambulatory or played from wheelchairs. A similar sport, poly hockey, uses a hard plastic puck, a smaller plastic version of the conventional ice hockey stick, and a playing area measuring 12×24 m at a maximum. Canada has further developed a version for power wheelchair users using a 3-inch plastic ball rather than a puck and following National Hockey League (NHL) rules. Sledge hockey (sled hockey in the United States) is played on a regulation-sized ice rink using a standard puck or small ball and short sticks called *pics*. Players are seated on a sledge, which is an oval-shaped frame with two skatelike blades and a runner. Pics are used to propel as well as to advance the puck or ball.

Equipment

Hockey sticks / pics	*Knee pads*
Puck / ball	*Elbow pads*
Goals	*Shin guards*
Helmet	*Sled / sledge*[36]

Quad Rugby

Quad rugby combines aspects of basketball, hockey, and soccer into an exciting sport developed for tetraplegic individuals. It is played with a volleyball on a regulation-size basketball court with goals at both ends measuring 8×1.75 m. Teams consist of four players in manual wheelchairs who play four 8-minute quarters. Players are classified from 0.5 to 3.5 in 0.5 increments based on increasing arm function and trunk control. The combined point value of players on the floor may not exceed 8.0 at any time. The ball must be advanced over midcourt within 15 seconds of possession, and the ball must be bounced or passed within 10 seconds. A goal is scored when two of the player's wheels cross the goal line with the volleyball under control. Penalties may result in loss of possession or a trip to the penalty box, depending on the infraction.

Equipment

Volleyball
Gloves
Straps (trunk, legs, feet)
Quad rugby wheelchair—must have antitippers

Racquetball

Racquetball may be either an ambulatory or a wheelchair sport. It is played on a regulation-sized racquetball court and follows the rules of the American Amateur Racquetball Association. There are novice, intermediate, open, junior, two-bounce, and multiple-bounce divisions. It is recommended that players using wheelchairs equip their chairs with roller bars or wheels under the footrest and with nonmarking tires. Racquetball is one of the few sports in which disabled and able-bodied players can play side-by-side.

Equipment

Standard racquet—a built-up grip or wrapping the handle to the player's hand may be required for those with grip difficulties.
Standard balls, lightweight sports wheelchair.[36]

Road Racing

As running has increased in popularity as a recreational and competitive sport, disabled athletes have formed their own running clubs and begun to participate in a variety of road races. Training is usually done on the road or a track. For the wheelchair road racer, rollers are also available. The racing chair is placed on the rollers allowing for free-wheeling and training indoors. The rules for road racing are no different between the able-bodied and disabled populations; whoever crosses the finish line first wins. Disabled athletes are placed in functional classes to make the competition more equitable. Power wheelchairs are not permitted in competition. Distances range from the 1-mile fun runs to full marathons. Many of the well-known marathons for able-bodied athletes now include one or more wheelchair divisions. The longest wheelchair race to date is the Midnite Sun

Wheelchair Marathon, which covers 367 miles from Fairbanks to Anchorage, Alaska.

Equipment

Sports wheelchair—customized racing wheelchairs are available for serious athletes; three-wheelers are most popular

Gloves[36]

Skiing and Slalom

In the past 30 years, adaptive skiing has grown immensely in popularity. With the advances in adaptive equipment, all disability groups can participate in this sport. Skiing techniques include three-track, four-track, and sit-skiing. Three-trackers use one ski and two outriggers, thus creating three tracks in the snow. Outriggers are essentially modified Lofstrand crutches with short skis attached with a hinge. They provide additional balance and steering maneuverability. Single-leg amputees and individuals with hemiplegia are often three-trackers. Four-trackers use two skis and two outriggers. In those with spasticity or poor leg control, a ski bra can be attached to the ski tips (Fig. 8–3). This prevents the ski tips from crossing. Individuals with muscular dystrophy, spina bifida, paraplegia, and cerebral palsy typically use four-track skiing. Sit-skiing uses a mono-ski or bi-ski and two outriggers (Fig. 8–4). All disability groups can sit-ski. A tether, which allows the instructor to slow the skier down, is required until the sit-ski is mastered. Tethers can also be beneficial during instruction in the ambulatory population (Fig. 8–5). Competitive racing includes slalom and downhill courses.

Equipment

Outriggers, skis, ski bra, ski boots.
Ski Hand/All-Terrain Ski Terminal Device—specialized terminal device for upper limb amputees.
Ski leg—a variety of ski-specific lower extremity prostheses are available.[36,38]

Soccer

There are few modifications to the actual game of soccer, and the rules of the US Soccer Federation are followed. The modifications include seven players on a team, a smaller field measuring 80 × 60 m, and occasionally a smaller goal. These modifications result from fewer participants in a given area. A smaller goal is indicated in the cerebral palsy population, in whom mobility impairments make a larger goal more difficult to defend. Crutches have been allowed

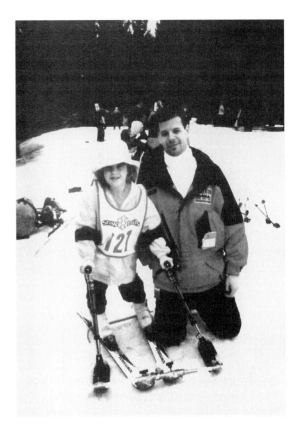

FIGURE 8–3. Four track skiing. Note that a simple ski bra can be fabricated with a dowel and heavy-duty (duct) tape.

for some competitors with lower extremity amputations who do not use a prosthesis.

Equipment

Regulation-sized soccer ball.
Super Sport—upper extremity prosthesis designed specifically for ball handling.[36]

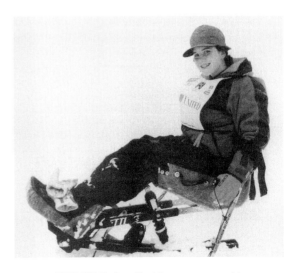

FIGURE 8–4. Sit-skier on a mono ski.

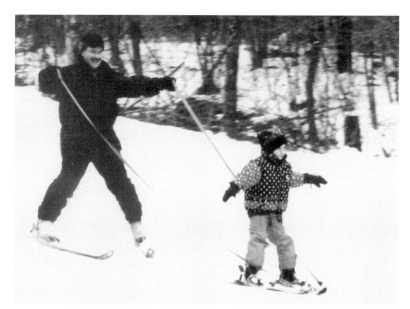

FIGURE 8–5. Ambulatory skier using a tether.

Softball

Dwarf softball is played according to the rules of the Amateur Softball Association without any modifications. The Special Olympics offers a variety of competitive events, including slow-pitch softball and tee-ball. Wheelchair softball is also available primarily for individuals with spinal cord injuries, amputations, cerebral palsy, or les autres conditions. It is played on a hard surface with the pitching strip 28 feet from home base and other bases 50 feet apart. Players must use a wheelchair with a foot platform and are not allowed to get out of their chairs. Ten players make up a team, and one of the players must be quadriplegic. The WS/USA point classification is used, and total team points on the field may not exceed 22. A larger ball is used, eliminating the need for a mitt which would interfere with propelling.

Equipment

Softball, mitt.
Prostheses—upper extremity terminal devices that fit into a mitt or substitute for a mitt are available. A set of interlocking rings can also be attached to the bottom of a bat allowing an adequate grip by a prosthetic hand.[36]

Swimming

Swimming is a universal sport in which all disability groups may participate. There are numerous competitive events offered across the United States. These include races of a variety of distances in freestyle, breast stroke, backstroke, butterfly, individual medley, freestyle relay, and medley relay. Classification systems have been developed by each disabled sports organization to divide participants into classes based on function. In addition, swimmers are grouped according to gender and age. Flotation devices are often recommended, although allowed in competition only in two USCPAA classes. Flotation devices include tire tubes, inflatable collars, waist belts, life vests, head rings, water wings, and personal flotation devices. The use and choice of device depend on swimming ability, swimming style, and experience.

Equipment

Flotation device, lift, or ramp.
Prosthetics—include swim fins attaching to lower extremity prosthetic sockets and swimming hand prostheses. These are generally not allowed in sanctioned competition.[36]

Table Tennis

Only slight modifications involving the delivery of the serve differentiate table tennis for the disabled from able-bodied competition, which follows US Table Tennis Association rules. The only equipment modifications allowed are to the paddle and, in the case of dwarf competition, floor raisers to make up for height differences. In recreational play, side guards may be added to the table to keep the ball in play longer.

Equipment

Velcro strap or cuffs—allow correct placement of the paddle in the player's hand.
Regulation-sized table, paddles, ball.[36]

Tennis

Wheelchair tennis is played on a regulation-sized tennis court as either a singles or doubles game. Players are allowed a maximum of two bounces before the ball must be returned. Scoring and other rules follow the US Tennis Association guidelines. Players are broadly divided into two groups: paraplegic and tetraplegic. Within these divisions, players compete in subdivisions based on their skill. This sport is open to all disability groups.

Equipment

Sport wheelchair, tennis racquet.
Straps (trunk, legs, feet).
Racquet holder—ace wrap or taping may provide additional support of grip strength if needed. Alternatively a racquet holder orthosis may be beneficial.[36]

Track and Field

Track and field events are some of the most popular of the adapted sports competitions and involve individuals from all disability groups. Track events may be ambulatory or at the wheelchair level. Ambulatory and wheelchair events range in distance from 10 m to a full marathon and take place on a typical track. Running, walking, and hurdles are all included in the ambulatory division. Power and manual wheelchair slalom races are available in the Special Olympics.

Field events typically include shot put, discus, javelin, long jump, and high jump. The USCPAA has also developed seven events for athletes who are more physically impaired. These include the distance throw, soft discus, precision event, high toss, thrust kick, distance kick, and club throw. In the distance throw, athletes throw a soft shot as far as possible. The soft discus is similar to the conventional discus except that the discus is made of a cloth material. For the precision event, six soft shots are thrown at a target with points awarded for accuracy. The high toss involves throwing a soft shot over a progressively higher bar. Athletes have three attempts to clear the height. In the thrust kick, athletes kick a 6-pound medicine ball away from them with their foot in constant contact with the ball. The distance kick is similar, although it uses a 13-inch rubber ball and allows the athlete to initiate a back swing with the foot before striking the ball. For the club throw, an Indian club is thrown as far as possible. As in other sports, participants are divided according to functional classification.

Equipment

Racing gloves.
Sport wheelchair—custom-designed racing chairs are available for the serious athlete.
Throwing chair—provides a stable platform from which athletes may throw.[36]

Recreation

Cycling

Cycling is immensely popular as both a recreational and a competitive activity. There are a variety of adaptations possible to make cycling accessible to a whole range of abilities. Children's tricycles may have blocks, straps, or shoe holders attached to pedals. Backrests and harnesses can be added to the seat to aid in positioning and stability. Adult-sized tricycles can be similarly adapted. Specialized terminal devices for upper limb prostheses make grasping handlebars easier, and both brakes can be controlled by one hand for safety. Arm-driven cycles with rowing or with push-pull drives assist individuals with lower limb impairment or absence. Recumbent cycles afford maximal trunk support for recreational use by those with poor balance as well as by able-bodied riders. Arm-driven units that attach to the front of a wheelchair frame are available with 3 to as many as 48 speeds. Finally, a variety of tandem cycles or tandem conversion kits are on the market. These range from simple tandems to hybrid hand and leg cycles that allow disabled and able-bodied to ride together. [36]

Outdoor Adventure—Land

Camping, mountaineering, hunting, and hiking are among the many outdoor adventure activities available to children with disabilities. The National Park Service maintains information on park accessibility and amenities across the United States. The Golden Access Passport is available to any blind or permanently disabled individual and allows free lifetime admission to all National Parks for the individual and accompanying passengers. It is obtained at any federal fee area and allows a 50% reduction in fees for recreation sites, facilities, equipment, or services at any federal outdoor recreation area.

Boy and Girl Scouts of America each run inclusion programs for children with disabilities. Opportunities also exist in dozens of adventure and specialty camps across the United States. Some are geared to the disabled and their families, allowing parallel or integrated camping experiences for disabled children. Participation requires few adaptations, and the Americans with Disabilities Act has been instrumental in improving awareness in barrier-free design for trails, campsites, and restrooms.

Outdoor Adventure—Water Sports

Rowing, sailing, canoeing, kayaking, and white-water rafting have become increasingly accessible. Modified seats and stabilizers have allowed even those with high tetraplegia to participate. Splints, gloves, straps, and elastic wraps have been devised for securing oars to the hands. Oars have also been modified for one-handed use or can be more easily grasped using specialized terminal devices. Prosthetic users generally wear suspension harnesses outside their clothing for quick doffing in the event of an emergency. Safety mandates that all participants wear flotation devices; helmets are also recommended. In colder water or climates, wet suits may be needed to prevent hypothermia. Padding of seats and lower limbs may be necessary for those with impaired sensation.

Adaptations similar to those for snow skiing have made water skiing accessible to the disabled. Sit-skis with trunk supports and stabilizing outriggers compensate for weakness or impaired balance, and attachments for tow ropes assist those with hand and arm impairments (Fig. 8–6).

Fishing

Fishing can be enjoyed by virtually anyone regardless of ability. One-handed reels, electric reels, and even sip-and-puff controls allow independent participation. A variety of options exist for grasping and holding rods as well. These range from simple gloves that wrap the fingers and secure with Velcro or buckles to clamps that attach directly to the rod, allowing a hand or wrist to be slipped in. Harnesses can attach the rod to the body or to a wheelchair, assisting those with upper limb impairments. There are devices that assist in casting as well for individuals with limited upper body strength or control. Depending on the level of expertise and participation of the fisherperson, simple or highly sophisticated tackle can also be had.[36,39]

Both land and sea fishing opportunities are accessible to the disabled. Piers are usually ramped and may have lowered or removable rails for shorter or seated individuals. Boats with barrier-free designs offer fishing and sightseeing tours at many larger docks. These offer variable access to one or all decks, toilet facilities, and shade. [36]

Scuba Diving

Freedom from gravity makes underwater adventure appealing to individuals with mobility impairments. Little adaptation to equipment is needed to allow older children and adolescents with disabilities to experience the underwater world (Fig. 8–7). Lower limb-deficient children may dive with specially designed prostheses or with adapted fins or may choose to wear nothing on the residual limb. They, similar to those with lower limb weakness or paralysis, may use

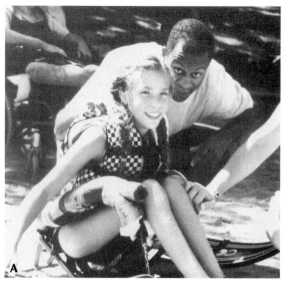
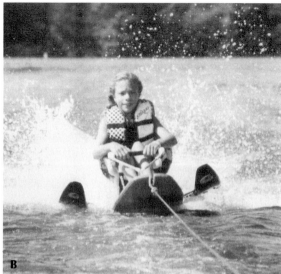

FIGURE 8–6. A, Water skiing on a sit-ski. Note the additional padding around the trunk and legs. B, Outriggers assist with balance, and a groove in the ski helps to guide and hold the tow rope.

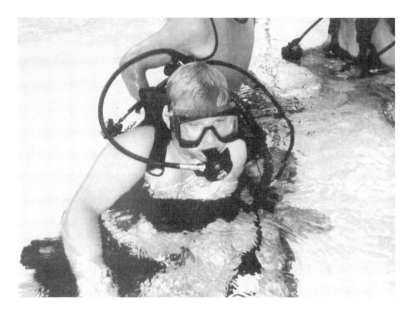

FIGURE 8–7. Scuba diving. Initial training is often done in a swimming pool.

paddles or mitts on the hands to enhance efficiency of the arm stroke. Of particular importance is the maintenance of body temperature, especially in individuals with neurologic disability, such as spinal cord injury or cerebral palsy. Wet or dry suits provide insulation for cool or cold water immersion. They also provide protection for insensate skin, which can be easily injured on non-slip pool surfaces, coral, and water entry surfaces.[36]

It is crucial that individuals receive proper instruction by certified dive instructors. Most reputable dive shops can provide information and referral. The Handicapped Scuba Association is an excellent reference as well (Appendix B). Disabled divers are categorized based on level of ability. They may be allowed to dive with a single buddy (as with able-bodied divers), two buddies, or two buddies, of which one buddy is trained in emergency rescue techniques. Although there is no particular exclusion from diving based solely on disability, there are a number of medical considerations that may preclude scuba diving, including certain cardiac and pulmonary conditions, poorly controlled seizures, and use of some medications. Discussion with the primary care physician and with dive instructors should precede enrollment or financial investment. Scuba diving has also been used as adjunctive therapy in acute rehabilitation programs.[40]

Conclusion

Whether for socialization, general fitness, or elite competition, sports and recreational pursuits are important components of a well-rounded lifestyle. Advances in attitudes, equipment, and technology have paved the way for participation by those with even the most profound disabilities. Appendices A and B provide resources for more detailed study.

Acknowledgment

The authors wish to thank Steve Ricker and the members of The Adaptive Adventure Sports Coalition (TAASC), 833 Eastwind Dr., Suite 1, Westerville, OH 43081, for their contributions of photographs used in Figures 8–2 through 8–6.

References

1. Guttman L: Textbook of Sport for the Disabled. Aylesbury, England, HM&M, 1976.
2. Brenes G, Dearwater S, Shapera R, et al: High density lipoprotein cholesterol concentrations in physically active and sedentary spinal cord injured patients. Arch Phys Med Rehabil 1986;67:445.
3. Dearwater SR, LaPorte RE, Robertson RJ, et al: Activity in the spinal cord-injured patient: An epidemiologic analysis of metabolic parameters. Med Sci Sports Exerc 1986;18:541.
4. Hooker SP, Wells CL: Effects of low- and moderate-intensity training in spinal cord injured persons. Med Sci Sports Exerc 1989;21:8.
5. Stotts KM: Health maintenance: Paraplegic athletes and non-athletes. Arch Phys Med Rehabil 1986;7:109.
6. Holland LJ, Steadward RD: Effects of resistance in flexibility training and strength, spasticity/muscle tone and range of motion of elite athletes with cerebral palsy. Palestra 1990;Summer:27.
7. Horvat M, French R, Henschen K: A comparison of the psychologic characteristics of male and female able-bodied and wheelchair athletes. Paraplegia 1986;24:115.
8. Valliant PM, Bezzubyk I, Daley L, Asu ME: Psychological impact of sport on disabled athletes. Psychol Rep 1985;56:923.
9. Brown M, Gordon WA: Impact of impairment on activity patterns of children. Arch Phys Med Rehabil 1987;68:828.

10. Margalit M: Leisure activities of cerebral palsied children. Isr J Psychiatry Relat Sci 1981;18:209.
11. Sherrill C, Hinson M, Gench B, et al: Self concepts of disabled youth athletes. Percept Motor Skills 1990; 70:1093.
12. Campbell E: Psychological well-being of participants in wheelchair sports: Comparison of individuals with congenital and acquired disabilities. Percept Motor Skills 1995;81:563.
13. DePauw KP: Horseback riding for individuals with disabilities: Programs, philosophy, and research. Adapted Physical Activity Quarterly 1986;3:217.
14. Cooke RE: Atlantoaxial instability in individuals with Down's Syndrome. Adapted Physical Activity Quarterly 1984;1:194.
15. Fox VM, Lawler VA, Luttges MW: Pilot study of novel test instrumentation to evaluate therapeutic horseback riding. Adapted Physical Activity Quarterly 1984;1:30.
16. Wingate L: Feasibility of horseback riding as a therapeutic and integrative program for handicapped children. Phys Ther 1982;62:184.
17. Bertoti DB: Effect of therapeutic horseback riding on posture in children with cerebral palsy. Phys Ther 1988;68:1505.
18. Biery MJ, Kauffman N: The effects of therapeutic horseback riding on balance. Adapted Physical Activity Quarterly 1989;6:221.
19. Basmajian JV: Exercises in water. In Basmajian JV (ed): Therapeutic Exercise, 5th ed. Baltimore, Williams & Wilkins, 1990.
20. Sweeney JK: Neonatal hydrotherapy: An adjunct to developmental intervention in an intensive care nursery setting. Phys Occup Ther Pediatr 1983;3:39.
21. Boyle A: The Bad Ragaz ring method. Physiotherapy 1981;67:265.
22. Dull H: WATSU: Freeing the Body in Water. Middletown, CA, Harbin Springs Publishing, 1993.
23. Campion MR: Hydrotherapy in Pediatrics. Oxford, Heinemann Medical Books, 1985.
24. Carter MJ, Dolan MA, LeConey SP: Designing Instructional Swim Programs for Individuals with Disabilities. Reston, VA, American Alliance for Health, Physical Education, and Dance, 1994.
25. Broach E, Dattilo J: Aquatic therapy: A viable therapeutic recreation intervention. Therapeutic Recreation Journal 1996;30:213.
26. Bar-Or O, Inbar O: Swimming and asthma: Benefits and deleterious effects. Sports Med 1992;54:397.
27. Adams MA, Chandler LS: Effects of physical therapy program on vital capacity of patients with muscular dystrophy. Phys Ther 1974;54:494.
28. Edlund LD, French RW, Herbst JJ, et al: Effects of a swimming program on children with cystic fibrosis. Am J Dis Child 1986;140:80.
29. Heikinaro-Johansson P, Vogler EW: Physical education including individuals with disabilities in school settings. Sport Sci Rev 1996;5:12.
30. Doll-Tepper G, DePauw KP: Theory and practice of adapted physical activity: Research perspectives. Sport Sci Rev 1996;5:1.
31. NCPERID (National Consortium for Physical Education and Recreation for Individuals with Disabilities): APE National Standards. Champaign, IL, Human Kinetics, 1991.
32. Standards for the Practice of Therapeutic Recreation and Self-Assessment Guide. Hattiesburg, MS, American Therapeutic Recreation Association, 1993.
33. DePauw KP, Gavron SJ: Disability and Sport. Champaign, IL, Human Kinetics, 1995.
34. Vanlandewijck YC, Chappel RJ: Integration and classification issues in competitive sports for athletes with disabilities. Sport Sci Rev 1996;5:65.
35. Steadward RD: Integration and sport in the Paralympic movement. Sport Sci Rev 1996;5:26.
36. Paciorek MJ, Jones JA (eds): Sports and Recreation for the Disabled, 2nd ed. Indianapolis, Masters Press, 1994.
37. Radocy B: Upper extremity prosthetics: Considerations and designs for sports and recreation. Clin Prosthet Orthop 1987;11:131.
38. Laskowski ER: Snow skiing for the physically disabled. Mayo Clin Proc 1991;66:160.
39. Stangler K: Accessing the great outdoors. Advance for Directors in Rehabilitation 1997;Oct:49.
40. Madorsky JG, Madorsky AG: Scuba diving: Taking the wheelchair out of wheelchair sports. Arch Phys Med Rehabil 1988;69:215.

Appendix A

Resources

Access to Recreation, Inc.
PO Box 5072-430
Thousand Oaks, CA 91359
800-634-4351

Disabled Outdoors magazine
2052 West 23rd Street
Chicago, IL 60608
708-358-4160

Exceptional Parent magazine
555 Kinderkamack Road
Oradell, NJ 07649
800-562-1973
web site, www.eparent.com *or*
www.familyeducation.com

Magalaner JL (ed): *Fodor's Great American Vacations for Travelers with Disabilities*
New York, Fodor's Travel Publications, 1994

Palaestra magazine (published in cooperation with AAHPERD)
PO Box 508
Macomb, IL 61455

Roth W, Tompane M: *Easy Access to National Parks: The Sierra Club Guide for People with Disabilities*
San Francisco, Sierra Club Books, 1992

Sports 'N Spokes magazine
Paralyzed Veterans of America
2111 East Highland Avenue, Suite 180
Phoenix, AZ 85016-4702

Webre AW, Zeller J: *Canoeing and Kayaking for Persons with Physical Disabilities: Instruction Manual*
Newington, VA,
American Canoe Association, 1990

Appendix B
Sports Organizations and Recreational Opportunities

American Athletic Association of the Deaf (AAAD)
3607 Washington Boulevard, Suite 4
Ogden, UT 84403-1737
801-393-7916 (TDD)
801-393-8710 (voice)
www.aaad.org

American Handcycle Association
1744 Pepper Villa Drive
El Cajon, CA 92021-1214
619-569-1986

American Sled Hockey Association
10933 Johnson Avenue South
Bloomington, MN 55437
612-881-2129

American Wheelchair Bowling Association (AWBA)
6264 North Andrews Avenue
Ft. Lauderdale, FL 33309
954-491-2886

American Wheelchair Table Tennis Association
23 Parker Street
Port Chester, NY 10573
914-937-3932

Disabled Sports USA (DS USA)
451 Hungerford Drive, Suite 100
Rockville, MD 20850
301-217-0960
www.dsusa.org/~dsusa/dsusa.html

Dwarf Athletic Association of America (DAAA)
418 Willow Way
Lewisville, TX 75067
214-317-8299
www.wws.net/usoda/daaa.htm

Eastern Amputee Athletic Association
2080 Ennabrock Road
North Bellmore, NY 11710
516-826-8340

Handicapped Scuba Association
1104 El Prado
San Clemente, CA 92672
714-498-6128
http://ourworld.compuserve.com/homepages/hsahdq

National Amputee Golf Association
2517 Hacienda Street
San Mateo, CA 94403
800-633-NAGA

National Foundation of Wheelchair Tennis
940 Calle Amenecer, Suite B
San Clemente, CA 92673
714-361-3663

National Ocean Access Project
PO Box 1705
Rockville, MD 20849-0705
301-217-9843

National Paralympic Committee
Disabled Sports Services, USOC
One Olympic Plaza
Colorado Springs, CO 80909
719-578-4818

National Wheelchair Basketball Association (NWBA)
Charlotte Institute for Rehabilitation
1100 Blythe Boulevard
Charlotte, NC 28203
704-355-1064

National Wheelchair Racquetball Association
2380 McGinley Road
Monroeville, PA 15146
412-856-2468

National Wheelchair Softball Association
1616 Todd Court
Hastings, MN 55033
612-437-1792

North American Riding for the Handicapped Association (NAHRA)
PO Box 33150
Denver, CO 80233
800-369-RIDE

Power Soccer
Bay Area Outreach Recreation Program
830 Bancroft Way
Berkeley, CA 94710
510-849-4663

US Association for Blind Athletes (USABA)
33 North Institute Street
Colorado Springs, CO 80903
719-630-0422
www.usaba.org

US Cerebral Palsy Athletic Association (USCPAA)
200 Harrison Avenue
Newport, RI 02840
www.uscpaa.org

US Disabled Ski Team
PO Box 100
Park City, UT 84060
801-649-9090

US Les Autres Sports Association (USLASA)
1475 West Gray, Suite 165
Houston, TX 77019-4926
713-521-3737

US Quad Rugby Association (USQRA)
5861 White Cypress Drive
Lake Worth, FL 33467
561-964-1712
www.quadrugby.com

US Rowing Association
201 S. Capitol Avenue, Suite 400
Indianapolis, IN 46225
317-237-5656

Wheelchair Athletics of the USA
2351 Parkwood Road
Snellville, GA 30278
770-972-0763

Wheelchair Sports USA (WS USA)
3595 E. Fountain Boulevard, #L-1
Colorado Springs, CO 80910
719-574-1150

Winners on Wheels (WOW)
2842 Business Park Avenue
Fresno, CA 93727
800-969-8255
www.wowusa.com

Chapter 9

Orthotics and Assistive Devices

Michelle A. Miller, MD
Liz Koczur, MPT
Carrie Strine, OTR/L
Denise Peischl, BSE
Richard Lytton, MA, CCC-SLP
Michael A. Alexander, MD

Knowledge of orthotic and assistive devices is an important component of rehabilitation practice. An understanding of normal upper and lower body movement is fundamental for appropriate recommendation and fabrication of an orthosis. Likewise, an understanding of normal communication behaviors is a prerequisite to the recommendation of an augmentative and alternative communication device.

An orthosis may be defined as any device applied to the external surface of an extremity that provides better positioning, immobilizes, prevents deformities, maintains correction, relieves pain, mobilizes joints, exercises parts, or assists or supports weakened or paralyzed parts.[16] Orthotic devices may be classified as static or dynamic, depending on the functional need and ability of the extremity. A static orthosis is rigid and supports the affected area in a particular position, whereas a dynamic orthosis allows some movement. They can be used to substitute for absent motor power, to allow optimal function, to assist motion, to provide for an attachment of devices, and to supply corrective forces to increase directional control.[16] Several variations of upper and lower extremity orthoses that have been proved to increase function for the user are available. Augmentative and alternative communication are discussed later. The keys to identifying the most appropriate orthosis or augmentative communication device are creativity and proper understanding of the anatomic, biomechanical, and communication needs of the patient.

The pediatric population adds a further challenge. Early development is heavily based on fine and gross motor skills. Infants and children use these skills to explore and manipulate their environment. Studies have indicated that the inability to master the environment independently

may lead to decreased socialization, learned helplessness, and a delay in normal development.[1,6] Therefore, an orthosis should allow and assist the growth of the child.

Several team members are involved in prescribing, fabricating, and fitting the orthosis or assistive communication device. The physician, often with input from the therapist, provides patient assessment and a prescription of the orthotic device.[21] The therapist and/or orthotist are instrumental in its fabrication and fitting. A team including a speech therapist, occupational therapist, special educator, and rehabilitation engineer is often beneficial for augmentative and alternative communication device recommendations. Lastly, the patient and family play an important role in its acceptance and usage. If the device is cumbersome and difficult to manage, it will be rejected and find a home on the top shelf in the closet.[4]

Upper and Lower Limb Orthoses

In choosing an orthosis, a few key principles should be kept in mind. The orthosis should enhance normal movement while decreasing the presence of abnormal postures and tone. It should be simple, lightweight, durable, and strong. It should be easy for the child to use and maintain. Lastly, it should augment functional independence. An orthotic device is not successful unless it helps to improve a child's quality of life. Tables 9–1 and 9–2 list some of the more common upper and lower extremity orthoses. Special considerations and limitations are also listed. For a more detailed discussion, please refer to the reference section. Specific recommendations for particular disease processes may be found in the respective chapters.

TABLE 9–1.   Upper Extremity Orthoses

Upper Extremity Orthosis	Common Name	Function	Special Considerations
Static			
Finger	Neoprene thumb abductor	Places thumb in abduction to promote functional use of the hand.	Will not overcome severe cortical thumb position.
	Static metal orthosis	Places thumb in abduction.	Not recommended for fluctuating edema in joint areas.
Hand	Short opponens	Places thumb in abduction and rotated under the second metacarpal. Wrist and fingers are freely mobile.	Allows full wrist flexion and extension. Should be worn at all times, removing only for hygiene and exercise.
Wrist-hand	Thumb spica	Immobilizes and protects thumb, positioning it in opposition. Provides stable post against which index finger can prehend.	Need to allow full MCP flexion of the fingers, especially index finger, and full IP flexion of thumb.
	Resting hand	Preserves a balance between extrinsic and intrinsic musculature and provides joint support when the hand is put at rest. Prevents deformity.	Should preserve MCP joint descent and palmar arch following contour of distal palmar crease. Pressure at MCP joint or proximal phalanx should be avoided because it may cause injury to the MCP joint.
	Wrist cock-up	Supports, immobilizes, or stabilizes wrist in extension. Increases mechanical advantage for grasp.	Must maintain full MCP flexion and CMC motion of thumb. Monitor area over styloid process for pressure changes if dorsal splint is used.
	Antispasticity ball	Positions wrist, abducts fingers and thumb, and maintains palmar arch in a reflex-inhibiting position.	Should not be used for minimal spasticity.
Elbow	Elbow extension	Increases extensor range of motion and prevents flexion.	Not recommended for severe flexor contracture or fluctuating tone in either flexor or extensor patterns.
Elbow-wrist-hand	Full elbow/hand	Promotes supination at forearm and provides long stretch of the limb near end range to decrease tone.	Not recommended for flexor tightness.
Shoulder	Humeral orthosis	Stabilizes the shaft of humerus circumferentially.	May shift position if not appropriately anchored by straps.
	Gunslinger	Supports the shoulder girdle and prevents shoulder subluxation.	Make sure the edges around base of splint do not cut into hip area. Check fitting both in standing and supine positions to accommodate shift of the splint.
Clavicle	Figure 8 harness strap	Proximally stabilizes shoulder girdle movement and limits shoulder flexion and abduction movement beyond 90°.	Must mark settings for appropriate fit due to increased adjustability. Keep a check on skin integrity around the underarm area.
Dynamic			
Hand	MCP flexion assist splint	Gradually lengthens or gently stretches soft tissue structures that limit joint flexion.	Ensure that applied traction is gentle to guard against soft tissue hemorrhages around joints, which may cause edema, pain, and increased scarring.
	MCP extension assist splint	Passively pulls proximal phalanx into extension while allowing active flexion.	Do not position the proximal phalanx in either radial or ulnar deviation when using dynamic traction.
	LMB finger spring—PIP extension assist	Gives dynamic traction of PIP joint without limiting motion at MCP joint. Assists in reducing tightness or contractures of PIP joint.	Not recommended for severe spasticity.
Elbow	Dynasplint	Brace adjusts to lock out undesired flexion and extension. Settings are adjusted in increments of 10°.	Not recommended for severe spasticity.
Power	Smart-WHO (wrist-hand orthosis)	Flexor-hinge hand orthosis which immobilizes thumb in opposition and semiflexes IP joints of index and middle fingers to allow index and middle fingers to move simultaneously toward thumb. Variations include using external power battery pack, SMA actuators, ratchet hand position, and shoulder-driven cables.[13]	Although design is lightweight and simple, actuator's bulkiness and unsightliness of of orthosis can be disadvantages.

MCP = metacarpophalangeal, CMC = carpometacarpal, LMB = lumbrical, PIP = proximal interphalangeal, IP = interphalangeal.

TABLE 9–2. Lower Limb Orthoses

Orthosis	Common Name	Function	Limitations
Solid ankle-foot orthosis	AFO, MAFO	Reduces tone, prevents joint contracture, and provides knee and ankle stability. Most appropriate for child with severe tone, ankle joint hypermobility, and rigid deformities.	Does not allow any ankle movement and therefore limits smooth progression from heel strike to push off.
Hinged or articulated ankle-foot orthosis	HAFO	Hinged AFO with plantarflexion stop and free motion into dorsiflexion allows tibia to translate over foot in stance. This orthosis allows foot to dorsiflex for balance reactions and improves ambulation on uneven surfaces and stairs. Posteriorly, dorsiflexion stop strap can be added to limit amount of dorsiflexion. Plantarflexion stop in 2–5° of dorsiflexion may assist to control genu recurvatum at knee.	Does not control "crouched" posture, allowing increased dorsiflexion and knee flexion. Children with strong extensor posturing may break ankle joint. May allow hindfoot to slip causing midfoot break if insufficient hindfoot dorsiflexion is present.
Anterior floor reaction or ground reaction ankle-foot orthosis	GRAFO	Limits "crouch" posture (stance posture with hip flexion, knee flexion, and ankle dorsiflexion). At heel strike, it encourages force up through anterior cuff, giving knee extension torque. Knee extension is maintained throughout stance.	Children with significant hamstring or hindfoot tightness or tone will not benefit from this orthosis.
Rear-entry hinged floor-reaction AFO		Dorsiflexion stop limits "crouch" posture while allowing for plantarflexion during loading phase of stance and at push-off.	Active dorsiflexion is required to restrict foot drag during swing.
Posterior leaf spring	PLS	The trimlines of this solid AFO are posterior to the malleoli. The slender posterior portion gives it flexibility to allow for some dorsiflexion in stance and plantarflexion at push-off.	Does not allow full motion into dorsiflexion or plantarflexion. For medial-lateral ankle stability and arch control, another orthosis may be more appropriate. Does not control foot deformity or extensor tone. Excessive torque on spring may cause skin problems.
Dynamic ankle-foot orthosis	DAFO	A supramalleolar orthosis which uses footboard to support arches of the foot. Provides medial-lateral ankle stability with control for pronation/supination. Allows some ankle dorsiflexion/plantarflexion.	Difficult to fit into shoes. Difficult for self-donning. Child may quickly outgrow this splint because it is finely contoured to the foot.
Knee hyperextension splint		Maintains neutral knee and limits knee hyperextension. Uses three points of pressure: superior-anterior surface of knee, inferior-anterior surface of knee, and posterior to knee joint.[7,11]	Controls only knee. Does not control extensor posturing well. It is bulky under clothes and difficult to sit with.
Swedish knee cage	KO	Controls genu recurvatum with same three points of pressure as above. Works same as a knee hyperextension splint. Uses metal uprights and straps instead of plastic material.[7]	Controls only knee. Difficult to fit it to smaller children and difficult to maintain correct positioning.
Knee-ankle-foot orthosis	KAFO	Molded plastic upper and lower leg components usually with a locked or unlocked hinged knee joint. Four most common knee locks are free, drop lock, bail lock, and dial lock. Free knee allows full motion at knee axis. Knee axis may be straight or offset. Offset axis has increased extensor moment at knee joint. Drop lock is metal collar that slides into place to maintain knee in extension. Bail lock is spring-loaded lock that has trip mechanism to unlock knee. Dial lock may be set in varying degrees of flexion; used to accommodate or decrease knee flexion contracture.[10]	Bulky and difficult to don/doff. Free knee at times allows too much motion. Drop lock requires fine motor control to lock and unlock. Child must be able to get knee fully extended to engage drop lock. Bail locks at times become easily disengaged. Dial locks do not allow free movement through available range.
Hip-knee-ankle-foot orthosis	HKAFO	Hip belt and joint. Hip and knee joints may be locked or unlocked. Able to progress child to increasing number of free joints at one time.	Bulky, difficult to don/doff. Difficult to manage clothing for toileting.

(Table continued on following page.)

TABLE 9–2.   Lower Limb Orthoses *(Continued)*

Orthosis	Common Name	Function	Limitations
Reciprocating gait orthosis	RGO	HKAFOs that are connected by cable system that links hip flexion on one side with hip extension on other. Assist children with active hip flexion and no hip extension to advance legs with a more normalized gait. Allow child to ambulate with reciprocal or swing-through gait.[10]	Bulky, expensive. Difficult to don/doff. Not appropriate for a child with hip and/or knee flexion contractures. Difficult to manage clothing for toileting.
Hip spica/hip abduction splint		Orthosis made of thermoplastic material and Velcro® to position newborn's legs in abduction and flexion. Used to maintain femoral head in acetabulum to mimic normal hip formation. Use helps to avoid hip subluxation and dislocation. Used from birth up to 1 year.	Requires frequent repositioning. May need frequent adjustments for growth. Difficult for caregivers to maintain appropriate fit.
Pavlick harness		Soft splint used for children with diagnosis of congenital hip dislocation. Generally used in first 9 months of age. Bilateral lower limbs are positioned with hips abducted and flexed to 90° in attempt to maintain hips in reduced position.	Careful positioning required. Caregivers must be vigilant in checking splint positioning.
Parapodium or Variety Village stander		This device allows child to stand without upper extremity support, freeing bilateral arms to do activities. Walking with this device and crutches can be quicker than with parapodium with swivel device.[12]	More energy expenditure than with swivel device. Children are unable to don/doff independently or to transfer independently from supine to stand and stand to supine. Device is heavy.
Parapodium with ORLAU swivel modification		This orthosis allows child to walk without use of gait aid and to use arms for other activities. Less energy expenditure than with parapodium and crutches.[12,22]	Same as above. Slower than walking with parapodium and crutches.
Twister cables		Cables are attached to a pelvic band and traverse lower limbs to attach on shoes or AFOs. These cables control for increased internal rotation. Work well with children with normal to floppy tone to control internal rotation.[10]	Do not work well with children with extensor spasticity. They may need to be frequently readjusted as child grows.

Shoe Inserts

Many orthopedic and neurologic pediatric disorders have sequelae that require orthotic management. Shoe inserts may be a viable option in many circumstances. Many commercially available products control differing levels of impairment in the hindfoot, midfoot, and forefoot. Heel cups help with shock absorption for joints, heels spurs, bursitis, and tendinitis. In the midfoot, orthoses help to maintain the arch of the foot in varying degrees of firmness. Numerous products are also available to control disorders of the forefoot and toes. Metatarsal bars are available to unload pressure from the metatarsal arch in patients with metatarsalgia. Pads are available to help to realign hammer and claw toes, cushion bunions and calluses and to protect toes from friction and irritation. A limitation of these commercially available products is that many do not come in pediatric sizes and must be modified to fit.

Orthoses for Positioning, Range of Motion, and Healing

Because of immobility, spasticity, and/or abnormal postures, many children are at risk for joint contractures, musculoskeletal deformity, and skin breakdown. Traditionally, caregivers have used pillows and towel rolls to maintain more appropriate postures. Bony areas such as the occiput, scapular spine, coccyx, femoral head, fibular head, and calcaneus are at greatest risk for skin breakdown from prolonged bedrest or maintenance of one position. Gel pads may be used to distribute weight over a larger area. The child may benefit from positioning pieces to maintain neutral positions and to decrease pressure on parts of the body. Foam wedges in various lengths and sizes are commonly used for back support to position a child in sidelying. An abduction pillow may be used to decrease scissoring and to increase hip abduction. Foam arm and leg elevators help to reduce edema, and foot splints and boots are available to maintain the foot in a dorsiflexed position with relief for the calcaneus to prevent pressure sores.

One recently developed product allows the caregiver a new flexibility with positioning. The Versa Form pillow (Fig. 9–1) is a semipermanent positioning support. These styrene bead bags are available in a variety of sizes and allow molding to a child in any position. A vacuum pump is required to remove air from the pillow to make it firm. The bead bags need to be reformed after several weeks of use. This new technology gives the practitioner flexibility to change a child's positioning frequently.

Adaptive Feeding Devices

Traditional approaches to fostering independence in self-feeding have been based on adaptation of eating utensils. The shape, thickness, or angle of the utensils was changed to accommodate the patient's limitations in range of motion, muscle strength, coordination, and endurance.[24] Examples include adding foam tubing to the handle to build up the grip and bending the utensil to improve the angle for food-to-mouth retrieval. This approach is especially helpful if shoulder range is limited. However, the degree of independence achieved with these methods has not always been optimal.

Over time, mechanical and electrical feeding devices that require less movement from the child and promote greater feeding independence have been developed.[9] Three feeding devices are commercially available. The most commonly used and readily available feeder is the Winsford feeder. A cheek switch with two modes—switch operation and plate rotation—operates this device. The child activates the switch to rotate the plate until food is in line with the pusher. The user then activates the pusher mode of the switch, pushing food onto the spoon. The spoon automatically lifts the food to mouth level. The cheek switch can be interchanged with a rocker switch, if deemed more appropriate. The movement, precision, and strength required to operate the device are minimal.

Another power feeding device available is the Handy-1, which was developed in England at the University of Keele and consists of an education robot and a tray. The child specifies food location by using a scanning system and switch selection. Although the Handy-1 has been relatively successful in the application of robotic technology to the eating task, its limitations are due to its size, difficulty of transport, and the types of food that it is able to accommodate. In addition, the price tag is high ($6000–$8000). However, it also offers other options for other

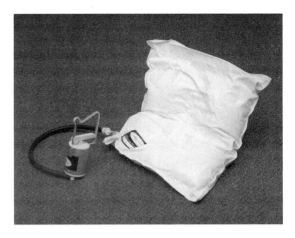

FIGURE 9–1. Versa Form pillow.

activities of daily living, such as shaving, drinking, and make-up application.

The Beeson feeder is no longer available for sale, but parts are still available for purchase and/or replacement. It is a powered device that tilts the plate and pivots the spoon toward the operator's mouth.

Mobility Aids

Transfer Aids

A number of patient care lifts are commercially available to assist caregivers and/or health care professionals with performing safe transfers for children. The Handi-Move (Fig. 9–2) is designed to ensure a strong, safe hold on the child's chest while leaving the back and seat entirely free. Two cup-shaped body supports hold the child, and the frame lifts automatically. Comfortable leg supports lift under the thighs to help maintain a natural sitting position. It is appropriate for anyone with poor-to-absent strength or sitting balance and ideal for lifting and lowering into a wheelchair or bath or onto a toilet. The system is motorized and can be fitted with either an electric hand control or an infrared remote control.

The Trans-Aid is similar to the Hoyer lift (Fig. 9–3). This lift is designed to transfer children from bed to wheelchair, off the floor, onto a toilet, into a car, and through an 18-inch doorway. Slings with heavy-duty support options are available to minimize further the effort of the caregiver while maximizing safety during transfer. Institutional lifters that offer a 400- and 600-lb weight capacity and portable home-care lifts that are lightweight and designed for home doorways and narrow halls are also available.

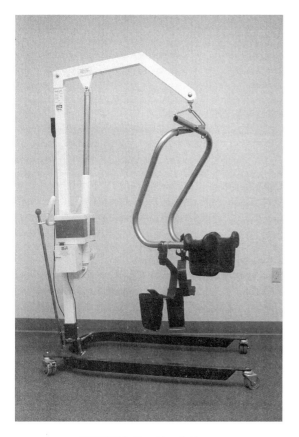

FIGURE 9–2.   Handi-Move.

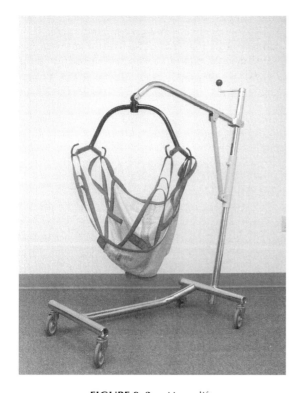

FIGURE 9–3.   Hoyer lift.

In addition to patient lifts, other smaller devices can assist children with ease of transfers. One option is a transfer board; another is an overhead trapeze bar attached to a frame over the bed. The most commonly used transfer board is constructed of maple wood and measures approximately 8 inches wide by 24 inches long. The BeasyTrans is made from an exceptionally strong duPont plastic and is ideal for all transfers (e.g., bed, car, bath bench, commode). The child glides laterally on a round seat that rotates 360° and allows reduced shear stress and friction across the buttocks. Lastly, trapeze bars may be attached overhead to bed frames to assist the child with bed mobility skills and positioning changes. The position is individually set and can be altered as needed. Typically, trapeze bars assist with supine-to-sitting transfers and initiation of side-to-side rolling. They are often appropriate initially but are soon removed after the child's strength and bed mobility skills improve.

Standers

Numerous passive standing devices are available. They offer many potential benefits for the child, including provision of sustained muscular stretch, maintenance of trunk and lower limb passive range of motion, facilitation of cocontraction of muscles, decrease of tone, and improvement in trunk and head control. Standers should be used a few times a day for as long as a total of 1 hour. The child should progressively work to increase tolerance in the standing position. However, passive standing should not take the place of the child exploring his or her environment and body.

In selecting a stander, the following points should be considered: head and trunk control, abnormal tone and posturing, ability for growth, long-term goal for standing, and family goals. Most standers, with the exception of the freedom stander, are cumbersome and heavy and do not fold easily for transport. The vertical stander is used most often for children with spinal dysfunction who have good head and trunk control. It is an upright stander that leaves the arms free to do activities. The parapodium, a type of vertical stander, is discussed in the orthosis part of this chapter. Three types of standers are discussed below: supine, prone, and upright.

Supine standers (Fig. 9–4) go from a horizontal position to approximately 90° upright, depending on the model. Laterals, kneepads, adduction/abduction supports, and head supports help to maintain the child's posture. Bilateral upper extremity strengthening can be performed in this position with or without a tray. However, the supine stander does not provide any upper extremity weight bearing. A further limitation is that it will not work to improve head and trunk control. The supine stander is recommended for a child with significant extensor tone and posturing and/or poor or absent head control. It is also preferred over the prone stander for the larger child because of the increased ease in positioning.

Prone standers (Fig. 9–5) support the child anteriorly. Postural support is supplied through trunk laterals, hip guides, abductor blocks, knee blocks, and shoe holders. Prone standers do come with a chin support to aid children who have limited head control or fatigue easily. However, the child should not be permitted to "hang" on the support; a supine stander is more appropriate if the child lacks fair head control. The stander can be used to improve antigravity head control and to promote bilateral upper extremity weight bearing. Its tray may serve as a functional surface for stimulation. The prone stander may not be appropriate for some children with increased extensor tone. In such cases, gravity increases the work required for neck and trunk extension as well as shoulder retraction, thus feeding into primitive posturing.

Upright standers maintain the child in an erect position through supports at the hips, knees, and trunk. Certain standers are available with a hydraulic or manual lift, making positioning of the larger child easier. A sling is placed under the child's buttocks to lift him or her upward into the standing frame. The upright stander mimics a normal standing position and permits the child to work on head control and upper extremity strengthening. It has no head support and only limited trunk support with a tray in front and a strap around the child's back. The lower extremity supports are limited and may not be enough for a child with increased tone.

Gait Aids

Gait aids are assistive devices designed to improve functional independence and/or to expand exercise options through standing and walking. In pediatrics, gait aids help children to explore and interact with their environment. Improved balance, decreased energy expenditure, decreased impact on joints, improved posture, and decreased pain are potential benefits of gait aids. The most common gait aids are canes, crutches, and walkers.

Canes are available in different sizes with a variety of handles and supports (e.g., straight

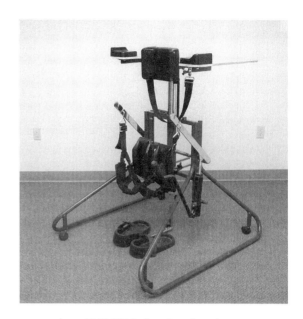

FIGURE 9–4. Grandstand.

cane vs. quad cane). A quad cane provides a better base of support, but a normal gait cycle is more easily mimicked using a straight cane. A hemicane is a combination of a cane and a walker. It has a four-point base and the largest base of support of all the canes. It gives the greatest amount of stability among the canes but also encourages the child to lean laterally when ambulating.

Crutches generally fall into two categories: axillary and Lofstrand. Axillary crutches are usually constructed of wood or aluminum and have limited adaptability. Some crutches may be modified to offer a forearm support to decrease

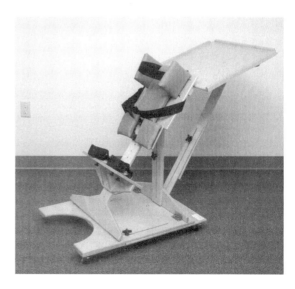

FIGURE 9–5. Prone stander.

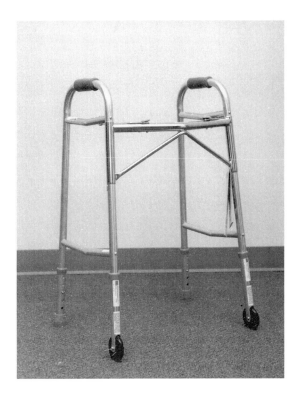

FIGURE 9–6.   Guardian forward walker.

weight bearing through wrists and hands. The child and family should be cautioned about possible nerve impingement from sustained axillary pressure with improper use. A Kenney crutch, not often used in the rehabilitation setting, is an axillary crutch without an underarm

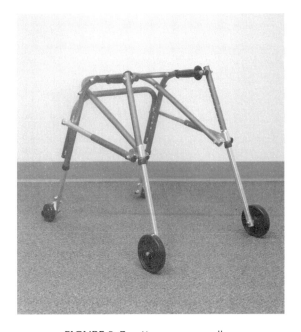

FIGURE 9–7.   Kaye reverse walker.

support. In place of the underarm support is a leather armband that fits around a child's arm.

Lofstrand crutches are much more flexible. They have a variety of forearm cuff styles, including circumferential or half cuff. Functional independence is increased with the use of Lofstrand crutches because the child is able to reach with his or her hands and the circumferential cuff will stay on the forearm. Half cuffs require less reliance on the cuff for balance, but they will not stay on the forearm if the handgrip is released. Handles may be wide and flat, pistol, or rounded. Rounded handles are the most commonly prescribed. The flat, wide handles may be helpful with tonal issues as well as carpal tunnel inflammation. Pistol grips provide grooves for finger placement. Newer varieties of Lofstrand crutches are lightweight for children who have limited strength or need shock absorption for their joints.

Another adjustable option for all crutches is the crutch tip. Crutch tips may be constructed with materials of various flexibilities and in different widths to make the crutches more stable. Tips may include a gel, which provides some shock-absorbent qualities. In addition, studded cups, which cover crutch tips, are available to facilitate ambulation in rain and snow.

Three varieties of walkers are appropriate for the pediatric population: forward, reverse, and gait trainers. Forward walkers, the tradiional type of walker, can be purchased with or without wheels (Fig. 9–6). Children can grip flat handles or use platforms on one or both sides to bear weight through the elbows and forearms. Forward walkers promote trunk flexion in many children.

Reverse walkers, also called posture-control walkers, promote an erect posture (Fig. 9–7). The child has increased extension at the trunk and hips when his or her hands are positioned to the sides or slightly in front. A pelvic support can be added to assist with lateral pelvic control and to facilitate trunk extension. Platforms also can be attached to allow forearm weight bearing. Reverse walkers are widely used in children. However, because of increased width, adult-sized children may have difficulty with accessibility. Other accessories available with some walkers are swivel wheels, forearm attachments, hip guides, hand brakes, baskets, and seats.

Gait trainers make ambulation a viable option for children who are unable to ambulate with other aids. A gait trainer is an assistive device that provides significant trunk and pelvic support. It consists of a metal frame with adjustable height metal uprights that support the trunk and arms. Adjustable height seats, which are either slings or a bicycle-type seat, are attached. The seat is not used to support the entire body weight but rather to keep the child erect. This gait device has been used to teach a more normal reciprocal gait pattern. It may function as a stepping stone to walking with a walker or crutches. Limitations of gait trainers include decreased transportability, difficulty with positioning, and decreased accessibility. They are wider and longer than traditional walkers. Gait trainers have a place in therapeutic rehabilitation—to provide a child independent means of ambulation when no other assistive device is appropriate and as a therapeutic tool toward ambulation with a more accessible assistive device. Accessories available with gait trainers are trays, wheel locks, harnesses, forearm supports, and differing lower extremity supports.[15]

Wheelchairs and Seating

The degree of limitation in mobility varies across a broad range for people with physical disabilities.[6] Over the years, technology related to wheelchair seating and mobility has enhanced the opportunities for people with disabilities. In particular, more wheelchairs are available to meet the diverse needs of children.[23]

To begin the process of matching the child's needs to a particular wheelchair, a thorough evaluation is recommended. Many factors contribute to choosing a particular seating and mobility device for children, including growth, specific disability, medical interventions, and prognosis of future functional and cognitive abilities. Assess the particular needs of the child, collect medical/surgical history, and perform a physical assessment. A multidisciplinary team approach usually works best. Once the evaluation is accomplished, educate the family about various wheelchairs relative to the child's goals. Simulate the child in as close to the final product as possible. Finally, determine the particular seating objectives for the child as well as the type of mobility base.[23]

Every child has a unique set of challenges that dictate how his or her rehabilitation needs will be met. Proper seating provides stability and support, decreases the likelihood of postural deformities, and enhances upper extremity control.[14] Within a wheelchair seating system, proper body alignment is maintained by using various seating and positioning components.[25] Seating systems, including both seat and back, may be linear, contoured, or molded. Of the three, only linear seating systems provide adjustability

that allows the seating system to grow as the child grows. Linear seating systems are the least conforming to the body and provide the least amount of pressure relief, but they are the easiest to fabricate. The basic materials consist of plywood for the base, foam (which varies in density) for comfort and minimal pressure relief, and a covering, usually Naugahyde. Positioners such as laterals, abductors, and adductors are easy to mount.

Contour systems, in contrast to linear systems, conform more closely to the actual shape of the body. In recommending a contour system, close attention should be given to the growth rate and potential medical interventions because the shape of the contour may not be an appropriate choice. Custom-molded systems provide maximal support and should be considered for children with fixed deformities. Molded systems do not change as the child grows unless remolding is performed, which is potentially time-consuming and costly. Although this system aids in controlling tone and nicely contours to most deformities, it has the reverse effect of limiting the child's freedom in the seating system.

For patients who lack sensation, a variety of cushions help to alleviate pressure and thus decrease the likelihood of skin breakdown. Cushions fall under several categories, including foam, gel, air, and water. Cushions should provide pressure relief under bony prominences and a stable support surface for the pelvis and the thighs and function effectively in different climates. They should be lightweight, especially if a person is transferring independently or is a self-propeller, and durable. Each type of cushion has advantages and disadvantages (Table 9–3).

Positioning Components

Within a wheelchair seating system, proper body alignment is maintained by using various positioning components. Lateral supports can be used to encourage midline trunk position

TABLE 9–3. Cushion Types

Foam	Gel	Air
Lightweight	Lightweight	Provides extremely good pressure relief
Provides stable base of support	Provides stable base of support	
Various densities can improve pressure-relieving qualities, but may be heavier	Various densities can improve pressure-relieving qualities, but may be heavier	Lightweight
		Can be unstable
Conforms to individual shape	Conforms to individual shape	Requires careful monitoring and maintenance

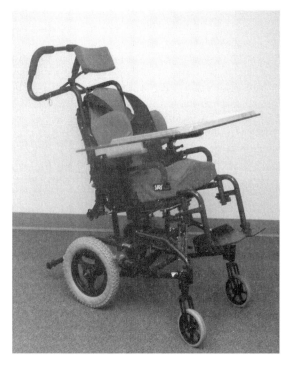

FIGURE 9–8. Tilt-in-space wheelchair.

when trunk control is poor. They also may be used to correct partially or delay the progression of scoliosis. Chest harnesses help to stabilize

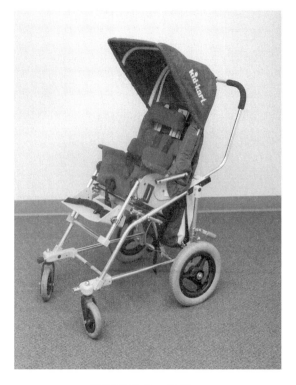

FIGURE 9–9. KidKart.

the trunk by anterior support as well as by preventing forward trunk flexion.

Positioning belts are used for pelvic alignment and stabilization. An improperly placed pelvic positioner is more detrimental than no positioner at all. The standard angulation of a pelvic positioning belt is at a 45° angle to the sitting surface.[5] Subasis bars are used primarily for high-tone patients. Proper placement and position of the bar are critical to the success of the product. Improper positioning may lead to skin breakdown.

Additional positioners include abductor pads that reduce or prevent increased adduction and help to provide proper leg alignment. Abductors are not to be used to block a child from "sliding" out of the wheelchair; this approach may cause injury to the perineal area.[1] Adductors decrease hip abduction and help to provide proper leg alignment. Shoe holders and a product called Ankle Huggers help to control increased extension or spasms in the lower limbs and correct or prevent excessive internal or external foot rotation.

Head position is important for many reasons, including proper visual input, control of tone, and proper alignment for feeding and swallowing. Headrests provide support and positioning for a patient with poor head control due to low tone, active flexion, or hyperextension. They provide posterior and, if necessary, lateral support. They also furnish safety in transport. The size and shape of the headrest depend on individual needs. Total head support can be achieved with the same headrest, which allows the child to move the head freely to explore his or her environment.

When proper seating and positioning components are in place, pediatric wheelchairs provide users with the opportunity to explore and experience the world around them. It encourages social integration and enhances the level of involvement in various school and home activities. Most wheelchairs can be divided into two main categories: dependent mobility and independent mobility. These categories represent the level of functional mobility that the child can achieve. Strollers, recliner wheelchairs, and tilt-in-space wheelchairs are typically recommended for people who need a temporary means of mobility or are incapable of independent mobility. Tilt-in-space chairs (Fig. 9–8) are recommended for people who need moderate-to-maximal positioning and have little tolerance for an upright position. They provide pressure relief by redistributing body weight. The tilt also can assist the caregiver in properly positioning the child in the wheelchair by allowing gravity to assist.

Strollers are typically used for younger children in whom independent mobility is less of an issue. Most strollers are also easily transportable (Fig. 9–9).

Independent mobility can be achieved by using a manual wheelchair or a power wheelchair. Functional abilities and mobility goals dictate the type of wheelchair recommended. Manual wheelchairs provide minimal-to-complete postural support. Manual wheelchairs are lightweight and have a multitude of features that can be adjusted or added to enhance efficient and effective use. Table 9–4 offers a comparative look at the various wheelchair components.

TABLE 9–4.   Wheelchair Characteristics

1. Frames

Rigid	Folding	Hemi-height	Tilt in Space	Recliner	One Arm Drive
(+) Efficient ride (+) Durable (+) Lightweight (−) Decreased shock absorption	(+) Shock absorption (+) Ease of transport (+) Ability to narrow chair (−) Less efficient propulsion	(+) Allows LE propulsion (+) May make transfer easier (+) Optimal height for peer interaction (−) May make transfers difficult (−) Compromise height at tables	(+) Pressure relief (+) May assist to help balance ± head control (+) Change position for respiration (−) Heavy (−) Difficult to break down	(+) Pressure relief (+) Seating for hip contractures (+) Limited tolerance for upright posture (+) Ease of breathing/feeding (−) Difficulty changing position with spasticity (−) Laterals and headrest move with changing position	(+) One functional UE (+) Sometimes difficult to manipulate

2. Armrests

Conventional	Height-adjustable	Flip-up	Swing Away	Arm Troughs
(+) Offers protection (−) Heavy (−) Hand function (−) Cosmesis	(+) Positioning assist (+) Offers protection (+) Ease of transfers (−) Bulky	(+) Hand function varies (+) Remains attached for quick availability (−) May be in bad position	(+) Durable (+) Cosmesis (+) Easiest to operate (+) Can change width via cushion (−) No protection (−) Must order side guards for protection	(+) Alignment of UE's with minimal AROM (−) Bulky

3. Footrests

	Hanger Angle		Types		
60 degrees	70 degrees	90 degrees	Tapered	Standard	Elevating
(+) Able to have large casters (+) Limited ROM (+) Increase depth without length (+) Taller person (−) Increased length of chair	(+) Reduces spasticity problems (+) Compromise	(+) Reduces turning radius (+) Reduces chair length	(+) Increased accessibility (+) Positioning (−) Decreased calf space	(+) Adequate calf space (−) Decreased accessibility	(+) Positioning—contractures (+) Edema (−) Increased chair weight (−) Increased length (−) Decreased accessibility (−) Elevating mechanism (−) Cumbersome

Footplates		Front Rigging			
Solid/platform	Angle-adjustable	High Mount	Flip-up	Fixed	Swing Away
(+) Folding frame more stable (+) Durable (−) Must remove to fold on folding frame	(+) Best positioning—ankle contractures (+) Reduce extensor thrust in lower limbs (−) Heavier	(+) Positioning for shorter legs	(+) Easier to move out of way (−) Not as durable	(+) More durable (+) Change seat depth without length (−) Transfers more difficult (−) Cannot reduce chair length	(+) Facilitate transfers (+) Greater accessibility (−) Must manipulate release mechanism

(Table continued on following page.)

TABLE 9–4. Wheelchair Characteristics *(Continued)*

4. Leg Straps

Toe Loop, Heel Loop, Calf Strap	Shoe Holders
(+) Maintain feet on footplates (+) Straps maintain position even with flexor spasticity (+) Straps may be used for WC/floor/WC transfer (−) May make transfer difficult	(+) Control increased extension or spasms in lower limbs (+) Excessive internal, external rotation (+) Prevent aggressive behavior for safety (−) Heavy (−) Cumbersome

5. Casters

Solid	Pneumatic	Semipneumatic	Size 6–8 inches	Size 3–5 inches
(+) No maintenance (+) Least rolling resistance (+) Energy efficient	(+) Most shock absorbent (+) Easier to maneuver over small objects	(+) No maintenance (+) Compromise	(+) Less rolling resistance (+) Increase footplate/ground clearance (+) Good on rough terrain (+) Tilt (+) Rugged terrain (+) Smoother ride	(+) Less shimmy (+) More responsive to quick turns (+) May aid in curb maneuverability (+) Increase footplate/caster clearance (+) Indoor use—tighter turns

6. Axles

	Axle Position			Axles	
Single Position	Multiposition	Amputee	Standard	Quick Release	Quad Release
(+) Durable (−) No adjustability	(+) Adjustability (−) Decreased durability	(+) Fits special population (−) Decreased durability	(+) Threaded (−) Cannot remove rear wheels	(−) Cannot remove rear wheels (+) Reduce size weight for transportability (−) Need good hand function (−) Durability	(+) Can remove rear wheels (+) Lower hand function (−) Durability (−) May accidentally disengage

7. Rear Wheels

Spoked	Mag
(+) Shock absorption (+) Lighter (−) Maintenance	(+) No maintenance (+) Decreased chance of finger injury (−) Heavier

8. Tires

Urethane	Pneumatic	Kevlar	Knobbie	High Pressure	Airless Inserts
(+) Good indoors (+) No maintenance (+) Durable (−) Rougher ride (−) Heavier	(+) Rough terrain (+) Good traction (+) Lighter (−) Maintenance	(+) Reinforced tire	(+) All terrain (+) Increased traction (+) Added flotation (−) Squeaks when new	(+) High pressure (+) Lighter (−) Need Presta Valve	(+) Flat free (+) Compromise (+) Low maintenance (−) One pound heavier

9. Push Rims

Aluminum	Friction Coated	Projection "Quad Knobs"
(+) No friction (+) Fine control (−) Cold in cold weather (−) Slippery if wet	(+) Impaired hand function (−) Chair width increased (−) Slippery if wet (−) Can cause burns (−) Coating wears	(+) Angle varies (+) Length varies (+) Number varies (−) Angle increases width (−) Decreased efficiency if pegs do not end up right position (−) Difficult to descend

10. Brakes

Push to Lock	Pull to Lock	Scissors	Extensions	Grade Aids
(−) May hit transfer surface and unlock (−) May hit hand when propelling	(+) Not as likely to unlock during transfer (+) Closer for transfers (+) Clear for propulsion	(+) Clear for propulsion (+) Clear for transfers (−) Difficult to manipulate (−) Less surface contact with camber	(+) Easier to reach (+) Easier to operate (−) Decrease brake durability (−) In the way (−) Toggle	(+) Prevents chair from rolling backwards (−) Difficult to propel forward (−) May engage inadvertently (−) Requires treaded tire (−) Prevents recovery from backward fall (−) Low durability

Although this is a list of manual wheelchair components, many features can be considered for power wheelchairs as well.

Power wheelchairs provide independent mobility when manual wheelchairs cannot be used. Technologic advances in electronics have enabled people with severe physical disability to operate a motorized wheelchair. Power wheelchairs may incorporate unique features that enhance function critical to health maintenance as well as social development. Power wheelchairs have pediatric sizes that are capable of raising the child from a seated to a standing position as well as elevating in the seated position using a "seat elevator" (Fig. 9–10).

Some power wheelchairs lower to floor level to allow the child to interact socially with peers. However, use of a power wheelchair may involve constraints. The family may not have the means to transport the wheelchair, or the power wheelchair cannot be used in the home because of limited physical space and accessibility. Funding also may prohibit acquisition of a power wheelchair. Another option for powered mobility for children may lie in three- or four-wheeled scooters. Scooters are usually less expensive than a power wheelchair but do not offer a great deal of positioning options. Although choices are limited for child-sized scooters, several can accommodate small children.

Car Seats

Car seats are a crucial component to consider in striving for safety for children during travel.[2] Several brands and models can be purchased commercially. There are two commonly used types: the Gorilla (Fig. 9–11) and the Columbia car seat. Both include deep seat depth, adequate positioning pads, safety straps, and an appropriate restraint system. The Carrie car seat comes complete with head support, harness and safety belt straps, and foot supports. At times, a child is sent home from the hospital in a spica cast or a cast that limits the fit for safe travel. The SpelCast is a car seat for children whose age requires that they travel in a car seat but who are unable to fit safely because of cast or splint wear. For children whose postures require more than a lap belt and shoulder harness, an Easy-On Vest is recommended. It can be used in upright sitting in the rear seat or in sidelying in the back seat. Models can accommodate ages 2–12 years, depending on size and weight. Another option is the Snug Seat, a stroller chair that also can be used as a car seat. It offers multiple positioning aids and easily disconnects from the stroller base.

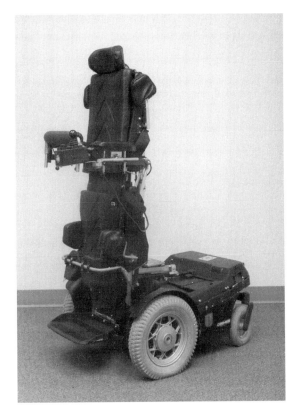

FIGURE 9–10. Chair-Man.

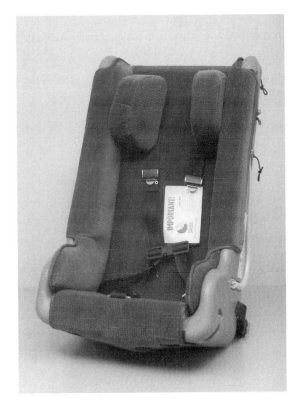

FIGURE 9–11. Gorilla car seat.

Children with tracheostomies should avoid using child restraint systems with a harness tray/shield combination or an armrest. On sudden impact the child may fall forward, causing the tracheostomy to contact the shield or armrest and possibly resulting in injury and a blocked airway. Five-point harnesses should be used for children with tracheostomies.[19]

Transport of wheelchair occupants can be a challenge for many, especially school bus supervisors. Research and accident data show that wheelchair tiedowns and occupant restraint systems (WTORS) reduce the possibility of injury by preventing the occupant's head from hitting the vehicle interior.[20] Several commercially available systems secure the wheelchair to the vehicle, including a four-point belt system, a "docking" station, and a T-bar configuration. It is also recommended that wheelchairs face forward to avoid collapsibility in collisions. In addition to the wheelchair seatbelt and shoulder or chest harness, the standard lap and shoulder belt anchored to the vehicle or the restraint system should be used.[2,3]

Adaptive Interfaces

With the level of human interaction incorporated into current technology, interface between a device and the child takes on a new meaning and new challenges. The success of a device is determined by the interface, which takes the form of various technologies. Depending on the physical abilities of the user, interfaces between the child and the product may look quite different. It may be a joystick or a head control used to operate a power wheelchair. It may be a palatal orthosis, as in the Tongue Touch KeyPad used to control not only a wheelchair but also a computer or home and office devices. Other adaptive interfaces include "sip-and-puff" systems, chin control devices, and other various switches configured to provide specific output, depending on the device to be controlled.

Other adaptive interfaces typically used to control the environment or access to a computer include voice activation and an eye-gaze system. Voice activation may use software such as Dragon Dictate. Eye gaze technology has been implemented in the EyeGaze System, a computer-based tool for explicitly measuring, recording, playing back, and analyzing what a person does with his or her eyes. The child can perform a broad variety of functions, including environmental control, playing games, typing, or operating a telephone. Although these technologies are sophisticated, they offer another means of accessing the environment and maximizing independence.

Recreational Equipment

An integral part of a child's life should be learning and self-exploration through recreational activities and play. Many tricycles now fit the needs of some physically challenged children. Special features include hand propulsion, wider seats, seatbelts, trunk supports, and chest straps. The Step-N-Go bicycle (Fig. 9–12) allows a rider to stand and pedal, making propulsion easier for children with extensor tone. A roller racer is a riding toy for children with lower extremity dysfunction. It sits close to the ground and is propelled by moving the handlebars from side to side. Electronic cars can be easily adapted with switches or a proportional joystick. Scooters can be propelled with arms or legs. Many mobility devices are commercially available. Further information about recreational equipment is available in the chapter on adapted sports and recreation.

Augmentative and Alternative Communication

All children, whether disabled or not, utilize a complex communication system that integrates spoken, written, and pragmatic social language skills. Augmentative and alternative communication (AAC) includes low- and high-technology devices that supplement these skills and facilitate language learning. Augmentative communications options are appropriate for all children whose natural speech and writing do not enable them to express themselves to all listeners in all environments and for all communication purposes. In addition, they are indicated when natural speech and writing do not sufficiently support continued speech, language, and academic learning and success. The cause of the communication impairment may be a motor speech disorder, such as dysarthria and dyspraxia; a cognitive and language disorder, such as global developmental delay, pervasive developmental disorder, autism, mental retardation, traumatic brain injury, cerebral palsy, and learning disabilities; or a neuromuscular disorder, such as muscular dystrophy and spinal cord injury.

Communication behaviors develop spontaneously in all children, regardless of the severity and multiplicity of their disabilities. Examples include vocalizations for satisfaction and dissatisfaction; eye gaze and eye contact; looking away from a person, place, or thing; idiosyncratic gestures; and other behaviors. Even when such communication behaviors are more "reflexive" or self-directed than intentionally interactive, parents, caregivers, and familiar listeners typically learn to recognize communicative information from their children's behaviors. The goal of AAC intervention includes introducing communication strategies that help the child develop systematic communications behaviors. Systematic communication helps listeners to understand more readily a child's communicative intent, helps to reduce the "twenty questions" guesses in which parents and caregivers typically engage, and helps the child and his or her listeners form a communication dyad. To achieve this goal, a set of communication symbols is introduced. The child learns the meaning of the symbols and communication systems within known, familiar, and functional routines of daily living. Communication systems may be simple, such as refrigerator magnets or homemade picture-magnets displayed on the refrigerator or on a cookie sheet for portability. Low-technology systems include communication notebooks, communication boards, and Picture Exchange Communication books. Simple speech output devices are also available.

The BigMack is a large single switch that can be programmed with a speech output message. By learning to press the BigMack at the beginning of a motivating activity such as eating or playing, the child learns to initiate the activity and communication. Passive participation and "learned helplessness" are replaced by intentional communication. The Cheap Talk and linked One-Step Communicators provide multiple speech output messages. They enable the child to incorporate spoken communication into several steps of a familiar routine and to start making choices within a routine. Examples include, "I need to go to the bathroom"; "I want to wash my hands"; "I need a towel"; "I'm done, can I go watch television?" Pressing a button on the side and speaking into the device program the BigMack, Cheap Talk, and One-Step Communicators quickly and easily.

Features of Various Devices

AAC devices and systems are differentiated by their configuration of features and capabilities. Low-technology AAC devices can be customized and created in almost any way that the AAC specialist, user, and family design. They may be constructed with a communication board format that takes up most of the surface of a wheelchair laptray or as multiple pages of a communication notebook. They may contain written words and letters, standardized picture symbols with captions, photographs, or even small three-dimensional objects. Low-technology communication systems do not contain speech

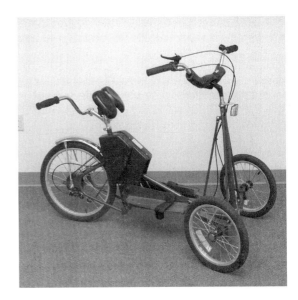

FIGURE 9–12.   Step-n-Go bike.

or written output, and the child is dependent on the listener to maintain attention throughout the communication interaction and to interpret the pictures, words, and pointing accurately. Low-technology and high-technology AAC systems can be analyzed according to the following features:

1. **Physical interface** refers to the physical keyboard or screen from which the user makes selections of symbols and vocabulary items and may include mechanical keys or flat areas of a screen or membrane keyboard. The overall size of the selection area is critical, as are the sizes and number of keys that may be displayed at once. Some screen-based devices are *dynamic display* devices in which the vocabulary items automatically change as the child selects symbols, which change the screen or keyboard displays. *Static display* devices utilize keyboards that contain fixed or static symbols and vocabulary items. Some devices have the keyboards and vocabulary items organized into changeable levels or overlays. Interface features also determine selection techniques such as direct selection through pointing to keys with a finger, light, mouse, or scanning with one or more switches.

2. **Communication output** may be speech output and may include synthesized speech or digitized speech. It also may be in the form of written output using built-in printers, external add-on printers, or text displays. Many devices also contain message displays that are intended for user feedback and enable the child to monitor and edit the message as he or she generates it, but before it becomes an expressed message.

3. **Language features** include how vocabulary items are represented. They may be represented visually through text or graphics or auditorily. Auditory systems provide lists to which the user listens before selecting the components of the message. Language features also include the language access and organization of a device. Vocabulary related to different functional topics or pragmatic categories may be located on different levels and pages, coded by alphanumeric or iconic coding systems, or accessed through word prediction. Finally, different devices have different storage capacities per vocabulary item, per message, or per total device.

Other features that are critical to different users include size and weight, type of power requirements, price, and purchasing information (Table 9–5).

Use for Language Development

The developing child concomitantly practices and learns receptive and expressive language and literacy skills. Disorders that affect oral-motor

TABLE 9–5. Available Augmentative and Alternative Communication Devices

Device	Physical Interfaces	Communication Output	Language Features
Alpha Talker	4, 8, 32 location keyboards Direct selection, scanning, optical pointer	Digitized speech	Designed for use with iconic Minspeak system including access to multiple "themes" from one overlay Messages can be programmed through symbol sequences for vocabulary expansion Can be used with multiple picture overlays or "levels"
Speak Easy	12 location keyboard Linear scanning External switches can directly access messages	Digitized speech	One level can be programmed at a time
Macaw	Multiple keyboards with different number of keys Direct selection, scanning	Digitized speech	Level-based with multiple overlays Messages can be programmed through symbol sequences for vocabulary expansion
DynaVox 2c, DynaMyte	Dynamic display with multiple screen displays and key arrays Direct selection, scanning, mouse	Synthesized speech Digitized speech On-screen visual display External printer option	Dynasym pictographic symbols Multiple screens which automatically link Supports spelling and word prediction
Vanguard	Dynamic display with multiple screen displays and key arrays, although "core vocabulary" is relatively fixed Direct selection, scanning, mouse	Synthesized speech Digitized speech On-screen visual display External printer option	Minspeak iconic symbol system Multiple screens which automatically link Supports spelling and word prediction
Light Writer	Alphanumeric keyboard Direct selection and scanning models available	Synthesized speech Text displays which face user and listener	Spelling with word prediction Alphanumeric coding of programmed messages
Co:Writer	Computer-based software, Windows and Macintosh compatible Keyboard, switch scanning, and mouse access (with supplemental programs)	Aid to writing and word processing Includes speech feedback options to user as a spelling, learning, and language processing aid	Word prediction based on frequency of use, recency of use, grammar, and word completion
Write:OutLoud	Computer-based software, Windows and Macintosh compatible Keyboard, switch scanning, and mouse access (with supplemental programs)	Aid to writing and word processing Includes speech feedback options to user as a spelling, learning and language processing aid	Talking word processing program for individuals with reading and learning disabilities
IntelliKeys	Computer-based software, Macintosh and Windows compatible Expanded keyboard with multiple key layouts and overlays, switch access	Can be used with other software to provide "talking pictures" for communication, language learning, and curriculum-based learning Can be used with any word processing, drawing, or other software	Supplemental software is available to support literacy learning, interaction, and communication

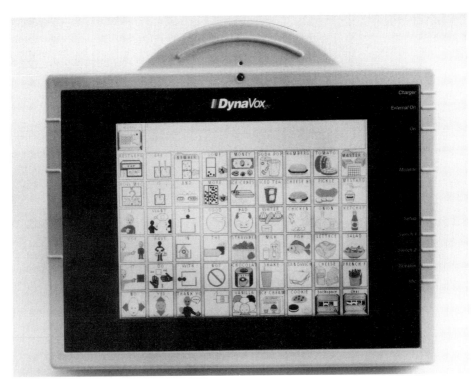

FIGURE 9–13. DynaVox 2c.

and expressive speech performance may disrupt a child's language-learning system. In such cases, an AAC system can serve both to supplement the child's functional communication and to support speech and language development.

The DynaMyte is one of the dynamic display devices. The keyboard is incorporated into a touch-sensitive screen and consists of different, but linking pages of symbol keys that represent single words, short phrases, and complete sentences. These elements may be combined into original utterances. Individual keys contain pictures, representational graphic symbols (such as Dynasyms in the DynaMyte and DynaVox2c [Fig. 9–13]), letters, or printed words. Individual screens may contain vocabulary related to semantic categories (e.g., fast foods, colors, numbers, toys, items used at work, cooking items), specific parts of speech (e.g., verbs, prepositions, adjectives), pragmatic language categories (e.g., greetings, slang expressions, conversational interactions, turn-taking), and other types of language organization (Fig. 9–14).

The DynaMyte and DynaVox 2c also contain syntactic markers so that one may easily change verb tenses, create regular and irregular plural nouns, and create adjectival and other syntactic forms to formulate sentences and passages. Using the DynaMyte, the child is able to create meaningful sentences that incorporate vocabulary related to verbs and actions, nouns, size, speed, color, and numbers that others understand. Children can participate actively and appropriately in school-based language learning activities; give others, more independently and intelligibly, complex information about likes, dislikes, and experiences; and initiate and maintain conversational topics.

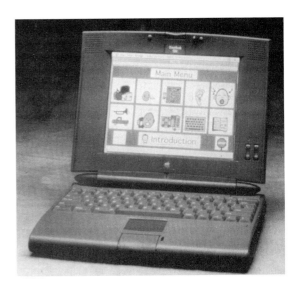

FIGURE 9–14. Speaking dynamically in a computer-based system.

Use in Acquired Disabilities

Children with acquired disabilities present a different constellation of learning styles, strengths, weaknesses, and preferences than children with congenital disabilities. People with spinal cord injuries retain their cognitive and language skills but may have insufficient respiratory support for effective use of speech in all environments. They may need new strategies and systems for producing written language. People with traumatic brain injury may have difficulty with new learning and organizational and executive cognitive functions. People who suffer strokes, anoxic brain injuries, or other neurologic insults may have global or localized deficits. Typically, children who used to speak but lost their speaking abilities are impatient with AAC devices and strategies and may not be satisfied until they can speak again.

It is important that all communicators utilize residual speech whenever it is functional; it is especially critical that AAC systems for people with acquired disabilities maximize the role of natural speech. Natural speech may be used primarily for initiation and attention-getting with a supplementary device used to communicate specific or complex information. Unaided natural speech may be the primary communication technique, supplemented by a speech amplifier in noisy environments. Frequently, people with acquired disabilities prefer "real" rather than synthesized speaking voices. AAC devices that utilize digitized speech can be programmed with the voices of age- and gender-appropriate cohorts so that a teen-aged girl speaks in the voice of an adolescent girl when she supplements her natural speech.

Digitized speech requires more computerized memory than synthesized speech and can be replayed only in the messages that were preprogrammed rather than combined into generative, original sentences. Therefore, digitized systems currently are not as flexible and powerful as devices that utilize synthesized speech. Digitized devices such as the SpeakEasy and the Easy Talk may contain limited memory, such as memory for one-minute of programmed speech. Others, such as the Macaw, the Alpha Talker, and the Digivox, contain memory for more extensive messages. Still others, such as the DynaVox 2c, the DynaMyte, and the DeltaTalker (Fig. 9–15), contain both synthesized and digitized speech capabilities. Some devices, such as the LightWriter, are small, portable, and powerful speech output systems based on spelling and preprogrammed messages using letter/abbreviation codes. They often are preferred by people with acquired communication impairments who have maintained many of their premorbid cognitive skills. Portable and lightweight speech amplifiers, such as the Voicette, can be carried by ambulatory users or mounted on wheelchairs. They can be adapted to be switch-activated so that people with limited motor skills can turn them on independently when they want their speech amplified and turn them off when they do not.

Technology, Literacy, and Disabilities

One of the skills most critical to success in school, work, and life in the community is the ability to read and write. Literacy learning for children with physical, cognitive, developmental, and learning disabilities should start as early as it does for typically developing children. Children with disabilities learn the patterns of language,

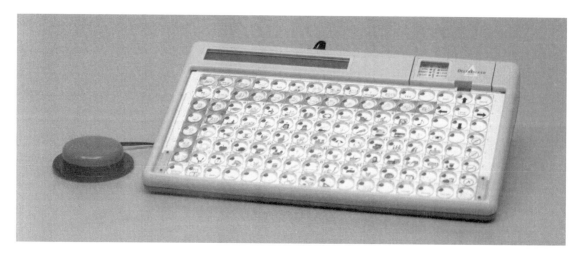

FIGURE 9–15.   Delta Talker. Note the single switch access.

the sequences of concepts and thoughts, the look of written language and printed words, and associations among ideas, pictures, and words by having their parents read to them. Opportunities for the richness of story book reading can be lost when a child has a significant disability and cannot turn a page, cannot "read" aloud a passage, or cannot memorize effectively. Augmentative communication and computer technology can help parents and children to overcome the barriers of their disabilities. For children who cannot speak, speech output communication aids are programmed with picture overlays and spoken passages of books. Children take turns with parents as they read "Good Night Moon" and initiate and complete the reading of each page of a Sesame Street book about numbers and number concepts. Simple adaptations can be made to help children turn pages. A tongue depressor or foam spacer glued to each page may be all that some children with physical disabilities need to turn pages independently. Others may gain independence and interdependence with the assistance of books on CD-ROM.

Older children who have already learned some reading and spelling skills may benefit from computer-assisted writing systems and strategies. People with fine motor disabilities may be able to use their handwriting for short tasks but may not have sufficient stamina or speed for longer tasks. Many children with attention deficits are unable to write longer passages and documents. They may effectively use handwriting for short writing tasks, a portable word processor such as an Alpha Smart 2000 or Laser PC5 for in-class tasks, and a desktop computer for longer and more sophisticated writing.

Clinicians and educators who have worked through the 1990s have seen a dramatic increase in the number of children and youth who are computer-literate because of their experiences with home and school computers. Children with language and motor impairments are often familiar with the arrangements of letters on a standard computer keyboard and frequently are expert mouse users. The Americans with Disabilities Act, technology transfer requirement of federally funded research and development projects, and standard competitive market practices have provided special access options for people within disabilities within the control panels of Windows and Macintosh operating systems. "Sticky Keys" settings can be made for one-handed and one-finger typists who have difficulty with entering simultaneous keystrokes. Similarly, keyboard and mouse speed settings can be adjusted to slow the computer response rate for people who have motor control and accuracy difficulties due to spasticity and athetosis.

Word prediction programs (Fig. 9–16) are used by people who write slowly for either motor or language processing reasons and people who have learning disabilities that limit their spelling, writing, and reading abilities. Many programs use multidimension prediction models to make the writing process more efficient. Words are displayed in prediction-lists according to frequency of use in the English language, recency of use in the child's writing patterns, syntactic models (in which verbs may be predicted to follow the word "to" and nouns and adjectives may be predicted to follow the word "the"), and word-completion models. In word-completion models, for example, words beginning with the letter "e" are presented after an initial "e" is typed.

Speech recognition or speech input technology took a great leap forward in 1997 with the release of Naturally Speaking. Before Naturally Speaking, speech recognition systems had at least one of several limitations. They were inherently slow and required speakers to "dictate" to their computers in speech patterns that contained acoustic separations and short pauses between words. Proficient users were able to achieve dictation and "typing" rates as high as 35 words per minute. Other speech recognition systems might achieve faster recognition patterns but had limited vocabularies of less than 1,000 words. Still others were designed to provide users with "speaking control" over computer functions such as opening files but no really flexible text input.

Naturally Speaking is a real-time system that enables a person to speak at a natural conversational pace and still provides access to a large and flexible vocabulary (30,000 active words, 230,000 total words). Although the child may speak at a natural pace, the speed and sophistication of the computer determine the rate at which the computer processes the speech and the rate at which the text appears on the screen. The text on the screen may be as much as a sentence or two behind the speaker with all but the fastest computers. Naturally Speaking and other systems also give users access to all computer operations, including mouse movements and mouse-button functions, through speech. Repetitive functions, such as selecting and opening a specific folder of documents, can be controlled through customizable macros such as "open social studies papers" to enhance independence and efficiency.

Computer access through on-screen keyboards, specialized mice, or speech recognition enables

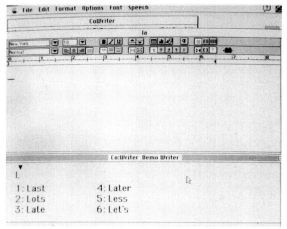

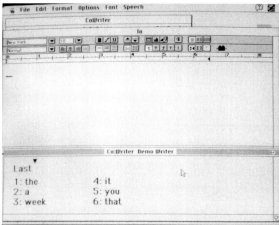

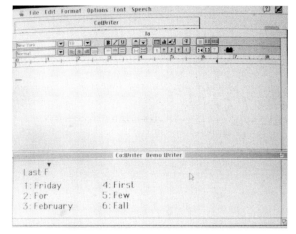

FIGURE 9–16. Co:Writer's word prediction screens.

children with disabilities to have the same opportunities to learn and communicate as their peers. It may enable them to engage in these activities in such a way that their disabilities are invisible to on-line communication partners.

National and International Resources

Many organizations offer specialized information and resources related to AAC and assistive technologies. Each offers a different perspective and a different assortment of assistance.

• The United States Society for Augmentative and Alternative Communication (USSAAC) is a national chapter of the international organization (ISAAC). Its members include people from all professions involved with AAC (including manufacturers and researchers) as well as consumers and family members. USSAAC may be contacted at USSAAC, PO Box 5271, Evanston, IL 60204, 847-869-2122, ussaac@northshore.net

• ISAAC offers journals and newsletters as well as information about AAC in countries around the world. ISAAC may be contacted at ISAAC, 49 The Donway West, Suite 308, Toronto, Ontario, M3C 3M9, Canada, 416-385-0351, isaac_mail@mail.cepp.org

• The American Speech-Language-Hearing Association (ASHA) includes a special interest division in AAC for speech-language pathologists. ASHA may be contacted at ASHA, 10801 Rockville Pike, Rockville, MD 20852, 301-897-5700, www.asha.org

• The Rehabilitation Engineering and Assistive Technology Society of North America (RESNA) is an interdisciplinary association for the advancement of rehabilitation and assistive technologies and includes a special interest group in AAC. RESNA may be contacted at RESNA, 1700 North Moore Street, Suite 1540, Arlington, VA 22209, 703-524-6686, www.resna.org

• Every state has a special project devoted to AAC and assistive technology. These projects were originally established by federal funding through the Technology-Related Assistance Act. They are known as Tech Act Projects. Directories are available from organizations such as USSAAC and RESNA.

• The Communication Aid Manufacturers Association (CAMA) offers packets of manufacturers catalogs and series of local workshops about AAC devices and their applications. CAMA may be contacted at CAMA, PO Box 1039, Evanston, IL 60204, 800-441-2262, cama@northshore.net

• Closing the Gap (CSUN) offers both conferences and publications. CSUN is an annual assistive technology conference at the California State University at Northbridge.

References

1. Alexander MA, Nelson MR, Shah A: Orthotics: Adapted Seating and Assistive Devices. In Molnar GE (ed): Pediatric Rehabilitation, 2nd ed. Baltimore, Williams & Wilkins, 1992.
2. American Academy of Pediatrics: Family Shopping Guide to Car Seats, 1996. Elk Grove Village, IL, American Academy of Pediatrics, 1996 [brochure].
3. American Academy of Pediatrics: Policy Statement: Transporting Children with Special Needs. American Academy of Pediatrics Safe Ride News Insert, Winter, 1993.
4. Bender LF: Upper extremity orthotics. In Kottke FJ, Stillwell GK, Lehmann J: Krusen's Handbook of Physical Medicine and Rehabilitation, 3rd ed. Philadelphia, WB Saunders, 1982.
5. Bergen AF, Presperin J, Tallman T: Positioning for Function: Wheelchairs and Other Assistive Technologies. New York, Valhalla Rehabilitation Publications, 1990.
6. Cook AM, Hussey SM: Assistive Technologies: Principles and Practice. St. Louis, Mosby, 1995.
7. Cusick BD: Management guidelines for using splints. In Cusick BD (ed): Progressive Casting and Splinting for Lower Extremity Deformities in Children with Neuromotor Dysfunction. San Antonio, TX, Therapy Skill Builders, 1990.
8. Demasco P, Lytton R, Mineo B, et al: The Guide to Augmentative and Alternative Communications Devices. Wilmington, DE, Applied Science & Engineering Laboratories, 1996.
9. Einset K, Deitz J, Billingsley F, Harris SR: The electric feeder: An efficacy study. Occup Ther J Res 1989;9:1.
10. Hennessey W, Johnson EW: Lower limb orthoses. In Braddom RL (ed): Physical Medicine and Rehabilitation. Philadelphia, WB Saunders, 1996.
11. Hylton NM: Postural and functional impact of dynamic AFOs and FOS in a pediatric population. J Prosthet Orthot 1989;2:40.
12. Lough LK, Nielsen D: Ambulation of children with myelomeningocele: Parapodium versus parapodium with ORLAU swivel modification. Devel Med Child Neurol 1986;28:489.
13. Makaran JE, Dittmer DK, Buchal RO, MacArthur DE: The SMART wrist hand orthosis (WHO) for quadriplegic patients. J Prosthet Orthot 1983;5:73.
14. Molnar GE: Orthotic management of children. In Redford JB, Basmajian JV, Trautman P (eds): Orthotics, Clinical Practice and Rehabilitation Technology. New York, Churchill Livingstone, 1995.
15. Paleg G: Made for walking: A comparison of gait trainers. Team Rehabil Rep 1997;July:41.
16. Schutt A: Upper extremity and hand orthotics. Phys Med Rehabil Clin North Am 1982;3:223.
17. Stern EB: Grip strength and finger dexterity across five styles of commercial wrist orthoses. Am J Occup Ther 1996;50:1.
18. Stratton M: Behavioral assessment scale of oral functions in feeding. Am J Occup Ther 1981;35:719.
19. Stroup KB, Wylie P, Bull MJ: Car seats for children with mechanically assisted ventilation. Pediatrics 1987;80:290.
20. Thacker J, Shaw G: Safe and secure. Team Rehabil Rep 1994;Feb:26.
21. Trombly CA, Scott AD: Occupational Therapy for Physical Dysfunction. Baltimore, Waverly Press, 1977.
22. Vogel LC, Lubicky JP: Ambulation with parapodia and reciprocating gait orthoses in pediatric spinal cord injury. Devel Med Child Neurol 1995;35:957.
23. Weber A: Kids on Wheels: Choices for Pediatric Wheelchairs. Advance for Directors in Rehabilitation. 1997, pp 10.
24. Weiner M: Brief or new—Feeding device for finger foods. Am J Occup Ther 1985;39:746.
25. Zolars A, Knezevich J: Special Seating: An Illustration Guide. Minneapolis, MN, Otto Bock Orthopedic Industry, 1996.

Chapter 10

Health Promotion in the Disabled Child: A Nursing Perspective

Joyce Harvey, RN, MSN, PNP
Judy Kerr, RN, MS, CRRN

Concept of Health Promotion

Providing for health promotion in the disabled pediatric population requires the blending of several nursing subspecialties. The principles of rehabilitation nursing and pediatric nursing are fundamental to promoting health within this population. Knowledge of pathophysiology as it relates to function in the neurologic, musculoskeletal, and other organ systems provides the framework of this chapter. Specific nursing interventions to be used in a variety of settings are outlined.

In 1995, the World Health Organization produced definitions related to disability that are consistently applied throughout this chapter. *Impairment* is defined as a loss or abnormality of psychological, physiologic, or anatomic structure or function at the organ level. A *disability* is the restriction or lack of ability to perform an activity in a normal manner. A *handicap* is a disadvantage because of impairment or disability that limits or prevents fulfillment of a normal role. The definitions provide a useful mechanism for separating problems of chronic illness from those related to disabilities.[1]

A trajectory perspective of chronic illness was described in 1991 by Corbin and Strauss.[2] The trajectory begins with the diagnosis of a chronic illness and ends with the phase called dying. Although it is evident that children with disabilities have chronic illness that can fit along that trajectory, the promotion of health for this group relies on the provider's ability to distinguish between aspects of a disability and of a chronic illness. Maximizing functional abilities cannot be accomplished without first making these distinctions. Preventing the complications of disability is equally reliant on a clear delineation between chronic illness and disability.[1]

Nursing Roles across Practice Settings

Children with disabilities are seen by nurses in a wide range of practice settings. School nurses and community health nurses interact with disabled children by enhancing their participation in both mainstream and adapted schools, in residential care centers, and in community environments. Family nurse-practitioners and pediatric nurse-practitioners encounter this population in general and specialty clinics. Hospital-based nurses encounter children with disabilities in emergency departments, intensive care, surgery, and rehabilitation. Home care nurses provide services to this population both on a long-term and on an intermittent basis. Finally, payer-based nurse case managers are challenged to coordinate the comprehensive care needs of this population.

In each of these settings, the nurse provider is charged with the responsibility of providing for care that recognizes the uniqueness of these children. Using the principles of anticipatory guidance, the nurse also provides families with information that allows for growth and development in as normal a curve as can be achieved given the physical, social, economic, and environmental constraints that exist for each individual. This chapter outlines general principles of care for the disabled child that can be applied across all practice settings.

Legal and Ethical Considerations

In 1920, the first Rehabilitation Act was passed by the U.S. Congress. This was followed over the years by a series of laws in the United States that promoted and protected the rights of disabled individuals. The Americans with Disabilities Act (ADA) is the most recent and most far-reaching of these laws. The full extent of the ADA is yet to be interpreted by the court systems in the United States. Running parallel to the legal rights of the disabled child are the ethical considerations that must be applied to each individual situation. The introduction of life-support systems to severely disabled children must be considered from a range of perspectives that are provided in ethics committees and forums. The ethical responsibilities of payers must also be addressed.[1]

Growth and Development

An overview of normal growth and development is provided in Chapter 2. Strategies for application of growth and developmental expectations are individualized and for the purposes of this chapter are functionally driven. There are no standard variances from the norm within any segment of the disabled pediatric population. It is this range of expectations that makes work with this population both rewarding and challenging. Anticipatory guidance allows positive outcomes. Normal growth and developmental curves can direct anticipatory guidance but cannot replace the intuitive knowledge of the expert nurse provider. Identifying potential barriers to the next step in development is the domain of the nurse working with the disabled child.[3,43]

Health Promotion

Cardiovascular System

Deconditioning and Endurance

Alterations in the cardiovascular system within the disabled pediatric population fall into two major categories. The first category relates to deconditioning and endurance. Children with acquired disabilities are faced with long-term hospitalizations and immobility, which contribute to decreased endurance and weakness. Postural hypotension secondary to immobility is usually amenable to a gradual increase in activity with attention to orthostatic changes. Generally, postural hypotension is short-lived and responds quickly to increased activity. Occasionally, children who have been on bed rest for an extended period of time require additional circulatory support of Ace wraps and abdominal binders. An individual child's tolerance to activity can be correlated to measures of apical heart rate, which should fall within the standards for age as listed in Table 10–1.[4]

Dysautonomic Effects

Dysautonomia results in cardiovascular system problems. Most frequently seen after a traumatic brain injury, disruptions of the autonomic nervous system can affect heart rate, blood pressure, and vasodilation. Although there is not always a clear cause for the dysautonomic response in the brain-injured pediatric patient, careful nursing assessment and intervention can eliminate potential triggers. Examples of conditions that can stimulate or exacerbate dysautonomia include pain, gastric distention, gastroesophageal reflux, and poor positioning. If exact triggers of the dysautonomia cannot be found, consultation with a physician is indicated so that pharmacologic management can be implemented. β-blockers and other medications can be helpful in controlling symptoms. Basic nursing measures of comfort, hydration, vital sign monitoring, and frequent position changes are helpful in preventing the complications of dysautonomia.[1,44]

TABLE 10–1.

Age	Heart Rate	Respiratory Rate	Significant Hypertension (mmHg)	Normal Caloric Requirements (No Catchup)
Newborn	140	30–80	>112/>74	108 kcal/kg/day
1 Yr	115–130	20–40	>112/>74	100 kcal/kg/day
2 Yr	110	20–30	>116/>76	100 kcal/kg/day
3 Yr	105	20–30	>116/>76	100 kcal/kg/day
4 Yr	105	20–30	>116/>76	100 kcal/kg/day
5 Yr	95	20–25	>122/>78	90 kcal/kg/day
10 Yr	85	15–20	>126/>82	70 kcal/kg/day
15 Yr		15–20	>136/>82	Varies with gender, 30–55 kcal/kg/day
Maintenance Fluid Calculation	Weight 1–10 kg	100 ml/kg		
	11–20 kg	1000 ml + 50/ml/kg (for each kg > 10)		
	> 20 kg	1500 ml + 20 ml/kg (for each kg > 20)		

A second dysfunction of the autonomic nervous system is seen in the spinal cord–injured child. Although autonomic dysreflexia is discussed in greater detail in Chapter 14 on spinal cord injury, it is important to note that children with spinal cord injuries above the T-6 level are at significant risk for complications of hypertension secondary to dysreflexia (hyperreflexia). All care providers of children with this type of disability need to be trained to assess the child for dysreflexia and to intervene appropriately. Caused by a noxious stimulus below the level of injury, the most likely precipitating factor of dysreflexia is a distended bladder. Facial flushing, pounding headache, bradycardia, hypertension (potentially life-threatening), and sweating above the spinal cord level are the most common presenting symptoms in the child with a spinal cord injury. Immediate intervention includes raising the head to decrease cerebral blood flow and concomitant risk of stroke, followed promptly by emptying the bladder. Monitoring the child for relief of symptoms after bladder intubation usually shows an end of the autonomic response. Symptoms that continue for more than 10–15 minutes after catheterization may indicate a bowel impaction. This must be addressed immediately with manual disimpaction using a topical anesthetic (dibucaine [Mupercainal] or lidocaine [Xylocaine]). All children at risk for dysreflexia should carry information for emergency medical personnel describing the treatment of unresolved dysreflexia.[5,6]

Venous Thrombosis

A consideration in the disabled pediatric patient facing long-term immobilization is the development of venous thrombosis and the more serious sequela of pulmonary embolism. This complication is generally rare before the onset of puberty. In the adolescent population, interventions may be similar to those used in immobilized adults, including assessment for swelling or redness, passive range of motion, compression stockings, and anticoagulant agents.[1]

Respiratory System

Incidence of Respiratory Disease

Alterations in respiratory functioning can be the primary cause of pediatric disability or can be seen as a complication of the primary disabling condition. Chronic respiratory failure in the disabled pediatric population represents a particular subset of patients whose lives have been successfully extended through the development of mechanical ventilators that can be used in a home setting. Chronic respiratory failure is defined as a condition that requires mechanical ventilation

for 28 or more consecutive days. Some patients are ultimately weaned from ventilator dependence, whereas others require lifelong technologic support. Because of the needs of third-party payers and economic decision making, there exists a legal definition of ventilatory dependency outlined in 1985 as a "condition which requires a ventilator for at least 6 hours per day."[7]

Chronic respiratory failure is almost always related to *pump* failure as opposed to acute respiratory failure, which generally derives from *lung* failure. Diseases that predispose to chronic respiratory failure include central nervous system problems affecting either the brain stem or the cervical spinal cord. Other problems can involve the accessory respiratory muscles and conditions that affect movement of the thorax deriving from motor unit dysfunction.[7]

Ventilator Dependency

A small group of patients can be successfully treated with negative pressure ventilation. Devices available include tank respirators, such as the iron lung, as well as more portable and adaptable cuirass devices. Maintaining an adequate seal between the thorax and the negative pressure device is critical to successful use of this device. Continuous positive airway pressure (CPAP) has also been explored and found to be successful in a small number of pediatric patients. Nasal airways have been used to maintain the positive pressure.[7,46,47]

Most children who are ventilator-dependent cannot be treated with negative pressure ventilators or with CPAP (Table 10–2) and require an artificial airway, generally a tracheostomy, for access to positive-pressure ventilation. In general, the ventilator of choice is the simplest device available, which at this writing is a volume cycled ventilator. The complexity of managing these children in the home, even with the use of the simplest positive-pressure ventilation is significant. An interdisciplinary home care team is required, which should include primary physicians, pulmonologists, home nurses, respiratory therapists, home health aides, social workers, vendors, and others. Families require extensive training and in-home support to maintain health both for the child and for the family unit. The decision to provide long-term ventilatory support must include an ethical and realistic consideration of the family's ability and willingness to maintain the complexities of care needs with available resources.

Family Training

Teaching families about managing the ventilator and the tracheostomy is most commonly

TABLE 10–2. Comparison between Positive-Pressure and Negative-Pressure Ventilators

Ventilator Type	Advantages	Disadvantages
Positive pressure	Readily available Easily adjustable Choice of mode Efficient ventilation in the presence of intrinsic lung disease Useful even with severe lung failure	Usually requires tracheostomy
Negative pressure	Limited variety of devices Devices are portable No need for tracheostomy	Less efficient with intrinsic lung disease Limited access to tracheobronchial secretions Predisposition to upper airway obstruction and sleep disruption Variable fit night to night Not suitable for 24-hr support Backup battery not always available Control mode only

Adapted from Mallory GB Jr, Stillwell PC: The ventilator-dependent child: Issues in diagnosis and management. Arch Phys Med Rehabil 1991;72:43.

coordinated by the nurse in the inpatient setting. The technical skills required are often easier to demonstrate on a doll, and the knowledge base is often easier to impart away from the bedside. Content of the teaching plan must be individualized based on the learner's cognitive, emotional, and psychomotor abilities. Mastery of skills is best measured by observed ability to solve unanticipated problems of real-life events with confidence. Specific procedures for ventilator care and tracheostomy management must adhere to the principles of infection control and patient comfort but are entirely driven by the requirements of the individual patient and types of equipment and supplies available and therefore are not outlined here.[8,9]

Gastrointestinal System

Alteration in Nutritional Intake

Maintaining adequate nutrition and hydration in the disabled child can be complicated by many factors, including impaired self-feeding skills, dysphagia, gastroesophageal reflux, dysmotility, behavioral food aversion, hyperphagia, and altered metabolic rates. Malabsorption factors are less commonly seen. Undernutrition in children with neurodevelopmental disabilities has been clearly shown to predispose this population to infection, skin breakdown, impaired brain growth and development, diminished attention span, and increased agitation. Undernutrition within the severely disabled pediatric population remains a significant contributing factor to morbidity and mortality.[10]

Decisions to supplement oral feeding with enteral feeds are based on assessment of the child's oral motor skill and efficiency and on the family's ability to assist the child in meeting nutritional needs orally. Some families forgo the surgical placement of a gastrostomy and continue to spend up to 8 hours per day engaged in oral feeding activities. Other families opt for more time-efficient alternatives. Both options are viable and should be supported by the nurse so long as the basic nutritional needs of the child are met. Skin-fold measures of body fat composition have been used to assess nutritional status in children who, because of musculoskeletal deformity, cannot otherwise be assigned to standard growth charts.[10,11]

Before the surgical placement of a gastrostomy tube, evaluation for esophageal reflux is recommended. Pharmacologic management of gastroesophageal reflux is often effective and can result in greater success with oral feeding programs. If gastroesophageal reflux is present and remains unresponsive to pharmacologic management, consideration of a surgical antireflux procedure, such as a Nissen fundoplication, is indicated. Antireflux procedures are not considered permanent. Often children outgrow their effectiveness within 2–3 years. Instruction to families after antireflux procedures should include information on decompressing the stomach (burping) as well as what to watch for as the child ages and may outgrow the procedure.[11]

Family Training

Teaching families about the management of gastrostomy tubes involves care of the gastrostomy site, tubes, and equipment as well as formula preparation. A variety of gastrostomy appliances are available. Devices that can be changed in the home setting and do not require a clinic visit to replace are preferred. Regardless of the specific appliance selected, families must be instructed in how to manage the accidental removal of the gastrostomy appliance or tube. Maintaining the integrity of the skin around the stoma requires diligent attention to hygiene. Mild soap and water are recommended for cleaning the gastrostomy site. Gastric content leakage can represent a particular difficulty and may indicate that the appliance needs to be resized or replaced. The development of granulation tissue around the gastrostomy site is sometimes seen in the early stages of healing and can be treated with silver nitrate topically. Previously mentioned attention to cleanliness at the os can prevent granulation tissue from forming. Because third-party payers do not consistently provide coverage for prepared formulas, families may need to be informed about the nutritional completeness of home-prepared formulas. Blenderizing family meals and diluting with milk or soy products is another alternative. Families must be provided with anticipatory guidance related to increasing caloric requirements as the child grows. Families are directed to remain in contact with an interdisciplinary team, which includes a clinical nutritionist.[12]

Children with feeding disorders are a particular challenge when they present with acute gastroenteritis. Anticipatory guidance to families related to this can greatly assist the family's coping mechanisms. Knowing how to recognize signs of dehydration, how to intervene, and when to contact a physician is of particular importance to families of this patient population. Diarrhea can be the result of an acute bacterial or viral infection, or it can result from feeding intolerance and food allergies. Families should recognize that diarrhea is not the primary risk, but rather that dehydration is what needs to be monitored. Constipation in this population is managed by adding fiber and increasing hydration and is generally less troublesome to families than diarrhea. Families should be taught to contact their health care provider if severe constipation is identified because paralytic ileus is a potential complication in chronic severe constipation.[4,13]

Oral Feeding with the Dysphagic Child

Dysphagia is to be considered with all disease processes affecting the neurologic system as well as with severe myopathies that present with weakness. Bottle-fed and breast-fed infants should be assessed for dysphagia and aspiration risk when they present with neurologic and musculoskeletal disorders that impair oral motor coordination. Patients in the inpatient setting should be considered at high risk for aspiration until specific testing rules out swallowing disorders. Oral feeding in a child with documented or suspected dysphagia must include proper upright posturing, adequate head control or support, observation of the phases of swallowing, and maintaining necessary equipment for suctioning should frank aspiration occur. Efficiency of oral feeding, including precise amounts taken over recorded periods of time, should be assessed and is helpful in deciding on surgical or endoscopic placement of gastrostomies.[14]

Alteration in Bowel Elimination

Neurogenic bowel dysfunction and toilet or habit training disorders represent the two primary causes of alterations in bowel elimination in the pediatric population. Neurogenic bowel problems are seen primarily in the spinal cord population, including both acquired and congenital spinal cord disease. Lower motor neuron bowel dysfunction is common in the spina bifida patient as well as in the lower spinal cord injury patient. Upper motor neuron bowel elimination is found primarily with tetraplegic spinal cord injury but is sometimes evident in severe traumatic brain injury. Mixed upper and lower motor neuron injuries can also have an effect on bowel elimination.[15]

Lower Motor Neuron Bowel

A lower motor neuron injury results in a flaccid rectal sphincter. This is most responsive to manual evacuation of stool from the rectum using an upright position on a commode or toilet. Sitting upright is important because gravity facilitates emptying of the bowel, and the 90-degree angle of sitting shortens the length of the colon. Suppositories are generally of no use because there is no innervation of the rectal sphincter and therefore no tone to stimulate. Digital stimulation is, for the same reason, generally not indicated. Stool softeners often create a greater problem with leaking stool and are generally not used. High-fiber diet and manual evacuation timed 30 minutes after each meal to maximize the effect of the gastrocolic reflex result in the best outcomes. Most patients use some sort of diaper or pad to protect against accidents. Rectal plugs have been used successfully by some patients. Continual stool leakage is common and often indicative of chronic constipation. When children present with chronic leakage, a careful assessment of bowel routines should be made. Diaries of bowel and dietary routines covering several days or weeks can help in diagnosing the problem. Children and families can become unaware of the odor associated with chronic bowel leakage. Although it is not always possible to achieve full continence with a lower motor neuron impairment, families and patients should be provided with interventions that will allow them to work toward that goal.[15]

Upper Motor Neuron Bowel

Upper motor neuron injury results in spared bulbocavernosus and anal reflexes, which can be stimulated to facilitate rectal evacuation. Digital stimulation with a finger or with a device manually stimulates the contraction of the anorectal musculature and the relaxation of the rectal sphincter resulting in defecation. There is no voluntary control of the reflexive evacuation. Bowel accidents secondary to dietary change or minor disruptions in routine can be anticipated and do not represent failure by the child or the caregiver. Anticipatory guidance directs parents and children to plan for occasional bowel incontinence. Irritant cathartics can be used to facilitate evacuation with an intact reflex arc. Medications that increase osmotic pressure in the intestinal tract and thereby increase stool water content can also be used to facilitate evacuation. Although these products can be useful in the initial phases of bowel training, use of digital stimulation alone is the objective of most upper motor neuron bowel programs.

Transition of bowel care from the parents to the child should be introduced conceptually as soon as the diagnosis of neurogenic bowel impairment is made. Developmental milestones guide the child and family to maximal independence in bowel elimination. It is important to distinguish between physiologic training of the bowel (with fluid, fiber, stimulation, medications, and timed evacuations) and the behavioral training of the parent and child. Regularity must be established by the family before responsibility can be shifted to the child. Psychological dependency issues within a family can greatly delay independence for the child who is otherwise physically and cognitively capable of independence in bowel management.[15]

Habit Training

Habit training is used in the disabled child who has a normal functioning bowel but for whom voluntary control is a primary obstacle. Children with traumatic brain injury and developmental disability respond well to habit training. High fiber content in diet and adequate hydration are combined with a closely followed daily routine. Most children establish a routine of early morning or early evening bowel elimination. Placing the child on the toilet 30 minutes after a meal gives families and caregivers an advantage in establishing habit training.

Constipation is a complication of ineffective bowel training both in habit training and in neurogenic bowel management. Chronic constipation is an indication that a full assessment of diet, hydration, daily routines, medication use, and neurologic function is needed. Occasional constipation is usually amenable to laxatives and enemas but can significantly disrupt family routines. Anticipatory guidance with families provides them with early signs and interventions for bowel irregularity.[45]

Urologic System

Bladder Function

The bladder has two primary functions: to store and to empty urine. The storage and passage of urine is termed *micturition* and is under both reflex and voluntary control. Normally the bladder wall expands slowly to fill with urine while maintaining a fairly low pressure until an appropriate urine volume is reached. The internal sphincter activity increases during bladder filling to allow for effective storage. When the bladder is full, sensory fibers are stimulated and send impulses to the sacral reflex center located at the S-2 to S–4 level of the spinal cord. From there, the impulses travel up the spinal cord to the micturition centers in the brain stem and frontal cortex. Efferent impulses from the brain stem move down the reticulospinal tract to the pelvic nerves. The pelvic nerves stimulate bladder contraction, closure of the ureter orifices, and internal sphincter (bladder neck) relaxation. When the internal sphincter relaxes, sensation of the need to void becomes apparent. The external sphincter comes under voluntary control in early childhood and is considered the "last line of defense for maintaining continence."[1] The external sphincter surrounds the distal portion of the urethra and comprises the skeletal muscles of the pelvic floor. Control of the external sphincter is regulated by impulses from the frontal cortex down the corticospinal tract to the pudendal nerve. Voluntary tightening of the external sphincter induces several cycles of bladder wall relaxation, internal sphincter contraction, and further urine storage before voiding or bladder emptying is essential. When the bladder empties, the wall of the bladder (the detrusor muscle) contracts, and both the internal and the external sphincter relax.[16]

Bladder dysfunction or neurogenic bladder may result from any injury or lesion that interrupts the normal neural pathways (central or peripheral) to the bladder. Classification of the neurogenic bladder may be anatomic, based on the location of the injury or abnormality, or functional, based on the patient's bladder and sphincter dysfunction identified via urodiagnostic studies.[16] Anatomic classifications help in understanding the pathophysiology of the bladder dysfunction and may direct an initial bladder program to prevent complications of dysfunction commonly seen with certain injuries or disabilities. A home program should be individualized and based on the child's bladder function as defined by a complete urologic workup. Urodiagnostic studies include postvoiding residuals, urinalysis and culture, renal ultrasound, voiding cystourethrogram, and urodynamics.[16,17]

In a core curriculum from the Association of Rehabilitation Nurses (ARN), a functional classification of neurogenic bladder developed by Lapides and Diokno (1976) is correlated with neurologic and urinary tract anatomy to provide an excellent background for planning appropriate bladder programs.[1] A summary of this schema incorporating nursing interventions follows.

Lapides and Diokno classified neurogenic bladders into five groups: (1) uninhibited, (2) reflex, (3) autonomous or areflexic, (4) motor paralytic, and (5) sensory paralytic.[18] An uninhibited neurogenic bladder may develop because of upper motor neuron injury either in the brain or corticoregulatory tract after a stroke, traumatic brain injury, or compression from a brain tumor. Inhibitory fibers fail to suppress detrusor contractions, resulting in a hyperreflexic bladder. The child may have difficulty with urgency, frequency, and nighttime wetting. Timed voiding may be effective in achieving continence. The child is reminded to void or is taken to the toilet to void every 2–3 hours. The goal is to empty the bladder before it is full enough to trigger reflex emptying at a less opportune time. The child should be encouraged to participate when developmentally appropriate. A child who is very young or has severe cognitive impairment may need to remain in diapers.

A reflex neurogenic bladder follows an upper motor neuron injury to both the sensory and the motor nerve tracts above S3–4. It may occur in patients who have spinal cord lesions above T12–L1 or who have experienced an ischemic event to the cord secondary to trauma, tumors, infection, or vascular malformations. Some children with spina bifida may demonstrate a reflex bladder dysfunction. Voiding is involuntary because of the lack of cerebral control and is incomplete because of bladder spasticity. The reflex arc remains intact and when stimulated triggers spontaneous voiding. Urodynamic studies show uninhibited contractions with decreased bladder capacity. In addition, detrusor-urethral sphincter dyssynergia may develop. Detrusor urethral sphincter dyssynergia occurs when there is an inappropriate contraction or failure of complete and sustained relaxation of the urethral sphincter during detrusor (bladder) contraction. This lack of coordination between the detrusor and external sphincter leads to increased intravesical pressures and subsequent upper tract involvement with vesicoureteral reflux, hydronephrosis, and possible renal damage. Bladder management for a child with a reflex bladder incorporates pharmacologic agents and clean intermittent catheterization. Credé or Valsalva maneuvers are discouraged in children with a reflex bladder because they may increase ureteral reflux.

The autonomous or areflexic bladder is characterized as flaccid with decreased sensation of fullness, weak or absent detrusor contractions, increased bladder capacity with high residual urine, and overflow incontinence. External sphincter activity may be present in an areflexic bladder, but it is not under voluntary control. These changes in bladder function are a result of lower motor neuron damage of both the motor and the sensory branches of the sacral reflex arc. Spinal cord lesions at or below T12–L1 or congenital lesions such as spina bifida may lead to an areflexic bladder. Achieving urinary continence in a child with an areflexic bladder may be quite difficult. Clean intermittent catheterization can provide continence if there is sufficient external sphincter activity. Valsalva maneuver, straining, or Credé maneuver may assist voiding and complete bladder emptying but presents an increased risk for ureteral reflux. Incontinence supplies, including diapers or an external collecting system, may be necessary.

The motor paralytic bladder occurs in patients who have suffered damage to the motor branch or ventral roots of S2–4. Characterized by loss of motor function with intact sensation, the child with a motor paralytic bladder may present with difficulty starting a stream, decreased force of urinary stream, or interrupted urinary stream. The child may need to strain to void. Bladder capacity is increased with high residual urine and overflow incontinence. A high bladder pressure may develop that increases the risk of upper urinary tract damage. Valsalva and Credé maneuvers or suprapubic stimulation (suprapubic tapping or jabbing over the bladder wall) may facilitate bladder contraction and emptying. These techniques may be combined with the use of a condom catheter or intermittent catheterization. Urodynamic studies are necessary in determining the appropriate treatment regimen.

The sensory paralytic bladder occurs when the sensory roots of the sacral reflex arc are disrupted. The child with a sensory paralytic bladder lacks the ability to sense fullness or bladder distention but may be able to void voluntarily. Timed voiding can maintain bladder continence and prevent prolonged periods of bladder distention. A loss of bladder tone from chronic bladder distention can further complicate bladder function if a normal voiding program is not initiated.

Intermittent Catheterization Programs

Clean intermittent catheterization is commonly used to help achieve urinary continence in children with a neurogenic bladder. The goal of intermittent catheterization is to prevent overdistention of the bladder from urinary retention and to provide dry continent periods between catheterization. The theory supporting a clean rather than sterile technique was introduced in the 1970s.[19] Lapides and colleagues[19] suggest that bladder distention results in an ischemic bladder wall hindering the bladder's defense against infection. Frequent emptying via catheterization prevents distention and flushes organisms from the bladder, therefore preventing infections. The success of clean intermittent catheterization in preventing urinary tract infections and upper tract deterioration is well documented.[20]

Most authors recommend catheterization at least five times a day. Fluids are discouraged late in the evening so that catheterization does not need to be performed during the night. An infant awakening for nighttime feeds may need to be catheterized at the time of the feeding. Use of latex-free catheters is recommended because recurrent use of latex products can result in latex sensitivity or allergy, especially in children with spina bifida. Harsh soaps should be avoided when cleaning the perineal area. Perfume-free diaper wipes or tap water can be

used. Good hand washing should be encouraged both before and after performing a catheterization. A variety of methods are recommended for cleaning the urinary catheter and appear to be equally effective. Storing the reusable catheter in a dry container is helpful in reducing bacterial contamination.[20,21] Guidelines for performing clean intermittent catheterization are provided in Table 10–3.

Family Training

Whenever possible, children should be involved in their bladder program. Mastering toileting skills is a normal developmental process for the 2–3-year-old; however, it may be delayed in a child who has suffered a brain injury or has a motor or sensory disability. In many cases, toileting must be relearned after an injury. Nurses can help develop a plan that is based on the individual needs of each child. Signs of readiness for toileting include the child's awareness of the need to urinate, dislike of wet or dirty diapers, ability to stay dry for at least 2 hours, ability to pull pants up and down, sense of social appropriateness, and interest or request to use the toilet. Adaptation to the bathroom and toilet may be necessary for the child to perform the toileting task independently.[22,23]

Children as young as 5 years old have also been taught to perform self-catheterization. Assessing the child's readiness and motivation to perform self-catheterization is essential. The child must possess certain psychomotor skills, including the ability to handle the catheter, to feel or see the urinary meatus, and to guide the tip of the catheter into the urethra. Cognitively the child must have some problem-solving skills to be able to sequence the steps correctly. With practice and patience on the part of both the teacher and the child, success is quite possible.

TABLE 10–3. Guidelines for Clean Intermittent Catheterization Programs

Supplies	Purpose of Procedure	Instructions
Clean, nonlatex urinary catheter of appropriate size	To empty the bladder at regular intervals to prevent bladder distention	Gather supplies Wash hands Have child in position of comfort with access to urethra
Disposable washcloth or cotton balls	To reduce the number or risk of bladder infections	Provide privacy
Soap and water; no harsh bactericidal soaps	To drain residual urine	Wash urethra with mild soap and water; rinse well with water
Container to collect urine	To control odors and prevent skin breakdown	Insert lubricated catheter with end positioned in cup or over toilet until urine begins to flow; then insert just a bit further. Hold in place until urine stops flowing
Container to store catheter	To achieve social continence and improve self-esteem	
Water-soluble lubricant		Remove catheter and wash catheter with water. Air dry. Store in clean container
Latex-free gloves if school or hospital staff performing procedure		Record amount of urine if directed by provider Report signs and symptoms of urinary tract infection (severe abdominal or flank pain, hematuria, foul-smelling urine, cloudy urine, fever)

Details of the approach in teaching self-catheterization to children are available.[17,23,24]

Other considerations to a bladder program include (1) maintaining adequate hydration, (2) maintaining skin integrity and perineal hygiene, (3) ensuring adequate bowel elimination, (4) eliminating intake of fluids or substances that have a dehydrating or irritating effect on the bladder (caffeinated drinks, aspartame, grapefruit juice), (5) identifying the symptoms of bladder infection, and (6) monitoring the child's compliance and response to pharmacologic regimens. Signs and symptoms of urinary tract infection include fever, abdominal or back pain, foul-smelling urine, decreased appetite, burning or irritation when voiding, hesitancy, increased incidence of autonomic dysreflexia, wetness between catheterization when the child was previously dry, increased spasticity, and vomiting. Children who are on an intermittent catheterization program may have white blood cells and bacteria in their urine, but they are not treated unless they are symptomatic, have ureteral reflux, or have bacteria counts greater than 100,000.[25]

Integumentary System

Assessing Skin

Assessing skin integrity and preventing skin breakdown is an essential skill for care providers. The skin should be inspected for color, hair distribution, nail characteristics, markings, and lesions. The skin should be palpated for temperature, texture, turgor, and capillary refill. Rashes, petechiae, or irritation can result from reactions to medications or skin products. Excessive moisture and excretions promote maceration and can cause chemical irritation. Other factors that increase the risk of skin breakdown that should also be assessed include immobility, sensory loss, altered metabolic or nutritional states, hypothermia or hyperthermia, decreased fatty tissue, altered level of consciousness, presence of shearing forces, friction or pressure, and poor compliance to daily skin care or pressure-relieving measures.[1]

Prevention of Breakdown

Prevention of skin breakdown is directed at limiting the impact of the aforementioned risk factors. Interventions may need to be adapted as the child's condition changes. In general, the skin should be kept clean and dry. Harsh soaps or preparations should be avoided. Skin moisturizers and skin barriers may be helpful when treating dry irritated skin. Children being treated with radiation therapy or for burns may require special skin care products to avoid further skin irritation. The nurse assists the patient and caregivers in learning pressure relief measures by turning, weight shifting, maintaining range of motion, and good body alignment. Friction and shearing injuries are avoided by limiting the patient's time in bed, using a lift sheet, and preventing stress on the sacral region from prolonged semiupright positions while in bed or in a chair. The nurse should encourage the patient to lie in the prone position and implement medical regimens for muscle spasms and spasticity. The nurse should initiate bowel and bladder programs or provide appropriate incontinence products to limit moisture and skin maceration. The child with sensory loss should be considered at increased risk, and insensate areas should be assessed frequently. The nurse should prevent injury by avoiding burns, sunburn, abrasions, and constrictive garments. Nutritional status should be assessed and optimal nutritional support promoted.[26–28]

Skin inspection should occur at least each morning and evening. Common pressure areas need to be checked after turning, respositioning, and removal of splints or braces. Hyperemic areas that remain red for more than 20 minutes after pressure relief, that do not blanch, or have delayed capillary refill time indicate that ischemic injury has occurred. This is the first sign or stage of a pressure ulcer. A stage II ulcer results in partial-thickness skin loss; is superficial; and presents clinically as an abrasion, blister, or shallow crater. A stage III ulcer is characterized as a deep crater with full-thickness skin loss involving damage of the subcutaneous tissue. It may extend down to, but not through, the underlying fascia. A stage IV pressure ulcer involves full-thickness skin loss with extensive destruction; tissue necrosis; or damage to muscle, bone, or supporting structures.[29]

Treatment of Skin Breakdown

When skin breakdown is present, a wound care program is implemented based on the grade, location, and general status of the wound. Children with recurrent pressure ulcers or patients admitted to the hospital with a high risk for developing skin breakdown should be placed on a pressure-reducing device, such as a low air-loss or air-fluidized bed. The use of a fluid mattress overlay was found to be effective and affordable for relieving pressure and preventing skin breakdown in pediatric patients.[28]

The development of pressure ulcers often interferes with the rehabilitation process and introduces the risk of infection, pain, restricted mobility, increased spasticity, depression, and even death.[30,31] The most serious and life-threatening complications of infection are bacteremia and osteomyelitis.[31] A wound that presents with malodorous drainage, fever, hypotension, increased heart rate, or change in mental status requires prompt evaluation and treatment for probable sepsis. Osteomyelitis should be considered whenever a stage III or IV ulcer fails to heal, especially one over a bony prominence.[31]

Neurologic System

The impact of long-term neurologic dysfunction secondary to traumatic injury or disability is immense. Children who have sustained a brain injury from trauma, hypoxia, hemorrhage, hydrocephalus, brain tumor, or congenital abnormality may have enduring cognitive or behavioral deficits. The brain lesion or injury may cause additional concerns, such as spasticity, seizures, sensorimotor impairment (loss of sight, hearing, smell, taste, swallow), or hypothalamic disturbances.

The rehabilitation team needs to define the child's level of cognitive functioning, pattern of behaviors, and developmental level before planning a successful transition home. Long-term goals are aimed at promoting an optimal level of function by reducing the effects of the child's deficits and promoting the child's strengths. A neuropsychological assessment of cognitive and behavioral function is usually initiated during the acute rehabilitation stay but may need to be completed after discharge. This evaluation provides valuable information to the family and school when transitioning the child back to the community. The inpatient rehabilitation team can also share their insights regarding the child's behavior and management strategies that have been effective during the child's stay. Parents often need guidance in setting limits and coping with difficult behaviors.

Caregivers should be instructed to notify their primary care provider if the child displays a sudden change in behavior, function, or level of awareness. Development of new deficits or recurrence of deficits that have previously improved may indicate growth of brain lesions, hemorrhage, onset of hydrocephalus, shunt malfunction, meningitis, or seizures. Other signs of increased intracranial pressure include headache, lethargy, vomiting (may be episodic), irritability, and enlarging head size and full fontanel in children less than 1 year old. Diplopia, paralysis of extraocular movements, and change in muscle tone may also occur. Late signs include bradycardia, widening pulse pressure, and unreactive pupils. A complete neurologic assessment,

brain computed tomography or magnetic resonance imaging, and electroencephalography may be indicated. Common pediatric illness, such as otitis and gastroenteritis, may alarm parents because the child may develop headache, fever, and vomiting. It is important to be supportive of these families when they seek medical attention. With time, parents become experts regarding their children, and they usually are sensitive to the differences between a minor illness or neurologic change.[30]

The incidence of seizures in the rehabilitation population varies tremendously. A study of early posttraumatic seizures in children found only 5% of children admitted with head injury experienced seizures. Risk factors included age less than 2 years, loss of consciousness for more than 24 hours, and presence of an acute subdural hematoma.[32] Late-onset seizures, up to 2 years after a traumatic brain injury, are reported by others. Patients who have a vascular malformation and who have experienced an intracranial or intraparenchymal bleed have a 25% chance of recurrent seizures.[30]

Primary interventions for seizure activity include the administration of anticonvulsant agents and maintaining safety precautions to protect the child from injury in the event of a seizure. The nurse should ensure that anticonvulsant medications are administered as prescribed and taken at time intervals to maintain therapeutic blood levels. During a seizure, the nurse records the onset, duration, and characteristics of the seizure. The nurse should maintain the use of a protective device (helmet, padded chair, or bed). The nurse should protect the child from injury by loosening restrictive devices or clothing, moving potentially harmful objects out of range, and reassuring the child. If loss of consciousness occurs, the child should be positioned to ensure an open airway and prevent aspiration. Emergency situations need to be recognized with prompt medical care made available if the child aspirates, if the child has prolonged apnea with a notable color change, or if the seizure is prolonged or recurrent.[22,30]

Initial treatment for children who present with seizures or who are at high risk for seizures is parenteral phenytoin or phenobarbital. Because these drugs can impair cognitive performance, carbamazepine (Tegretol) or valproic acid (Depakene) are preferred as soon as oral medications are tolerated.

Hypothalamic Dysfunction

Hypothalamic and pituitary injuries can result in diabetes insipidus or the syndrome of inappropriate antidiuretic hormone secretion

(SIADH). Both disorders are managed acutely by controlling fluids and electrolytes and by monitoring serum electrolytes and osmolarity. Persistent diabetes insipidus may be treated with subcutaneous vasopressin or intranasal DDAVP (desmopressin). SIADH is often treated with fluid restrictions, making it difficult to promote adequate nutrition in children requiring enteral feedings.[30,33] Consultation and close follow-up with the endocrinology team are important for both inpatient and home management of diabetes insipidus and SIADH.

A rare complication of traumatic brain injury and spina bifida is temperature instability. Central fever is usually secondary to lesions in the anterior hypothalamus and to generalized decerebration. It can also result from drug fever. Cooling blankets and tepid sponge baths can be used to reduce body temperature. Pharmacologic modalities include morphine, neuroleptic medications, dopamine agonists, dantrolene sodium, and prostaglandin inhibitors. Lesions in the posterior hypothalamus can cause hypothermia. Maintenance of body temperature secondary to hypothalamic lesions is dependent on the environment; therefore interventions include dressing warmly, adapting the room temperature, and preventing chills or drafts.[33]

A child with a spinal cord injury at the thoracic level may present with impaired body temperature. Spinal cord injury above the thoracolumbar pathway of the sympathetic nervous system results in loss of function in the hypothalamic thermoregulatory mechanisms. The body is unable to control temperature below the level of the lesion because of absence of vasoconstriction, loss of ability to shiver to conserve body heat, and loss of sweating to dissipate heat.

Family members should be instructed to assess for altered body temperature and to apply preventive measures and intervention as needed. The family should know how to obtain an appropriate measure of body temperature. Prevention of fever and infection should be stressed. Environmental control measures to prevent hyperthermia and hypothermia should be discussed. The child should not be exposed to extreme hot or cold conditions. On warm days, the child should remain in a cool house or in the shade and be dressed appropriately. Exercise should be limited and fluid input increased. On cold days, the child should be dressed in layers or remain inside with proper heating. Chills should be avoided. Family members should seek medical attention when fever or hypothermia does not respond to attempts to normalize the temperature or if the child's level of responsiveness has decreased.

Neuromuscular System

Spasticity is diagnostic of an upper motor neuron injury of the corticospinal or extrapyramidal tracts. Characterized by muscle tightness or rigidity, spasticity may interfere with active or passive movement and activities of daily living. Clinical signs associated with spasticity include increased resistance to passive stretch, increased deep tendon reflexes, impaired voluntary control of muscles, difficulty relaxing muscles once movement has stopped, difficulty initiating rapid movements, and poorly coordinated movements.[34] Continued spasticity can be painful and lead to contractures, scoliosis, and hip dislocation.

Treatment of spasticity requires a multidisciplinary approach and may include oral medications, physical therapy, orthopedic surgery, intrathecal baclofen, nerve blocks, or neurosurgery. Management usually follows a progressive approach, beginning with noninvasive therapies and, if unsuccessful, moving to more invasive procedures.

Physical modalities used by therapists, nurses, and families to improve range and inhibit abnormal postural and reflex tone include daily range of motion, prolonged stretching, positioning, serial casting or splinting, application of ice or heat, and electrical stimulation.[34,35] In addition, care providers need to assess and eliminate conditions that exacerbate spasticity, such as pressure sores and infections.

The most significant advances in the treatment of spasticity have been the use of botulinum toxin (Botox), intrathecal baclofen, and selective posterior rhizotomy surgery. Although these measures are more invasive, results are longer-lasting and may reduce the need for corrective orthopedic procedures and high-dose drug regimens. Details of these procedures are presented elsewhere; however, several nursing considerations should be mentioned.

Intrathecal baclofen is administered directly into the spinal fluid by a pump that is implanted under the skin in the abdomen. Pump refills are necessary every 2 to 3 months and may be performed by trained nursing staff. The risks of pump placement include wound or cerebrospinal fluid infection, spinal fluid leaks, and rarely drug toxicity.[36,37]

Botulinum toxin is injected into the belly of the target muscle, where it performs its blocking effect. The reduction of spasticity after botulinum toxin injection is specific to the muscles injected and the dose of toxin administered. Adverse effects of botulinum toxin are minimal. Excessive weakness of injected muscles may occur, but this subsides with time.[36]

The primary neurosurgical procedure for treating spasticity in children is selective posterior rhizotomy. The risks of surgery include cerebrospinal fluid leak, infection, bladder dysfunction, hypotonia, weakness, or sensory loss. The child must lie flat for 48–72 hours postoperatively to allow the dural closure to heal and to prevent a cerebrospinal fluid leak. Although there are some initial restrictions in hip flexion and rotation, the child can be mobilized soon after surgery and begin an acute rehabilitation program.[38]

Anticipatory Guidance

The rehabilitation nurse has an important role in preparing a patient and family for their transition back home and to the community. Interventions that assist families with changes in function and behavior have been discussed throughout this chapter. In addition to providing instruction regarding impaired levels of function and potential complications of injury or disability, nurses need to provide anticipatory guidance regarding normal developmental concerns, including sleep, safety, and discipline.

Sleep

Making time for school, play, therapy, feedings, skin care, toileting, and other care needs fills the child's day quickly. It is important for care providers to schedule enough time for the child to rest and sleep. Most children require 10–11 hours of sleep at night. Daytime naps decrease in length and frequency as the child grows from an infant to preschooler. Most children no longer nap after the age of 4 years. Adolescents rarely get enough sleep and should be allowed 9 hours of sleep at night.[39] Children with an exacerbation of a chronic illness such as juvenile rheumatoid arthritis or sickle cell disease fatigue easily and may require rest periods during the day.[40] Parents should be instructed that children with motor disabilities consume more energy during physical activities and need additional rest.

Pain, discomfort, or medications may affect the child's ability to fall asleep or sleep through the night. Check the skin for irritating rashes or pressure from clothing. Readjust braces or appliances as needed. Assess medication regimens and possible side effects that may disrupt sleep. Some medication, such as diphenhydramine (Benadryl), chloral hydrate, phenobarbital, or diazepam, may have a paradoxical effect and make the child agitated and hyperactive, preventing sleep. Medication schedules and treatments should be arranged to avoid interrupting the child's bedtime routine or waking the child during the night. In addition to helping the child sleep, families will have a much easier time continuing this schedule at home.

A bedtime routine and sleep schedule can be developed during the child's hospital stay. Parents should be encouraged to continue their home routine if possible. Occasionally, previous bedtime rituals are not successful or are not possible in the acute setting. The rehabilitation team, parents, and possibly the patient should work together to develop a bedtime program that is acceptable. A consistent routine that includes a pleasant but quiet activity is helpful. Scary or painful events should be avoided before bed. A special toy or blanket from home is helpful for the hospitalized child. Some children have difficulty transitioning from alert to quiet states and may require being wrapped and held or slowly rocked to sleep.[36,39] The nurse should assess the child's daytime sleep pattern. Some children have an irregular sleep-wake cycle and take long or frequent naps during the day. Preventing daytime naps can improve the duration and quality of sleep at night.[40]

Safety

Safety practices and injury prevention are important in children who have sustained a previous traumatic injury. The degree of precaution indicated for children with disabilities or after traumatic injury must be tailored to the child's motor ability, behavioral style, and awareness of potential hazards. Children who have sustained a traumatic brain injury are particularly vulnerable to future injury as a result of neuropsychological and behavioral deficits resulting in poor judgment, overactivity, impulsivity, and perceptual deficits.[41]

Specific safety precautions include keeping the home and school environment free of clutter and sharp-angled furniture, placing barriers at stairways and steps, installing grab bars or railings for stairways and bathrooms, and checking assistive equipment (wheelchairs, highchairs) for safety. Caregivers should be instructed in proper body mechanics to avoid injury during lifting and transfers. Families should also plan ahead for special emergency and evacuation needs in the event of power failure or natural disaster. All temporary caregivers should be aware of the child's special needs and know whom to contact in the event of a problem.

Families should be reminded of safety and injury prevention measures that apply to all children. The American Academy of Pediatrics Committee on Accident and Poison Prevention has developed injury prevention guidelines based on the developmental level of the child, which can be adapted for the rehabilitation population.[42]

Discipline

Alterations in behavior and personality should be anticipated after a traumatic injury or prolonged hospitalization. The child may have changes in temperament, including apathy, poor motivation, and being socially withdrawn. Other children may be hyperactive, irritable, impulsive, aggressive, or inattentive.[41] Early guidance and counseling with parents should encourage limit setting and reinforcement of normal household rules. A behavioral management program often needs to be initiated while the child is hospitalized for acute rehabilitation because problem behaviors may interfere with therapy and nursing care. Consultation with a pediatric psychologist is often helpful in developing a behavioral program that benefits the child and care providers. Behavior problems often become more evident to families after discharge. It is important to discuss behavioral concerns with parents at follow-up visits and to advise the family and school regarding behavior modification regimens and discipline.

Transitions

Transitions are often difficult for families and children who are dealing with a chronic disability. Initial transitions occur as the child is discharged home, but new challenges must be met as the child progresses through school, adolescence, and young adulthood. It is extremely important for the rehabilitation team to foster the necessary skills and support services to help the child make a successful transition at each developmental stage. Family support groups and foundations are available for many specific conditions or for families of children with disabilities in general. These parent groups may also help to facilitate links to community services and programs. As more young children survive acute injuries and are living with long-term disabilities, practitioners must also begin to take a role in caring for this population as they become adults. Assisting families to find adult providers and providing for continuity of care may be a long-term goal for the rehabilitation nurse.

References

1. McCourt A: The Specialty Practice of Rehabilitation Nursing: A Core Curriculum. Glenview, IL, Association of Rehabilitation Nurses, 1993.
2. Johnson K (ed): Advanced Practice in Rehabilitation. Glenview, IL, Association of Rehabilitation Nurses, 1997.
3. Revell G: Understanding the child with special health care needs. J Pediatr Nurs 1991;6:258.
4. Burns C, Barber N, Brady M, et al: Pediatric Primary Care. Philadelphia, WB Saunders, 1996.
5. Erickson R: Autonomic hyperreflexia. Arch Phys Med Rehabil 1980;61:431.
6. Braddom R, et al: Autonomic dysreflexia. Am J Phys Med Rehabil 1991;70:234.
7. Mallory GB Jr, Stillwell PC: Ventilator-dependent child: Issues in diagnosis and management. Arch Phys Med Rehabil 1991;72:43.
8. Barnes L: Tracheostomy care: Preparing parents for discharge. J Matern Child Nurs 1992;21:293.
9. Buzz-Kelly L, et al: Teaching CPR to parents of children with tracheostomies. J Matern Child Nurs 1993;18:158.
10. Eyman RK, et al: Survival of profoundly disabled people with severe mental retardation. Am J Disabled Child 1993;147:329.
11. Vane D, Harmel R, King D, et al: The effectiveness of Nissen fundoplication in neurologically impaired children with gastroesophageal reflux. Surgery 1985;84:4.
12. Huddleston K, et al: Preparing families of children with gastrostomies. Pediatr Nurs 1991;17:153.
13. Barkauskas V, et al: Health and Physical Assessment. St. Louis, Mosby, 1994.
14. Sullivan P: Gastrostomy and the disabled child. Dev Med Child Neurol 1992;34:547.
15. Edwards-Becket J, et al: The impact of spinal pathology on bowel control in children. Rehabil Nurs 1996;21:292.
16. Cardenas DD, Hooton TM: Urinary tract infection in persons with spinal cord injury. Arch Phys Med Rehabil 1995;76:272.
17. McLaughlin JF, Murray M, Zandt KV, et al: Practical procedures: Clean intermittent catheterization. Dev Med Child Neurol 1996;38:446.
18. Lapides J, Diokno AC: Urine transport, storage, and micturition. In Lapides J (eds): Fundamentals of Urology. Philadelphia, WB Saunders, 1976.
19. Lapides J, Diokno AC, Silber SJ, et al: Clean intermittent self catheterization in the treatment of urinary tract disease. J Urol 1972;107:458.
20. Moore KN: Intermittent catheterization: Sterile or clean. Rehabil Nurs 1991;16:15.
21. Lavallee DJ, Lapierre NM, Henwood PK, et al: Catheter cleaning for re-use in intermittent catheterization: New light on an old problem. Sci Nurs 1995;12:10.
22. Kurtz LA, Dowrick PW, Levy SE, et al: Handbook of Developmental Disabilities: Resources for Interdisciplinary Care. Gaithersburg, MD, Aspen Publishers, 1996.
23. Segal ES, Deatrick JA, Hagelgans NA: The determinants of successful self-catheterization programs in children with myelomeningocele. J Pediatr Nurs 1995;10:82.
24. Brown JP: A practical approach to teaching self-catheterization to children with myelomeningocele. J Enterostomal Ther 1990;17:54.
25. Cardenas DD, Mayo ME, King JC: Urinary tract and bowel management in the rehabilitation setting. In Braddom RL (ed): Physical Medicine and Rehabilitation. Philadelphia, WB Saunders, 1996.
26. Baggerly J, DiBlasi MD: Pressure sore prevention in a rehabilitation setting: Implementing a programmatic approach. Rehabil Nurs 1996;21:234.
27. Basta S: Pressure sore prevention education with the spinal cord injured. Rehabil Nurs 16:6, 1991.
28. Garvin G: Wound and skin care for the PICU. Crit Care Nurs Q 1997;20:62.

29. ACHCPR, Agency for Health Care Policy and Research: Treatment of Pressure Ulcers: Clinical Practice Guidelines, No. 15, AHCPR Publication No. 95-0652. Rockville, MD, Agency for Health Care Policy and Research, Public Health Service, US Department of Health and Human Resources, 1994.

30. Hanak M: Rehabilitation Nursing for the Neurological Patient. New York, Springer, 1992.

31. Salcido R, Hart D, Smith AM: The prevention and management of pressure ulcers. In Braddom RL (ed): Physical Medicine and Rehabilitation. Philadelphia, WB Saunders, 1996.

32. Ong LC, Dhillion MK, Selladurai BM, et al: Early post-traumatic seizures in children: Clinical and radiological aspects of injury. J Pediatr Child Health 1996;32:173.

33. Bontke CF, Boake C: Principles of brain injury rehabilitation. In Braddom RL (ed): Physical Medicine and Rehabilitation. Philadelphia, WB Saunders, 1996.

34. Albany K, Atrice M, Barry MJ, et al: Intrathecal Baclofen Therapy: Guidelines for the Physical Therapist. Minneapolis, MN, Medtronic Inc, 1996.

35. Geralis E: Children with Cerebral Palsy: A Parents' Guide. Woodbine House Inc, USA, 1991.

36. Albright AL: Treating spasticity: Today's choices require careful consideration: Part III. Exceptional Parent 1997;Feb:28.

37. Rawlins P: Intrathecal baclofen for spasticity of cerebral palsy: Project coordination and nursing care. J Neurosci Nurs 1995;27:157.

38. Brucker JM: Selective dorsal rhizotomy: Neurosurgical treatment of cerebral palsy. J Pediatr Nurs 5:105, 1990.

39. Ferber R: Solve Your Child's Sleep Problems. New York, Simon & Schuster, 1985.

40. Jackson PL, Vessey JA: Primary Care of the Child with a Chronic Condition, 2nd ed. St. Louis, Mosby, 1992.

41. Michaud LJ, Duhaime AC, Batshaw ML: Traumatic brain injury in children. Pediatr Clin North Am 1993;40:553.

42. Stain JE: AAP periodicity guidelines: A framework for education patients. Pediatrics 74(5 pt 2):924, 1984.

43. Broughton B: Chronic childhood illness. Rehabil Nurs 1995;20:318.

44. Jaffe K (ed): Pediatric Head Injury. J Head Trauma Rehabil 1986;1:4.

45. Leibl B: Dietary fiber and long-term large bowel response in enterally nourished nonambulatory profoundly retarded youth. J Parenter Enter Nutr 1990;14:371.

46. Miller M, et al: Ventilator assisted youth: Appraisal and nursing care. J Neurosci Nurs 1993;25:287.

47. Storgion S: Care of the technology-dependent child. Pediatr Ann 1996;25:12.

Chapter 11

Cerebral Palsy

Dennis J. Matthews, MD
Pamela Wilson, MD

Cerebral palsy is a disorder of movement and posture that results from a nonprogressive lesion or injury of the immature brain.[1,2] The definition includes a heterogeneous spectrum of clinical syndromes characterized by alteration in muscle tone, deep tendon reflexes, primitive reflexes, and postural reactions.[3,4] These neurologic abnormalities often produce characteristic abnormal patterns of movement that are recognized as the hallmarks of cerebral palsy.[5,6] Although the essential diagnostic sign is a motor deficit, the possibility that there may be other associated symptom complexes of cerebral dysfunction is implicit in the stipulation of central nervous system pathology.[2]

Epidemiology

Cerebral palsy is the leading cause of childhood disability.[7,8] The reported incidence varies but is approximately 2–3 per 1000 live births.[9,10] Nelson and Ellenberg[11] found a prevalence rate of 5.2 per 1000 neonatal survivors at 12 months of age but reported resolution in up to half of these children by age 7 years. More recent studies report an overall prevalence rate of 1.5–2.0 per 1000 live births.[12]

Advances in medical care and technology raised the hopes of reducing morbidity among neonatal survivors. Despite marked improvements in maternal and perinatal care, the prevalence has remained relatively constant. This is partially explained by higher survival rates for more immature, smaller, and premature infants with medical complications.[9,10,13] Paneth and Kiely[14] concluded that the overall prevalence of cerebral palsy has not changed from the 1950s and that a school-age rate of 2 per 1000 live births is a reasonable estimate for industrial countries.

Cause

The origin of the brain injury resulting in cerebral palsy may occur during the prenatal, perinatal, or postnatal period. Overwhelming evidence suggests that in approximately 70% to 80%, cerebral palsy is prenatal in origin.[12,15–19] A higher proportion of children with cerebral palsy had growth retardation, dental enamel abnormalities, and abnormal dermatoglyphic patterns and a greater than expected prevalence of other congenital anomalies or dysmorphic features.[20] The risk is multifactorial (Table 11–1), and a large proportion remains unexplained.

Prenatal factors may lead to premature birth or intrauterine growth retardation of both term and preterm infants. Prematurity remains the most common antecedent of cerebral palsy.[2,10,21–23] The combination of immaturity, fragile brain vasculature, and the physical stresses of prematurity combine to predispose these children for compromise of cerebral blood flow.[24] The blood vessels are particularly vulnerable in the watershed zone next to the lateral ventricles in the capillaries of the germinal matrix. Different degrees of bleeding result in intraventricular hemorrhage: grade 1, isolated to the germinal matrix; grade 2, intraventricular hemorrhage with normal ventricular size; grade 3, intraventricular hemorrhage with ventricular dilation; and grade 4, intraventricular hemorrhage with parenchymal hemorrhage.[25]

The outcome of the infant with intraventricular hemorrhage depends, in large part, on the degree of associated parenchymal injury. There is only an approximate relationship between the quantity of intraventricular blood and neurologic outcome.[25] Infants with minor degrees of hemorrhage have only a slightly increased risk of major neurologic sequelae, but risk increases to 90% with severe hemorrhage and periventricular hemorrhagic infarction.[26,27] Volpe[26] has postulated five basic subtypes of hypoxic-ischemic neuropathology:

1. *Parasagittal cerebral injury:* This principal lesion of the term infant involves bilateral cortical

TABLE 11–1. Risk Factors Associated with Cerebral Palsy[2,19]

Prenatal	Congenital malformations
	Socioeconomic factors
	Maternal intrauterine infections
	Reproductive inefficiency
	Toxic or teratogenic agents
	Maternal mental retardation, seizures, hyperthyroidism
	Placental complications
	Multiple births
	Abdominal trauma
Neonatal	Prematurity < 32 weeks' gestation
	Birth weight < 2500 gm
	Growth retardation
	Abnormal presentations
	Intracranial hemorrhage
	Trauma
	Infection
	Bradycardia and hypoxia
	Seizures
	Hyperbilirubinemia
Postnatal	Trauma
	Infection
	Intracranial hemorrhage
	Coagulopathies

and adjacent subcortical white matter necrosis of the superior medial and, particularly, the posterior aspects of the cerebral convexities. The necrosis occurs within the border watershed zones. Injury to this region involves the motor cortex that subserves proximal extremity function, with the upper extremities more severely affected than the lower extremities. This pattern of weakness is appreciated readily when the homunculus topography of injury is considered. The most frequent long-term consequences of injury to this region are spastic quadriplegia (Fig. 11–1).[28]

2. *Periventricular leukomalacia:* Periventricular leukomalacia occurs in the preterm infant involving bilateral white matter necrosis adjacent to the external angles of the lateral ventricles affecting the centrum semiovale and optic and acoustic radiations. The periventricular white matter resides within the border zones between the penetrating branches of the major vessels and is exquisitely sensitive to decreases in cerebral perfusion.[29,30] This region of white matter is traversed by descending fibers of the motor cortex. The fibers subserving function of the lower extremities are more likely to be affected by moderate lesions, and because of extension laterally into the centrum semiovale and corona radiata with the more severe lesions, upper extremity involvement occurs as well.[26] In the corona radiata, descending fibers from the motor cortex are arranged with those subserving the lower extremities located medially and those to the upper extremities laterally. Therefore, smaller lesions cause spasticity in the legs, whereas larger lesions affect both the lower and the upper extremities. The long-term manifestations include spastic diplegia and spastic quadriplegia, with visual and cognitive deficits in more severe injury (Fig. 11–2).[31,32]

3. *Focal and multifocal ischemic brain necrosis:* Focal and multifocal ischemic brain necrosis is characterized by injury to all cellular elements caused by an infarction within a vascular distribution. The middle cerebral artery is the most common vascular territory affected, with the left side twice as commonly involved as the right.[33,34] Neuropathologic sequelae include porencephaly, multicystic encephalomalacia, and hydranencephaly. The long-term neurologic manifestations reflect the location and extent of the primary lesion and include spastic hemiplegia, spastic quadriplegia, and seizures (Fig. 11–3).

4. *Status marmoratus:* Status marmoratus is the rarest lesion and is characterized by neuronal injury within the basal ganglia (thalamus, caudate nucleus, globus pallidus, and putamen).[26] The condition rarely occurs in isolation and invariably is associated with one of the other neuropathologic subtypes. In its isolated

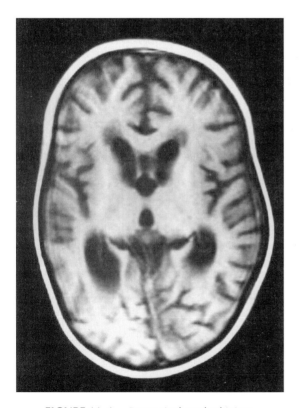

FIGURE 11–1. Parasagittal cerebral injury.

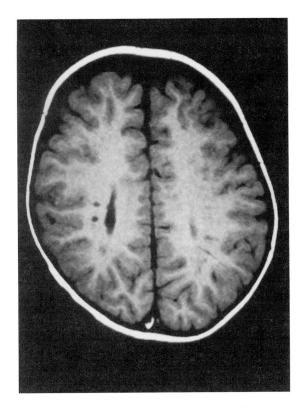

FIGURE 11–2. Periventricular leukomalacia.

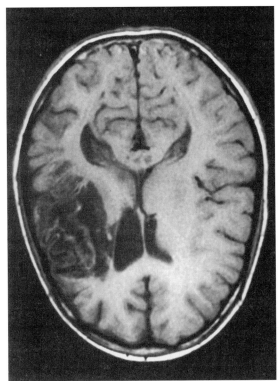

FIGURE 11–3. Multifocal ischemic brain necrosis.

form, the long-term neurologic manifestation is chorcoathctosis (Fig. 11–4).

5. *Selective neuronal necrosis:* Selective neuronal necrosis is the most common variety of injury observed in hypoxic-ischemic encephalopathy. Invariably, it coexists with one or more of the other lesions. Specific neurons are vulnerable, including CA 1 region (Sommers sector) and subculum of the hippocampus; the lateral geniculate body and thalamus of the diencephalon; caudate nucleus, putamen, and globus pallidus of the basal ganglia; and the fifth and seventh cranial nerve motor nuclei within the pons and the dorsal vagal nuclei.[26] The pathogenesis appears to be related to oxygen deprivation and excitotoxic amino acids.[35] The long-term sequelae include mental retardation and seizures.

The genesis of hypoxic-ischemic cerebral injury in most cases of cerebral palsy is prenatal.[26,36–38] The timing of the insult is critical to the evolution of a specific lesion. Cerebral ischemia before the 20th week of gestation results in a neuronal migration deficit; between the 28th and 34th week, in periventricular leukomalacia; and between the 34th and 40th week, focal or multifactorial cerebral injury.[26] Factors that have been associated with prenatal hypoxic-ischemic cerebral injury include multiple pregnancy, maternal

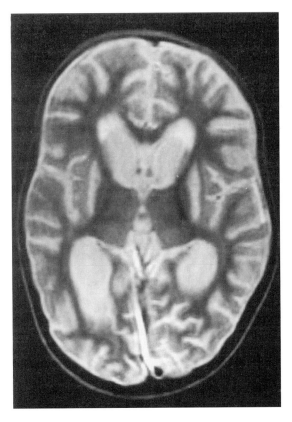

FIGURE 11–4. Status marmoratus.

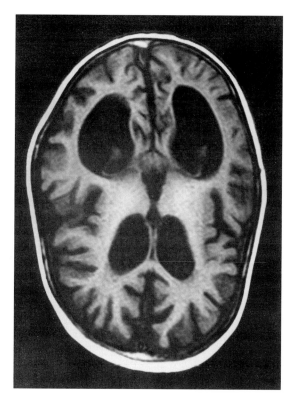

FIGURE 11–5. Selective neuronal necrosis.

bleeding, and maternal drug use; most frequently the cause is idiopathic (Fig. 11–5).[16,39–41]

Frequently the exact cause of cerebral palsy cannot be determined. There are complex interactions among the components of the developing nervous system, and interference in these interactions can result in a wide variety of pathophysiologic disorders and clinical conditions. Evidence continues to support a multifactorial cause of cerebral palsy.

Classification of Cerebral Palsy

Classification of cerebral palsy is a complex process incorporating information on a variety of disorders grouped together under a large umbrella term. Historically, neurologic involvement was used as the method to delineate various levels of involvement in the cerebral palsy patient. Current trends, however, are trying to incorporate a more functional basis for classification.

There have been multiple systems developed over the years, including Little's in 1862 and Sachs' in 1891. Little used three categories, which included *hemiplegic rigid*, *paraplegic*, and *generalized rigid*.[42] Little's disease or the paraplegic variety is known today as *spastic diplegia*. Sachs classified children according to

cause and clinical involvement.[43,44] Many classification strategies used today are based on neuroanatomy, body distribution, functional parameters, and severity of the disorder. These different systems are presented; however, it may be that a combination of these is the best method of classifying the child with cerebral palsy.

Neurologic Classification

Crothers and Paine[42] developed a system in 1959 that used a spastic and extrapyramidal model. A modification of this system is the most frequently used classification method used by clinicians today. Because cerebral palsy may manifest itself differently as the child ages, earlier classifications may need to be changed as the child matures. The modified neurologic classification system divides the patients into the following categories:

1. Spastic (pyramidal) cerebral palsy
2. Dyskinetic (extrapyramidal) cerebral palsy
3. Mixed types

Spastic Types

The spastic cerebral palsy disorders tend to be the most commonly occurring. This group accounts for approximately 75% of the children affected, whereas the other 25% is divided into the dyskinetic and mixed types.[45] Children in this spastic subgroup typically manifest signs of upper motor neuron involvement.[19,46] These may include the following:

- Hyperreflexia
- Clonus (newborns may normally have a few beats of clonus)
- Extensor Babinski response (abnormal after 2 years of age)[4]
- Persistent primitive reflexes
- Overflow reflexes such as a crossed adductor

The spastic group can be further subdivided into the topographic distribution or the part of the body that is involved:[48]

- Monoplegia—one limb, either an arm or leg
- Diplegia—primarily lower extremities are involved
- Triplegia—three extremities involved
- Quadriplegia—all four extremities and trunk involved
- Hemiplegia—one side of body involved, including arm and leg

As most clinicians are well aware, it is often quite difficult to categorize exactly individuals into these topographic subdivisions. Following are descriptions of each category with related information:

Spastic monoplegia
Isolated upper or lower extremity involvement
Rarely seen
Usually mild clinical presentation
Often the presentation of a misdiagnosed hemiplegia

Spastic diplegia (Fig. 11–6)
Term first used by Freud; also known as Little's disease
History of prematurity common; in this group of preterm infants who eventually develop cerebral palsy, 80% evolve into the spastic diplegic type[49]
History of intraventricular hemorrhages, particularly in the 28–32-week-old infant
More complex multifactorial cause in the term infant, although in 28% no identifiable risk factors present[50]
Magnetic resonance (MR) imaging may show periventricular leukomalacia or posthemorrhagic porencephaly[51,52]
History of early hypotonia followed by spasticity[53]
Developmental delays most pronounced in the gross motor sector
Lower extremity spasticity caused by damage to pyramidal fibers within the internal capsule
Mild coordination problems in the upper extremities
Upper motor neuron signs in the lower extremities
Diplegic gait pattern, including spastic adductors, gastrocnemius, and hip flexors
Contractures associated with spasticity
Eye findings, including strabismus in 50% and visual deficits in 63%[53,54]
Seizures present in 20–25% of this group[50,53]
Cognitive impairment present in approximately 30% of this population[45]
Vasomotor signs common in affected extremities

Spastic triplegia
Three extremities involved, classically bilateral lower extremities and one upper extremity
Spasticity in involved limbs
Mild coordination problems in noninvolved limb
Upper motor neuron signs in involved limbs
Scissoring and toe walking
Similar features to the spastic quadriplegic

Spastic quadriplegia (Fig. 11–7)
All extremities involved; patterns include truncal hypotonia with appendicular hypertonia or total body hypertonia
Classically, individuals with more involvement in the upper extremities than the lower extremities categorized into double hemiplegia
History of a difficult delivery with evidence of perinatal asphyxia common
Approximately 50% prenatal in origin; 30%, perinatal; 20%, postnatal[55,56]

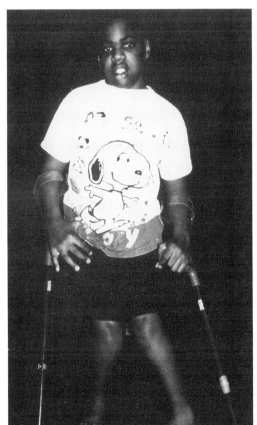 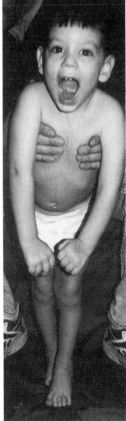

FIGURE 11–6 (Left). Child with spastic diplegia.

FIGURE 11–7 (Right). Child with spastic quadriplegia.

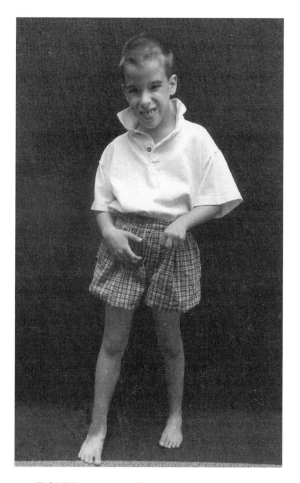

FIGURE 11–8.   Child with spastic hemiplegia.

MR imaging in preterm children showed periventricular leukomalacia; full-term children had *term-type lesions* and brain anomalies[51,52]

Opisthotonic posturing may begin in infancy, often persisting in the severely involved

Oromotor dysfunction, pseudobulbar involvement, and risk for aspiration

Feeding difficulties common; many require gastric tube placement

Significant cognitive involvement in high percentage of children

Spasticity and persistent primitive reflexes

Upper motor neuron signs in all limbs

High incidence of visual impairment

Usually most severely involved children

About half have seizures[53]

Vasomotor signs common in involved limbs

Spastic hemiplegia (Fig. 11–8)

One side of the body involved: arm generally more than leg

Most cases congenital (70–90%); 10–30% acquired causes, including vascular, inflammatory, and traumatic events[57]

MR imaging evidence of unilateral lesions in 66%: middle cerebral artery infarcts, hemibrain atrophy, and posthemorrhagic porencephaly[51,52]

In term infants, cause usually due to prenatal events[58]

In premature infants, asymmetric periventricular leukomalacia may be common cause[45]

Hemiparesis usually evident by 4–6 months of age[45]

Hypotonia may be first indicator of this type of cerebral palsy

Slightly higher incidence of right-sided involvement[49,53]

Cranial nerves may be involved and generally present as facial weakness

Often growth retardation of the affected side, which can result in a shorter leg or arm[59,60]

Spasticity in hemiplegic side

Upper motor neuron signs in hemiplegic side

Hemiplegic gait pattern

Sensory deficits on the ipsilateral side in 68%; stereognosis, graphesthesia, two-point discrimination, and joint position may also be involved[57,61,62]

Visual deficits in approximately 25% of individuals with hemiplegia, including homonymous hemianopsia along with convergent strabismus[61,63]

Some cognitive impairment in 28% of cases of congenital hemiplegia[58]

Perceptual motor deficits fairly common, causing learning difficulties[57]

Vasomotor instability common, including both coolness and edema[57]

Seizures relatively common, occurring about 33% of cases[58]

Children often have weakness of the ipsilateral trapezius, but the sternocleidomastoid on that side is normally functioning[64]

Dyskinetic Types

Dyskinetic disorders are characterized by extrapyramidal movement patterns. These abnormal responses are secondary to abnormal regulation of tone, defects in postural control, and coordination deficits.[63] The movement patterns can be divided into hyperkinetic and dystonic groups. Dyskinetic movements are defined as follows:

1. *Athetosis*—slow, writhing, involuntary movements particularly in the distal extremities; both agonist and antagonist muscles are active; intensity may increase with emotions and purposeful activity.

2. *Chorea*—abrupt, irregular, jerky movements usually occurring in the head, neck, and extremities.

3. *Choreoathetoid*—combination of athetosis and choreiform movements; generally large-amplitude involuntary movements; dominating pattern is the athetoid movements.

4. *Dystonia*—slow, rhythmic movements with tone changes generally found in the trunk and extremities; abnormal postures.

5. *Ataxic*—unsteadiness with uncoordinated movements; often associated with nystagmus, dysmetria, and a wide-based gait.

The child with extrapyramidal disorders is generally hypotonic at birth. Classic movement patterns emerge sometime between 1 and 3 years of age.[42] Severely affected children have persistent hypotonia for the longest time.[65] The upper extremities are more frequently involved than the lower limbs. Movement patterns typically increase with stress or purposeful activity and can change from hour to hour depending on fatigue and other factors. During sleep, the muscle tone is normal, and the involuntary movement stops. The term *tension athetosis* is used when moving the limb increases tone. Deep tendon reflexes are usually normal to slightly increased, and some spasticity can be present.[57] These children and adults are usually thin with a small percentage of body fat. They generally have a low incidence of contractures, although scoliosis may develop.

Pseudobulbar involvement presents with dysarthria, swallowing difficulty, drooling, and oromotor dyskinesias. Speech patterns are affected by problems with coordinating the muscles of articulation and difficulty with breath control. The characteristic speech pattern demonstrates difficulty initiating speech and articulating some words. Once vocalization has started, there is variability in speech rate along with explosive phrases or words.

Because these children manifest such a loss of motor and speech control, they are often pigeonholed into the severely impaired range when evaluating intelligence. This group of children falls into the normal intelligence range 78% of the time.[42] There is a high incidence of sensorineural hearing loss in this population.[66] Hearing loss has been associated with hyperbilirubinemia and neonatal jaundice. Dental enamel dysplasia can be used as a clue that a child was exposed to high levels of bilirubin. The overall incidence for this group has been reduced with the current treatment for Rh incompatibility and the availability of blood volume exchange techniques.

Mixed Types

Mixed types classification includes descriptions from both spastic and dyskinetic classifications. For example, a spastic-athetoid child has a predominant dyskinetic movement pattern with an underlying component of spasticity.

Functional Systems

Alternative classification systems based on functionality and severity of cerebral palsy have evolved over the years. The most simple of these systems uses a mild, moderate, and severe description. The mild group has no limitations in ordinary activities, the moderate group has definite difficulties in activities of daily living and may require assistive devices or bracing, and the severe group has moderate-to-severe limitations in activities of daily living.[44] A newer functionally based system has been proposed to standardize gross motor function in the child with cerebral palsy. This system was developed by Palisano and colleagues[67] at McMaster University and is referred to as the *Gross Motor Function Classification System*. Based on the premise of rating a child on functional skills, such as sitting and walking, the individual is classified into one of five groups. These groups were developed to emphasize abilities and limitations:

Level I—walks without restrictions: limitations in more advanced gross motor skills
Level II—walks without assistive devices: limitations walking outdoors and in the community
Level III—walks with assistive mobility devices: limitations walking outdoors and in the community.
Level IV—self mobility with limitations: children are transported or use power mobility outdoors and in the community.
Level V—self mobility is severely limited even with the use of assistive technology

Evaluation of the Child with Cerebral Palsy

History

The history is a key component in evaluating the disabled child. Information obtained can guide one in understanding cause, determining underlying medical problems, determining function, and developing a medical treatment plan. A thorough history comprises the following components:

Prenatal history
Information on pregnancy
Exposure to toxins, alcohol, or drugs
Gestational age (prematurity)
Acute maternal illnesses
Prenatal care
Fetal movements
Trauma or radiation exposure
Family history
Familial diseases
Perinatal history
Delivery type and presentation of child
Birth weight
Apgar scores
Complications

Intubation time, use of surfactant
Intraventricular hemorrhage, shunts
Feeding, tone, resting position
General nature of child: calm, jittery, consolable
Developmental history
Developmental milestones
Current gross motor function, including head
control, trunk control, rolling, crawling, bunny
hopping, standing, and walking
Current fine motor function, including handed-
ness, hand to mouth, bimanual activity, grasp,
play, writing, and activities of daily living
Current language, including babbling, words,
stringing words together, body parts, count-
ing, alphabet, and receptive language skills
Current social and personal skills
Persistent reflexes
Tone and patterns
General information
Nutrition; feeding style; oral skills; all growth
parameters, including height, weight, and
head circumference
Medications and allergies
Past surgeries
Seizures
Visual disturbances, including strabismus, ne-
glect, esotropia, and correction
Hearing
General health, respiratory illnesses
Immunizations
Contractures
Equipment
Positioning devices
Bathing equipment
Wheelchair and seating
Adaptive devices
Communication devices
Computers and peripherals
Environmental control units
Transportation system
Education
Early intervention program
School environment and educational style
Special service, including Individual Education
Plan
Adaptive physical education
Recreation

Clinical Examination

Musculoskeletal Examination

The musculoskeletal examination is both a
static and a dynamic evaluation of the child.
The static evaluation is geared toward isolating
each joint and assessing passive range of motion
along with tone and spasticity. The dynamic
evaluation is oriented toward observing movement, function, and gait.[68]

Dynamic Evaluation

In general, with the dynamic evaluation, it is
best in the young child to start with observation

and then proceed to a more hands-on approach.
The examination starts even before the child
enters the clinic. Observing how the child uses
mobility coming into the examination room is a
key evaluation tool. Important information can
be assessed in both the ambulatory and the
wheelchair-dependent individual.

Gait Assessment. The gait cycle is broken
down into two phases: swing phase and stance
phase. Within each phase, the biomechanics can
be broken down into components of gait. In evaluating a child, it is necessary to analyze what each
joint in the lower extremity is doing during these
phases. In reviewing the hip, watch for excessive
hip flexion, hip adduction, and femoral anteversion. At the knee, note flexion and extension
along with varus or valgus stress. The foot should
be observed for equinus or toe walking, along
with dynamic varus or valgus of the hindfoot.

Typical gait abnormalities are as follows:

Spastic diplegia
Scissoring gait pattern
Hips flexed and adducted
Knees flexed with valgus
Ankles in equinus
Hemiplegia
Weak hip flexion and ankle dorsiflexion
Overactive posterior tibialis
Hip hiking or hip circumduction
Supinated foot in stance phase
Upper extremity posturing
Crouch
Tight hip flexors
Tight hamstrings
Weak quadriceps
Excessive dorsiflexion in both diplegic and quad-
riplegic individuals

Static Evaluation

For the static evaluation, the child should be
placed on an examination table, although in a
young child parts may be done from the parent's
lap.[69]

Hip Assessment

Tests for Hip Contracture. The *Thomas
test* is done by bringing both legs up to the chest
to stabilize the lumbar spine. One leg at a time
is extended until there is resistance in hip extension or movement in the pelvis. The measurement is taken by the angle of the femur and
the table.

The *Ely test* is done in a prone position with
the examiner's hand on the buttock. The lower
leg is quickly flexed, and if the buttock rises off
the table, this indicates a spastic or tight quadriceps (Fig. 11–9).

The *Staheli test* is done with the patient in a
prone position with the legs dangling over the

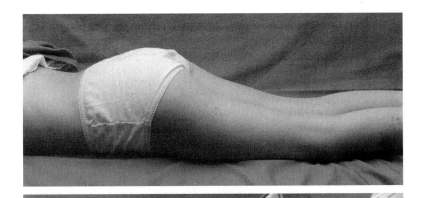

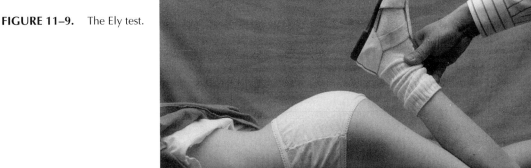

FIGURE 11–9.   The Ely test.

edge of the table. The pelvis is stabilized, then one leg at a time is extended until there is anterior movement of the pelvis. The angle is measured by the femur and a horizontal line.

Test for Adductor Contracture.   Range of motion should be evaluated in both flexion and extension. If range of motion is less in extension, this may be related to a spastic gracilis muscle.

Test for Both Internal and External Rotation.   Testing should be done both in flexion and extension. Excessive internal rotation suggests femoral anteversion.

Leg Length Evaluation.   Measurements of actual leg lengths should be taken from the anterior-superior iliac spine to the medial malleolus. When knee contractures are present, the measurements should be broken into two segments using the medial joint space in the knee as an additional anatomic point. If the pelvifemoral angles are asymmetric because of contracture or adductor spasticity, the measurements are from the greater trochanter to the medial malleolus. These measurements allow the clinician to differentiate between apparent and actual leg length discrepancies.

Knee Assessment

Test for Hamstring Contracture.   The popliteal angle is measured by stabilizing the contralateral leg on the table, then flexing the ipsilateral hip to 90 degrees. The lower leg is extended until resistance is felt. The angle can then be measured from either the tibia and the line of full extension or the 90-degree position to full extension.

Evaluation of the Position of the Patella.   The clinician should look for a high-riding patella, or patella alta, or a low-riding patella, called patella baja.

Test for Posterior Capsular Tightness.   Testing is done with the legs extended on the examination table. The knees are extended until there is resistance.

Foot and Ankle Assessment

Test for Gastrocnemius/Soleus Contracture.   The Silfverskiold test of ankle dorsiflexion is done in both a flexed and an extended knee position. If the ankle range of motion is greater in flexion, the gastrocnemius is the site of contracture.

Evaluation of the Posterior Tibialis and Peroneal Muscles.   A spastic posterior tibialis can cause varus of the heel along with plantar flexion. A spastic peroneus can cause a valgus deformity.

Test for Tibial Torsion.   Tibial torsion can be evaluated either in a sitting or a prone position. In prone, the thigh-foot angle is evaluated with the knee flexed to 90 degrees. In a sitting position, the femoral condyles are lined up, and a line is drawn through the malleoli.

Back Assessment.   Posture is evaluated in either standing or sitting position. The spine is palpated for curves or rib humps. If scoliosis is present, the spine should be tested for mobility. The pelvis should be checked for obliquity.

Upper Extremity Assessment.   Evaluation of the upper extremity begins with observation of how a child uses the upper limbs spontaneously. The observer should be aware of asymmetries, spasticity, and abnormal postures. Measurements should be obtained both passively and actively when evaluating range of motion. Testing of the hand should evaluate thumb position, wrist position, and finger extension. When testing active finger extension, the clinician should place the wrist in a neutral or extended position. Functional testing is also recommended along with a complete sensory evaluation.

Neurologic Examination

In evaluating the nervous system, there must be an understanding of the normal maturation and development of children. Often what is found is that reflexes and patterns persist past the age when they should normally be suppressed by the nervous system. A systematic approach to examining the nervous system should include these components along with the general neurologic evaluation.

Tone Assessment.   Tone has been described as ranging from hypotonic to rigid in children. In assessing tone, it is necessary to feel the movement of a joint through passive range of motion. When evaluating tone, the clinician should be careful to position the head in neutral because tonic neck reflexes may influence the evaluation. If the movement has a velocity-dependent component, by definition this muscle has spasticity. Spasticity can be classified on an Ashworth scale. Other descriptors can be used to describe tone, such as *fluctuating*, *rigid*, *dystonic*, and *clasp knife*.

Postural and Reflex Assessment.   Each child should be evaluated for normal and abnormal reflexes. Reflexes are suppressed in a predictable pattern during normal development, and if they persist this may indicate damage to

the central nervous system.[65] Reflexes important for assessing central nervous system development are as follows:

1. Moro reflex
2. Asymmetric tonic neck reflex
3. Neck righting reflex
4. Vertical suspension
5. Grasping reflexes
6. Tonic labyrinthine reflex
7. Protective reflexes
8. Symmetric tonic neck reflex

Laboratory Tests and Diagnostic Imaging

The use of laboratory and diagnostic imaging assists the clinician in categorizing and predicting clinical course. In evaluating metabolic diseases and some genetic diseases, it is necessary to obtain blood and urine samples. Routine testing includes thyroid functioning, lactate and pyruvate, organic and amino acids, and chromosomes. Blood pH is a useful indicator of perinatal asphyxia, which can provide needed information and indicate severity of the perinatal event.[70] Evaluation of the cerebrospinal fluid may also assist in determining asphyxia. Protein levels within the cerebrospinal fluid can be elevated along with an elevated lactate-to-pyruvate ratio.[71]

Neuroimaging techniques have been pivotal in the diagnostic evaluation by providing insight into pathology and physiology. The most commonly used test for the premature infant is the real-time cranial ultrasound study. This technique provides useful information about the ventricular system, basal ganglia, and corpus callosum.[72] It provides diagnostic information on intraventricular hemorrhage and hypoxic-ischemic injury to the periventricular white matter.[63,73] It allows the clinician to follow the classic changes in the brain associated with periventricular leukomalacia. This is an initially echodense area that converts to an echolucent area at about 2 weeks of age.[63] Computed tomography (CT) has a wide spectrum of uses in this population. CT is helpful in diagnosing congenital malformations, intracranial hemorrhages, and periventricular leukomalacia in the infant.[63] MR imaging studies have limited use in the premature infant and are the most beneficial after the child is 2–3 weeks old. This is the study of choice for following white matter disease because it allows visualization of myelin on T2 images and visualization of the sulci.[74] In the older child, if imaging studies are needed, MR imaging is the best diagnostic test. Positron-emission tomography (PET) is an experimental tool used to define blood flow and glucose metabolism.

These parameters can be abnormal in both the acute and the chronic stages of injury.[73,75] Single-photon emission computed tomography (SPECT) is another experimental tool used to document cerebral perfusion. Using radioactive tracers, areas of the brain that are injured or hypoperfused show a decreased radioactive pattern.[74] One of the newest techniques for evaluating asphyxia is ^{31}P magnetic resonance spectroscopy. MR spectroscopy measures phosphorus-containing compounds in the brain. By comparing the MR signal ratios of phosphocreatine to inorganic phosphorus, it is possible to find indications of cerebral asphyxia. Studies have shown that the deeper cortical layers are involved with ischemic injury.[76]

Evoked potentials are tests used to evaluate the brain's responses to external stimuli. They have been used successfully in evaluating the anatomic pathways of the auditory and visual systems. Children with severe perinatal asphyxia may have damaged auditory and visual pathways, which alter the amplitude and latencies of the evoked studies.[2] Even if the information shows that the pathways are intact, there is no way to know if a child can interpret the information, as in cortical blindness. Visual evoked responses use a flash or pattern shift stimuli, and information is obtained from the occipital lobes.[73] In premature infants with unshunted hydrocephalus, there is a prolonged latency,[26] and it is useful in diagnosing demyelinating disease, leukodystrophies, and silent optic neuritis.[77] Brain stem auditory evoked response tests use an external clicking system to evaluate cranial nerve VIII, the cochlear nucleus, the superior olivary nucleus, and the inferior colliculus. This test can be done in premature infants with a gestational age as young as 26 weeks. The response in the brain stem is abnormal in perinatal asphyxia and hyperbilirubinemia.[77] The electroencephalogram (EEG) measures electrical activity on the surface of the brain. It is a useful tool in evaluating severe hypoxic-ischemic injury. The classic pattern, as described in Volpe and Hill's summary of previous work,[73] states that initially there is marked suppression of amplitude and slowing followed by a discontinuous pattern of voltage suppression, interposed with bursts of high-voltage sharp and slow waves at 24 to 48 hours.[77] If an EEG pattern shows burst suppression, the prognosis is poor, but if it rapidly normalizes, the prognosis is promising.[77]

Clinical Course and Functional Prognosis

Cerebral palsy is by definition a nonprogressive lesion of the immature brain, but the clinical course is anything but static. As can be expected in a group of syndromes as diverse in their manifestations as cerebral palsy, the differences in clinical course are considerable.[42,53,78] The clinical course is characterized by changing function and dysfunction over the years of growth and development. The natural history can be envisioned as a summation of competing favorable and adverse developmental lines represented by the preserved innate potential, on the one hand, and by the organic deficits and their secondary consequences, on the other.[2]

One of the most frequently observed symptoms is abnormal muscle tone. Abnormal tone is manifested as either a decreased or increased resistance to passive movements. It is not unusual for most children to have an early period of hypotonia.[42,53,78,79] Spasticity and dyskinesia tend to evolve gradually with an apparent intensification of clinical signs as part of the natural history.[2] Later, changing clinical manifestations are related to the secondary musculoskeletal sequelae resulting from muscle imbalance. These tend to occur earlier in children with moderate and severe disability, affecting mobility and function.

The child with hemiplegia exhibits definite hand preference usually before 1 year of age compared with normal handedness by age 2 years. These children often have an asymmetric crawl or do not crawl at all. The affected upper extremity is often held with the shoulder adducted, elbow flexed, forearm pronated, wrist flexed, hand fisted, and thumb in the palm. Impaired sensation is frequent, including abnormalities of two-point discrimination and position sense, astereognosis, graphesthesia, and topagnosia.[80,81] Growth disturbance is usually commensurate with the extent of spasticity. Most children become independent in activities of daily living but may need some aids. Almost all children with hemiplegia become ambulatory. They have an unequal stride length, flexed hip and knee, and frequently an equinus. Often a heel-cord contracture requires a tendon lengthening. Growth discrepancy rarely exceeds 2.5 cm.

After a period of hypotonia, the child with spastic diplegia manifests spasticity in the lower extremities with little or no functional limitation in the upper extremities. There is a late attainment of gross motor skills, especially in standing and walking. In a prospective study of children, maintenance of sitting by 2 years was a good predictive sign of eventual ambulation, and children who did not sit by age 4 years did not ambulate.[82–84] Posture and gait frequently change over time. Early extensor hypertonicity may revert to excessive flexor tone at a later age. The classic *scissoring* is simultaneous hip adduction, knee hyperextension, and plantar flexion of the lower extremities (see Fig. 11–7). The hips must be monitored for coxa valga and subluxation. This condition can require intervention, including motor point blocks and surgery, to facilitate motor control and ambulation. Gait training usually requires orthoses and walkers or crutches. With increasing age, a *crouched* posture may develop and affect the energy efficiency of ambulation (see Fig. 11–6).

Children with spastic quadriplegia present wide variations in severity of functional limitations, clinical course, and final functional outcome. The severity of motor involvement directly affects the delay in developmental milestones. After a period of initial hypotonia, these children frequently develop excessive extensor spasticity. Extensor tone persists for variable lengths of time, and the longer the delay in resolution, the poorer the prognosis.[53] Children with spastic quadriplegia must be closely monitored for hip dislocation and scoliosis. Spastic muscle imbalance results in persistence of infantile coxa valga and femoral anteversion.[69] Subluxation, acquired acetabular dysplasia, and eventual hip dislocation particularly occur in the severely affected, nonambulatory child.[69,85] Dislocation may lead to pain and impaired function.

About one-fourth of children with spastic quadriplegia have only mild involvement with minimal or no functional limitation in ambulation, self-care, and other activities.[2] Approximately one-half are moderately impaired, so complete independence is unlikely, but still they are able to function satisfactorily. Only about one-fourth are so severely disabled that they require care and are nonambulatory. Maintenance of sitting by 2 years and suppression of obligatory infantile reflexes by 18 months are good prognostic indicators of eventual walking.[83]

The child with dyskinetic cerebral palsy may show increased tone and opisthotonus as a newborn.[79] This is usually followed by a period of hypotonia that persists for a longer period than in the spastic types. The child frequently demonstrates a persistence of the Moro and asymmetric tonic neck reflexes.[2,79] The writhing involuntary movements are first noted in the hands and fingers. With time, these involuntary movements tend to change in quality, resembling dystonia, choreoathetosis, or other types of dyskinesias.[2] Abnormal movements are usually evident in all affected extremities by 18 months. In adolescents, these movements may give way to dystonia. The upper extremities are frequently more involved than the lower extremities. Involvement of the face and oropharyngeal musculature often causes dysphagia, drooling, and dysarthria.

Neuromuscular dysfunction is often severe, and its functional consequences reflect spastic paresis and dyskinetic incoordination.[2] Approximately one-half of children attain walking, most of them after age 3 years.[83] In ambulatory children, upper extremity function is generally adequate for performing activities of daily living. Nonambulatory children usually need assistance and are at risk for hip dysplasia and scoliosis.

Associated Deficits

Although motor deficit receives the most attention, the central nervous system damage is not confined to the motor areas. There are many associated problems that can significantly change the ultimate functional outcome (Table 11–2). Associated disabilities alone can often produce significant developmental delay. When seen in association with severe motor dysfunction, they have an additional adverse effect on the rate of development.

Mental retardation is the most serious associated disability. The overall incidence of mental retardation is approximately 30–50%.[2,23,86] Severe-to-profound mental retardation comprises about one-half of the retarded group. Approximately one-third of cases with mental retardation have mild cognitive deficits. The child with athetosis is usually superior to children with the other types. The greatest retardation is seen in the rigid, atonic, and severe spastic quadriplegic cerebral palsy.

TABLE 11–2.   Associated Problems in Cerebral Palsy

Mental retardation	50% incidence; most common in rigid, atonic, and severely spastic quadriplegia
Seizures	50% incidence; most frequent in hemiplegia and spastic quadriplegia
Oromotor	Difficulty sucking, swallowing, and chewing; poor lip closure, tongue thrust, drooling, dysarthria; most common in spastic quadriplegia, dyskinetic
Gastrointestinal	Reflux, constipation
Dental	Enamel dysgenesis, malocclusion, caries, gingival hyperplasia
Visual	Strabismus, refractory errors; hemianopsia in hemiplegia
Hearing impairment	Infection (TORCH), medications, bilirubin encephalopathy
Cortical sensory deficit	Hemiplegia
Pulmonary	Deficient ventilation; bronchopulmonary dysplasia in premature infants; microaspirations with oromotor dysfunction

Approximately one-half of children with cerebral palsy have a seizure disorder.[2,79,87,88] These disorders occur most frequently in postnatally acquired hemiplegia (70%), congenital hemiplegia (50%), and spastic quadriparesis (50%). Seizures are rare in children with diplegia and athetosis.[88] The clinical manifestations of epilepsy include various kinds of generalized and focal, minor motor or partial seizures.[2,79] Grand mal with tonic-clonic manifestations is the most frequent type in spastic quadriplegia. Focal motor seizures may occur in hemiplegia. An uncontrolled seizure disorder may further delay development, especially in the cognitive area.

Some children with cerebral palsy, particularly those who are severely affected, may have oromotor problems. This may lead to difficulty sucking, swallowing, and chewing. The motor incoordination is manifested by poor lip closure, retraction or thrusting of the tongue, and decreased tongue movements. Videofluoroscopy can be used to evaluate swallowing effectiveness and protection of the airway from aspiration.[19,89] These feeding difficulties can contribute to undernutrition and malnutrition. Supplemental feedings with gastrostomy tubes or buttons to improve nutrition and growth may be required. Insidious microaspiration may occur.

Gastrointestinal symptoms are frequent in children with cerebral palsy.[90] Gastroesophageal reflux often requires medical management. Frequent emesis producing undernutrition may require surgical correction. Constipation, exaggerated by immobility and abnormal diet and fluid intake, can be managed with standard medical treatments.[19,91] Bowel and bladder management is usually related to dysfunction of central neuromotor control and cognitive developmental status of the child.

Drooling, a significant problem in about 10% of children with cerebral palsy, can cause social embarrassment and affect the quality of social integration.[17] It can result from dysfunctional oromotor activity, oral sensory problems, inefficient and infrequent swallowing, and poor head control. Management may include feeding and oral stimulation, behavior modification programs, medication (scopolamine patches), or surgery.[17,19,79] Pseudobulbar palsy is manifested by defective speech in addition to feeding and drooling difficulties. The dysarthria may be so severe as to preclude functional speech. Augmentative, nonverbal communication training for both spoken and written language is the method of choice when there is a profound speech production deficit.

Dental problems occur frequently in children with cerebral palsy. Depending on the cause, the precipitating factors may also affect tooth enamel development.[79,92] Motor problems and oral sensitivity make brushing and oral hygiene difficult. Dental malocclusion is twice as frequent in children with cerebral palsy as in nondisabled children.[92] The combination of enamel dysplasia, mouth breathing, and poor hygiene leads to caries and periodontal diseases. Some anticonvulsants may also cause gingival hyperplasia.

Pulmonary problems are common in children with cerebral palsy. Defective control of the respiratory muscles may compromise the efficiency of pulmonary ventilation. When the pseudobulbar palsy is associated with poor ventilation and ineffective cough, these children frequently develop recurrent aspiration pneumonia. Bronchopulmonary dysplasia in the premature infant compounds the problem. There are frequent recurrent acute and chronic respiratory infections in children with severe handicaps. Chronic pulmonary disease as a result of insidious microaspirations is a major cause of shortened life expectancy in the severely disabled group.

Defective or slow language often reflects an intellectual disability.[2,17,42,93] Disorders of verbal and written language may be encountered. Speech defects due to impaired coordination of articulation, phonation, and respiration may range from slightly distorted sound production to complete mutism. Nearly all children with dyskinesia have dysarthria. Lack of speech caused by severe oromotor dysfunction must be differentiated from lack of language as a result of cognitive impairment.

Communication disorders may be related to hearing impairments, defective motor control of speech production, central language dysfunction, or cognitive deficit.[2] The characteristic hearing loss is a sensorineural impairment.[94] They are most frequently caused by congenital nervous system infections.[94] Ototoxic drugs are an increasingly rare cause of hearing loss. Improvements in detecting and treating these conditions have significantly reduced their incidence.[19]

Prediction of the long-term functional outcome in the first few years of life is difficult. The interactions of motor dysfunction, associated disabilities, natural history, and the effect of treatment modalities all affect outcome. Certain skills are helpful in establishing an ultimate motor prognosis. Seventy-five percent of children with cerebral palsy ambulate. Those who cannot sit by age 2 years or ambulate by age 7 years rarely walk.

About 90% of children with cerebral palsy survive to adulthood.[94,95] Mental retardation, seizures, and wheelchair dependency are factors reducing the likelihood of living independently.[95–97]

Positive prognostic factors for employment include mild physical involvement, good family support, vocational training, and good employment contracts.[94] Bleck[69] noted that positive factors for independent living are regular schooling, completion of secondary school, independence in mobility and the ability to travel beyond the home, good hand skills, living in a small community, and having spasticity as the motor dysfunction. Life expectancy is reduced by immobility and severe or profound retardation.[98]

Therapeutic Management

Management of cerebral palsy requires an understanding of the interaction of biologic and environmental factors with normal development. By integrating a basic knowledge of the child's anatomic-physiologic abnormalities with a clear concept of the interaction between structure and experience, the physician working with the child, the family, and the rehabilitation team seeks to encourage the development of the handicapped child to a maximal level of motor, intellectual, and social function.[79]

Children with cerebral palsy often have multisystem involvement. Rehabilitation management requires numerous professionals using a variety of techniques and methods. Periodic reassessment and programmatic updating are essential.[2,19,79] The major goals of the rehabilitation program are anticipatory treatment of potential complications and fostering the acquisition of new skills.[2]

Early Intervention

Once the diagnostic assessment is completed, a rehabilitation intervention strategy can be developed. The goals are to improve function, develop compensatory strategies, and encourage functional independence.[2] To achieve an optimal development, management programs should begin as early as possible.[2,79,99–103] Early intervention implies a system of programs that work with the infant and young child and the family to prevent or minimize adverse developmental outcome.[100,105,106]

The rationale for early intervention is that the program provides improved infant-caregiver interaction, family support for coping, parental education for handling a child at home, and treatment to promote motor and other developmental skills. Public Law 99-457 (IDEA: Individuals With Disabilities Education Act) mandated early intervention for children 0 to 3 years old who demonstrate developmental delay. IDEA clearly identifies the family as central to the

goals of early intervention. The team acts not only to treat the child, but also to empower the family by identifying their strengths and needs.

Management in infancy includes careful positioning and alignment to prevent exaggeration of abnormal reflexes and posture. Proper handling techniques and selected sensorimotor experiences not only produce movement patterns, but also the resultant responses increase the child's experiences, thereby becoming the basis for learning and building blocks of future motor activity. Instruction of the parents in the therapeutic methods used to increase sensorimotor experiences allows these techniques to be incorporated into the daily activities of the child.

Early intervention may produce its most significant effect by making the parents feel more comfortable, accepting, involved, and less guilty about their child. Through instruction and demonstration, the parents learn how to work within the functional capabilities of the child. These programs provide the parents with guidance and support through specific skill development and activities with their child.

The intervention team frequently represents a blend of the educational and medical models. The direct therapy model of service delivery can occur as a part of an interdisciplinary, multidisciplinary, or transdisciplinary treatment in a center- or home-based program.[2,19,79,100,106] Therapists provide hands-on treatment services. In the consultation model, the treatment team assessment data, intervention techniques, strategies, and goals agreed on with the family are implemented by the caregiver, reducing the number of individuals handling the child.

Although early intervention programs are generally accepted, it is not clear who should be targeted, what type of intervention should be provided, and what is the optimal timing for this intervention. There is no evidence that early intervention prevents disability or produces changes in brain organization, especially in the presence of central nervous system damage.[100,104] There is evidence that these strategies do minimize secondary complications and do support the families.[100,104]

The committee on Children With Disabilities of the American Academy of Pediatrics[107] has noted that passage of Public Laws 94-142 and 99-457 demonstrates a national commitment to the concept that early services are critical for children with disabilities. Future studies documenting successful outcomes need to include cognitive and motor development; the child's acceptance into the family; interpersonal skills; "stabilizing rather than curing" health problems; and building capacities, even within the context of significant limitation, to maximize the potential for independence and productivity in adult life. The effectiveness of early services must increasingly relate not only to the specific outcomes of the child, but also to the family's adaptation to the child's disability, to improvement in their coping abilities, and to the general strength of the family unit. Resources for the young child with special health care needs should include social, educational, and health services delivered through a variety of agencies, preschool facilities, and medical and other health programs. The emphasis of all services should be focused on integrating the child into appropriate community supports and activities.

Therapeutic Exercise

A number of therapy systems have influenced the management of children with cerebral palsy. Most of these methods have developed empirically from clinical observation, and a theoretical framework was devised later to explain the possible neurophysiologic principles.[2,100,108] Few therapists adhere strictly to a single therapy system but use an eclectic approach of many techniques and methods individualized for the child.

Phelps combined a treatment for poliomyelitis with movement patterns and inhibition of abnormal tone.[2,79,100,108] The child is conditioned to exercises accompanied by song. Phelps recommended extensive bracing, withdrawing support as motion is performed with a minimum of tension, overflow, and substitution. Muscle tone was reduced by using special chairs and sitting devices. There was an emphasis on self-help skills and development of balance and position sense.

Deaver recommended extensive bracing, limiting all but two motions of an extremity.[2,79,100,108] As motor control was achieved, braces were removed. Voluntary motion was emphasized for the performance of activities of daily living, especially bed and wheelchair skills. Many assistive devices were used to facilitate performance of these skills.

Expanding on the ideas of Temple Fay, Doman and Delacato recommended a program following the evolutionary process.[2,79,100,108,109] This controversial method uses a series of set patterns repeated many times during the day, attempting to train cerebral dominance and normalization of function. Proponents believe that the treatment promotes normal development in undamaged areas of the brain and externally imposes patterns of movement in areas controlled by the damaged brain.[109] The program also focuses on neurologic organization, sensory stimulation, language, reading, and respiratory control.

Rood[110] places equal emphasis on the sensory and motor systems. She advocates activating muscles through sensory receptors. Specific stimulation techniques are used to activate, facilitate, or inhibit motor responses. Rood's overall goal is to activate movement and postural responses at an automatic level while following the developmental sequences.

The most widely used method is that developed by Bobath and Bobath.[111–113] The main goals of the neurodevelopmental treatment are to normalize tone, inhibit abnormal primitive reflex patterns, and facilitate automatic reactions and subsequent normal movement. These goals are accomplished by the therapist providing *key points of control* throughout the body. Theoretically the child experiences normal kinesthetic feedback. They emphasize the family involvement and carryover of handling techniques in the home environment. As the child ages, the emphasis shifts to activities of daily living.

Vojta[114] is a method frequently used in Europe, which bases treatment on activation of postural development and equilibrium reactions to guide normal development. The therapist develops a treatment plan based on reflex locomotor patterns and proprioceptive input and then teaches the parents a home program. The treatment can be uncomfortable and cause the children to cry, limiting its acceptance in the United States.

Conductive education, originated by Peto in Hungary, is based on the theory that the difficulties of the child with motor dysfunction are problems of learning.[115] The goal of treatment is the ability to function independently in the world without aids. Participants, selected for their ability to learn, are usually treated in group settings that provide incentive of competition and allow more intensive therapy than does individual treatment. They are instructed by *conductors* who are trained in all facets of rehabilitation. Functional goals are broken down into small steps. Children initiate the activities on their own, with direct conscious action aided by mental preparation.

A review of the literature recommending each of these methods produces many questions. Most methods evolved empirically from clinical observations. The validity of the claimed neurophysiologic theories is unproven.[2,79,100,108] Review of the efficacy of specific methods or programs indicates inconsistent but small positive effects for children with motor deficits.[2,79,100,108] Generally, there is inadequate research with respect to design, random assignment to group, a lack of control groups, and blind observation procedures. There is also a lack of validity and reliability of outcome results, and no proper assessment tools were used to measure clinically important functional changes.

Rigid adherence to any one system of treatment is unjustified.[2,79,100] A mode of intervention should be selected that is most appropriate for each child and family at a particular time. Well-selected components of each method can be used to produce the best individualized therapeutic approach.

Functional Training

The applicability of traditional exercises is limited in infants and preschool children because of the need for cooperative participation. Mobility of the joints and soft tissues is maintained by movement through full range of motion. Limitation of range of motion is of greatest importance when it interferes with function. It is easier to prevent tightness by repeated activities than to correct it after it has developed. Stretching to increase motion should be slow and gentle with the child relaxed. It should stop just short of pain, although the child may experience some discomfort.

Children with cerebral palsy are often weak. When the aim is to increase strength, progressive resistive exercise and isometric and isokinetic training programs can be used for those who demonstrate adequate cooperation. For the younger child, age-appropriate play, adaptive toys, and games can serve the same purpose. Strengthening knee extensor muscles resulted in increased force production, improved stride length, and less crouching.[116] The program improved function and quality of life.

Training of postural and motor control should follow the developmental sequence. Postural reactions can and should be trained in all positions when possible and developmentally appropriate. Generally, head and trunk control should be established first, but failure to attain this goal does not prevent the child from working on upper extremity use. Good supported sitting with adequate head and trunk control permits the child to practice and experience upper extremity movements. Training of balance should progress from symmetric to asymmetric patterns. It is important that the child also develop the ability to change postures because inability to move in and out of a position frequently limits the versatility of movement behavior required for independent activities.

To develop optimal motor performance, individual voluntary motor control must be established.[2,69,79] A skilled performance uses all synergists of a motion optimally and with minimal interference by antagonist. This performance can be accomplished only if the child learns the correct movement pattern and can successfully repeat the performance. Discrete, voluntary movements can be accomplished only under direct control. Once basic control has been established, therapy can be directed toward coordination.[100] This training requires an accurate perception of motion, precision of movement, and repetition of the precise pattern. It may be necessary to break the activity into individual components. As the precise pattern is repeated, the motor performance becomes both coordinated and automatic, the highest level of movement control.

With children, it is important to encourage performance at a level of success. Activities must be selected just below peak performance. It is absolutely essential that each therapeutic session should end in success and interval goals be achieved in the period of time planned for the therapy. Short-term goals are then combined into a sequence of movements and should result in continuing functional activity at the end of the therapy.[100]

Gross motor abilities and hand dexterity are physical determinants for planning a program in activities of daily living.[2,79] When complete independence is not realistic, the child should be encouraged to learn part of the task. Compensatory functional techniques and adaptive devices are aids to independence. No functional training is successful unless the child is expected to perform in all situations of life.

Orthoses and Durable Medical Equipment

Orthoses are prescribed to provide support, limit motion, improve function, and delay or prevent deformity. The specific goals are to prevent contracture, provide optimal joint alignment, provide selective motion, protect weak muscles, control abnormal tone and related deviations, enhance function, and protect tissues postoperatively.[2] Orthoses are frequently required for both the upper and the lower extremities. Opinions differ as to when to start and what type of orthosis to use. The decision depends on the age of the child, motor control, type of deformity, orthotic design, and short-term and anticipated long-term functional prognosis (see Chapter 9).

The ankle-foot orthosis (AFO) and its variants are the most frequently prescribed braces. The AFO can be used to control spastic equinus, promote alignment of the hindfoot, and control midfoot and excessive knee extension in stance. Solid AFOs are used if restriction of ankle motion is desired. Children who would benefit from freedom of movement at the ankle can be fitted with a hinged AFO.

Upper extremity orthoses are frequently used to maintain a functional joint position. They can be used for passive support in the spastic child for activities of daily living or as a training device to substitute for poor motor control. An orthosis allows the child the opportunity to practice a functional skill or motor activity with the hand positioned optimally.

Frequent reevaluation of the orthotic device is necessary. Orthoses are not all bad or all good. To use orthoses effectively requires an understanding of the limitation of each orthosis and the potential function of the child.

Assistive devices and durable medical equipment should be considered in the context of functional prognosis. These are used to attain function not otherwise possible. In addition to wheelchairs and mobility aids, there are a wide variety of individual aids for activities of daily living, communication, education, recreation, and vocation (see Chapter 9).

The early introduction of independent mobility for children with cerebral palsy has become increasingly advocated. Increased mobility and exploration of one's environment has been demonstrated to improve self-esteem.[117] Selection of the most appropriate device requires an understanding of the features and limitations of each device, patient and family needs, functional goals and prognosis, and economic restrictions and requirements (see Chapter 9).

Management of Spasticity

Management of tone and posture has received much attention in children with cerebral palsy. The mainstay of treatment is through the application of modalities.[2,79,100] Primarily, this has been through therapeutic exercise.[79,118] Regular and daily range of motion can help prevent or delay contractures and can reduce the severity of increased muscle tone for several hours. Therapeutic exercise includes a variety of treatment techniques that are used to decrease or inhibit tone. The use of heat and cold has been shown to have a short-term use and is impractical for long-term use.[119] Casting and splinting can improve range of motion. Casting for 2 or 3 weeks can decrease tone and improve range of motion for 3 to 4 months.[120,121] Biofeedback may modulate spasticity, but no long-term usefulness has been documented.[122,123] Cyclical use of functional electrical stimulation was found to decrease upper extremity contractures, improve motor activity of the agonist muscles, and reduce tone in the antagonist. These tone

effects generally last only for hours.[124–127] Therapeutic electrical stimulation has been advocated.[128] There are reports of improved strength and motor control, but few validated studies are available.

Management of spasticity in children with cerebral palsy includes an increasingly wide assortment of medications (Table 11–3). Response to these drugs is often unpredictable, and occasionally the side effects preclude long-term use. Reappraisal and monitoring of efficacy and complications are essential. The most commonly used antispasticity medications are benzodiazepines, dantrolene, baclofen, clonidine, and tizanidine. These medications may decrease spasticity, but generally they do not improve coordination. A new innovative approach has been the use of intrathecal baclofen, which has been shown to reduce spasticity and improve function. The long-term efficacy and complications have not been established in children.[129,130]

Spasticity has also been treated with phenol intramuscular neurolysis and botulinum A toxin (Botox) intramuscular blocks, which reduce spasticity for 3 to 6 months.[131–134] These procedures are used to improve range of motion, alter selected muscle tone and strength for training motor control, or reduce deformity. Botox has been increasingly used in selected muscles of the upper extremity with encouraging results.[135]

Several neurosurgical procedures have been recommended for tone management. Stereotaxic ablation of selected thalamic nuclei and chronic electrical stimulation of the cerebellum or posterior columns have been unsuccessful in the child with cerebral palsy.[136,137] Selective posterior rhizotomy of roots L-2 to L-5 has had success in children with velocity-dependent spasticity.[138–141] Reduction in tone, as recorded by the modified Ashworth scale, is improved.[140–143] Gait analysis studies have shown an improved availability of range of motion at the knee and hip, resulting in an increased stride length.[144,145] Careful selection is critical because the weakness produced may reduce the level of functional independence.

Orthopedic Surgery

In the overall plan of rehabilitation, there is an important role for judiciously used and well-timed surgical treatment.[69] Nearly all children with cerebral palsy develop an abnormality of form and function. Surgery may be indicated to improve function and appearance and to prevent or correct deformities. The fundamental goal of orthopedic surgery should reflect a functional approach to the problems of alignment.[69,146] The purpose of and expectations for surgery must be

TABLE 11–3. Medications for Management of Spasticity

Medication	Site of Action	Mode of Action	Dose	Side Effects	Precautions	Comments
Baclofen	GABA receptors in spinal cord	Decreases release of excitatory neurotransmitters from afferent terminals	Start with 2.5–5.0 mg bid; increase by 2.5–5.0 mg q 3–5 d; max: 20 mg qid	Weakness, fatigue, confusion, constipation	May lower seizure threshold; abrupt withdrawal may precipitate seizures or hallucinations	Drug of choice for MS and SCI
Baclofen: intrathecal	GABA receptors in spinal cord	Decreases release of excitatory neurotransmitters from afferent terminals	Test dose 50 μg; pump dose 27–800 μg/d	Weakness, fatigue, confusion, constipation, cardiorespiratory depression	May lower seizure threshold; abrupt withdrawal may precipitate seizures or hallucinations, cardiorespiratory arrest	Approved for MS, SCI, CP, TBI
Dantrolene	Intrafusal and extrafusal muscle fibers	Decreases release of calcium from sarcoplasmic reticulum	Start with 0.5 mg/kg bid; increase by 0.5 mg/kg q 5–7 d; max: 12 mg/kg/d to 400 mg	Weakness, fatigue, drowsiness, diarrhea	Hepatotoxicity (2%); frequent liver function tests	Drug of choice for spasticity of cerebral origin
Benzodiazepines	Receptors of brain stem, reticular formation, spinal cord	Increases GABA binding, potentiating presynaptic inhibition	Start with 1–2 mg bid; increase by 1–2 mg q 2–3 d; max: 20 mg qid	Drowsiness, fatigue, impaired memory and recall	Tolerance and dependence; CNS depression	Most helpful in incomplete SCI
Clonidine	α₂-agonist in brain, brain stem, substantia gelatinosa of spinal cord	Inhibits short latency of motor neurons; augmentation of presynaptic inhibition	Start with 0.1-mg patch for 7 d	Bradycardia, hypotension, depression	Blood pressure and pulse monitoring	Effective in reducing spasms and resistance to stretch
Tizanidine	α₂-adrenergic receptors both spinally and supraspinally	Prevents release of excitatory amino acids from presynaptic terminal of spinal interneurons; may facilitate glycine, an inhibitory neurotransmitter	Start with 2–4 mg at bedtime; increase 2 mg q 2–4 d; max: 36 mg	Dry mouth, sedation, dizziness	Orthostatic hypotension, hallucination, elevated liver function tests	MS, SCI, stroke
Botulinum A toxin	Presynaptic acetylcholine neuromuscular junction	Prevents release of acetylcholine	1–12 units/kg depending on size of muscle; 50 units per site; no more frequent than 3 mo	Weakness, cramping, pain	Antibody formation, respiratory arrest	Dystonia, torticollis, blepharospasm, strabismus
Phenol	Peripheral nerve; motor end plate	Denatures protein and disrupts myoneural junctions	4–6% aqueous solution; max: 20 ml	Pain, skin irritation, peripheral neuropathy	Anesthesia, cardiac arrhythmia	Targeted muscles

GABA, γ-Aminobutyric acid; bid, twice a day; qid, four times a day; q, every; max, maximum; CNS, central nervous system; MS, multiple sclerosis; SCI, spinal cord injury; CP, cerebral palsy; TBI, traumatic brain injury.

Modified from Stempien LM, Gaebler-Spira D: Rehabilitation of children and adults with cerebral palsy. In Braddom RL (ed): Physical Medicine and Rehabilitation. Philadelphia, WB Saunders, 1996.

clear to all involved with the care of the child. Goal-oriented management requires that the child's problem be analyzed consistent with the priorities and needs for independent living.

Spastic muscle imbalance and deforming forces can be decreased or altered by tendon lengthening or transfer. The skeletal complications of spastic muscle imbalance can be anticipated long before their appearance and may be avoided by early soft tissue surgery. These procedures are not always successful in preventing bony deformities necessitating osteotomy or arthrodesis.

Postural alignment for sitting requires a level pelvis and a reasonably straight spine.[147–149] Excessive pelvic obliquity reduces the sitting surface area and causes excessive pressure on the bony prominences of the pelvis.[147–149] Close monitoring of the pelvis, hips, and spine is required, including serial radiographs to anticipate potential deformities.[150] Abnormal muscle imbalance can be controlled with early soft tissue releases. Fixed contractures may require a release most frequently of the adductor longus; gracilis; and occasionally the iliopsoas, sartorius, and rectus femoris. Postoperative management includes casting or splinting for 3–6 weeks.

If the hip progresses to subluxation or dislocation, a more extensive procedure is required involving the femur and perhaps the acetabulum. Frequently, excessive anteversion and a valgus orientation necessitate a varus derotational osteotomy. Postoperative management after a varus derotational osteotomy and, if required, an acetabular augmentation requires 6–8 weeks of immobilization. Rehabilitation plays an important role after cast removal.[69,146,151] Goals are to improve range of motion, strength, and motor control and to reduce pain and spasticity. This usually takes twice the time of immobilization to be accomplished.

Pelvic alignment is also influenced by the hamstrings, which pull the pelvis into a posterior pelvic tilt producing sacral sitting. Release of the hamstrings can partially correct the constant sliding out of the chair.[19,146,152] Postoperative management includes prolonged splinting to delay or prevent recurrence.

The prevalence of structural scoliosis and kyphosis in cerebral palsy differs between ambulatory and nonambulatory individuals. Mechanisms that influence the development and progression of scoliosis include asymmetric muscle imbalance, posture, and biomechanical and structural factors.[19,153] Careful monitoring including serial radiographs until spinal growth ceases is required to design the most appropriate management program. Orthoses of various types appear to be effective, especially to delay or control the rate of progression when used in conjunction with exercise.[154] Electrical stimulation of the spinal muscles has had intermediate results.[69,100] Surgical treatment is indicated when scoliosis is progressive despite adequate orthotic use or a severe degree of curvature, usually greater than 40 degrees.[155,156] The specific technique and instrumentation, along with a review of the risk of anesthesia, infection, blood loss, neurologic compromise, and pseudarthrosis, should be considered before surgery.[156]

Knee flexion deformities may be due to spastic and contracted hamstring muscles or secondarily due to weakened triceps surae muscles. They are often accompanied by a hip flexion deformity in the crouched-gait pattern. When the knee flexion deformity is greater than 40 degrees, the energy efficiency of ambulation is reduced.[69,157–159] Surgical techniques include hamstring tenotomy, transfers, or lengthening. Postoperative management includes range of motion, strengthening, and gait training.

Deformity of the foot in cerebral palsy is due to spastic muscle imbalance.[69,108,160] Alleviation of deforming muscle forces for preventive purposes is an important aim. Appropriately timed surgery to treat the fixed equinus foot deformity allows better heel strike desirable for stance.[69,160] All surgical techniques are designed to reduce the increased stretch reflex and lengthen the muscle. Increasingly the percutaneous technique is being used with 3 to 6 weeks of immobilization, followed by a weight-bearing program and consideration to use orthoses. Other foot deformities include varus, valgus, and metatarsal abnormalities. Surgical correction involves lengthening or transfers of tendons, arthrodesis, or osteotomies.[69,108,160,161] Postoperative management includes 6 to 8 weeks of immobilization, usually non–weight bearing, followed by orthoses.

Surgery to improve ambulation remains problematic.[69,108,161] Difficulty in predicting outcomes for the ambulator has led to caution in recommending orthopedic surgery. The use of gait analysis has refined identification of the components of the gait cycle and the combined effect of contractures on gait dynamics.[162] Adductor myotomies in combination with hamstring lengthenings can create a better base of support for a more upright posture and reduced scissoring gait.[162] Rectus femoris transfers and lengthenings have decreased the problem of stiff-knee gait after hamstring release.[163,164] Orthopedic surgery can affect the alignment and structure, but central control of balancing reactions remains the same after surgery.

Upper extremity surgery is uncommonly done to improve hand function.[69,165] Surgical management of the spastic upper extremity requires an understanding of dynamic muscle imbalance, tendons and ligamentous contractures, and bony abnormalities. Analysis of the child must include documentation of adequate hand sensation, including light touch, two-point discrimination, and proprioception. Botulinum A toxin block of selected muscles has aided in the selection of the surgical procedure. The child should also have adequate cognitive and emotional stability to comprehend the goals of the operation and to cooperate in the restoration of hand function postoperatively. Goals are to improve function and appearance of the hand.

Thumb deformities are common in cerebral palsy. Most frequent is a thumb-in-palm deformity resulting from spasticity of the adductor pollicis and flexor pollicis longus muscles. Management includes tendon lengthening, release of contracted muscles, Z-plasty of the web space, and arthrodesis of the metacarpophalangeal joints. Flexor carpi ulnaris transfer has a role in reducing the wrist flexion deformity.[69,108,165] Pronator teres tenotomy can improve active supination. Surgery of the elbow is considered if fixed contractures affect function and involves tendon lengthening, capsulotomy, and skin Z-plasty. Postoperative splinting should include adequate extension to prevent excessive stretch of the nerve and vessels. Orthopedic surgical techniques are rarely applied to the shoulder.

Psychosocial Issues

The process of growing up with a disability has an impact on the individual and how the family functions in society. Parents initially must deal with the loss of their idealized child. An already demanding job of raising a child is confounded by the disability. Parents often need to function in a variety of different roles, as well stated by this parent: "We've learned a lot. I sometimes feel like a doctor, therapist, nurse, teacher, chauffeur, inventor, builder, computer expert, communication expert—so many things that I sometimes forget I'm still a mom."[46] The classic patterns of dealing with grief are routinely experienced. Parents who are able to move through the grieving process quickly attribute this to communication, education, and support. The child with the disability not only has to struggle with the physical impairments, but also the social implications of his or her disability. In accepting the disability, a child needs to develop a sense of self-esteem. They need to

explore and learn about their relationships to the world around them. A physical disability can affect this task of early learning and lead to impaired social skills. Hints from parents on how to nurture this development include the following:

1. Do not overprotect the child; let the child learn his or her limitations.
2. Be honest with the child.
3. Set realistic goals for the child.
4. Let the child make choices.
5. Use discipline and encourage self-esteem.
6. Cheer the child on.[46]

The transition from home to school can be a difficult time. Formal educational experiences should begin with early interventional programs. These programs are designed to enhance environmental exposures along with providing therapy and can be home-based or center-based. Once children are age appropriate, there is a transition into the community-based school system. This may be accomplished in the local school, a regional school, or at a home school. Children during this time may become more socially isolated because it is often difficult to include them in all regular activities. The move for full inclusion may positively affect this process. The law requires that all children with a disability are entitled to an *Individual Education Plan*. The transition into high school can be a stressful time but also a time of emotional maturation. The child may become more independent or more regressed. Things such as drooling and incontinence take on a negative social perspective, whereas active participation and group activities enhance social interactions. The key to dealing with the disabled individual is accepting the limitations while accentuating the abilities. With inclusion of the disabled into school programs, the able-bodied students can be exposed to a unique segment of the population. Through education, a mutual respect for each person's individuality can emerge. Leisure and recreational activities are also an important part of developing social interactions (see Chapter 8).

Aging with Cerebral Palsy

The topic of aging with a disability has only recently emerged as an area of extensive research. Previously, individuals with cerebral palsy were believed to have a shortened life expectancy. Studies show that during the first 10 years, there is about a 10% mortality rate and at 30 years a 13% mortality rate.[96] These aging studies are ongoing to follow the population over a longer period of time.

Medical concerns related to aging with cerebral palsy are often confounded by a lack of accessible health services, transportation issues, inadequate knowledge about disabilities by providers, inadequate insurance, and provider attitudes.[166] Although there are specific issues related to aging with a disability, in general, health-related problems appear to occur at about the same rate as in the able-bodied population.[167] There are, however, some medical issues specifically related to aging with cerebral palsy. In evaluating the musculoskeletal problems of the adult, it is necessary to incorporate information on surgeries, limitations in movement, pain, and other relevant information into the evaluation. One of the most common complaints is cervical neck pain. This occurred in 50% of the spastic population but increased to 75% in the dyskinetic population.[167] Radiographic studies of patients with athetoid cerebral palsy show earlier disc degeneration along with a more rapid progression of their disease. They also have a higher incidence of cervical canal narrowing.[168] Other problems encountered included noncervical back pain, pain in weight-bearing joints, contractures, overuse syndromes, and a high incidence of carpal tunnel syndrome.[166,167,169] Fractures were more common in ambulators.[167] Scoliosis has a much higher incidence in nonambulatory individuals. Other areas specifically related to the aging process included gastrointestinal and dental problems. The gastrointestinal issues include ongoing constipation and persistent reflux. Dental problems were found to occur frequently as a result of poor follow-up, and drooling persisted into adulthood.[170]

Sexuality and reproductive functioning in the disabled community has emerged as a complex area of study. Sexuality is a natural human experience that integrates all facets of an individual's personality.[171] A disability does not infer that a person is not able to develop sexual potential. There is limited information available specifically about fertility in men and women with cerebral palsy, but current data imply that this group is capable of near-normal reproduction. There is information on pregnancy and delivery in mild to moderately involved women with cerebral palsy. In this group, the obstetric outcomes were about the same as the general able-bodied population with a slightly higher incidence of elective termination and cesarean section.[172] There is no difference between degree of disability and level of sexual activity.[173] Women with cerebral palsy may also experience an increase in spasticity and incontinence during their menstrual cycles.[174]

Vocational Rehabilitation in Cerebral Palsy

Vocational rehabilitation was established to educate and train disabled individuals to compete in the work environment. It employs a counselor-client relationship to explore viable options for training or placement. Vocational testing includes general intelligence, work interests, aptitudes, and existing work skills.[175] Information obtained from these tests is compiled into an individualized rehabilitation/habilitation plan. This plan identifies which services or adaptations are needed to employ the disabled client. There are a variety of employment situations available depending on the needs of the client. These include sheltered workshops, day programs, home-based programs, traditional job placement, and supported employment.[175] A study showed the following predictors of successful and unsuccessful employment for individuals with cerebral palsy:[94]

Unemployable/unable to work
  IQ less than 50
  Nonambulatory and non-oral
  Required assistance using hand
Sheltered employment
  IQ between 50 and 79
  Ambulation with or without assistive devices
  Speech hard to understand to normal
  Hand use normal to requiring assistance
Competitive
  IQ greater than 80
  Ambulation with or without assistive devices
  Speech hard to understand to normal
  Hand use normal to requiring assistance

Legislation to protect the rights of the disabled has been enacted over the last 30 years (see Table 2–1). These public laws have been developed to provide education and accessibility to the disabled community. They are a first step toward integration of the disabled into all aspects of the world community.

References

1. Bax MCO: Terminology and classification of cerebral palsy. Dev Med Child Neurol 1964;6:295.
2. Molnar GE: Cerebral palsy. In Molnar GE (ed): Pediatric Rehabilitation. Baltimore, Williams & Wilkins, 1985, p 481.
3. Blasco PA: Primitive reflexes: Their contribution to the early detection of cerebral palsy. Clin Pediatr 1994; 33:388.
4. Harris SR: Early neuromotor predictors of cerebral palsy in low birth weight infants. Dev Med Child Neurol 1987;29:508.
5. Illingworth RS: The diagnosis of cerebral palsy in the first year of life. Dev Med Child Neurol 1966;8:178.
6. Bobath K, Bobath B: The diagnosis of cerebral palsy in infancy. Arch Dis Child 1956;31:408.

7. Nicholson A, Alberman E: Cerebral palsy: An increasing contributor to severe mental retardation? Arch Dis Child 1992;62:1050.
8. Stanley FJ: Cerebral palsy trends: Implications for perinatal care. Acta Obstet Gynaecol Scand 1994;73:5.
9. Grether JK, Cummins SK, Nelson KB: The California cerebral palsy project. Pediatr Perinatol Epidemiol 1993;6:339.
10. Cummins SK, Nelson KB, Grether JK, et al: Cerebral palsy in four northern California counties, births 1983 through 1985. J Pediatr 1993;123:230.
11. Nelson KB, Ellenberg JH: Children who outgrew cerebral palsy. Pediatrics 1982;69:529.
12. Pharoah POD, Cooke RWI: A hypothesis for the aetiology of spastic cerebral palsy—the vanishing twin. Dev Med Child Neurol 1997;39:292.
13. Bhushan VB, Paneth N, Kiely JL: Impact of improved survival of very low birth weight infants on recent secular trends in the prevalence of cerebral palsy. Pediatrics 1993;91:1094.
14. Paneth N, Kiely J: The frequency of cerebral palsy. In Stanley F, Alberman E (eds): The Epidemiology of Cerebral Palsies. Clinics in Developmental Medicine Series. Philadelphia, JB Lippincott, 1984.
15. Nelson KB, Ellenberg JH: Antecedents of cerebral palsy. Am J Dis Child 1986;315:81.
16. Taft LT: Cerebral palsy. Pediatr Rev 1995;16:411.
17. Stanley FJ, Blair E: Cerebral palsy. In Pless IB (ed): The Epidemiology of Childhood Disorders. New York, Oxford University Press, 1994.
18. Stanley FJ: Prenatal determinants of motor disorders. Acta Paediatr 1997;422(Suppl):92.
19. Stempien LM, Gaebler-Spira D: Rehabilitation of children and adults with cerebral palsy. In Braddom RL (ed): Physical Medicine and Rehabilitation. Philadelphia, WB Saunders, 1996.
20. Stanley FJ: The aetiology of cerebral palsy. Early Hum Dev 1994;36:81.
21. Ellenberg JH, Nelson KB: Cluster of perinatal events identifying infants at high risk for death or disability. J Pediatr 1988:113:546.
22. Batshaw ML, Eicher PS: Cerebral palsy. Pediatr Clin North Am 1993;40:537.
23. Kuban KC, Leviton A: Cerebral palsy. N Engl J Med 1994;330:188.
24. Bozynski M, Nelson M, Genaze D, et al: Cranial ultrasonography and the production of cerebral palsy in infants weighing ≤ 1200 grams at birth. Dev Med Child Neurol 1988;30:342.
25. Papile L, Munsick-Bruno G, Schaefer A: Relationship of cerebral intraventricular hemorrhage and early childhood neurologic handicaps. J Pediatr 1983;103:273.
26. Volpe JJ: Neurology of the Newborn. Philadelphia, WB Saunders, 1995.
27. Guzzeta F, Shackelford GD, Volpe S, et al: Periventricular intraparenchymal echodensities in the premature newborn: Critical determinants of neurological outcome. Pediatrics 1986;78:995.
28. Lou HC, Henricksen L, Bruhn P, et al: Focal cerebral dysfunction in developmental learning disabilities. Lancet 1990;335:8.
29. Takashima S, Tanaka K: Development of cerebral vascular architecture and its relationship to periventricular leukomalacia. Arch Neurol 1978;35:11.
30. Rorke LB: Anatomical features of the developing brain implicated in pathogenesis of hypoxic-ischemic injury. Brain Pathol 1992;2:211.
31. Koeda T, Takeshita K: Visuoperceptual impairment and cerebral lesions in spastic diplegia with preterm birth. Brain Dev 1992;14:239.
32. Perlman JM, Risser R, Broyles RS: Bilateral cystic periventricular leukomalacia in the premature infant: Associated risk factors. Pediatrics 1996;97:822.
33. Rogers B, Msall M, Owens T, et al: Cystic periventricular leukomalacia and type of cerebral palsy in preterm infants. J Pediatr 1994;125:S1.
34. Perlman JM, Rollins NK, Evans D: Neonatal stroke. Pediatr Neurol 1994;11:281.
35. McDonald JW, Johnson MV: Physiological and pathological roles of excitatory amino acids during nervous system development. Brain Res Rev 1990;15:41.
36. Paneth N, Stark RI: Cerebral palsy and mental retardation in relation to indicators of perinatal asphyxia. Am J Obstet Gynecol 1983;47:960.
37. Blair E, Stanley FJ: Intrapartum asphyxia—a rare cause of cerebral palsy. J Pediatr 1988;112:515.
38. Torfs CP, Van der berg BJ, Oeschali FW: Prenatal and perinatal factors in the etiology of cerebral palsy. J Pediatr 1990;116:615.
39. Sher MS, Belfar H, Martin J, Painter MJ: Destructive brain lesions of presumed fetal onset: Antepartum causes of cerebral palsy. Pediatrics 1991;88:898.
40. Zupan V, Gonzales P, Lacaze-Masmonteil, et al: Periventricular leukomalacia: Risk factors revisited. Dev Med Child Neurol 1996;38:1061.
41. Perlman JM: Intrapartum hypoxic-ischemic cerebral injury and subsequent cerebral palsy: medicolegal issues. Pediatrics 1997;99:851.
42. Crothers BS, Paine RS: The Natural History of Cerebral Palsy. Cambridge, Harvard Press, 1959.
43. Alberman E: Describing the cerebral palsies: Methods of classifying and counting. In Stanley F, Alberman E (eds): The Epidemiology of the Cerebral Palsies. Clinics in Developmental Medicine Series. Philadelphia, JB Lippincott, 1984.
44. Sachs B, Hausman L: The proper classification of the cerebral palsies of early life. Am J Med Sci 1926;171:376.
45. Uvebrandt P: Hemiplegic cerebral palsy. Acta Paediatr Scand 1988;345(Suppl):1.
46. Gersh E: What is cerebral palsy? In Geralis E (ed): Children with Cerebral Palsy. New York, Woodbine House, 1991.
47. Paine RS, Oppe TE: Neurologic Examination of Children. Clinics in Developmental Medicine. London, William Heinemann, 1966.
48. Nelson K, Swaiman K, Russman B: Cerebral palsy. In Swaiman K (ed): Pediatric Neurology: Principles and Practice. St Louis, Mosby, 1994.
49. McDonald AD: Cerebral palsy in children of very low birth weight. Arch Dis Child 1963;38:579.
50. Veelken N, Hagberg B, Hagberg G, Olow I: Diplegic cerebral palsy in Swedish term and preterm children: Differences in reduced optimality, relations to neurology and pathogenetic factors. Neuropediatrics 1983;14:20.
51. Okumura A, Hayakawa F, Kato T, et al: MRI findings in patients with spastic cerebral palsy: I. Correlation with gestational age at birth. Dev Med Child Neurol 1997;39:363.
52. Okumura A, Hayakawa F, Kato K, et al: MRI findings in patients with spastic cerebral palsy. Dev Med Child Neurol 1997;39:369.
53. Ingram TT: Pediatric Aspects of Cerebral Palsy. Edinburgh, ES Livingston, 1964.
54. Uggetti C: Cerebral visual impairment in periventricular leukomalacia: MR correlation. Am J Neuroradiol 1989;17:979.
55. Edebol-Tysk K, Hagberg B, Hagberg G: Epidemiology of spastic tetraplegic cerebral palsy in Sweden: II. Prevalance, birth data and origin. Neuropediatrics 1989;20:46.

56. Edebol-Tysk K, Hagberg B, Hagberg G: Epidemiology of spastic tetraplegic cerebral palsy in Sweden: I. Impairments and disabilities. Neuropediatrics 1989;20:41.
57. Brett E, Scrutton D: Cerebral palsy, perinatal injury to the spinal cord and brachial plexus birth injury. In Brett E (ed): Pediatric Neurology. New York, Churchill Livingstone, 1997.
58. Perlstein M, Hood P: Infantile spastic hemiplegia. Pediatrics 1954;14:436.
59. Roberts C, Vogtle L, Stevenson R: Effect of hemiplegia on skeletal maturation. J Pediatr 1994;125:824.
60. Holt KS: Growth disturbances. In Holt KS (ed): Hemiplegic Cerebral Palsy in Children and Adults. Clinics in Developmental Medicine. London, William Heinemann, 1961.
61. Tizard J, Paine R, Crothers B: Disturbances of sensation in children with hemiplegia. JAMA 1954;155:628.
62. Skatvedt M: Sensory, perceptual and other non-motor deficits in cerebral palsy. Little Club Dev Med 1960;1:115.
63. Menkes J: Perinatal Asphyxia and Trauma. In Menkes J (ed): Textbook of Child Neurology. Baltimore, Williams & Wilkins, 1995.
64. Marcus J: The spinal accessory nerve in childhood hemiplegia. Arch Neurol 1989;46:60.
65. Paine RS, Oppe TE: Neurologic Examination of Children. Clinics in Developmental Medicine. London, William Heinemann, 1966.
66. Kyllerman M, Bager B, Bensch J, et al: Dyskinetic cerebral palsy. Acta Paediatr Scand 1982;71:543.
67. Palisano R, Rosenbaum P, Walter S, et al: Development and reliability of a system to classify gross motor function in children with cerebral palsy. Dev Med Child Neurol 1997;39:214.
68. Jones E, Knapp R: Assessment and management of the lower extremity in cerebral palsy. Orthop Clin North Am 1987;18:725.
69. Bleck EE: Orthopedic Management of Cerebral Palsy. Philadelphia, MacKeith Press, 1987.
70. Freeman J, Nelson K: Intrapartum asphyxia and cerebral palsy. Pediatrics 1988;82:240.
71. Svenningsen N, Siesjo B: Cerebrospinal fluid lactate/pyruvate ratio in normal and asphyxiated neonates. Act Paediatr Scand 1972;61:117.
72. Levene M: Periventricular haemorrhage. In Levene M, Williams J, Fawer C: Ultrasound of the Infant Brain. Clin Devel Med 1985;92.
73. Hill A, Volpe J: Hypoxic-ischemic cerebral injury in the newborn. In Brett E (ed): Pediatric Neurology. New York, Churchill Livingstone, New York.
74. Volpe J: Positron emission tomography in the newborn: Excessive impairment of regional blood flow with intraventricular hemorrhage and hemorrhagic intracranial involvement. Pediatrics 1983;72:589.
75. Johnson M, Pennock J, Bidder G, et al: Serial imaging in neonatal cerebral injury. Am J Neuroradiol 1987;8:83.
76. Moorcraft J, Bolas N, Ives N, et al: Spatially localized magnetic resonance spectroscopy of the brains of normal and asphyxiated newborns. Pediatrics 1991;87:273.
77. Holmes G, Rowe J, Hafford J, et al: Prognostic value of the electroencephalogram in neonatal asphyxia. Electroencephalogr Clin Neurophysiol 1982:53:60.
78. Scherzer A, Tscharnuter I: Early Diagnosis and Therapy in Cerebral Palsy. New York, Marcel Dekker, 1990.
79. Matthews DJ: Nonprogressive diseases of the central nervous system. In Kaplan PE, Matterson RS (eds): The Practice of Rehabilitation Medicine. Springfield, IL, Charles C Thomas, 1982.
80. Lesny I, Stehlik A, Tomasek J, et al: Sensory disorders in cerebral palsy: Two-point discrimination. Dev Med Child Neurol 1993; 35:402.
81. Van Heest AE, House J, Putman M: Sensibility deficiencies in the hands of children with spastic hemiplegia. J Hand Surg Am 1993;18:278.
82. Bleck EE: Locomotor prognosis in cerebral palsy. Dev Med Child Neurol 1975;17:18.
83. Molnar GE, Gordon SU: Cerebral palsy: Predictive value of selected clinical signs of early prognostication of motor function. Arch Phys Med Rehabil 1976;57:153.
84. Sala DA, Grant AD: Prognosis for ambulation in cerebral palsy. Dev Med Child Neurol 1995;37:1020.
85. Laplaza FJ, Root L, Tassanawipas A, et al: Femoral torsion and neck-shaft angles in cerebral palsy. J Pediatr Orthop 1993;13:192.
86. McCarty SM, McCarty SM, James PS: Assessment of intelligence functioning across the life span in severe cerebral palsy. Dev Med Child Neurol 1986;28:369.
87. Sussova J, Seidl Z, Faber J: Hemiparetic forms of cerebral palsy in relation to epilepsy and mental retardation. Dev Med Child Neurol 1990;32:792.
88. Krageloh-Mann I, Hagberg G, Meisner C, et al: Bilateral spastic cerebral palsy. Dev Med Child Neurol 1993;35:1031.
89. Rogers B, Arvedson J, Buck G, et al: Characteristics of dysphagia in children with cerebral palsy. Dysphagia 1994;9:60.
90. Drvaric DM, Roberts JM, Burke SW, et al: Gastroesophageal evaluation in totally involved cerebral palsy patients. J Pediatr Orthop 1987;7:187.
91. Agnarsson U, Warde C, McCarthy G, et al: Anorectal function of children with neurological problems. Dev Med Child Neurol 1993;35:903.
92. Herman SC, McDonald PE: Enamel hypoplasia in cerebral palsy children. J Dent Child 1963;30:46.
93. Eicher PS, Batshaw ML: Cerebral palsy: The child with developmental disabilities. Pediatr Clin North Am 1993;40:537.
94. Robinson R: The frequency of other handicaps in children with cerebral palsy. Dev Med Child Neurol 1973;15:305.
95. Evans PM, Evans SJW, Alberman R: Cerebral palsy: Why we must plan for survival. Arch Dis Child 1990;65:1329.
96. Crichton JU, MacKinnon M, White CP: The life expectancy of persons with cerebral palsy. Dev Med Child Neurol 1995;37:567.
97. Murphy KP, Molnar GE, Lankasky K: Medical and functional status of adults with cerebral palsy. Dev Med Child Neurol 1997;37:1075.
98. Eyman RK, Grossman HJ, Chaney RH, et al: The life expectancy of profoundly handicapped people with mental retardation. N Engl J Med 1990;323:584.
99. Kong E: Very early treatment of cerebral palsy. Dev Med Child Neurol 1966;8:198.
100. Taggart P, Matthews DJ: Developmental intervention and therapeutic exercise. In Molnar GE (ed): Pediatric Rehabilitation. Baltimore, Williams & Wilkins, 1990.
101. Shonkoff JP, Hauser-Cram P: Early intervention for disabled infants and their families: A quantitative analysis. Pediatrics 1987;80:650.
102. Low NL: A hypothesis why early intervention in cerebral palsy might be useful. Brain Dev 1980;2:133.
103. Harris S: Efficacy of early intervention in pediatric rehabilitation. Phys Med Rehabil Clin North Am 1991;2:725.
104. Harris S: Evaluation the effects of early intervention. AAJOC 1993;147:12.
105. Turnbull JD: Early intervention for children with or at risk of cerebral palsy. Am J Dis Child 1993;147:54.

106. The Infant Health Program: Enhancing the outcomes of low birth weight, premature infants. JAMA 1990; 263:3035.

107. American Academy of Pediatrics: Committee on Children with Disabilities: Pediatric services for infants and children with special needs. Pediatrics 1993;92:163.

108. Matthews DJ: Controversial therapies in the management of cerebral palsy. Pediatr Ann 1988;17:762.

109. Doman R, Spitz E, Zuckman E, et al: Children with severe brain injuries. JAMA 1960;174:257.

110. Rood M: Neurophysiological mechanisms utilized in the treatment of neuromuscular dysfunction. Am J Occup Ther 1956;10:220.

111. Bobath B: A neurodevelopmental treatment of cerebral palsy. Physiotherapy 1963;49:242.

112. Bobath K, Bobath B: Motor Development in the Different Types of Cerebral Palsy. London, Heinemann, 1975.

113. Bobath K: Neurophysiological Basis for Treatment of Cerebral Palsy. Lavenham, Spastics International, 1980.

114. Vojta V: The basic elements of treatment according to Vojta. In Scrutton D (ed): Management of the Motor Disorders of Children with Cerebral Palsy. Oxford, Blackwell Scientific Publications, 1984.

115. Hari M, Tillemans T: Conductive education. In Scrutton D (ed): Management of Motor Disorders of Children with Cerebral Palsy. Oxford, Blackwell Scientific Publications, 1984.

116. Kramer J, MacPhail A: Relationship among measures of walking efficiency, gross motor ability and isokinetic strength in adolescents with cerebral palsy. Pediatr Phys Ther 1994;6:3.

117. Butler C: Effects of powered mobility on self-initiated behaviors of very young children with locomotor disability. Dev Med Child Neurol 1986;28:325.

118. Little JW, Merritt JL: Spasticity and associated muscle tone. In Delisa J (ed): Rehabilitation Medicine: Principles and Practice. Philadelphia, JB Lippincott, 1988.

119. Katz RT: Management of spasticity. In Braddom R (ed): Physical Medicine and Rehabilitation. Philadelphia, WB Saunders, 1996.

120. Cusick B: Splints and casts: Managing foot deformity in children. Phys Ther 1988;68:1903.

121. Ricks NR, Eilert RE: Effects of inhibitory casts and orthoses on bony alignment of foot and ankle during weight-bearing in children with spasticity. Dev Med Child Neurol 1993;66:1522.

122. Basmajian J: Biofeedback in therapeutic exercise. In Basmajian J: Therapeutic Exercise. Baltimore, Williams & Wilkins, 1984.

123. O'Dwyer NJ, Neilson P, Nash J: Reduction of spasticity in cerebral palsy using feedback of the tonic stretch reflex. Dev Med Child Neurol 1994;36:770.

124. Carmick J: Clinical use of neuromuscular electrical stimulation for children with cerebral palsy: Part 1. Lower extremity. Phys Ther 1993;73:505.

125. Carmick J: Clinical use of neuromuscular electrical stimulation for children with cerebral palsy: Part 2. Upper extremity. Phys Ther 1993;73:514.

126. Dubowitz L, Finnie N, Hyde SA, et al: Improvement of muscle performance by chronic electrical stimulation in children with cerebral palsy. Lancet 1988;1:587.

127. Hazelwood ME, Brown JK, Rowe PJ, Salter PM: The therapeutic use of electrical stimulation. Dev Med Child Neurol 1994;36:661.

128. Pape K, Kirsch SE, Galil A, et al: Neuromuscular approach to the motor deficits of cerebral palsy. J Pediatr Orthop 1993;13:628.

129. Penn RD: Intrathecal baclofen for spasticity of spinal origin: A seven-year experience. J Neurosurg 1992; 77:236.

130. Albright AL: Intrathecal baclofen in cerebral palsy movement disorders. J Child Neurol 1996;11:S29.

131. Easton JKM, Ozel T, Halpern D: Intramuscular neurolysis for spasticity in children. Arch Phys Med Rehabil 1979;60:155.

132. Cosgrove AP, Corry IS, Graham HK: Botulinum toxin in the management of the lower limb in cerebral palsy. Dev Med Child Neurol 1994;36:386.

133. Koman LA, Mooney JF, Smith BP, et al: Management of spasticity in cerebral palsy with botulinum-A toxin. J Pediatr Orthop 1994;14:299.

134. Koman LA, Mooney JF, Smith BP: Neuromuscular blockade in the management of cerebral palsy. J Child Neurol 1996;11:S23.

135. Corry IS, Cosgrove AP, Walsh EG, et al: Botulinum toxin A in the hemiplegic upper limb: A double-blind trial. Dev Med Child Neurol 1997;39:185.

136. Cooper I, Riklan M, Amin I, et al: Chronic cerebellar stimulation in cerebral palsy. Neurology 1976;26:744.

137. Trejos H, Araya R: Stereotactic surgery for cerebral palsy. Stereotact Func Neurosurg 1990;54:130.

138. Peacock WJ, Staudt LA: Functional outcomes following selective posterior rhizotomy in children with cerebral palsy. J Neurosurg 1991;74:380.

139. Abbott R, Johann-Murphy M, Shiminski-Maher T, et al: Selective dorsal rhizotomy: Outcome and complications in treating spastic cerebral palsy. Neurosurgery 1993;33:851.

140. Peter JC, Arens LJ: Selective posterior lumbosacral rhizotomy for management of cerebral palsy: A ten-year experience. S Afr Med J 1993;83:745.

141. Abbott R: Sensory rhizotomy for the treatment of childhood spasticity. J Child Neurol 1996;11:S36.

142. Kinghorn J: Upper extremity functional changes following selective posterior rhizotomy in children with cerebral palsy. Am J Occup Ther 1992;46:502.

143. Hays RM, McLaughlin JF, Stephens KF, et al: Electrophysiological monitoring during selective dorsal rhizotomy, and spasticity and GMFM performance. Dev Med Child Neurol 1998;40:233.

144. Adams J, Cahan L, Perry J, et al: Foot contact pattern following selective dorsal rhizotomy. Pediatr Neurosurg 1995;23:76.

145. Wright FV, Sheil EMH, Drake JM, et al: Evaluation of selective dorsal thizotomy for the reduction of spasticity in cerebral palsy: A randomized controlled trial. Dev Med Child Neurol 1998;40:239.

146. Matthews DJ, Stempien LM: Orthopedic management of the disabled child. In Sinaki M (ed): Basic Clinical Rehabilitation Medicine. St. Louis, Mosby, 1993.

147. Hoffer M, Abraham E, Nickel V, et al: Salvage surgery of the hip to improve sitting posture of mentally retarded, severely disabled children with cerebral palsy. Dev Med Child Neurol 1992;14:51.

148. Rang M, Douglas G, Bennet G, et al: Seating for children with cerebral palsy. J Pediatr Orthop 1981;1:279.

149. Koop S: Orthopedic aspects of static encephalopathy. In Miller G, Ramer J (eds): Static Encephalopathies of Infancy and Childhood. New York, Academic Press, 1992.

150. Moreau M, Drummond D, Rogala E, et al: Natural history of the dislocated hip in spastic cerebral palsy. Dev Med Child Neurol 1979;21:749.

151. Mathias A: Management of cerebral palsy: Physical therapy in relation to orthopedic surgery. Phys Ther 1967;47:473.

152. Hoffer M: Management of the hip in cerebral palsy. J Bone Joint Surg 1986;68A:629.

153. Rinsky LA: Surgery of spinal deformity in cerebral palsy. Clin Orthop 1990;32:347.

154. Zimbler S, Craig C, Harris J, et al: Orthotic management of severe scoliosis in spastic neuromuscular diseases—results of treatment. Orthop Trans 1985; 9:78.

155. Allen BL, Ferguson RL: L-rod instrumentation for scoliosis in cerebral palsy. J Pediatr Orthop 1982;2:87.

156. Lonstein JE, Akbarnia B: Operative treatment of spinal deformities in patients with cerebral palsy or mental retardation. J Bone Joint Surg 1983;65A:33.

157. Mullaferoze P, Voro P: Surgery in lower limbs in cerebral palsy. Dev Med Child Neurol 1972;70:490.

158. Hadley N, Chambers C, Scarborough N, et al: Knee motion following multiple soft-tissue releases in ambulatory patients with cerebral palsy. J Pediatr Orthop 1992;12:324.

159. Hoffinger SA, Rab GT, Abou-Ghaida H: Hamstring in cerebral palsy crouch gait. J Pediatr Orthop 1993; 13:722.

160. Fulford GE: Surgical management of ankle and foot deformities in cerebral palsy. Dev Med Child Neurol 1988;82:48.

161. Dormans JP: Orthopedic management of children with cerebral palsy. Pediatr Clin North Am 1993;40:645.

162. Gage JR: Gait analysis in cerebral palsy. Clin Dev Med 1991;121:177.

163. Gage JR, Perry J, Hicks RR, et al: Rectus femoris transfer to improve knee function of children with cerebral palsy. Dev Med Child Neurol 1987;29:159.

164. Ounpuu S, Muik E, Davis RB, et al: Rectus femoris surgery in children with cerebral palsy. J Pediatr Orthop 1993;13:331.

165. Hunter JM, Mackin EJ, Callahan AD: Rehabilitation of the Hand: Surgery and Therapy. St. Louis, Mosby, 1995.

166. Gans B, Mann N, Becker B: Delivery of primary care to physically challenged. Arch Phys Med Rehabil 1993; 74:15.

167. Murphy KP, Molnar G, Lankasky K: Medical and functional status of adults with cerebral palsy. Dev Med Child Neurol 1995;37:1075.

168. Harada T, Ebera S, Anwar M, et al: The cervical spine in athetoid cerebral palsy. J Bone Joint Surg 1996; 78B:613.

169. Kim H, Diamond M, Johnson M: The prevalence of carpal tunnel syndrome in adults with cerebral palsy. Arch Phys Med Rehabil 1997; 78:1025.

170. Gaebler DJ, Elliot-Scanlon G: Cerebral palsy in adults over 40: Lifestyle issues related to aging. Arch Phys Med Rehabil 1997;77:979.

171. Ducharme S, Gill K, Biener-Bergman S, et al: Sexual functioning: Medical and psychological aspects. In Delisa J (ed): Rehabilitation Medicine: Principles and Practice. Philadelphia, JB Lippincott, 1988.

172. Winch R, Bengtson L, McLaughlin J, et al: Women with cerebral palsy: Obstetrical experience and neonatal outcome. Dev Med Child Neurol 1993;35:974.

173. Nosek MA, Rintala D, Young ME, et al: Sexual functioning among women with physical disabilities. Arch Phys Med Rehabil 1996;77:107.

174. Turk M, Geremski C, Rosenbaum P, et al: The health of women with cerebral palsy. Arch Phys Med Rehabil 1997;78:S10.

175. Blake D, Scott D: Vocational Rehabilitation. In Braddom RL (ed): Physical Medicine and Rehabilitation. Philadelphia, WB Saunders, 1996.

Chapter 12

Spina Bifida

Gabriella E. Molnar, MD
Kevin P. Murphy, MD

Spina bifida is the second most common disability in childhood following cerebral palsy. It represents a group of neural tube defects caused by congenital dysraphic malformations of the vertebral column and spinal cord[1-4] and often is associated with other anomalies of the central nervous system and, at times, of mesodermal structures. Neonatal neurosurgery and advances in the treatment and rehabilitation of the spectrum of clinical manifestations have increased the survival of children and adults with spina bifida.

Epidemiology. Extensive epidemiologic studies during the past three decades demonstrated differences in the incidence of neural tube defects by geographic location and reported a trend of declining frequency.[5] On a worldwide scale, the highest incidence is in the British Isles, Ireland, Wales, and Scotland, and the lowest in Japan.[6] A recent survey from Scotland found decreased prevalence from 5.63/1,000 births in 1964–1968 to 1.04/1,000 births in 1979–1989.[7] In the United States the rate of neural tube defects declined from 1.3/1,000 births in 1970 to 0.6/1,000 births in 1989.[8] Both studies concluded that the decline preceded the availability of prenatal screening. Therefore, antenatal detection and consequent termination of pregnancy can be held only partially responsible for the trend of decreasing rate. In the United States there is a higher incidence in families of Irish, German, or Hispanic ancestry and lower among Asians and Pacific Islanders than in the general population at large.[9,10]

Etiology. The etiology of spina bifida is complex; both polygenic inheritance and environmental influences seem to contribute in a mulifactorial manner.[1-6] Increased familial incidence and recurrence rate and a slightly greater number of affected females than males point to a genetic etiology.[11,12] The recurrence rate is 2.4–5% after the birth of one child with spina bifida and doubles after two affected children.[13]

Although studies of chicken and mouse models with neural tube defects similar to those in humans demonstrated genetic abnormalities, the exact genes responsible in humans have not been identified.[14] The malformations are attributed to abnormal interaction of several regulating and modifying genes in early fetal development.[15] The female-to-male prevalence ratio was 1.2 in two United States Surveillance Systems.[10]

Several environmental risk factors have been implicated, including low socioeconomic class,[16] midspring conception, and maternal obesity.[17] In utero exposure to anticonvulsant drugs, specifically valproic acid[18,19] or carbamazepine,[20] was found to increase the risk of spina bifida. On the other hand, extensive investigations demonstrated that folic acid periconceptually and during early pregnancy significantly reduces the occurrence and recurrence of neural tube defects.[21-23] The U.S. Public Health Service recommends a daily intake of 0.4 mg folic acid for all women of childbearing age.[24] Heat exposure, in the form of maternal febrile illness or as a result of high environmental temperature (e.g., hot baths during the first trimester), is another more recently proposed teratogenic agent of unknown mechanism.[25,26]

Prenatal Diagnosis. Pregnant women with a positive familial history, a previous child with spina bifida, or exposure to teratogenic agents should undergo routine and, if warranted, repeated prenatal screening tests.[2-4,27] Measurement of alpha-fetoprotein (AFP) and acetylcholinesterase in the maternal serum and amniotic fluid and fetal ultrasound are methods of prenatal diagnosis.

AFP is a component of fetal serum globulin. Under normal circumstances it is excreted into the amniotic fluid through fetal urine and eventually absorbed into the maternal serum. Open neural tube defects allow leakage of fetal cerebrospinal fluid, leading to elevated AFP in the amniotic fluid by the 13th–15th postconceptual week. The usual time for maternal serum AFP testing is between 16 and18 weeks of gestation.[27] AFP testing provides reliable detection in approximately 80% of cases. However, anterior abdominal wall defects or fetal death may lead to false-positive results. False-negative measurements also have been reported.[3] By the 16th–18th postconceptual week amniocentesis does not pose a fetal risk and may be considered as a confirming test; its accuracy is nearly 100% in open neural tube defects.[28] Elevated amniotic fluid AFP and, even more specifically, acetylcholinesterase isoenzyme, which is elevated only in conjunction with an open spina bifida lesion, determine the diagnosis.[28] As is the case with maternal serum examinations, amniocentesis does not detect closed neural tube defects without leakage of fetal cerebrospinal fluid.

Fetal ultrasound between 16 and 24 weeks of gestation is an additional diagnostic method reported to have over 90% reliability in some studies.[29] It also may demonstrate other associated central nervous system malformations—for example, cerebellar compression due to Arnold-Chiari malformation, the so-called banana sign, or diastematomyelia.[2] Vertebral anomalies without actual dysraphism may create false-positive impression on fetal ultrasound. False-negative results reportedly decrease with advancing gestational age.[30]

When prenatal diagnosis is established, some families may choose to terminate pregnancy. The frequency of this decision varies in different reports.[31,32] Elective cesarean section has been recommended by some studies to decrease the possibility of further damaging the protruding spinal sac during vaginal delivery.[33] Despite some suggestions that muscle weakness is less severe after cesarean section than with vaginal delivery, no differences in the level of paralysis were demonstrated.[34]

Pathogenesis.   Theories about the pathogenesis of neural tube defects relate to embryonic development of the central nervous system.[1–4,35,36] Neurulation of the anterior and posterior neuropores occurs during the third-to-fourth weeks after conception.[2,35,36] Spina bifida cystica, craniorachischisis, and anencephaly are anomalies thought to develop during this stage. The postneurulation phase takes place during the fourth-to-seventh postconceptual weeks and consists of canalization and retrogressive differentiation of the most caudal portion of the spinal cord. Defects occurring at this stage are skin-covered lesions, often associated with malformations of the conus, filum terminale, or tumors in the caudal spinal canal.[36] Another theory proposes that overgrowth of neuroectodermal tissues at

the site of spinal defect is either the cause or the result of failed neural fold fusion.[35,37] Secondary reopening due to focal mesodermal/ectodermal tissue necrosis, possibly from vascular compromise, also has been suggested.[38] According to the hydrodynamic theory, which postulates a different mechanism for secondary opening, the responsible factor is a malformation of the rhombic roof of the fourth ventricle that prevents drainage of the cerebrospinal fluid to the subarachnoid space and leads to increased pressure within the ventricles and spinal canal and eventual rupture of the cord.[39,40]

Clinical Types.   Neural tube defects with absent or faulty midline closure of the spinal cord and vertebral canal have a variety of clinical manifestations. The two major types are spina bifida occulta and spina bifida cystica or aperta.

In spina bifida occulta dysraphism affects primarily the vertebrae, but the neural and meningeal elements are not herniated to the surface.[1–4] In normal development, fusion of the vertebral arches is incomplete at birth. It proceeds postnatally, although closure of the posterior vertebral structures may remain incomplete and is detectable in 5–36% of adults as an incidental finding without evidence of spinal cord dysfunction.[41] In contrast, the distinguishing feature of spina bifida occulta is the presence of associated malformations of the spinal cord, nerve roots, and/or other contents of the spinal canal.[1–3,42] A rather frequent warning sign reported in 50% of cases is the presence of a pigmented nevus, angioma, hirsute patch, dimple, or dermal sinus on the overlying skin.[2,43] Spina bifida occulta usually occurs in the lumbosacral or sacral segments. At an early age, some cases with less extensive spinal cord involvement are or may appear asymptomatic. However, such children need careful observation for progressive symptoms that may develop during the growing years from tethered cord, expanding fibrolipomatous tumor or other malformations within the spinal cord or canal[1–3,44] (Fig. 12–1). Unlike the cystic form of neural tube defects, spina bifida occulta is not associated with Arnold-Chiari malformation.[2]

In spina bifida cystica contents of the spinal canal herniate through the posterior vertebral opening. The protruding sac may be nonepithelialized or covered partially or completely by a modified or normal skin layer. Incomplete skin coverage leads to leakage of cerebrospinal fluid. In meningocele the herniation consists of a meningeal cyst filled with cerebrospinal fluid. In the absence of other underlying malformations neurologic signs are normal. However, as in the case of spina bifida occulta, observation for possible progressive signs is indicated for the same reasons. Meningoceles are not associated with hydrocephalus.[2,3] In myelomeningocele the sac also contains dysplastic neural tissues. A malformed neural placode and abnormal rootlets may be exposed on the nonepithelialized surface with leakage of the cerebrospinal fluid. Clinical symptoms include motor paralysis and sensory deficit; their level depends on the anatomic location and extent of spinal cord malformation. Bowel and bladder function is affected. Arnold-Chiari type II malformation is present in almost all cases and is complicated by hydrocephalus in over 90%.[1–4,35] Myelomeningocele affects an overwhelming majority of the group with spina bifida cystica; true meningocele occurs in less than 10% of cases.[3] Approximately 75% of lesions affect the lumbar or lumbosacral segments. The remainder are located in the thoracic or sacral area but only rarely at the cervical level.[3,4,35]

Clinical Signs and Course

The spinal cord defect associated with central nervous system and other malformations creates multisystemic symptoms with various health problems and potentially life-threatening consequences. Motor and sensory deficits vary according to the level and extent of the spinal cord anomaly.[2–4] Motor paralysis is usually of the lower motor neuron type. When the spinal cord malformation is extensive and located at a higher segmental level, most lower extremity muscles are involved; the legs are flail and atonic. Lesions that preserve some innervation of the lower extremities are associated with partial flaccid weakness and abnormal joint position consistent with the paralytic muscle imbalance. Because deep tendon and superficial reflexes depend on an intact peripheral reflex arc, absent reflexes correspond to the segmental spinal cord lesion. A combination of flaccid and spastic paralysis is reported in 10–40% of cases.[2–4,35,45,46] Spasticity may be either distal or proximal to the level of dysplastic spinal cord malformation.[47–49] Distal spasticity tends to occur mostly in high thoracic lesions when a caudal portion of the spinal cord below the malformed segments is at least partially preserved. Isolated from its central connections, it gives rise to upper motor neuron signs, hyperactive deep tendon and spinal reflexes, and increased tone. Because spinal reflexes are not under voluntary control, such movements are not useful for functional purposes.[45,47] Presence or gradual development of proximal spasticity above the level of the spinal cord dysplasia may be related to tethering, Arnold-Chiari type II malformation that

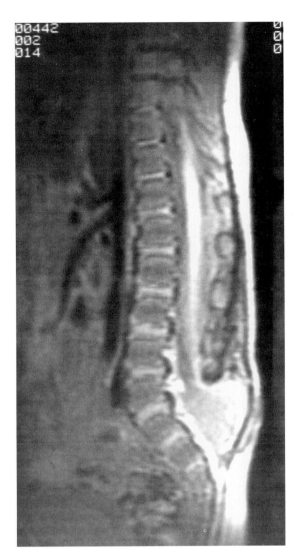

FIGURE 12–1. Initially asymptomatic spina bifida occulta with sacral lipoma; bladder incontinence and constipation from tethering onset at 5 years. Symptoms resolved after surgical release of tethering and resection of lipoma. No recurrence at 4-year follow-up. (From Molnar GE: Spina bifida: Clinical correlations of associated central nervous system malformations. Phys Med Rehabil State Art Rev 1991;5:288, with permission.)

exerts pressure on the cervical cord, decompensating hydrocephalus, ventriculitis, syringohydromyelia or coexistent anoxic encephalopathy sustained before or at birth.[35,48–50] In some cases muscle function innervated from higher segments may be absent or impaired, whereas other muscles subserved by more distal spinal cord level are active. At times, neurologic signs are asymmetric. Both types of clinical manifestations reflect an anatomically irregular spinal cord anomaly instead of a clearcut transverse lesion. Sensory deficit is present in the dermatomes

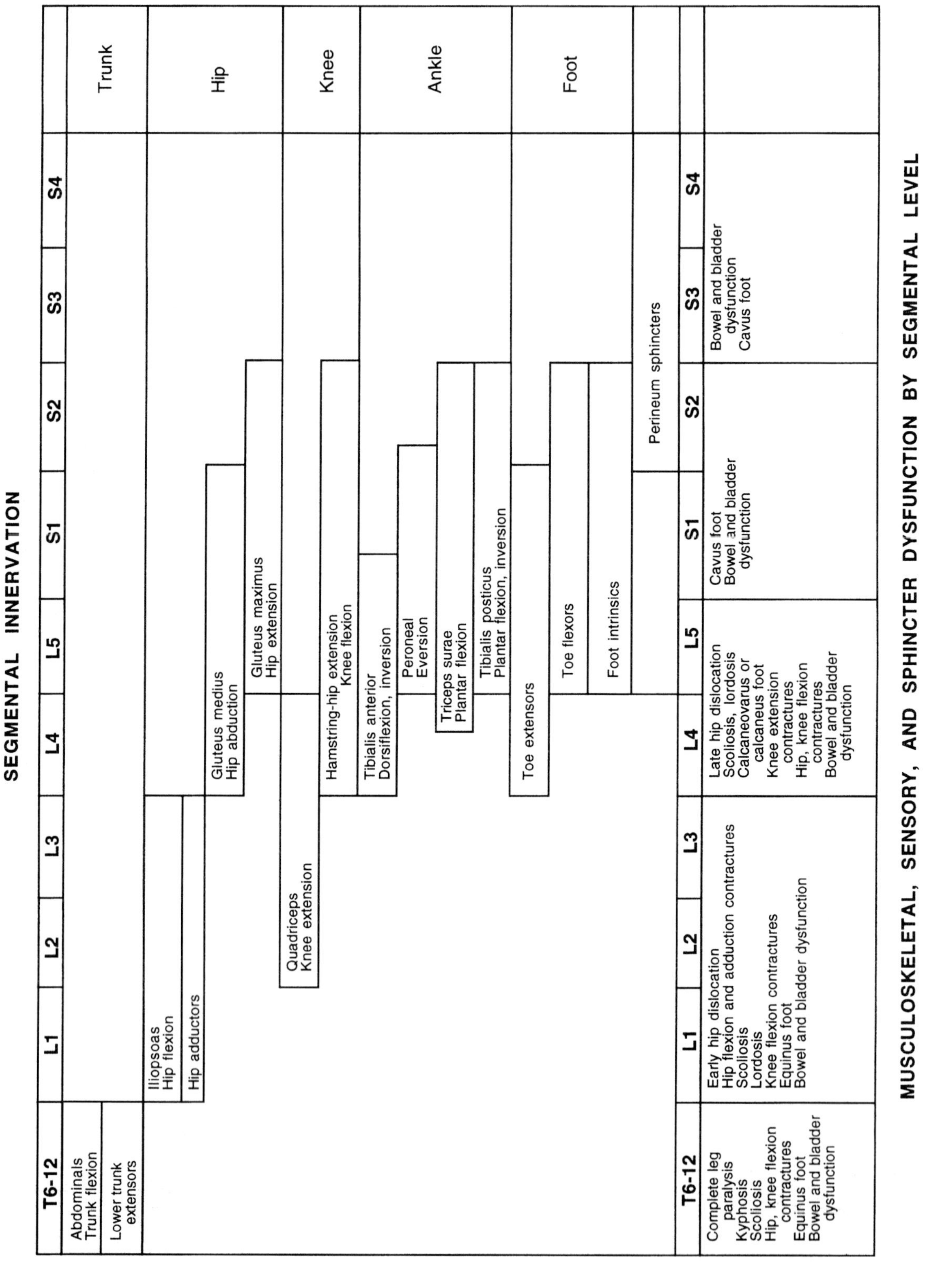

SEGMENTAL INNERVATION

	T6-12	L1	L2	L3	L4	L5	S1	S2	S3	S4	
	Abdominals Trunk flexion										Trunk
	Lower trunk extensors										
		Iliopsoas Hip flexion									Hip
		Hip adductors									
					Gluteus medius Hip abduction						
						Gluteus maximus Hip extension					
			Quadriceps Knee extension								Knee
					Hamstring-hip extension Knee flexion						
					Tibialis anterior Dorsiflexion, inversion						Ankle
						Peroneal Eversion					
						Triceps surae Plantar flexion					
						Tibialis posticus Plantar flexion, inversion					
					Toe extensors						Foot
						Toe flexors					
						Foot intrinsics					
								Perineum sphincters			

MUSCULOSKELETAL, SENSORY, AND SPHINCTER DYSFUNCTION BY SEGMENTAL LEVEL

T6-12	L1	L2	L3	L4	L5	S1	S2	S3	S4
Complete leg paralysis Kyphosis Scoliosis Hip, knee flexion contractures Equinus foot Bowel and bladder dysfunction	Early hip dislocation Hip flexion and adduction contractures Scoliosis Lordosis Knee flexion contractures Equinus foot Bowel and bladder dysfunction			Late hip dislocation Scoliosis, lordosis Calcaneovarus or calcaneus foot Knee extension contractures Hip, knee flexion contractures Bowel and bladder dysfunction		Cavus foot Bowel and bladder dysfunction		Bowel and bladder dysfunction Cavus foot	

FIGURE 12-2. Segmental innervation and dysfunction.

that would be innervated by the defective spinal cord segments and nerve roots. It may or may not affect all sensory modalities equally or in the same distribution. A rather characteristic dissociation of sensory deficits that may develop above the original spinal cord level includes impaired pain and temperature perception with sparing of other modalities seen in syringohydromyelia.[2,3] The segmental locations of motor and sensory deficits are usually similar but may differ. Again, such dissociated motor and sensory dysfunction indicates the anatomic irregularity of spinal cord malformation. Because of the distal innervation of the bladder and bowel, neurogenic bladder and bowel dysfunction are present in all levels of lesions.

Prevention and correction of musculoskeletal deformities are serious clinical concerns. In general, one can distinguish two types of joint abnormalities: (1) static, rigid deformities present at birth or (2) deformities developing over the years, more progressive in nature as a result of neurogenic muscle imbalance or improper positioning. Congenital deformities are attributed to intrauterine position with absent movements or to additional malformation, sometimes resembling and denoted as arthrogrypotic deformity. A common example of congenital deformity is equinus foot.[51] Contractures developing after birth are related to unbalanced action of opposing muscle groups on a particular joint, such as calcaneus foot.[51] An example of deformity related to positioning is hip and knee flexion contractures due to continuous sitting in a nonambulatory child. During the growing years, complications affecting various organ systems may ensue, mainly from neurogenic bladder dysfunction or central nervous system malformations.

In the following discussion clinical signs of motor paralysis are described by spinal cord level primarily for didactic purposes. However, as pointed out earlier, both motor and sensory deficits may be different, incomplete, or asymmetric. Figure 12–2 shows segmental innervation, preserved muscle function, and musculoskeletal complications in various levels of spinal cord malformation.

Thoracic Lesions. Thoracic defects spare the upper extremities. Intercostal, abdominal, and back musculature weakness varies with location of spinal cord dysfunction. Although the diaphragm is functioning, respiratory difficulties may arise with increased ventilatory demands in upper thoracic lesions. Kyphosis and kyphoscoliosis result from trunk weakness and are enhanced if vertebral anomalies are present.[51] The legs are flaccid or may show signs of spasticity when some portion of the distal spinal cord

is preserved. Lack of volitional movements and positions assumed under the effect of gravity lead to lower extremity deformities. In complete flail paralysis the usual lower extremity posture in the supine position is partial hip external rotation, abduction, and ankle plantarflexion from gravity, resulting in tightness or eventual contractures of these muscle groups. From sitting hip, knee flexion, and equinus foot deformities develop. Hip flexion contractures with compensatory lumbar lordosis increase any preexisting kyphosis or kyphoscoliosis.

L1–L3 Segments Spared. Hip flexors and adductors are innervated. Knee extensors are functioning but not at full strength. Other lower extremity movements are absent. With this distribution of muscle imbalance, hip flexion and adduction contractures are inevitable and lead to a serious musculoskeletal complication of early paralytic hip dislocation. Pelvic obliquity in asymmetric hip pathology enhances scoliosis. Gravity-related equinus foot deformity develops in the absence of muscle activity at the ankles and feet.

L4–L5 Segments Spared. Innervation of the knee extensors is now complete; hip abductors and extensors remain weakened. Therefore, coxa valga and acetabular dysplasia are still a concern, although hip dislocation develops more slowly and later at L4–L5 segmental levels. Newborns with a well-defined lesion sparing L4 lie in a typical position of hip flexion, adduction, and knee extension that enables identification of the level of neurologic deficit on visual observation (Fig. 12–3). When the L5 segment is spared, the gluteus medius and maximus and hamstrings gain strength. Knee extension contracture is less likely. However, late hip dislocation is still a possibility. Because the tibialis anterior is partially innervated and unopposed by its plantarflexion and everter antagonists, calcaneovarus foot deformity develops. When the L5 segment is intact, the peroneus muscles have partial innervation, eliminating the varus, inversion component. Although the plantarflexors are not completely denervated in lesions that spare L5, they are still too weak to counteract the strong forces of ankle dorsiflexors. The characteristic foot position is calcaneus attitude (Fig. 12–4). In less well-defined lesions there may be valgus or calcaneovalgus deformity.

Sacral Lesions. Active plantarflexion is stronger, and some toe movements are present. However, in lower sacral lesions the intrinsic foot muscles remain weak, resulting in pes cavus with high arch and clawing of the toes (Fig. 12–5).

Sensory Deficit. Partial or complete absence of different sensory modalities predisposes

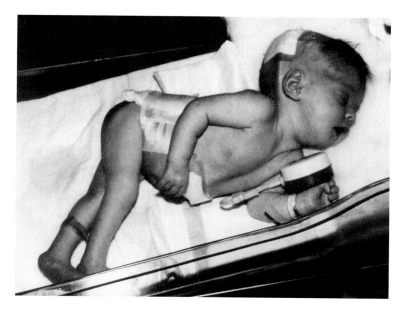

FIGURE 12–3. L4 segment-spared lumbosacral myelomeningocele newborn. Hip flexion adduction, knee extension contractures, mild calcaneus feet. Neurosurgical closure of spina bifida cystica and VP shunt for hydrocephalus.

the skin to injuries because the child does not perceive pressure, pain, trauma, or heat.[2-4,35] Decubitus ulcers tend to develop in static positions from muscle imbalance or fixed deformities, particularly over areas of prominence and weight bearing. The lower back, perineum, feet, heels, and toes are sites of predilection, but any area with sensory loss may be affected. Scoliotic or kyphotic prominence over the posterior trunk is also an area prone to skin breakdown.[51] Pressure ulcers tend to recur, become infected, and usually heal slowly, even in the absence of infection. The possibility that a neurotrophic factor may contribute to delayed healing seems to be supported by observations that decubiti of several years' duration resolve shortly after release

of the tethered cord.[52] Longstanding ulceration with deep soft tissue necrosis may extend to the underlying bone, causing acute or chronic osteomyelitis. For example, in decubitus ulcer with calcaneus deformity, weight bearing is primarily on the anesthetic heel, and a deep ulcer eventually leads to osteomyelitis of the os calcis.

Other Consequences of Denervation. In severe extensive paralysis signs of vasomotor dysfunction may be present in the form of decreased skin temperature and slight bluish discoloration over the involved area.[35] The trophic effect of denervation includes decreased or asymmetric lower extremity growth resulting in severe or unequal lower extremity weakness.[4,51] Neuropathic Charcot joints may develop.[53] Osteoporosis

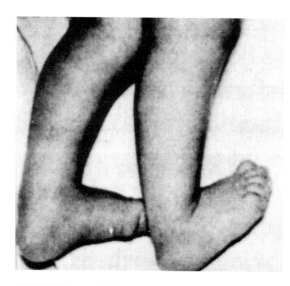

FIGURE 12–4. Calcaneus foot deformity in a newborn.

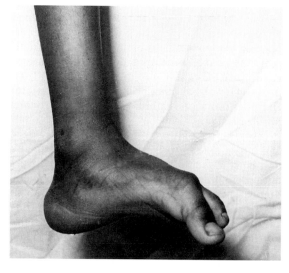

FIGURE 12–5. Cavus foot, claw toes with sacral lesion.

TABLE 12–1. Associated Central Nervous System Malformations

Spinal cord	Brain stem (cont.)	Ventricular system
Tethering	Herniation into cervical spinal	Hydrocephalus
Distal focal abnormalities	canal	Aqueductal stenosis, forking, atresia
Thick, short filum terminale	Abnormalities of nuclear structures	**Forebrain**
Supernumerary fibrous bands	Dysgenesis, hypoplasia, aplasia,	Polymicrogyria
Lumbosacral tumors—lipoma,	defective myelination	Abnormal nuclear structures
fibrolipoma, fibroma dermoid,	Hemorrhage, ischemic necrosis	Heterotopia—subependymal
epidermoid cyst, teratoma	Syringobulbia	nodules
Bony vertebral ridge	**Cerebellum**	Heterotaxia
Diastematomyelia, diplomyelia,	Arnold-Chiari type II malformation	Prominent massa intermedia
split cord	Elongated vermis, inferior	Thalamic fusion
Brain stem	displacement	Agenesis of olfactory bulbs
Arnold-Chiari type II malformation	Herniation into cervical spinal canal	and tracts
Kinking, inferior displacement	Abnormal nuclear structures	Attenuation/dysgenesis of
of medulla	Dysplasia, heterotopia, heterotaxia	corpus callosum

is an inevitable consequence of extensive lower motor neuron paralysis and is further increased during long immobilization, such as casting after orthopedic procedures.[4,51] Osteoporotic fractures with no history of trauma and no pain because of sensory deficit may occur in the course of normal daily activities and handling. Localized, painless swelling, redness, and warmth on palpation in the lower extremity of a child with a history of recent immobilization and cast removal are typical signs that should arouse the suspicion of osteoporotic fracture. Weight-bearing by passive standing has been proposed for nonambulatory children to decrease osteoporosis and fractures. However, the beneficial effect of such attempts has not been demonstrated in terms of reduced fracture rate.[4,54]

Associated Central Nervous System Malformations. Extensive neuropathologic studies showed that neural tube defects are associated with a high incidence of gross and microscopic malformations of the forebrain and hindbrain.[55] Additional anomalies in the spinal cord or canal may further complicate the original local dysraphic defect.[1–3,35,56] A knowledge of these abnormalities should help clinicians to understand the implications of a progressive course and other clinical symptoms that cannot be explained by the focal spinal cord malformation.[2,3,35,57] Table 12–1 lists associated anomalies by anatomic location.

Spinal Cord. Tethered cord is a term for abnormal attachment of the spinal cord at its distal end.[35] Under normal circumstances, by the second-to-twelfth postnatal month the conus medullaris ascends from its earlier distal position to L1–L2 vertebral level.[58] In neural tube defects focal anatomic abnormalities interfere with this process. Examples include thickened and shortened filum terminale, supernumerary fibrous bands, persistent membrana reuniens, dural sinus, diastematomyelia, entrapment by

lumbosacral tumors, and adhesions in the scar tissue of repaired myelomeningocele.[35] Benign lumbosacral tumors generally associated with neural tube defects are lipoma or fibrolipoma, whereas teratomas have a potential for malignant transformation. Epidermoid tumor or dermoid cyst may undergo further cystic expansion.[2,3,35,59] (Fig. 12–6).

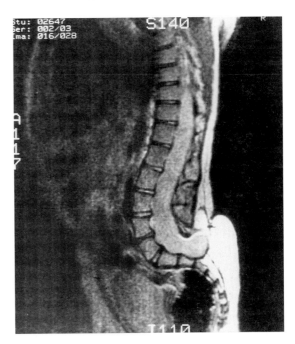

FIGURE 12–6. Lipomeningocele and myelodysplasia repaired at birth. Initial motor and sensory deficit L5 segment. Progressive lower extremity spasticity, sensory deficit ascending to L1, severe back pain and regression of ambulation onset at 6 years. MRI shows intramedullary tumor, which at surgery proved to be an epidermoid cyst filled with thick sebaceous material, partial postoperative relief of symptoms. (From Molnar GE: Spina bifida: Clinical correlations of associated central nervous system malformations. Phys Med Rehabil State Art Rev 1991;5:289, with permission.)

Diastematomyelia, a postneurulation defect, is a sagittal cleavage of the spinal cord. When the split cords have separate dural coverage, the term *diplomyelia* is used. A bony vertebral ridge or fibrous septum protruding into the clefted cord is present in most cases and may act as a fulcrum for tethering.[2,35]

In nearly all cases of myelomeningocele, magnetic resonance imaging (MRI) shows a low-lying spinal cord, but in the majority of cases this anatomic tethering remains asymptomatic.[35,50,60–62] Neurologic deterioration is attributed to enhanced tension due to increasing length discrepancy between the spinal cord and vertebral column during growth and mechanical stretching related to physical activities that produce a hypoxic effect on the spinal cord.[35,63] Neuroradiologic procedures are now under development to demonstrate decreased cord mobility and thus to distinguish a low-lying cord from true traction syndrome.[64–66] Somatosensory evoked potential studies were found to be helpful for detecting abnormal tethering in some but not all reports.[67–69] Symptomatic tethered cord syndrome may develop in all forms of neural tube defects and at any age. However, it is most frequent in myelomeningocele and diastematomyelia. Clinical signs tend to become evident around 6 years of age and also correlate with height.[50,70] Symptoms may develop insidiously. Loss of motor function may manifest as increasing lower motor neuron weakness or spasticity. Ambulatory children may have greater difficulties with walking. Spasticity may lead to new joint deformities. Deteriorating upper extremity function and an ascending sensory deficit are other suspicious signs.[2,3,35] Back pain radiating to the legs, especially if it occurs in radicular distribution and is intensified by neck flexion, are another indication of tethering.[35] Slowly developing bladder and bowel dysfunction in a previously asymptomatic child or deterioration of already impaired control is a common and often the earliest sign.[35,71,72] Scoliosis, which may be related to various other factors, is of debatable significance as a diagnostic sign of tethered cord syndrome.[35,73,74] The treatment of symptomatic tethered cord syndrome is neurosurgical release for cord untethering or, in the presence of tumor, its resection or reduction. Results of surgery range from resolution of symptoms to additional dysfunction. Unsatisfactory outcomes are attributed to longstanding irreversible spinal cord compromise or additional damage of the deeply embedded neural elements in the scar or tumor tissue. Retethering is reported in 10–15% of cases.[35]

Syringomyelia is a tubular cavitation in the spinal cord parenchyma lined with glial cells. The term *hydromyelia* was used in the past to differentiate a fusiform dilatation of the central canal, which in turn is lined with ependymal cells.[75] The estimated incidence of syringohydromyelia is 5–40%,[76] but autopsy studies, which are biased toward more severe cases, showed an even higher frequency.[55] The origin of syringohydromyelia is increased cerebrospinal fluid pressure as a result of obstructed flow through the rhombencephalic roof of the fourth ventricle and/or at the foramen magnum.[55] Several theories elaborated other possible mechanisms contributing to enhanced pressure within and around the spinal cord.[77] The syrinx may be located anywhere along the spinal cord, medulla, or pons but seems to have a predilection for the cervical area.[2,3,78] There may be single or multiple cavities of variable length and size. MRI is the standard diagnostic procedure for detecting syringohydromyelia[76] (Fig. 12–7). Progressive early scoliosis above the level of the initial neurologic deficit and unexplained by local vertebral anomalies has been recognized as one of the first signs.[35,79] Sensory and motor symptoms correlate with the location and extent of the syrinx. Progressive upper or lower motor neuron paralysis of the legs, trunk, and upper extremities leads to deterioration of sitting, ambulation, and arm

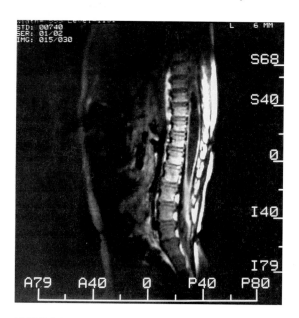

FIGURE 12–7. MRI with large thoracolumbar syringohydromyelia in myelomeningocele repaired at birth. Initial sensory and motor deficit at L4–L5 level. Rapidly developing thoracic scoliosis, loss of sitting, complete lower extremity paralysis, and ascending sensory deficit to T10 level between 10 and 12 months of age. (From Molnar GE: Spina bifida: Clinical correlations of associated central nervous system malformations. Phys Med Rehabil State Art Rev 1991;5:292, with permission.)

function; wasting of intrinsic hand muscles; and joint deformities. Sensory dysfunction affects several modalities. Disassociation of sensory deficits may develop with impairment of pain and temperature perception, whereas other modalities subserved by uncrossed posterior column fibers are spared.[2,3,35] Trophic and vasomotor signs are characteristic of such disassociated sensory deficit. Symptoms often develop insidiously and tend to occur in the second decade.[2,3] The current treatment is syringopleural shunt, which allows drainage of the cerebrospinal fluid and decompression of the syrinx.[35]

Cerebellum and Hindbrain. The most common hindbrain anomaly in neural tube defects is the Arnold-Chiari type II malformation[2,3,35,80] (Fig. 12–8). MRI is a reliable neuroradiologic method to demonstrate this abnormality. The malformation includes caudal displacement or herniation into the cervical spinal canal of the medulla, lower pons, elongated fourth ventricle, and cerebellar vermis.[2,3,35,81] There may be kinking or elongation of the medulla. Suggested mechanisms include herniation due to distal traction from a tethered cord or proximal downward forces from hydrocephalus and increased intracranial pressure. Another proposed explanation is cerebrocranial disproportion due to the abnormally small posterior fossa or to overgrowth and crowding of the hindbrain.[2,3,35,57] Because these anatomic abnormalities interfere with the outflow of cerebrospinal fluid, Arnold-Chiari type II malformation is always associated with hydrocephalus. About 80–90% of patients with myelomeningocele have Arnold-Chiari type II malformation. The highest incidence is in lumbosacral lesions.[3] However, it was estimated that only 20% have clinical signs of brain stem dysfunction.[81,82] Signs of bulbar compromise arise from compression of the herniated hindbrain. Caudal displacement of the medulla may lead to traction neuropathy of the cranial nerves. Symptoms may be evident at birth or develop in the first 2–3 months of life. Less frequently clinical signs occur in later childhood or adulthood.[81] The density of anatomic structures and variety of neurophysiologic functions located in the medulla explain the spectrum of clinical symptoms.[2,81] The most severe form is central ventilatory dysfunction, which was described in 5.8–30% of cases in two different studies.[2,83] Stridor, laryngeal nerve palsy with vocal cord paralysis, upper airway obstruction, periodic breathing, central and sleep apnea, and aspiration are typical signs. Aggressive measures of ventilatory and airway support are necessary in such cases. Dysphagia and extraocular motion abnormalities indicate involvement of other

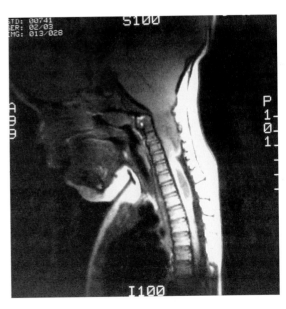

FIGURE 12–8. Arnold-Chiari type II malformation. Kinking and downward displacement of the medulla and upper cervical cord; elongated cerebellar vermis with herniation into the cervical spinal canal; low cervical syringohydromyelia. Myelomeningocele with L3 motor and sensory deficit repaired at birth; VP shunting. Child has not developed bulbar or upper extremity symptoms by 2½ years of age. (From Molnar GE: Spina bifida: Clinical correlations of associated central nervous system malformations. Phys Med Rehabil State Art Rev 1991;5:295, with permission.)

cranial nerves.[80–82,84–86] Severe dysphagia and aspiration may require gastrostomy feeding. Neurosurgical treatment is decompression of the high intracranial pressure by shunt revision, posterior fossa craniotomy, and cervical laminectomy.[35] Despite successful initial treatment, problems may recur within 2–3 years.[80] At times partial cranial nerve palsies persist for life. Central respiratory dysfunction is the most frequent single cause of death in myelodysplasia; one study reported a mortality rate of 50%.[29,50] Hemorrhages, infarcts, and necroses in the brainstem found on autopsies are manifestations of ischemic compression.[55]

Neuropathologic studies also showed signs of brain stem dysgenesis in the form of defective myelination, reduction in cell number, hypoplasia, or aplasia of the olivary, basal pontine, and cranial nerve nuclei, most often of the hypoglossal and vagal nerves. These observations suggest that an embryonic dysgenetic process also may play a role in hindbrain abnormalities, including the Arnold-Chiari type II malformation[55] (Fig. 12–9). As mentioned earlier, syringohydromyelia may affect the medulla. A lesion in this location is designated syringobulbia and is evident

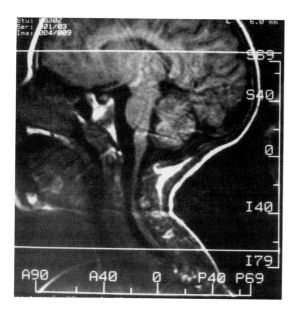

FIGURE 12–9. Atrophy of brain stem and upper cervical cord. Neonatal signs of transient vocal cord paralysis and severe dysphagia requiring gastrostomy. Paresis of the right arm and right Horner syndrome with partial resolution over 7 years. No symptoms of respiratory dysfunction. L5 myelomeningocele closed at birth. (From Molnar GE: Spina bifida: Clinical correlations of associated central nervous system malformations. Phys Med Rehabil State Art Rev 1991;5:296, with permission.)

on MRI. It may be the cause of any of the above described symptoms of bulbar dysfunction. The brainstem is a relay site for auditory pathways. Abnormal brain stem auditory evoked responses (BAERs) occur in many cases, even with compensated hydrocephalus and asymptomatic Arnold-Chiari type II malformation, perhaps as a result of intrinsic dysgenesis. Therefore, abnormal BAERs alone are not considered sensitive indicators of decompensating hydrocephalus. For the pyramidal tracts the brainstem is a locus of transit. Hemiparesis or quadriparesis may develop with brain stem compromise.[2–4,35] Such symptoms are more likely to become evident in older children or adults than in infants or young children. Craniolacunae, a mesodermal anomaly of the calvarial skull in Arnold-Chiari type II malformation, are evident on regular radiogram. They are considered to reflect severe underlying central nervous system involvement. Improvement of craniolacunae was noted after successful shunting.[35]

As described above, the gross anatomic cerebellar abnormality is an integral part of Arnold-Chiari type II malformation. In addition, neuropathologic studies demonstrated microscopic cerebellar dysplasias, which seem to reflect disturbed neuronal migration and were found in

conjunction with all levels of meningomyelocele.[55] Such abnormalities included (1) heterotopias with well-formed but displaced cerebellar folia, (2) heterotaxias with disordered combinations of mature and germinal cells, and (3) various other aberrations of cellular architectonics.

The cerebellum has an important role in upper extremity coordination. Impairment of fine hand function is well documented in meningomyelocele. It was found in 67% of thoracic lesions and in 23–29% of lumbosacral lesions.[4,87,88] Tremulous or ataxic hand movements are usual manifestations. Control of ocular motility—specifically saccadic eye movements, visual fixation, and pursuit—is also related to cerebellar function. Long-term follow-up of several hundred children with spina bifida found a high rate of ophthalmologic problems, strabismus, lateral rectus palsy, and nystagmus. Only 29% had completely normal visual function.[85,86]

Ventricles. Abnormalities of the fourth ventricle were described in conjunction with Arnold-Chiari type II malformation. Enlargement of the third ventricle from hydrocephalus is an almost universal feature of myelodysplasia and always accompanies Arnold-Chiari type II malformation.[2–4,35,89] It is caused by obstructed flow of cerebrospinal fluid, which normally circulates from the ventricular system to the subarachnoid spaces of the brain and spinal cord and ultimately is absorbed in the subarachnoid villi of the dural sinuses. In communicative or constrictive hydrocephalus, interference with cerebrospinal fluid circulation occurs at the outlet foramina of the fourth ventricle and in the crowded posterior fossa and cervical canal, as noted earlier with Arnold-Chiari type II malformation. In noncommunicating hydrocephalus, aqueductal abnormalities, such as stenosis, forking or atresia, either as congenital malformation or secondary to increased intracranial pressure, compromise cerebrospinal fluid flow between the third and fourth ventricles.[2–4,35] Neuroultrasound detects hydrocephalus in utero and postnatally while the anterior fontanelle is open. Computed tomographic (CT) scan and MRI are diagnostic methods thereafter. Serial examinations are indicated when deterioration is suspected. Neurosurgical treatment, which has undergone many modifications since its inception, is ventriculoperitoneal shunt.[4,35,89] About 85–90% of children with myelomeningocele require shunting, and one-third require shunt revision. Infection is the most frequent shunt complication, followed by obstruction. Hydrocephalus is usually present at birth and becomes symptomatic during the first week.[4,35] Severe cases are associated with craniomegaly, craniotabes, bulging fontanelles, widely separated cranial sutures, distended scalp veins, and sunset sign of the eyes. Subtle or more evident symptoms of medullary compromise may be concurrent signs. In newborns and infants disproportionate enlargement in head size, somnolence, irritability, poor feeding, and vomiting indicate decompensating hydrocephalus. Older children may complain of headaches. Papilledema, diplopia, optic atrophy, and even transient blindness may occur with rapidly progressive decompensating hydrocephalus or shunt malfunction.[4,35,90] One study reported a 70% correlation between ophthalmologic signs and proven episodes of decompensated hydrocephalus with increased intracranial pressure.[4,35] Insidious, slowly progressive hydrocephalus becomes symptomatic in several months or years with more subtle signs, such as personality changes, decline in school performance, increasing difficulties with fine hand function, and eye-hand coordination.[4,35]

Forebrain. Malformations of the forebrain range from gross anatomic to microscopic anomalies.[55] Polymicrogyria, a term for cerebral gyri of small size and increased number with shallow, disorganized sulci, has been reported in 40–65% of cases with or without hydrocephalus (Fig. 12–10). Heterotopias, found in 40% of cases, are aberrant neural tissues in the form of subependymal nodules located mostly in the lateral ventricular walls. Microscopic studies also showed disordered cortical lamination, neuronal hypoplasias of the thalamus, and, in a few cases, complete or partial agenesis of the olfactory bulbs and tracts, suggestive of neuronal migration defects. Thinning and attenuation of the corpus callosum occur in hydrocephalus.[55] Recent studies also demonstrated true agenesis of the corpus callosum. However, unlike in other specific syndromes of callosal agenesis, this defect was also associated with malformed cingulate gyrus and septum pellucidum. Recent observations found that left-hand preference was more frequent among children with progressive hydrocephalus. This disorder of lateralization may be attributable to corpus callosum dysfunction.[91] The contribution of forebrain malformations to cognitive and perceptual dysfunction in children with myelodysplasia is currently unknown.

Other Malformations. Neural tube defects are also associated with an increased rate of malformations unrelated to the central nervous system. Vertebral fusion, hemivertebra, or other morphologic vertebral anomalies above the level of dysrhaphic defect contribute to progressive kyphosis and scoliosis.[92] Absence, bifurcation, or reduction of the ribs increases thoracic deformities. Malformations of the urinary system also

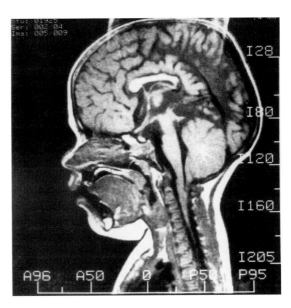

FIGURE 12–10. Polymicrogyria and agenesis of the splenium of corpus callosum. Normal intelligence, superior reading skill. L4–L5 myelomeningocele closed at birth. (From Molnar GE: Spina bifida: Clinical correlations of associated central nervous system malformations. Phys Med Rehabil State Art Rev 1991;5:302, with permission.)

may be present—for example, renal hypoplasia, horseshoe configuration, solitary kidney, ureteral, or lower tract anomalies that may accelerate deterioration of renal status and neurogenic bladder dysfunction.[4,35]

Neurogenic Bladder Dysfunction. The urinary bladder and sphincters are controlled by both autonomic and somatic nerves.[93] Parasympathetic cholinergic innervation arises from S2–S4 spinal segments. Efferent motor fibers generate detrusor contraction for bladder emptying. Afferent parasympathetic fibers convey stretch sensation from the bladder and internal sphincter contributing to coordinated contraction and relaxation on voiding. Sympathetic adrenergic innervation from the T10–T12 segments acts to inhibit detrusor contraction, tightens the internal sphincter, and thereby helps with urinary retention and storage. Somatic innervation of bladder function is from S2–S5 through the pudendal plexus. Efferent fibers control voluntary contraction of the external sphincter, pelvic floor, and perineal musculature for volitional urinary retention whereas afferent fibers provide sensation for the external sphincter and posterior urethra. With relaxation of the smooth muscle detrusor and contraction of the internal and external sphincters urine is retained in the bladder. Detrusor contraction and simultaneous relaxation of both sphincters lead to voiding.[93] Supraspinal integration of both autonomic and somatic innervation is most likely in the nucleus caeruleus of the pons and frontal cortex. In addition, experimental animal studies have shown that the hypothalamus, septum pellucidum, and paracentral lobules are also involved in cerebral integration of continence and voiding.[93]

Physiologic bladder function has three stages: (1) filling, (2) opening, and (3) voiding. Under normal circumstances and with detrusor stability, intravesical/detrusor pressures show no significant rise during the filling phase. The overactive, unstable, or hyperreflexic detrusor is associated with uninhibited contractions during the filling phase, sometimes triggered by cough, sneezing, or postural changes.[94,95] It is seen with uninhibited bladder in spasticity and results in voiding without volition.[96] The hyporeflexic or areflexic detrusor is associated with impaired lower motor neuron control.[94,95] Detrusor pressure in children during peak voiding is generally 40 cm H_2O or less and in adults less than 70 cm H_2O. Straining, Valsalva maneuvers, and Crede maneuvers may increase bladder pressure. When used judiciously, they may help with voiding in case of a hypotonic detrusor, provided that outlet resistance is not increased.[97] Bladder sensation may be classified as normal, hypersensitive, reduced, or absent. The last two abnormalities are usually seen in spina bifida. Under normal circumstances most children and adults experience a sensation of bladder filling around one-third of normal bladder capacity. The formula for calculating age-appropriate bladder volume in children is age + 2 × 30 in cc or age + 2 in ounces. In spina bifida disturbed bladder sensation interferes with perception of bladder filling.

The complex autonomic and somatic neurologic control of coordinated detrusor and sphincter mechanism may be interrupted in several different ways.[94,95,97] In hypotonic bladder detrusor, contractions are weak or absent, intravesicular pressure is low, dribbling is usual, and emptying is incomplete. Bladder volume is increased. Overdistention of the flaccid bladder eventually leads to retrograde flow and dilatation of the upper urinary tract from reflux. This type of bladder is common in sacral lesions.[98] Hypertonic or spastic bladder develops when the voiding reflex arc is intact, and detrusor contractions are uninhibited because of loss of central control.[99] Intravesicular pressure is high and results in increased retrograde pressure reflux to the upper urinary tract. Eventually, the bladder wall becomes thickened with small capacity. Hypertonic bladder is most likely to be present in thoracic lesions. In addition to detrusor dysfunction, the sphincter mechanism is also affected. Incontinence occurs when outflow resistance is weak, although intravesical pressure may be normal, or when sphincter closure is inadequate against enhanced detrusor activity with high intravesical pressure. Detrusor sphincter dyssynergia is a specific severe disturbance of voiding function in which bladder and sphincter contractions occur simultaneously, leading to high intravesical pressure, consequent reflux, and dilatation of the upper urinary tract.[97]

Urodynamic study is a means to demonstrate disturbances in the biomechanical and hydrodynamic aspects of urinary tract function.[93] Multichannel computerized monitoring during the filling and voiding phases measures intraabdominal intravesical, detrusor-generated, and urethral pressures in cm H_2O, flow velocity in ml/sec and, by using surface electrodes, pelvic floor electromyographic (EMG) activity (Figs. 12–11, 12–12, and 12–13). Intravesical pressure

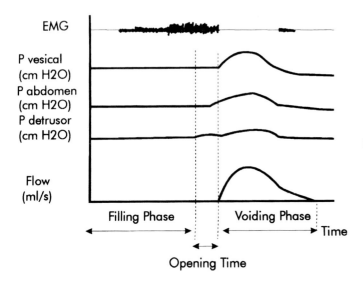

FIGURE 12–11. Normal urodynamic study.

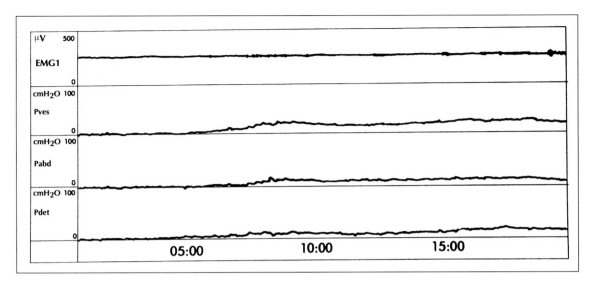

FIGURE 12–12.   Urodynamic study—hypotonic bladder.

is a sum of intraabdominal and intravesical pressures. Important information from urodynamic study is bladder wall compliance, which is calculated by the ratio of volume change to intravesical pressure change. A compliance ratio of less than 10 is believed to be abnormal, although definite standards for children have yet to be established.

Urinary incontinence is present in 95% of children with spina bifida. It may be a dysfunction of urine storage due to inadequate outflow resistance, hypotonic enlarged bladder with overflow incontinence, small capacity spastic bladder, or a combination of these factors. Urinary tract infections are common and used to be one of the major causes of morbidity and mortality. In the

presence of reflux, pyelitis and pyelonephritis develop, enhancing the seriousness of infection. Hydronephrosis occurs with reflux more often in the high-pressure bladder. Intravesical pressure of over 40 cm H_2O was found to result in upper tract dilatation in 81% of children.[100] Calculosis of the urinary tract is frequent with infections, particularly with the urea-splitting *Proteus* bacteria.[97] Deteriorating kidney function is the eventual consequence of hydronephrosis and infections. Renal function is further complicated in the presence of malformed or solitary kidneys.

Neurogenic Bowel Dysfunction.   The colon, rectum, and internal anal sphincter are controlled by autonomic nerves.[4,35] Parasympathetic innervation is from S2–S4, whereas

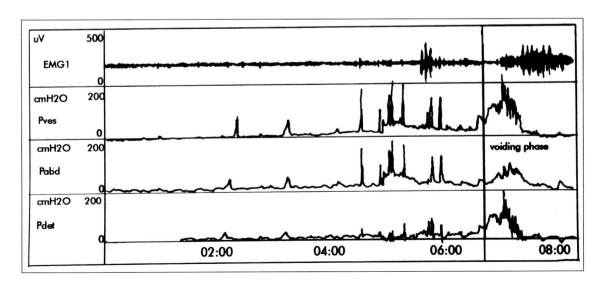

FIGURE 12–13.   Urodynamic study—spastic bladder detrusor—sphincter dyssynergia.

sympathetic fibers arise from the lower thoracic and lumbar segments. Voluntary somatic motor and sensory nerve supply for the external anal sphincter is from S2–S4 through the pudendal plexus. Coursing through the spinal cord, these nerves have direct connections with the integrating supraspinal centers in the pons and cerebral cortex. Colon peristalsis propels feces into the rectum. Gastrocolic reflex increases peristalsis for about 30 minutes after food intake.[4] Rectal fullness initiates an autonomic stretch reflex with relaxation of the internal anal sphincter and creates a sensation of pre-defecation urge. In contrast, the voluntarily controlled external sphincter remains contracted to retain feces. When the situation warrants, this action is further enhanced by voluntary contraction of the levator ani, gluteal, and other thigh muscles. The anorectal reflex is a coordinated opposing muscle activity whereby relaxation of the internal anal sphincter is associated with contraction of the external sphincter. The reflex may be elicited by sensory stimulation of the perianal skin. Defecation occurs when the external sphincter is voluntarily relaxed.[4] Most children with myelodysplasia have a patulous anus, absent cutaneous reflex response, and perianal sensory deficit, which indicate involvement of S2–S4 segments and lead to fecal incontinence. In lesions above L2 an intact spinal reflex arc can maintain perineal sphincter tone, despite absent rectal sensation.[93,101] Dysfunction of autonomic innervation of the colon, rectum, and internal anal sphincter creates additional problems with bowel motility and stool consistency. The resulting diarrhea or constipation further complicates fecal incontinence and bowel training.

Obesity. Excessive weight is a frequent problem among children with myelodysplasia. Obesity is attributed to reduced daily energy expenditure because (1) muscle paralysis and associated growth reduction decrease lean body mass and (2) physical activity level is lower than in nondisabled children of similar age.[4,35] In higher-level lesions energy expenditure becomes proportionately lower. As a rule, obesity is calculated from weight/height ratio. In myelodysplasia diminished growth and difficulties with measuring exact height in the presence of spinal and/or lower extremity deformities make the use of stature for this calculation less valid. Extensive investigations demonstrated that substituting arm span for height and measuring subscapular skin fold thickness are more reliable indicators of overweight in this group.[4,102,103] Obesity increases the risk of decubiti and upper extremity stress with physical activities and eventually leads to further restriction of activity

level. It creates problems with self-image, social adaptation, and acceptance. Discussion of weight and dietary control should be a proactive measure, initiated in infancy to prevent overweight because correction of obesity is often unsuccessful.[4] The recommended general guidelines include (1) 10–20% reduction in calculated caloric needs and (2) a diet low in fat and carbohydrates, and high in protein and bulk fiber content with proper vitamin supplementation.[4,103,104]

Precocious Puberty. The pathogenesis of precocious puberty with hydrocephalus is thought to be premature activation of the hypothalamic-pituitary-gonadal axis from increased pressure on the hypothalamus.[105–108] It is reported to occur in 10–20% of cases in myelomeningocele with hydrocephalus.[106,107] Clinical diagnosis is based on breast and testicular enlargement before 8–9 years instead of the usual age of 11–11.6 years. Examinations of serum luteinizing and follicular-stimulating hormones are confirmatory laboratory studies. An associated symptom is advanced bone age resulting in short stature. Treatment with gonadotropin-releasing hormone analogs produced good results in several studies by reducing the signs of precocious puberty, including cessation of menstruation and resumption of growth in height.[105,106]

Intellectual Function. On psychological testing children with myelomeningocele as a group show a shift to the left in IQ scores compared with their able-bodied peers.[4,35] Scores in the high average range and above are about four times less common, whereas low scores show an approximately threefold increase.[109] Intellectual functioning correlates inversely with the neurologic level of spinal cord dysfunction.[110] Thoracic lesions are associated with a high rate of low scores. Children with low lumbar or sacral lesions are more likely to have higher or above average function.[110] More severe physical deficit with greater restriction of early motor exploration and learning has been suggested as a possible factor in the intellectual discrepancies related to the level of spinal cord dysfunction.[4] The more extensive association of higher lesions with cerebral anatomic and microscopic anomalies may be additional contributors of unknown significance. In early reports hydrocephalus was proposed as a cause of intellectual deficit. However, recent investigations indicate that hydrocephalus alone does not exclude normal cognitive function, but its complications, such as infections, bleeding, and shunt malfunction, have a deleterious effect.[111,112] Concentration and attention deficits are thought to be related to hydrocephalus. A widely observed trend among children is higher test scores on verbal tasks compared with performance IQ, which involves visual and visual-motor integration.[4,35,110] The so-called cocktail party syndrome[113] describes children with deceptively good verbal facility that creates the impression of higher intellectual functioning than is found on formal psychological testing.

Several considerations explain the lower performance scores on visual perception and visual motor tasks. A recent MRI study found progressive widening of the posterior occipital horns of the lateral ventricles without enlargement of the anterior horns in children with spina bifida and hydrocephalus.[114] The close correlation between this finding and the presence of visual perceptual deficits suggests that posterior horn dilatation affects the adjacent visual cortex and pathways and that visual perceptual dysfunction may be preventable by more adequate shunting. Abnormalities of extraocular muscle function and their correlation with shunt malfunction, described in many studies, also may play some role in visual perceptual dysfunction. Scores on tasks requiring visual motor integration are affected by difficulties with upper extremity fine coordination, which are well documented among these children.[4,110,115] Substitution of special motor-free tests for the customary methods that involve hand use may eliminate some of this bias.

Treatment

Team Approach.   Primary care for the usual childhood illnesses and preventive health maintenance remain the responsibility of pediatricians. However, proper management of the problems particular to the disability requires a team of specialists.[4,35] Details of treatment by various specialists are beyond the scope of this discussion. Nevertheless, certain aspects are highlighted because realistic plans for overall rehabilitation must be coordinated with all modes of treatment.

After the birth of the child, parents and family need to be informed about the diagnosis and its implications. Cautious predictions may be given in terms of prognosis for anticipated functional abilities and limitations, including self-care and ambulation. Considering the many issues involved, participation of several medical specialists is necessary. It is emphasized that the child will require careful follow-up by specialists and that at certain times one specific aspect of treatment may take temporary precedence over others. Future bracing, physical therapy, and orthopedic surgery are mentioned as anticipated modalities of treatment for the physical handicap. Discussions and instructions about the child's care and handling at home require several sessions so that the family members are not overwhelmed by the amount and apparent complexity of information. They should be encouraged to ask questions at the initial and all subsequent meetings. Although one should be frank in presenting the problems that the parents and child will face, they should be discussed with compassionate optimism. Etiology and implications for subsequent pregnancies should be discussed with referral to further genetic counseling if the parents so desire. The frequency of follow-up visits after the infant is discharged from the neonatal unit depends on presence or absence of complications. When the course is benign, the interval of visits may be extended from 3–4 months in the first 1–2 years to every 6 months or longer thereafter.

Neurosurgical Treatment.   Involvement of the neurosurgeon begins either prenatally, if spina bifida is detected,[116,117] or at birth. Neonatal neurosurgical treatment has gone through many changes during the past several decades. The original approach of delaying closure for the open spinal defect until 3–6 months of age resulted in a high mortality rate due to infection and was replaced in the 1960s by immediate nonselective surgery in all neonates.[117a] Based on reviews of childhood survival rates and quality of life in survivors after universal immediate neonatal surgery, selective closure was advocated in the 1970s.[117a] The proposed criteria for not performing immediate surgery on neonates were (1) complete paralysis of both legs consistent with lesions at L1 or above; (2) significant hydrocephalus with enlarged head present on the first day of life; (3) severe spinal deformity, kyphosis, or scoliosis at birth; (4) serious associated malformations of other organ systems, such as congenital heart disease; and (5) evidence of cerebral birth injury.[117a] Selective closure remains a controversial ethical issue and has not become a standard practice.

Neurosurgical repair of a cystic lesion is usually performed on the first day of life. A ventriculoperitoneal shunt is inserted if hydrocephalus is present at birth or develops after repair of myelomeningocele.[4,35] Ninety-five percent of children are likely to have hydrocephalus, and 75–85% require shunting. The average revision rate of shunt procedure is 30–50% in the first year and 50–75% in the second year; nearly all are revised once by 5 years of age.[118] Spontaneous arrest of hydrocephalus was said to occur in approximately 25% of children after 5 years. However, most neurosurgeons believe that a child with hydrocephalus that required shunting will remain shunt-dependent.[35]

Continuing neurosurgical follow-up is required not only for hydrocephalus but also for other possible central nervous system complications that need surgical treatment. MRI assists in anticipating such a course and clarifies the nature of pathology in case of progressive symptoms.[119] For syringohydromyelia the current neurosurgical procedure is syringopleural shunting. Surgical untethering is the treatment for cord traction syndrome. An expanding intraspinal tumor or cyst needs resection. In diastematomyelia removal of the bony vertebral spur may be necessary.[35]

Urologic Treatment. Urologic assessment and treatment of bladder dysfunction start in the neonatal period and continue throughout life. The primary aims are (1) to control incontinence, (2) to prevent and control infections, and (3) to preserve kidney function.

During infancy and early childhood the modified voiding alert system provides an objective way to assess accurately the frequency of dribbling and wetness.[120] Continuous dribbling and lack of significant bladder dilatation are the usual signs of a hypotonic bladder with weak or absent sphincter activity, whereas a distended bladder indicates urinary retention, most probably with hypertonic bladder or detrusor sphincter dyssynergia. Investigations of bladder and kidneys in the neonate should include an abdominal ultrasound, which demonstrates bladder size, hydronephrosis, or renal malformation.[97,121–123] Ultrasound also estimates post-voiding residual urine, although catheterization gives a more exact measurement. When residual urine is ≥ 20 cc, intermittent catheterization is started. Urodynamic study gives additional objective information about the hydrodynamics of bladder and sphincter function.[124,125] In 36 neonates with myelodysplasia, urodynamic studies showed detrusor sphincter dyssynergia in 50%, coordinated sphincter activity in 25%, and no external sphincter activity in 25%.[123] Detrusor sphincter dyssynergia can be demonstrated only by urodynamic study. Blood urea nitrogen, serum creatine, and urine culture are obtained in neonates. Voiding cystourethrography should be performed in the first few months of life to detect vesicoureteral reflux with increased risk for upper tract deterioration and hydronephrosis or in the presence of bladder infection or pyelonephritis.[93,97,121] About 15–20% of children have vesicoureteral reflux at birth. Dimercaprol succinic acid (DMSA) scan or radionuclide scanning with diethylenetriamine pentaacetic acid (DPTA) gives a better measurement of renal function itself.[97] Intravenous pyelography is generally deferred until 2 years of age and can identify renal and ureteral abnormalities.[97] These diagnostic tests are periodically repeated at a frequency depending on previous findings and course of urinary tract dysfunction.

Pharmacologic treatment is aimed at improving bladder dynamics. Anticholinergic medications, oxybutynin, benzoic acid, or propantheline bromide can decrease detrusor contractions and enlarge storage capacity by improving bladder wall compliance. Alpha-adrenergic agents, such as ephedrine, may help to increase outflow resistance by tightening the bladder neck. Urinary infections must be treated with appropriate antibiotics. In the presence of vesicoureteral reflux prophylactic treatment is advisable, using nitrofurantoin, 1–2 mg/kg/day, or trimethoprim, 0.25 ml/kg/day, generally at bedtime.[4,35]

The introduction of clean intermittent catheterization (CIC) in 1972 has transformed the lives of many children with neurogenic bladder.[126–128] Achievement of continence with this method alone was reported in more than one-half of children in some studies.[4,35,128] Improvement in infection rate and renal function also was demonstrated.[128] Although chronic bacilluria may accompany CIC, it is considered an indication of actual infection only in the presence of pyuria and other abnormal signs.[129] At around 5–6 years of age, most children can achieve independent self-catheterization.[35,130] Because of anatomic differences, boys usually learn the technique more easily than girls. Along with appropriate dexterity, visual perception and cognitive skills, the child must have reasonable emotional maturity.[4,35] Encouragement from family and school personnel, as well as proper environmental setting, is essential. To ensure continence, catheterization has to be performed at 4-hour intervals. The total daily time requirement is estimated at about 1–1½ hours.[131]

When conservative intervention is unsuccessful for controlling incontinence and other consequences of neurogenic bladder, various urologic surgical procedures may be considered. To prevent reflux, particularly in the presence of recurrent infections and gradual urinary tract deterioration, the options include ureteral reimplantation, bladder augmentation, or suprapubic vesicostomy.[4,35] For augmentation cystoplasty the ileum or colon is used, but this procedure eliminates any bladder reflex action and continuing CIC may be needed.[4,35,132] The Mitrofanoff procedure uses the appendix, which is mobilized on a vascular pedicle to create a catheterizable conduit between the bladder and anterior abdominal wall.[132–135] Control can be achieved through the use of a flutter valve mechanism that prevents external leakage. Suprapubic vesicostomy may be considered as a temporizing measure for older children and adults prior to complex surgery involving the bladder and bowel system. Ileal conduit was the first urinary diversion procedure, but follow-up studies showed a disappointingly high rate of renal deterioration, calculosis, hydronephrosis, and the need for undiversion.

The artificial urinary sphincter has revolutionized the management of severe incontinence.[136–138] It consists of a hydraulic device with cuff, balloon, pump, and control assembly. The cuff provides circumferential urethral compression with force governed by the regulating balloon. Urine flows from the balloon to the cuff placed subcutaneously in the scrotum or labium major. On squeezing the balloon fluid flow is reversed, contents of the urethral cuff empty into the balloon, and urethral pressure is decreased for emptying. The device may have mechanical problems, and complications with infection and erosion may arise. Artificial urinary sphincter may be considered for older schoolchildren who can also perform self-catheterization. The family and child must be motivated and reliable.

Achievement of urinary continence is a landmark of success in the management of spina bifida, but it should not occur at the expense of compromising kidney function. In a random sample, 38% of respondents who used normal voiding straining, bladder expression, or CIC were reliably dry compared with 71% of respondents who had undergone some form of urinary diversion.[139] Changes such as deterioration in previously achieved control need to be investigated for urologic and neurologic causes. Many children can be treated conservatively, but surgical options should be offered when clear indications are present. Transition to adolescence and adulthood may require alternative management more suitable for the person's lifestyle and independence.

Orthopedic Treatment. Orthopedic surgery is closely interrelated with conservative modalities to treat the motor dysfunction. Congenital musculoskeletal deformities or deformities secondary to unbalanced muscle action require surgical correction.[51,140] The goals of orthopedic treatment are to maintain a stable spine with the best possible correction and to achieve proper anatomic alignment of lower extremity joints. Although in most cases the time for surgery does not arise until early school age or later, orthopedic follow-up is necessary from infancy through adolescence.

Deformities of the spine may be congenital, paralytic, or a combination of both.[4,51,140] Scoliosis, kyphosis, and lordosis often occur in combination and deteriorate over the years. Progression of scoliosis is fastest during the adolescent growth spurt. Spinal deformities are most frequent in thoracic lesions (80–100% by 14–15 years). Their incidence decreases in lumbar lesions, but they are present even in sacral level paralysis at a rate of 5–10%.[51,140] Hip dislocation and pelvic obliquity are often coexistent findings in paralytic scoliosis. Initial treatment is an orthosis with a bivalved body jacket or Milwaukee brace. Congenital spinal deformities are generally rigid and more difficult to brace. Pressure ulcers over prominent areas must be avoided. Obesity may interfere with the use of spinal orthosis. Orthotic treatment does not provide complete or permanent correction. It is a temporary measure to delay more rapid progression of the deformity and to allow the surgeon to select the optimal time for operative intervention, based on the child's age and progression of scoliosis. Long spinal fusion at an early age results in stunted growth of the torso. It is usually recommended around 11 years in girls and 2 years later in boys because children with spina bifida attain spinal growth earlier than able-bodied peers.[51] A rapidly progressive scoliosis may necessitate earlier surgery because correction tends to be less adequate with severe curvature. Several techniques of bony fusion and internal fixation are available. Postoperatively the child wears a spinal orthosis, usually for 6–12 months, until solid fusion is achieved.[51] A kyphectomy may be necessary when the deformity is severe. Complications of surgery include lack of complete fusion, subsequent loss of correction, infection, and pseudarthrosis.

A serious problem affecting the hip is paralytic subluxation or dislocation.[4,140–142] In lumbar lesions the mechanical imbalance between active hip flexion and adduction with absent or weak abductor and extensor function produces persistence of the fetal coxa valga and a dysplastic, shallow, slanted acetabulum. Hip abduction splint or Pavlik harness is used in the first 2 years in an attempt to counteract the abnormal mechanical forces.[51] Soft tissue surgical procedures are aimed at ameliorating the paralytic muscle imbalance. Adductor release combined with posterolateral iliopsoas and external abdominal oblique muscle transfer posterior to the greater trochanter attempts to restore more balanced muscle action by providing active hip abduction and extension.[51,140] As a rule, bilateral, flexible dislocated hips do not need surgery. In patients with severe acetabular dysplasia and coxa valga, acetabuloplasty and proximal femoral varus osteotomy are necessary. Because these procedures are major and not uniformly successful, surgery is recommended only for children who have a good prognosis for ambulation, as indicated by strong bilateral quadriceps function.[51,140–142] A severe hip flexion contracture or hip flexion combined with abduction external rotation deformities due to iliotibial band and tensor fasciae latae contractures in thoracic lesions are released by surgery if they interfere with comfortable sitting or lying in bed.

Knee flexion contracture is most common in thoracolumbar lesions. Its origin is often unclear, although it may be related to intrauterine position, continuous sitting without proper range-of-motion exercises postnatally, spastic hamstrings, or progressive crouch posture on standing and walking.[140] Knee extension contracture, although less frequent, develops from muscle imbalance with strong quadriceps and weak hamstrings and is seen mostly in lesions that spare the L4 segment.[51,143]

Rigid club foot is usually congenital and associated with a thoracic or upper lumbar lesion.[51,144] Muscle imbalance accounts for foot deformities in lower lumbar and sacral lesions, which may include calcaneus feet with a varus or valgus component or cavus feet with flexion deformities of the toes.[51,140,145,146] Bony deformities of the ankles and feet, such as tibial torsion, vertical talus, and pes varus or valgus with wedging and consequent asymmetric epiphyseal growth, enhance the effect of paralytic deformities.[51,140,147] Early treatment is orthosis or progressive casting when the deformity is mobile. Posterior transfer of the tibialis anterior is performed after 5 years of age for calcaneus foot.[51,145,146] Equinus deformity is treated with Achilles' tendon lengthening. Flexor tenodesis or transfer and plantar fasciotomy are options to correct severe claw toe deformity and pes cavus.[51,140] Additional soft tissue releases, tendon transfer, or capsulotomy may be necessary, particularly when a varus or valgus component is also present. If soft tissue surgery does not produce satisfactory results, the surgeon may consider a bony procedure—for example, subtalar fusion, epiphysiodesis, triple arthrodesis, or talectomy.[51] Possible complications after immobilization and surgery are osteoporotic fractures and heterotopic ossifications.[148,149]

Latex Allergy.   Although the existence of latex allergy has been known for some time, its increased incidence in children with spina bifida was realized only recently.[150,151] Clinical signs are skin rash, angioedema, and, in severe cases, bronchospasm and other symptoms of anaphylactic reaction.[150,151] Predisposing factors are atopic disposition with known allergies to other substances,[152,153] multiple surgical procedures,[153–155] and previous frequent exposure to latex-containing gloves, nonsurgical equipment,

or toys. One study found latex sensitization in 59% of children with spina bifida and 55% in children who had multiple surgeries for other diagnoses.[153] Diagnostic tests for latex allergy include serum IgE antigens specific for rubber,[154] skin pinprick test (SPT),[152] and radioallergosorbent testing (RAST).[150] Because latex allergy develops over time,[150] negative tests do not rule out future sensitization. Therefore, the recommendation is for children with spina bifida to avoid all exposure to latex-containing objects, catheters, and other medical or nonmedical equipment in all aspects of daily life as well as at surgery, including dental treatment. Parents must be informed about existing or potential latex allergy to reinforce these precautions vigorously and consistently.

Rehabilitation.   The role of rehabilitation is to develop and implement a comprehensive intervention plan that enables the child to attain maximal level of function in all areas. This process must be coordinated with treatment by other specialists.

Musculoskeletal System.   Conservative management of potential or existing musculoskeletal deformities begins in the newborn and should continue as part of daily care thereafter. Passive range-of-motion exercise (PROME) is applied to all joints below the level of paralysis with special emphasis on joints with evident muscle imbalance. The infant should not lie constantly in one position but should be moved and turned frequently. This practice must be taught to parents not only to mitigate contractures, including those related to gravity, but also to avoid breakdown of the anesthetic skin. For the same reason, splints must be used with great precaution, removed frequently to check for skin irritation, and adjusted or discontinued if such problem occurs. PROME and splints are advisable after surgical correction of deformities to maintain joint mobility gained by the procedure. Strengthening exercises are sometimes beneficial for partially innervated muscles or after surgical muscle transfer for improving strength or function. It is also part of ambulation training with upper extremity assistive devices.

Examination of motor function in the neonate is based primarily on observation of spontaneous movements, presence or absence of deep tendon and infantile reflexes, habitual postures, passive joint motion, and tone. For example, consistently maintained hip flexion, particularly when passive extension is incomplete, is a sign of hip extensor weakness. Palpation of muscle bulk is helpful because atrophy may be evident with severe or complete paralysis in particular muscles. In assessing motor and sensory function, the presence of spinal reflex withdrawal or triple flexion of hip, knee, and ankle should not be mistaken for voluntary motion and preserved sensation, particularly in high spinal lesions. A normal asymmetric tonic neck reflex elicited in the arms without response in the legs suggests lower extremity paralysis.

Motor Development. During the first half year of life motor development may be close to normal unless the infant has complications of hydrocephalus, significant cognitive deficit, or severe urinary tract infections. In the absence of these adverse factors most children attain some head control and develop hand play. In the second half of the first year when gross motor development accelerates and active participation of the trunk and extremities is expected, delays become obvious. Provision of adaptive equipment for assisting in early motor milestones and exploratory behavior is important. Lack of such experience leads to early sensory motor deprivation and may affect subsequent development beyond the extent of organic deficit.[4,110]

A child with midthoracic deficit cannot sit because of trunk weakness and paralyzed legs. By 1 year some children learn to use their arms to pull themselves to a sitting position and maintain it by leaning on their hands.[4] To free the upper extremities for play and exploration, an adapted firm but well-padded seating arrangement with trunk support is needed. A lesion at T12 gives trunk control, but help is still needed to assume and maintain sitting because of weakness around the hips. Children with a midlumbar lesion can sit by themselves, usually with some delay, but assume a position of increasing lordosis that needs corrective support. When L4–L5 segments are spared, there is no physical reason to prevent or delay the onset of sitting.

Rolling over and prone progression are considerably delayed in thoracic lesions and in patients with complete paralysis of the legs. Nevertheless, unless other significant complications are present, most of these children develop compensatory ways for turning over, usually around 18 months of age. They initiate rolling from the shoulder and upper trunk. The paralyzed lower part of the body is turned over either by momentum or by passive movement of the legs with the hands. The urge to move around is present in children of this age. Youngsters with paralyzed legs or additional trunk weakness drag themselves around by their arms in flat prone position on the floor and inevitability develop abrasions, ulcers, and infections of the anesthetic skin. A low spina bifida caster cart[156] should be provided to avoid such problems and to allow mobility, access to toys, and play activities that usually take place on the floor at this age. A hand-operated caster cart is considered around 1 year. The age for using a motorized version depends on the child's emotional and cognitive development. Many children with midlumbar deficit and all children with L5 or sacral lesions get up on their hands and knees to crawl. Sensory deficit over the knee, shin, and dorsum of the foot requires protective padding.

Ambulation and Gross Mobility. Children with thoracic lesions require an assistive device for passive standing; the device is generally started at 12–18 months of age.[4,156,157] The parapodium was the first easy-to-apply and stable innovative device for this purpose. It allows both standing and sitting. Because arm support is not necessary for standing, the child can use the hands to play.[158] A thoracolumbosacral orthosis may be added in case of scoliosis. Young children are able to use a parapodium with a walkerette or crutches for limited exercise ambulation. Because the size of the baseplate increases with height, ambulation becomes more cumbersome. In the Orlau swivel walker an attachment to the baseplate converts lateral trunk movements to forward propulsion. This adaptation lowers the energy requirement for walking compared with the parapodium, although ambulatory function remains at household level.[159]

Orthoses that allow reciprocal gait pattern are used in lower thoracic and upper lumbar lesions. The hip guidance orthosis extends above these joints and has rocker soles.[160] With the use of crutches or walkerette, pressing down on one arm raises the contralateral foot, which is moved forward and down by gravity. The hip guidance orthosis enhances function and efficiency of ambulation of children with T11–L3 deficits from 6–15 years of age. The reciprocal gait orthosis (RGO), which is most effective in the presence of some active hip flexion, has undergone several modifications.[157] The latest design is the isocentric RGO (IRGO). The principle used in this orthosis is that mechanical tension created by forward stepping or hip flexion generates an extension moment at the contralateral hip. The device has a hip abduction joint to allow diaper change and a two-step hip joint release mechanism that enables sitting but also prevents sudden collapse when the lock is released.[158,161] In most cases the outcome of ambulation with RGO is at the household or exercise level and is accomplished after 3 years of age. Energy requirement is close to that of wheelchair locomotion[162]

Midlumbar lesions are associated with various degrees of knee extension strength, which was found to be an important factor to achieve walking. Upper extremity assistive devices are necessary to compensate for hip extensor weakness. Orthotic choices include the hip-knee-ankle-foot (HKAFO) orthosis, when hip instability interferes with knee alignment, and the KAFO with special adaptations to correct knee flexion tendency in the upright position.[157] For some children with L3-sparing, an AFO eventually may be adequate. Because of the many variations frequent reassessment and adjustment of orthosis are needed. Functional household and limited community ambulation are feasible.

Children with low lumbar lesions pull to stand and cruise near the expected age. In most cases, they walk by around 2 years. Gait is characterized by Trendelenburg lurch and gastrocnemius limp. Stationary standing is usually more difficult because of anteroposterior ankle instability with triceps surae weakness. In low lumbar or sacral lesions different types of ankle orthosis or shoe modifications may be warranted depending on the presenting foot deformity.[157] A floor reaction orthosis may be used for the nonfixed calcaneus foot to increase knee extensor moment and to control the tendency for flexed knee posture during standing and walking.[163] Functional community ambulation is a realistic expectation in most cases.

Generally a mental age of 2–3 years is a prerequisite to learn principles of crutch walking. Higher neurosegmental lesions require more upper extremity strength and coordination. Youngsters with upper lumbar or low thoracic lesions seldom have the physical ability for the task until they are 4–5 years old. A walkerette provides more stability and is easier to handle than crutches. It may be the first choice in the early stage of training to use upper extremity ambulatory aids. Reverse or posterior walker is preferred because it encourages better erect posture.

Ambulatory outcome has been addressed in several studies.[4,164–166] There is general agreement that all children and adults with sacral lesions achieve functional community ambulation. With low lumbar lesions functional community ambulation was reported in 38% of children[164] and 95% of patients between 15 and 31 years.[165] Approximately one-third of patients who have high lumbar lesions attain some degree of community ambulation.[164,165] With thoracic lesions similar achievements ranged from a surprisingly high 33%[165] to none.[164] In a statistical analysis of 206 patients and average follow-up of 10 years, sitting balance and motor level were identified as early predictors of walking.[167] As a practical clinical guideline, strong quadriceps muscles are considered a necessity for eventual ambulation. Deformities of the spine and lower extremities and obesity are unfavorable factors.[166] Because young children are motor-oriented, walking is a primary interest in preschool and early school ages. However, priorities change with age, and growth in stature further increases the already high energy demands of walking. For these reasons many children who were partial ambulators choose to give up walking for full-time wheelchair use around adolescence.[4]

Training in wheelchair use can begin during the second year, particularly for youngsters who are not expected to become functional ambulators. Children with spina bifida require special adaptation and seating for the purpose of positional support and protection of the anesthetic skin. The child, parents, and caretakers must be instructed about the importance of frequent weight shifting and precautions during transfer to prevent skin damage. Manual wheelchair is adequate for independent mobility in young children. An electric wheelchair is recommended at school age for children with adequate cognitive function and emotional maturity. Details of wheelchairs and various seating systems are discussed in Chapter 9.

Bladder and Bowel Training.   Dysfunctional bladder and bowel affect the whole family both physically and psychologically. The degree of success in achieving continence is of vital importance for self-esteem, independent living, and social acceptance of persons with spina bifida. Methods of management for bladder dysfunction include CIC and pharmacologic and surgical treatment, which were discussed earlier in this chapter.

Bowel training must be pursued as one of the major goals of rehabilitation.[4,168–171] Anocutaneous and bulbocavernosus reflexes have some (although not uniformly consistent) correlation with bowel dysfunction.[4,101,168] Absence of these reflexes is generally a sign of decreased rectal motility to expel stool and lack of sphincter tone to retain feces. Overdistention of the colon and rectum with chronic constipation or obstipation also results in loss of rectal motility. With incomplete emptying, however, stress incontinence or continuous leakage may occur. High fiber diet and appropriate fluid intake help to make the stool more bulky and firm, thereby aiding with evacuation. Manual evacuation timed about 30 minutes after meals uses the gastrocolic reflex for bowel emptying. The Crede maneuver or straining while the child is sitting on the toilet may reinforce stool passage and emptying. In the presence of the anocutaneous reflex, contraction of the rectal sigmoid is likely to occur with the use of digital stimulation or a rectal suppository such as Dulcolax. Fecal softeners, lactulose, docusate, or suppositories may be helpful on an intermittent basis if digital stimulation has not produced results.

In severe constipation with palpable stool in the abdomen, a colonic cleansing enema should be considered.[172] Organic anatomic bowel obstruction should be ruled out by abdominal radiographs before this procedure is done. In most difficult cases, an enema may be needed every other day to establish some intestinal rhythm. The antegrade continence enema (ACE)[173] creates a continent, catheterizable appendicocecostomy through the abdominal wall. Tap water enemas delivered through the surgical conduit have a high success rate in facilitating regular evacuation and fecal continence.

Anorectal manometry[174,175] and biofeedback offer encouraging results in the presence of anocutaneous reflex and intact or partial rectal sensation. Responses of the internal anal sphincter to rectal distention are measured by inflating a rectal balloon. Rectal sensation is considered normal when a balloon volume of 10 ml or less is perceived. Associated activity of the external anal sphincter is documented by EMG. Biofeedback training consists of repeated sessions of successive inflation and deflation of the rectal balloon. As in the management of bladder incontinence, a competent rehabilitation nurse is mandatory for training in bowel control. Education of the family and other persons in regular contact with the child is essential for achieving satisfactory compliance and results.

The overall outcome of bowel training varies in different surveys.[4,131,168,169,171] The most promising results were reported in 44 children over 5 years of age: 66% achieved continence with only rare accidents; 19% achieved good control (mostly younger children with less than 1 weekly episode of soiling); and only 6% remained incontinent.[176] For further details about bladder and bowel training and the role of the rehabilitation nurse, the reader is referred to Chapter 11.

Self-Care. Acquisition of developmental skills, particularly self-care, should be monitored and encouraged. Many children function below expectation in activities of daily living (ADLs) despite normal intelligence and adequate upper extremity control for performing age-appropriate self-care skills.[177,178] In most cases this problem is related to confusion on the part of the parents about proper expectation and excessive, although well-intentioned help in all physical activities for the child with a motor handicap. Visual motor and fine hand coordination problems are rarely significant enough to account for the delays. The

family must be advised about the importance of fostering the child's independence from an early age and the impact of their attitude on both physical and emotional development. If the problem persists, an occupational therapy evaluation should be arranged to demonstrate to parents what can be expected and what the child can actually do and, if warranted, to recommend adaptations. Occupational therapy is necessary in extensive lower extremity paralysis and thoracic lesions to learn techniques of dressing and other ADLs adapted to the home environment and other functional situations. Such sessions include training the child as well as the parents.

Education. Early intervention programs with parental participation are an additional resource for training the family and child. Referral to a preschool program, which is legally mandated for children with disabilities from 3 years of age, is the next step in preparation for formal education. An ideal program combines opportunities in motor and self-care activities, social interaction, communication skills, and cognitive tasks. On entering formal education, intellectual capacity should determine class placement. Children with cognitive deficits require special education. Severe motor dysfunction or special physical needs should not interfere with mainstreaming and academic education for children who have good intellectual capacity. A motorized wheelchair is recommended at this age to increase speed and efficiency of gross mobility. As a group, youngsters with spina bifida tend to score lower in arithmetic, spelling, and graphomotor skills than able-bodied peers.[4] In some cases such difficulties may call for continuing regular educational placement and part-time remedial classes for specific identified problems. Use of a computer is helpful when graphomotor skills are impaired. Several reports examined the influence of integrated vs. special education. Despite differences in study design and variables, the emerging trend seems to be better psychological, social, and academic achievements relative to expectations for age and actual IQ in children attending integrated school.[4,35,110]

For maximal effectiveness and communication within the team and with the family, pediatrician, and outside agencies involved in the child's care and education, it is advisable that one physician should act as the liaison and assume the responsibility for coordinating the child's management. Pediatric physiatrists with training and knowledge in the diagnosis and treatment of motor disabilities, neurogenic bladder and bowel dysfunction, and child development are well suited for this role.

Emotional Social Adjustment and Intervention. Many children with spina bifida experience low self-esteem, feelings of insecurity, self-doubt, and social isolation.[179] In the early school years anxiety and fearfulness are more frequent than among able-bodied children. Physical appearance is a significant concern among girls. Emotional problems increase with age, including adolescent depression, and do not necessarily correlate with the severity of motor deficit.[4,35,180] Bowel and bladder control are most important for social acceptance.

Research into family dynamics shows increased stress related to daily care, treatment demands, medical complications, expenses, and career compromise.[181] Self-doubts about parenting competence correlate with the child's disability.[182] Overprotective parenting is seen in many cases. Family environment and social experiences are the strongest influences shaping personality and emotional development and preparedness for adult life. A positive correlation was found between adult functioning and family environment that encouraged independence, assertiveness, self-sufficiency, and achievement-oriented behavior.[183]

Preoccupation with medical issues often diverts the physician's attention from psychosocial concerns. The family and child, on the other hand, may be reluctant to voice their concerns. It is the physician's responsibility to initiate discussion of such matters and to provide informative guidance. Referral to community resources, such as the Spina Bifida Association of America (SBAA); meeting other families; and information about available social, sports, and recreational activities offer a variety of opportunities for the child and parents. The SBAA has many informative publications for parents about different aspects of diagnosis and management.

Long-term Outcome

Most youngsters complete high school, and approximately 50% continue with further education.[184,185] In a U.S. survey, independent living was achieved by 30–60%; one third lived with their family; and only a small number were in institutions.[4,184] Data from England indicated that nearly 90% of adults live with their family.[186] The employment rate is in the range of 25–50% and depends on intelligence, academic qualifications, behavior, continence, and severity of physical disability.[4,184,187,188]

Marriage and reproductive capacity have been studied in both females and males.[189] Conception is possible in women, but problems related to shunt and urinary dysfunction require special care during pregnancy. Vaginal delivery is preferable in case of ventriculoperitoneal shunt, although cesarean section may be necessary for women with an underdeveloped pelvis.[190] The frequency of premature labor is increased. Male sexual functioning is present in L5 and sacral deficits,[191] with reproductive potential related to lower and less severe lesions.[192] Genetic counseling is advisable because the incidence of spina bifida in offspring with one affected parent is 4%.[190] The wide spectrum of problems presented by adults with spina bifida led to the recent trend of establishing multidisciplinary facilities, similar to those for children, that in the past were not available for adults.[193,194]

Twenty-two- to 28-year follow-up of a complete cohort with nonselective closure found a survival rate of 79% at 1 year, 66% at 5 years, and 52% at 26 years. Urologic causes were responsible for nearly 40% of deaths between the ages of 5 and 30 years.[195] Calculations based on these data indicated that during this age span the survival rate falls steadily by 3% for every 5 years.[196]

Conclusion

The range of problems in myelodysplasia requires a multidisciplinary treatment team. Specific concerns of comprehensive functional rehabilitation are prevention of deformities, training in self-care and adaptive function, achievement of independent mobility, control of bowel and bladder dysfunction, promoting emotional and social adjustment, and educational and vocational guidance. Treatment of the child and training of the family are of equal importance.

The Spina Bifida Association of America (SBAA) may be contacted at 4590 MacArthur Blvd, NW, Suite 250, Washington, DC 20007-4226, or by telephone at 202-944-3285 for information and publication orders.

References

1. Swaiman KF, Wright FS (eds): The Practice of Pediatric Neurology, 2nd ed. St. Louis, Mosby, 1982.
2. Aicardi J: Diseases of the nervous system in childhood. Clinics in Developmental Medicine, no 115/118. New York, Cambridge University Press, 1992.
3. Menkes JS: Textbook of Child Neurology. Philadelphia, Lea & Febiger, 1990.
4. Shurtleff DB (ed): Myelodysplasias and Extrophies: Significance, Prevention and Treatment. New York, Grune & Stratton, 1986.
5. Mortimer EA: The puzzling epidemiology of neural tube defects. Pediatrics 1980;65:636.
6. Laurence KM: The genetics and prevention of neural tube defects and uncomplicated hydrocephalus. In Emery AEH, Rimoin DL (eds): Principles and Practice of Medical Genetics. New York, Churchill Livingstone, 1990.

7. Omran M, Stone DH, et al: Pattern of decline in prevalence of anencephaly and spina bifida in a high-risk area. Health Bull 1992;50:407.
8. Yen IH, Khoury MJ, et al: The changing epidemiology of neural tube defects, United States, 1968–1989. Am J Dis Child 1992;146:857.
9. Chatkupt S, Skurnick JH, et al: Study of genetics, epidemiology and vitamin usage in familial spina bifida in the United States in the 1990s. Neurology 1994;44:65.
10. Lary JM, Edmonds LD: Prevalence of spina bifida at birth—United States, 1983–1990; A comparison of the surveillance systems. MMWR 1996;45:15.
11. Carter CO: Clues to the etiology of neural tube malformation. Dev Med Child Neurol 1974;32(Suppl):3.
12. Wiswell TE, Tuttle DJ, et al: Major congenital neurologic malformations. A 17-year survey. Am J Dis Child 1990;144:61.
13. Cowchock S, Ainbender E, et al: The recurrence risk for neural tube defects in the United States: A collaborative study. Am J Med Genet 1980;5:309.
14. Morrison K, Papapetrou C, et al: Genetic mapping of the human homologue (T) of mouse T (Brachyury) and a search for allele association between human T and spina bifida. Hum Mol Genet 1996;5:669.
15. George TM, McLone DG: Mechanisms of mutant genes in spina bifida: A review of implications from animal models. Pediatr Neurosurg 1995;23:236.
16. Nevin NC, Johnston WP, et al: Influence of social class on the risk of recurrence of anencephalus and spina bifida. Dev Med Child Neurol 1981;23:155.
17. Watkins ML, Scanlon KS, Mulinare J, et al: Is maternal obesity a risk factor for anencephaly and spina bifida? Epidemiology 1996;7:507.
18. Lindhout D, Schmidt D: In utero exposure to valproate and neural tube defects. Lancet 1986;1:1392.
19. Lammer EJ, Severe LE, Oakley GP: Teratogen update: Valproic acid. Teratology 1987;35:165.
20. Rosa FW: Spina bifida in infants and women treated with carbamazepine during pregnancy. N Engl J Med 1991;324:674.
21. Medical Research Council Vitamin Study Research Group: Prevention of neural tube defects. Lancet 1991;338:131.
22. Sarwark JF: Spina bifida. Pediatr Clin North Am 1996;43:1151.
23. Czeizel AE, Dudas I: Prevention of the first occurrence of neural tube defect, by periconceptual vitamin supplementation. N Engl J Med 1992;327:1832.
24. Centers for Disease Control and Prevention: Recommendations for the use of folic acid to reduce the number of cases of spina bifida and other neural tube defects. MMWR 1991;11:1.
25. Milunski A, Ulcickas M, et al: Maternal heat exposure and neural tube defects. JAMA 1992;268:882.
26. Sanford MK, Kissling GE, et al: Neural tube defects etiology: New evidence concerning maternal hyperthermia, health and diet. Dev Med Child Neurol 1992;34:661.
27. Milunsky A (ed): Genetic Disorders and the Fetus: Diagnosis, Prevention and Treatment, 2nd ed. New York, Plenum Press, 1986.
28. Report of Collaborative Acetylcholinesterase Study: Amniotic fluid acetylcholinesterase electrophoresis as a secondary test in the diagnosis of anencephaly and open spina bifida in early pregnancy. Lancet 1981;328:321.
29. Nicolaides KH,van den Hof MC, et al: Ultrasound screening for spina bifida: Cranial and cerebellar signs. Lancet 1986;333:77.
30. Watson WJ, Chescheir NC, et al: The role of ultrasound in evaluation of patients with elevated maternal serum alpha-fetoprotein: A review. Obstet Gynecol 1991;78:123.
31. Cragan JD, Roberts HE, et al: Surveillance for anencephaly and spina bifida and the impact of prenatal diagnosis—United States 1985–1994. MMWR 1995;44:1.
32. Omran M, McLoone P, et al: Factors limiting the effectiveness of prenatal screening for anencephaly and spina bifida in a high-risk area. Paediatr Perinat Epidemiol 1993;7:461.
33. Luthi DA, Wardinsky T, et al: Cesarean section before the onset of labor and subsequent motor function in infants with myelomeningocele diagnosed antenatally. N Engl J Med 1991;324:662.
34. Hill AE, Beattie F: Does cesarean section delivery improve neurologic outcome in open spina bifida? Eur J Pediatr Surg 1994;4(Suppl 1):32.
35. Rekate HL (ed): Comprehensive Management of Spina Bifida. Boston, CRC Press, 1991.
36. Lemire RJ: Neural tube defects. JAMA 1988;259:558.
37. Padget DH: Neuroschisis and human embryonic maldevelopment: New evidence of anencephaly, spina bifida and diverse mammalian defects. J Neuropath Exper Neurol 1970;29:192.
38. Stevenson RE, Kelly JJ, et al: Vascular basis for neural tube defects: A hypothesis. Pediatrics 1987;80:102.
39. Gardner WJ: Hydrodynamic mechanism of syringomyelia: Its relationship to myelocele. J Neurol Neurosurg Psychiatry 1965;28:247.
40. Gardner WJ: Myelocele: Rupture of the neural tube? Clin Neurosurg 1968;15:57.
41. Sutow WW, Pryde AW: Incidence of spina bifida in relation to age. Am J Dis Child 1956;91:211.
42. James CCM, Lassman LP: Spinal Dysraphism: Spina Bifida Occulta. London, Butterworth, 1972.
43. Belzberg AJ, Myles ST, Trevenen CL: The human tail and spinal dysraphism. J Pediatr Surg 1991;26:1243.
44. Yamane T, Shinoto A, et al: Spinal dysraphism: A study of patients over 10 years of age. Spine 1991;16:1295.
45. Stark GD, Baker GCW: The neurological involvement in myelomeningocele. Dev Med Child Neurol 1967;9:732.
46. Stark GD, Drummond M: The spinal cord lesion in myelomeningocele. Dev Med Child Neurol 1971;25(Suppl 13):1.
47. Gutkelch AN: Studies in spina bifida cystica: Anomalous reflexes in congenital spinal palsy. Dev Med Child Neurol 1964;6:264.
48. Mazur JM, Stillwell A, et al: The significance of spasticity in the upper and lower limbs in myelomeningocele. J Bone Joint Surg 1986;68B:213.
49. Park TS, Cail WS, et al: Progressive spasticity and scoliosis in children with myelomeningocele: Radiologic investigation and surgical treatment. J Neurosurg 1985;62:367.
50. Hays RM, Erickson D, et al: Tethered cord syndrome in myelomeningocele: Analysis of clinical features for early diagnosis. Arch Phys Med Rehabil 1989;70:45.
51. Mayfield JK: Comprehensive orthopedic management in myelomeningocele. In Rekate HL (ed): Comprehensive Management of Spina Bifida. Boston, CRC Press, 1991, p 113.
52. Srivasta VK: Wound healing in trophic ulcers in spina bifida patients. J Neurosurg 1995;82:40.
53. Brocklehurst G (ed): Spina Bifida for the Clinician. Philadelphia, JB Lippincott, 1976.
54. Schafer MD, Dias LS: Myelomeningocele: Orthopedic Treatment. Baltimore, Williams & Wilkins, 1983.
55. Gilbert JN, Jones KI, et al: Central nervous system anomalies associated with myelomeningocele, hydrocephalus and Arnold-Chiari malformation: Reappraisal of theories regarding the pathogenesis of posterior neural tube closure defects. Neurosurgery 1986;18:559.
56. Azimullah PC, Smit LM, et al: Malformations of the spinal cord in 53 patients with spina bifida studied by magnetic resonance imaging. Childs Nerv System 1991;7:63.

57. Molnar GE: Spina bifida: Clinical correlation of associated central nervous system malformations. Phys Med Rehabil State Art Rev 1991;7:63.

58. Wilson DA, Prince JR: MR imaging determination of the location of conus medullaris throughout childhood. Am J Roentgenol 1989;152:1029.

59. Pierre-Kahn A, LaCombe J, et al: Intraspinal lipomas with spina bifida. J Neurosurg 1986;65:756.

60. Just M, Schwarz M, et al: Magnetic resonance imaging of dysraphic myelodysplasia. Childs Nerv System 1986; 4:149.

61. O'Neill P, Stack JP: Magnetic resonance imaging in the preoperative assessment of closed spinal dysraphism in children. Pediatr Neurosurg 199;16:240.

62. McEnery G, Borzyskowski M, et al: The spinal cord in neurologically stable spina bifida: A clinical and MRI study. Dev Med Child Neurol 1992;34:342.

63. Yamada S, Iacono RP, et al: Pathophysiology of the tethered cord. Neurosurg Clin North Am 1995;6:311.

64. Naidich TP, Radkowski MA, et al: Real-time sonographic display of caudal spine anomalies. Neuroradiology 1986;28:512.

65. Johnson DL, Levy LM: Predicting outcome in the tethered cord syndrome: A study of cord motion. Pediatr Neurosurg 1995;22:115.

66. Boor R, Schwarz M, et al: Tethered cord after spina bifida aperta: A longitudinal study of somatosensory evoked potentials. Childs Nerv System 1993;9:328.

67. Li V, Albright AL, et al: The role of somatosensory evoked potentials in the evaluation of spinal cord retethering. Pediatr Neurosurg 1996;24:126.

68. Kothbauer K, Schmid UD, et al: Intraoperative motor and sensory monitoring of the cauda equina. Neurosurgery 1994;34:702.

69. Peterson MC: Tethered cord syndrome in myelomeningodysplasia: Correlation between level of lesion and height at time of presentation. Dev Med Child Neurol 1992;34:604.

70. Herman JM, McLone DG, et al: Analysis of 153 patients with myelomeningocele or spinal lipoma reoperated upon for a tethered cord: Prevention, management, and outcome. Pediatr Neurosurg 1993;19:243.

71. Fone PD, Vapnek JM, et al: Urodynamic findings in tethered cord syndrome: Does surgical release improve bladder function? J Urol 1997;157:604.

72. Vernet O, Farmer JP, et al: Impact of urodynamic studies on the surgical management of spinal cord tethering. J Neurosurg 1996;85:555.

73. McLone DG, Herman JM, et al: Tethered cord as a cause of scoliosis in children with a myelomeningocele. Pediatr Neurosurg 1990;16:8.

74. Reigel DH, Tchernoukh AK, et al: Change in spinal curvature following release of tethered cord associated with spinal bifida. Pediatr Neurosurg 1994;20: 30.

75. Gardner WJ: Hydrodynamic mechanism of syringomyelia: Its relationship to myelocele. J Neurol Neurosurg Psychiatry 1965;28:247.

76. Samuelson L, Bergstrom K, et al: MR imaging of syringohydromyelia and Chiari malformation in myelomeningocele patients with scoliosis. Am J Neurol 1987; 8:539.

77. Ball MJ, Dayan AD: Pathogenesis of syringomyelia. Lancet 1972;ii:799.

78. Tashiro K, Fukazawa T, et al: Syringomyelic syndrome: Clinical features in 31 cases confirmed by CT myelography or magnetic resonance imaging. J Neurol 1987; 235:26.

79. Hall PV, Lindseth RE, et al: Myelodysplasia and developmental scoliosis: A manifestation of syringomyelia. Spine 1976;1:48.

80. Park TS, Hoffman JH, et al: Experience with surgical decompression of the Arnold-Chiari malformation in young adults with myelomeningocele. Neurosurgery 1983;13:147.

81. Bell WO, Charney EB, et al: Symptomatic Arnold-Chiari malformation: Review of experience with 22 cases. J Neurosurg 1987;66:812.

82. Charney EB, Rorke LB, et al: Management of Chiari II complications in infants with myelomeningocele. J Pediatr 1987;111:304.

83. Hays R, Jordan R, et al: Central ventilatory dysfunction in myelodysplasia. An independent determination of survival. Dev Med Child Neurol 1989;31:366.

84. McLone DG: Results of treatment of children born with a myelomeningocele. Clin Neurosurg 1983;30:407.

85. Gaston H: Ophthalmologic complications of spina bifida and hydrocephalus. Eye 1991;5:279.

86. Lennerstrand G, Gallo JE, et al: Neuro-ophthalmologic findings in relation to CNS lesions in patients with myelomeningocele. Dev Med Child Neurol 1990;32:423.

87. Mazure JM, Menelaus MB, et al: Hand function in patients with spina bifida cystica. J Pediatr Orthop 1986;5:442.

88. Dahl M, Ahlsten G, et al: Neurological dysfunction above the cele level in children with spina bifida cystica: A prospective study of three years. Dev Med Child Neurol 1995;37:30.

89. Dias MS, McLone DG: Hydrocephalus in the child with dysraphism. Neurosurg Clin North Am 1993;4:715.

90. Cedzich C, Schramm J, et al: Reversible visual loss after shunt malfunction. Acta Neurochirurg 1990; 105:121.

91. Wassing HE, Siebelink BM, et al: Handedness and progressive hydrocephalus in spina bifida patients. Dev Med Child Neurol 1993;35:788.

92. Mandell GA, Maloney K, et al: The neural axis in spina bifida: Issues of confusion and fusion. Abdom Imag 1966;21:541.

93. Mundy AR: Clinical physiology of the bladder, urethra, and pelvic floor. In Mundy AR, Stevenson TP, et al (eds): Urodynamics: Principles, Practice and Application. Edinburgh, Churchill Livingstone, 1984.

94. Borzykowsky M, Mundy AR (eds): Neuropathic bladder in childhood. Clin Devel Med 1990;120.

95. Lewis MA, Shaw J, et al: The spectrum of spinal cord dysraphism and bladder neuropathy in children. Eur J Pediatr Surg 1997;1(Suppl):35.

96. Mayo ME: Lower urinary tract dysfunction in cerebral palsy. J Urol 1997;147:419.

97. Bailey RR: Urologic management of spina bifida. In Rekate HL (ed): Comprehensive Management of Spina Bifida. Boston, CRC Press, 1991, p 185.

98. Stone AR: Neurologic evaluation and urologic management of spinal dysraphism. Neurosurg Clin North Am 1995;6:269.

99. Abrams P, Blaivas JG, et al: Standardization of terminology of lower urinary tract function. International Continence Society Committee on Standardization of Terminology. New York, Alan R. Liss, 1988.

100. McGuire EJ, Woodside JR, et al: Prognostic value of urodynamic testing in myelodysplastic patients. J Urol 1981;126:205.

101. Agnarsson U, Warde C: Anorectal function of children with neurologic problems: Spina bifida. Dev Med Child Neurol 1993;35:893.

102. Shurtleff DB, Lamers J, et al: Are myelodysplastic children fat? Anthropometric measures: A preliminary report. Spina Bifida Ther 1982;4:1.

103. Mita K, Akatak K, et al: Assessment of obesity of children with spina bifida. Dev Med Child Neurol 1993;35: 305.

104. Roberts D, Sheperd RW, et al: Anthropometry and obesity in myelomeningocele. J Paediatr Child Health 1991;27:83.
105. Brauner R, Fontoura M, et al: Growth and puberty in children with congenital hydrocephalus. In Bannister CM, Tew B (eds): Current Concepts in Spina Bifida and Hydrocephalus. Clin Devel Med 1991;122.
106. Trollman R, Strehl E, et al: Precocious puberty in children with myelomeningocele: Treatment with gonadotropin releasing hormone analogues. Dev Med Child Neurol 1998;40:38.
107. Elias RE: Precocious puberty in girls with myelodysplasia. Pediatrics 1994;3:521.
108. Dahl M, Proost L, et al: Early puberty in boys with myelomeningocele. Eur J Pediatr Surg 1997;1(Suppl):50.
109. Appleton PE, Minchom P, et al: The self-concept of young people with spina bifida: A population-based study. Dev Med Child Neurol 1994;36:198.
110. Tew B: The effects of spina bifida and hydrocephalus upon learning and behavior. In Bannister CM, Tew B (ed): Current Concepts in Spina Bifida and Hydrocephalus. New York, Cambridge University Press, 1991.
111. Mapstone TB, Rekate HL, et al: Relationship of cerebrospinal fluid shunting and IQ in children with myelomeningocele. Childs Brain 1984;11:12.
112. McLone DG, Czyzewski D, et al: Central nervous system infections as a limiting factor in the intelligence of children born with myelomeningocele. Pediatrics 1982;70:338.
113. Hadenius AM, Hagberg B, et al: The natural prognosis of infantile hydrocephalus. Acta Paediatr 1962;51:117.
114. Ito J, Saijo H, et al: Neuroradiological assessment of visuoperceptual disturbance in children with spina bifida and hydrocephalus. Dev Med Child Neurol 1997;39:385.
115. Muen WJ, Bannister CM: Hand function in subjects with spina bifida. Eur J Pediatr Surg 1997;1(Suppl):18.
116. Bannister CM: The role of fetal neurosurgery in the management of central nervous system abnormalities. In Bannister CM, Tew B (eds): Current Concepts in Spina Bifida and Hydrocephalus. New York, Cambridge University Press, 1991.
117. Maresh MJA: Fetal abnormality management group. In Bannister CM, Tew B (eds): Current Concepts in Spina Bifida and Hydrocephalus. New York, Cambridge University Press, 1991.
117a. Lorber J: Selective treatment of myelomeningocele: To treat or not to treat. Pediatrics 1974;53:307.
118. Brocklehurst G: Spina bifida for the clinician. Clin Devel Med 1976;57.
119. Hawnau JM: Diagnostic Imaging in Spina Bifida and Hydrocephalus. New York, Cambridge University Press, 1991.
120. Murphy KP, Kliever EM, et al: The voiding alert system: A new application in the treatment of incontinence. Arch Phys Med Rehabil 1994;75:924.
121. Gaum LD, Wese FX, et al: Radiologic investigation of the urinary tract in the neonate with myelomeningocele. J Urol 1982;127:510.
122. Chiaramonte RM, Horowitz EM, et al: Implications of hydrocephalus in the newborn with myelodysplasia. J Urol 1986;136:427.
123. Bauer SB: Early evaluation and management of children with spina bifida. In King LR (ed): Urologic Surgery in Neonates and Young Infants. Philadelphia, WB Saunders, 1988.
124. Bauer SB, Hallett N, et al: Predictive value of urodynamic evaluation in newborns with myelodysplasia. JAMA 1984;242:650.
125. Sidi AA, Dykstra DD, et al: The value of urodynamic testing in the management of neonate with myelodysplasia: A prospective study. J Urol 1986;135:90.
126. Lapides J, Diokno AC, et al: Clean intermittent self catheterization in the treatment of urinary tract disease. J Urol 1972;107:458.
127. Diokno AC, Sonda LP, et al: Fate of patients started on clean intermittent self catheterization therapy ten years ago. J Urol 1983;129:1120.
128. Enrile GB, Crooks JK: Clean intermittent catheterization for home management of children with myelomeningocele. Clin Pediatr 1986;19:143.
129. Kass EJ, Koof S, et al: The significance of bacilluria in children on long term intermittent catheterization. J Urol 1981;126:223.
130. Kass EJ, McHugh T, et al: Intermittent catheterization of children less than six years old. J Urol 1979;121:792.
131. Lie HR, Lagergren J, et al: Bowel and bladder control of children with myelomeningocele: A Nordic study. Dev Med Child Neurol 1991;33:1053.
132. Keating MA, Rink RC, et al: Appendicovesicostomy: A useful adjunct to continent recoordination of the bladder. J Urol 1991;149:1091.
133. Ducat JW, Snyder HM: Continent urinary diversion: Variations on the Mitrofanoff principle. J Urol 1986;136:58.
134. Horowitz M, Kuhr CS, et al: The Mitrofanoff catheterizing channel: Patient acceptance. J Urol 1995;153:771.
135. Sumfest JM, Burns MW, et al: The Mitrofanoff principle in urinary reconstruction. J Urol 1993;150:1875.
136. Barrett DM, Furlow WL: Artificial urinary sphincter in children. In Kelalis PP, King LR, et al (eds): Clinical Pediatric Urology, vol. 1, 2nd ed. Philadelphia, WB Saunders, 1985.
137. Gonzalez R, Sheldon CA: Artificial sphincters in children with neurogenic bladder: Long-term results. J Urol 1982;128:1270.
138. Nurse DE, Mundy AR: One hundred artificial sphincters. Br J Urol 1995;154:759.
139. Malone PS, Wheeler RA, et al: Continence in patients with spina bifida: Long-term results. Arch Dis Child 1994;70:107.
140. Menelaus MB: The Orthopedic Management of Spina Bifida Cystica. Edinburgh, Churchill Livingstone, 1986.
141. Fraser RK, Bourke HM, et al: Unilateral dislocation of the hip in spina bifida: A long-term follow-up. J Bone Joint Surg 1995;77B:615.
142. Kalman BA, Bhandari M, et al: Function of dislocated hips in children with lower-level spina bifida. J Bone Joint Surg 1996;78B:294.
143. Sandhu PS, Broughton NS, et al: Tenotomy of the ligamentum patellae in spina bifida: Management of limited flexion range at the knee. J Bone Joint Surg 1995;77B:832.
144. Broughton NS, Graham G, et al: The high incidence of foot deformity in patients with high level spina bifida. J Bone Joint Surg 1994;76B:548.
145. Rodrigues RC, Dias LS: Calcaneus deformity in spina bifida: Results of anterolateral release. J Pediatr Orthop 1992;12:461.
146. Stotts NS, Zionts LE, et al: Tibialis anterior transfer for calcaneus deformity: A postoperative gait analysis. J Pediatr Orthop 1996;16:792.
147. Fraser RK, Menelaus MB: The management of tibial torsion in patients with spina bifida. J Bone Joint Surg 1993;75B:495.
148. Parsch K: Origin and treatment of fractures in spina bifida. Eur J Pediatr Surg 1991;1:298.
149. Bouchard J, D'Astous J: Postoperative heterotopic ossification in children: A comparison of children with spina bifida and cerebral palsy. Can J Surg 1991;34:454.
150. Pearson ML, Cole JS, et al: How common is latex allergy? A survey of children with myelodysplasia. Dev Med Child Neurol 1994;36:64.

151. Tosi LL, Slater JE, et al: Latex allergy in spina bifida patients: Prevalence and surgical implications. J Pediatr Orthop 1993;13:709.

152. Michael T, Niggerman B, et al: Risk factors for latex allergy in patients with spina bifida. Clin Exp Allergy 1996;26:934.

153. Porri F, Pradal M, et al: Association between latex sensitization and repeated latex exposure in children. Anesthesiology 1997;86:599.

154. Kelly KJ, Pearson ML, et al: A cluster of anaphylactic reactions in children with spina bifida during general anesthesia: Epidemiologic features, risk factors, and latex hypersensivity. J Allergy Clin Immunol 1994;94:53.

155. Cremer R, Hoppe A, et al: The influence of shunted hydrocephalus on the prevalence of allergy to latex in patients with spina bifida. Eur J Pediatr Surg 1997;7(Suppl 1):47.

156. Pomatto RC: The use of orthotics in the treatment of myelomeningocele. In Rekate HL (ed): Comprehensive Management of Spina Bifida. Boston, CRC Press, 1991.

157. Molnar GE: Orthotic management of children. In Redford JB, Basmajian JV, Trautman P (eds): Orthotics, Clinical Practice and Rehabilitation Technology. New York, Churchill Livingstone, 1995.

158. Motloch WM: Device design in spina bifida. In Murdoch G (ed): Advances in Orthotics. Baltimore, Williams & Wilkins, 1976.

159. Lough LK, Nielsen DH: Ambulation of children with myelomeningocele: Parapodium vs parapodium with ORLAU swivel modification. Dev Med Child Neurol 1986;28:489.

160. Rose GK, Stallard J, et al: Clinical evaluation of spina bifida patients using hip guidance orthosis. Dev Med Child Neurol 1981;23:30.

161. Motloch W: Principles of Orthotic Management for Child and Adult Paraplegia and Clinical Experience with the Isocentric RGO. International Society for Prosthetics and Orthotics, 1992,II:28.

162. Flandry F, Burke S, et al: Functional ambulation in myelodysplasia: The effect of orthotic selection on physical and physiologic performance. J Pediatr Orthop 1986;6:662.

163. Yang GW, Chu DS, et al: Floor reaction orthosis: Clinical experience. Orthot Prosthet 1986;40:33.

164. Hoffer MM, Feiwell E, et al: Functional ambulation in patients with myelomeningocele. J Bone Joint Surg Am 1973;55:137.

165. Stillwell A: Walking ability in mature patients with spina bifida. J Pediatr Orthoped 1983;3:184.

166. Asher M: Factors affecting the ambulatory status of patients with spina bifida cystica. J Bone Joint Surg 1983;65A:350.

167. Swank M, Dias LS: Walking ability in spina bifida patients: A model for predicting future ambulatory status based on sitting balance and motor level. J Pediatr Orthop 1994;14:715.

168. King JC, Currie DM, et al: Bowel training in spina bifida: Importance of education, patient compliance, age and anal reflexes. Arch Phys Med Rehabil 1993;75:243.

169. Roberts CS: Bowel management in spina bifida: Perspectives and issues. BNI Q 1988;4:17.

170. White JJ, Suzuki M, et al: A physiologic rationale for the management of neurologic rectal incontinence in children. Pediatrics 1972;49:888.

171. Dietrich S, Okamoto G: Bowel training for children with neurogenic dysfunction: A follow-up. Arch Phys Med Rehabil 1982;63:166.

172. Scholler-Gyure M, Nesselaar C, et al: Treatment of defecation disorders by colonic enemas in children with spina bifida. Eur J Pediatr Surg 1996;6(Suppl 1):32.

173. Koyle MA, Kaji DM, et al: The Malone antegrade continence enema for neurogenic and structural fecal incontinence and constipation. J Urol 1995;154:759.

174. Rao SC, Patel RS: How useful are manometric tests of anorectal function in the management of defecation disorders? Am J Gastroenterol 1997;92:469.

175. Sangwan YP, Coller JA, et al: Relationship between manometric anal waves and fecal incontinence. Dis Rectum 1995;38:370.

176. Caldamone AA, Dixon MSJR: Current Trends in Urology, vol 3. Baltimore, Williams & Wilkins, 1985.

177. Sousa JC, Gordon LH, et al: Assessing the development of independence of daily living skills in patients with spina bifida. Dev Med Child Neurol 1976;18(Suppl 37).

178. Sousa JC, Telzrow RW, et al: Developmental guidelines for children with myelodysplasia. J Am Phys Ther Assoc 1983;63:21.

179. Appleton PL, Minchom PE, et al: The self-concept of young people with spina bifida: A population-based study. Dev Med Child Neurol 1994;36:198.

180. Appleton PL, Ellis NC, et al: Depressive symptoms and self-concept in young people with spina bifida. J Pediatr Psychol 1997;22:707.

181. Holmbeck GN, Gorley-Ferguson L, et al: Maternal, paternal and marital functioning in families of preadolescents with spina bifida. J Pediatr Psychol 1997;22:167.

182. Havermans T, Eiser C: Mother's perception of parenting a child with spina bifida. Child Care Health Dev 1991;17:259.

183. Loomis JW, Javornisky JG, et al: Relations between family environment and adjustment outcomes in young adults with spina bifida. Dev Med Child Neurol 1997;39:620.

184. Dunne KB, Shurtleff DB: The adult with myelomeningocele: A preliminary report. In McLaurin RL (ed): Spina Bifida: A Multidisciplinary Approach. New York, Praeger, 1986.

185. Smith AD: Adult spina bifida survey in Scotland: Educational attainment and employment. Z Kinderchir 1983;38(Suppl 2):107.

186. Lonton AP, O'Sullivan AM, et al: Spina bifida adults. Z Kinderchir 1983;38(Suppl 2):110.

187. Tew B, Laurence KM, et al: Factors affecting employability among young adults with spina bifida and hydrocephalus. Z Kinderchir 1990;45(Suppl 1):34.

188. Lonton AP, Laughlin AM, et al: The employment of adults with spina bifida. Z Kinderchir 1984;39(Suppl 2):132.

189. Cass AS, Bloom AB, et al: Sexual function in adults with myelomeningocele. J Urol 1986;136:425.

190. Rietberg CO, Lindhout D: Adult patients with spina bifida cystica: Genetic counseling, pregnancy and delivery. Eur J Obstet Gynecol Reprod Biol 1993;52:63.

191. Sandler AD, Worley G, et al: Sexual functioning and erection capability among young men with spina bifida. Dev Med Child Neurol 1996;38:823.

192. Decker RM, Furness PD, et al: Reproductive understanding: Sexual functioning and testosterone levels in men with spina bifida. J Urol 1997;157:1466.

193. Begeer IH, Staal-Screinemachers AL: The benefit of team treatment and control of adult patients with spinal dysraphism. Eur J Pediatr Surg 1996;6(Suppl 1):15.

194. Morgan DJ, Blackburn M, et al: Adults with spina bifida and/or hydrocephalus. Postgrad Med J 1995;71:17.

195. Hunt GM, Poulton A: Open spina bifida: A complete cohort reviewed 25 years after closure. Dev Med Child Neurol 1995;37:19.

196. Hunt GM, Palmer C: The median survival time in open spina bifida. Dev Med Child Neurol 1997;39:568.

Chapter **13**

Traumatic Brain Injury

Linda E. Krach, MD
Robert L. Kriel, MD

Epidemiology and Costs of Brain Injury in Children

Acquired brain injury is a major cause of disability, death, and expense in the United States. The incidence of concussions of all severities in the population at large is in the range of 148–270 per 100,000 for males and 70–116 for females.[1,2] Transportation-related accidents (motor vehicle, pedestrian, and bicycle accidents) account for approximately one half of these injuries, followed by falls, assault, firearms, and recreational activity.[2] Approximately 20% with brain injury die, usually before reaching the hospital, and approximately 15% are classified as severe, usually resulting in disability. The male predominance of brain injury is evident in all epidemiologic reports, as is the striking rise in incidence beginning at age 15, when motor vehicle operation and assaults peak.

Traumatic injury is the leading cause of death in the United States in children more than 1 year of age.[3] Approximately 10 per 100,000 children die each year from brain injury, which is about five times the rate of death for leukemia, the next leading cause of death.[1] The annual incidence of traumatic brain injury (TBI) for children is approximately 185 per 100,000 per year: 235 for boys and 132 for girls. The leading causes of pediatric brain injury are transportation-related (39%), falls (28%), sports and recreational activities (17%), and assault (7%).[4] In the 15% of brain-injured children who had serious damage, motor vehicle accidents and assault were responsible for more than half.

The costs of brain injury are enormous. With conditions resulting in long-term disability, costs are both direct, relating to inpatient and outpatient medical expenses, and indirect, which result from the patient's or family members' reduced employment level. As might be expected, medical charges largely depend on the severity of the brain injury. In a series of 127 primarily

adult patients with brain injury, investigators found that mean inpatient charges were $17,015 for mild cases and $133,467 for severe ones.[5] These patients also incurred follow-up medical expenses for the first 4 years after injury ranging from $2323 to $54,701 for mild and severe injuries. The authors projected that for the United States, medical costs for all brain-injured patients exceed $8 billion during the first 4 posttraumatic years. Much greater costs are incurred if indirect costs are also considered, which include loss of income and resulting decrease in tax revenue. Indirect costs, generally thought to exceed direct costs, are more difficult to document. Somewhat lower figures have been presented for pediatric brain injury. Jaffe and colleagues[7] reported a median cost for hospitalized children of $598 for mild, $12,529 for moderate, and $53,332 for severe TBI. In addition, 20 of 96 brain-injured children required inpatient rehabilitation. These children incurred median costs of $23,896 (mean $49,259).

Mechanisms of Injury

The damage caused by TBI typically occurs as a result of more than one mechanism and can be divided into primary and secondary causes. Primary injuries are those due to the direct impact or to the initial deceleration or shearing forces applied to the brain. Secondary injury occurs as a result of the sequelae of the initial injury and contributes to additional damage.

Primary Injury

Direct impact results in primary injury. This may be cerebral contusion underlying an area of impact, epidural hematoma associated with skull fracture, cerebral laceration from depressed skull fracture, or injury secondary to penetration of the brain due as a result of a gunshot wound or object entering the skull.[8-10] Penetrating injury most typically results in focal lesions.[9,10] In general, the presence or absence of skull fractures is not indicative of the severity of brain damage.[11,12] Direct-impact injuries are generally focal in nature.

Deceleration forces and shearing result in more generalized injury. They are essentially a result of the brain moving within the rigid skull, which is stopped by an impact or other restraining force. A classic example of this type of injury is contrecoup. *Contrecoup* is a cerebral contusion that occurs distant to the point of impact against an object. With the impact, the head is stopped, but the brain continues to move within the skull, and contusion occurs against a bony ridge or wall of the skull.[13] Shearing injuries also result in damage away from any point of impact and include diffuse axonal injury and multiple punctate hemorrhages. Most individuals with TBI have elements of both impact-related and deceleration-related injury.[8,14]

Secondary Injury

Secondary injury can result from a number of causes. Anything that interferes with cerebral perfusion or oxygenation can cause damage. These include hypotension, hypoxia, increased intracranial pressure because of cerebral edema, acute hydrocephalus, or mass lesion. Midline shift or herniation may lead to infarction because of pressure or traction on cerebral vessels.[8,10,15]

Children are particularly likely to develop diffuse cerebral edema. This edema may result in decreasing level of responsiveness. Diffuse cerebral edema is associated radiographically with small ventricles and obliterated cisterns as well as a loss of the white/gray matter differentiation.[16] Because the brain is confined within the rigid skull after the sutures fuse, edema leads to increased pressure within the skull. Cerebral blood flow depends on the perfusion pressure. Perfusion pressure is essentially the difference between the arterial pressure and the mean intracranial pressure. Increases in intracranial pressure can result in decreased blood supply and therefore further injury.[10]

Acute management of TBI focuses largely on the prevention of secondary damage. Efforts are made to control the intracranial pressure through fluid and electrolyte management, hyperventilation, and controlling the intensive care unit (ICU) environment. Maintenance of normal blood pressure and oxygenation are additional goals.[14] Although steroids are often used in the management of acute brain injury, there is no conclusive evidence of their benefit.[17] Experimental protocols exist that attempt to minimize the damage resulting from primary injury. These include drugs that are free radical scavengers, excitatory amino acid antagonists, and gangliosides. As yet no direct clinical applications have been done.[8,15]

The influence of age on mechanism of injury has been examined. In young children, it has been suggested that incomplete myelinization may result in a greater risk of shearing injury. Also, their relatively large heads supported on small, weak necks may increase the likelihood of injury because of increased rotational forces.[18] Some authors have suggested that young children and toddlers are at greater risk to develop cerebral edema.[18,19] Nonaccidental injury in young children is a result of acceleration-deceleration forces and is generally associated with retinal hemorrhages, fractures, and multiple injuries of varying severities.[14,20]

Growing Skull Fracture

Children who are very young at the time of trauma may develop a unique entity, a growing skull fracture. These result from the arachnoid protruding through a dural tear, resulting in a cyst that can contribute to a widening skull deficit that usually requires operative repair.[13,21] Although an arachnoid cyst is not always present, there is always a tear of the dura.[22] Magnetic resonance (MR) imaging findings consistent with growing skull fracture include skull fracture with tissue of the same intensity of the underlying brain within the margins of the fracture.[22]

Associated Injuries

Because a significant number of TBIs are due to motor vehicle accidents or other high-speed/high-energy accidents, it is not uncommon to find other concurrent injuries. Almost one-half of all children who sustain a TBI sustain another injury as well.[23] These associated injuries can complicate the acute management or affect the long-term outcome. Approximately 5–10% also sustain spinal cord injury.[24] Brachial plexus injuries because of traction, fractures because of impact, perforated viscus, and liver or spleen laceration have all been reported. Sometimes fractures or ligamentous injuries are diagnosed later when the child is sufficiently responsive to give an indication of discomfort. Sobus and colleagues[25] reported that of 60 children with TBI, 16 had a total of 25 fractures, and 19 had 24 areas of soft tissue injury diagnosed on transfer to rehabilitation that had not been detected in the acute care setting. These children were unable to indicate the presence of pain.

Injury Severity

Glasgow Coma Scale

Several classifications of brain injury severity have been proposed. Each has its merits and drawbacks. The Glasgow Coma Scale (GCS) has found wide clinical application and has the advantage of being determined within hours of injury. A score of 8 or less is considered to be coma and classified as severe injury, 9–11 as moderate injury, and 12–15 as mild injury.[26] Although the GCS was initially formulated to aid in acute triage and in neurosurgical management, many studies have correlated outcome with initial scores. There is, however, wide patient-to-patient variability. Adaptations of the GCS have been made to facilitate evaluation of children (Table 13–1).[27–29] Other refinements of the scale include the number of days until a patient returns to GCS 6 or 15. Also, some have noted that the GCS later in the postinjury course, particularly the motor component at 72 hours after injury, has proven to be a better predictor of disability.[6,30,31]

Posttraumatic Amnesia and Children's Orientation and Amnesia Test

The duration of posttraumatic amnesia (PTA) is another commonly used indicator of severity. Compared with the GCS, PTA has the merit of a longer period of patient observation. There is general agreement that the duration of PTA is directly correlated with the severity of injury.[32] There is no generally accepted and easily applied method, however, for determining the duration of PTA in children. This is especially problematic in young children, and assessment must be adapted as appropriate for the individual's age.[33]

TABLE 13–1. Glasgow Coma Scale for Young Children: Modification of Scoring of Verbal Responses*

Verbal Score	Adult and Older Child	Young Child
5	Oriented	Smiles, oriented to sound, follows objects, interacts
4	Confused, disordered	Cries but consolable, interacts inappropriately
3	Inappropriate words	Cries but is inconsistently consolable, moaning
2	Incomprehensible sounds	Inconsolable crying, irritable
1	No response	No response

* Scoring of eye opening and motor responses same as for adults.

Modified from Simpson DA, Cockington RA, Hanieh A, et al: Head injuries in infants and young children: The value of the paediatric coma scale. Childs Nerv Syst 1991;7:183.

The Children's Orientation and Amnesia Test (COAT) has been helpful in this respect.[34] Although this test should be useful in prospective outcome studies of children without profound injury, it has a major disadvantage because it takes from 5–10 minutes to administer and therefore has not become a routine on most services. It has also been shown to be sensitive to nontraumatic impairment. For example, children receiving special education services sometimes fall within the impaired range.[35]

Duration of Unconsciousness

Duration of unconsciousness is another measure of severity and also has the advantage of longer observation than GCS. It is generally easier to recognize than the duration of amnesia in children and is more easily determined in retrospective chart review. This is the most appropriate measure in series of more severely injured children who are unconscious many weeks, many of whom never regain recent memory. Severity ratings as determined by these alternative criteria are summarized in Table 13–2.

Although most outcome studies have correlated outcome with only one index of brain injury severity,[18,36–38] McDonald and colleagues[39] have compared 10 measures. In that report, the number of days to reach age-adjusted 75% performance on the COAT, the number of days to reach GCS 15, initial total GCS scores, and duration of unconsciousness were most predictive of outcome. The intercorrelations of these brain injury indices were also quite high. In general, these indices could be used interchangeably, and one severity measure predicted most outcomes almost as well as use of multiple ones.

Common Motor Deficits

There is a wide spectrum of motor deficits that may be seen after TBI. This spectrum results from the variable nature of the injury itself and the combination of focal and diffuse damage.

Focal Damage

Obviously, if there is a penetrating or focal injury involving the motor area, a hemiparesis may result. Depending on the precise location of the damage, hemiparesis may be more pronounced in the upper or lower extremity.

Diffuse Damage

The diffuse nature of TBI has resulted in a constellation of motor impairment that is familiar

TABLE 13–2. Rating of Severity of Brain Injury

	Mild	Moderate	Severe	Profound
Initial Glasgow Coma Scale	13-15 with no deterioration	9-12 with no deterioration	3-8	
Posttraumatic Amnesia	< 1 hr	1-24 hr	> 24 hr	
Duration of Unconsciousness	< 15–30 min	15 min–24 hr	1–90 days	> 90 days

to clinicians who work with these problems. These include difficulties with balance, coordination, and speed of response. Despite these impairments, however, a significant number of children achieve functional mobility. In a study by Boyer and Edwards,[40] at 1 year after injury, 46% of their patients walked independently without assistive device, and 27% walked with orthoses or assistive device. Overall, 79% had independent mobility.

Swaine and Sullivan[41] have examined early motor recovery after TBI in 16 adolescents and adults who had a GCS score of 8 or less for at least 6 hours. Assessments included evaluation of muscle tone, range of motion, abnormal and voluntary movement, primitive reflexes, equilibrium and protective responses, and specific motor skills. There were differential patterns of recovery and differential rates of recovery among the subjects, which is to be expected considering the heterogeneous nature of TBI.

Chaplin and colleagues[42] evaluated motor performance in children after TBI. Fourteen children with TBI who were unconscious for 24 hours or longer were compared with 14 age-matched and sex-matched children. The Bruininks-Oseretsky Test of Motor Proficiency was administered at least 16 months after injury. Children with TBI scored significantly poorer on the Gross Motor Composite, including all subsets—running speed, balance, bilateral coordination, and strength. Also, they scored lower on the fine motor subtest for upper-limb speed and dexterity. Most of these subtests involve timed tasks. Chaplin and colleagues also found a correlation between the Gross Motor Composite score and the time since injury. They concluded that this correlation supports continuing long-term improvement in skills after TBI.

Others have also noted impaired fine motor skills after TBI. Again the speed component of the assessment on these tasks may account for some of the impairments that were observed. Long-term impairment of finger tapping has also been described.[43] Practice of activities requiring fine motor coordination improves skills, even long after injury.[44]

Balance

Balance is commonly abnormal after TBI. Cochlear and vestibular function may be impaired. True vertigo may be present as well as clinical evidence of impaired balance. Meclizine may be of benefit.[45] When postural instability is assessed quantitatively, long-term impairment of static and dynamic control of posture is often found after TBI.[46,47] It may be related to latency of response and asymmetric stance.[48] It was also suggested that specific training may be helpful.[49]

Tremor

Another motor impairment is tremor, which frequently is more pronounced proximally and increases with effort and movement. Lesions have been noted in varying areas. Treatment with medications typically used for tremor may be of benefit.[50,51]

Dystonia

Dystonia has been reported as a rare motor impairment and more commonly seen in those injured as children than as adults.[52,53] Interval between injury and onset of dystonia varies. No consistent picture is seen on neuroimaging study. Multiple pharmacologic interventions have been tried with little effectiveness.

Spasticity and Rigidity

Diagnosis. Muscle tone abnormalities are common after TBI. The type of problems noted varies depending on the time since injury as well as the severity of injury. Cause of acquired brain injury also influences the type of problem that is most commonly noted. Spasticity has been noted in 38% and combined spasticity and ataxia in 39% of children and adolescents 1 year after injury.[36] Spasticity results from an upper motor neuron injury and is manifested by increased deep tendon reflexes and a velocity-dependent resistance to movement.[54] After TBI, individuals may also have difficulty with rigidity, dystonia, or posturing. Rigidity or dystonia is seen especially when there has been secondary injury due to hypoxia or ischemia.[55]

Physical Management. It is important to treat spasticity when it interferes with function or results in a tendency to develop contractures. Several treatment approaches exist. Range of motion itself may be helpful to reduce tone temporarily.[56] Also, one may begin with positioning options, including but not limited to splinting and weight bearing, if tolerated, as well as the use of neutral warmth, gentle shaking, and reflex inhibition.[57] If a child has a tendency to assume a total extension posture, positioning in side-lying with hips flexed beyond 90 degrees and neck flexion may assist in interrupting the extension pattern. If active posturing is present, one must be careful in the use of splints and casts because constant pressure against the splint or cast may result in the development of an ischemic ulcer.[57]

Pharmacologic Management. In addition to positioning, splinting, and casting, the use of botulinum toxin and phenol motor point blocks may be helpful. Early after injury, with severe posturing and intolerance of splinting, botulinum toxin may be a helpful adjunct in attempting to maintain range of motion. It is reversible, so if there is significant motor recovery, there is no permanent effect of the injection. There may be functional gains with the longer-term use of botulinum toxin.[58] Phenol blocks tend to be used later after injury when there is residual difficulty with increased tone. If severe deformity exists, surgical tendon or muscle lengthening may need to be considered.[55]

Enterally administered pharmacologic agents may also be beneficial in decreasing abnormal muscle tone and posturing. Their potential side effects may limit their effectiveness in this population. This is especially true of the sedating effects of baclofen and benzodiazepines. Dantrolene sodium may also produce sedation. Alpha-adrenergic agonists, such as clonidine and tizanidine, have also been reported to decrease tone.[54,59,60] The effectiveness of all of these medications is variable.

Early after injury, when posturing may be a problem, chlorpromazine has been of assistance. It has the significant potential to sedate.[54] Bromocriptine has also been effective in reducing posturing early postinjury.

Intrathecal baclofen has been shown to be effective in the treatment of spasticity of cerebral origin, particularly cerebral palsy.[61,62] The authors have found intrathecal baclofen to be helpful in the reduction of spasticity and dystonic rigidity in a few individuals with traumatic and anoxic brain injuries. Further investigation of this intervention in TBI would be helpful to evaluate its long-term efficacy.

Common Sensory Deficits

Anosmia

Anosmia is a common consequence of TBI. A partial loss of the sense of smell, microsmia, has also been reported. There have been efforts to locate and quantify the deficits using radiographic studies. Most patients with impaired olfaction showed damage to the olfactory bulbs and tracts, temporal lobes, or subfrontal areas. There is usually poor recovery from anosmia.[63,64] Impairment in the sense of smell may have social and safety implications. Those with anosmia must be cautioned to use other senses to look for dangers, such as a gas burner left on, fire hazard, or similar problems. Teenagers and young adults may need to be advised about the use of fragrance when they cannot receive any feedback about its strength.

Hearing Impairment

Hearing impairments and impairments of vestibular function are also commonly noted. Vestibular impairments have already been briefly mentioned in the discussion on balance. Hearing impairment may occur secondary to several causes: central processing deficit, peripheral nerve damage, cochlear injury, or disruption of the middle ear structures. Cognitive impairments that are common after TBI often interfere with the child recognizing the difficulty. It is important for clinicians to have a high index of suspicion and initiate screening for hearing impairment.

Central auditory processing impairment occurs with damage to tracts or cortical tissue. In such individuals, pure tone audiometry is normal, but other studies, such as speech discrimination or late wave forms of brain stem auditory evoked potentials, are abnormal.[65] Central auditory impairment is difficult for most families to understand. Their intuitive conclusion is that hearing is related to the ear, so they frequently anticipate that intervention such as a hearing aid may be helpful.

Hearing loss may be conductive in nature because of disruption of the ossicles or because of cerebrospinal fluid or blood in the middle ear. Both these types of injuries are frequently associated with fractures of the temporal bone. Problems related to fluid in the middle ear usually resolve spontaneously. Surgical exploration and repair of ossicular disruption may be indicated.[66]

Sensorineural hearing loss may also be seen. There may be trauma to the eighth cranial nerve or injury to the labyrinthine capsule or labyrinthine concussion, which may result in loss of hearing because of the transmission of high-energy vibration and a pattern similar to the hearing loss after prolonged noise exposure.[66] Injuries to the labyrinthine capsule and the eighth cranial nerve are frequently associated with basilar skull fracture.

Visual Impairment

Because of the complexity of the visual system, a variety of visual impairments may be seen. Impairments may result from injury to cranial nerves, eyes, optic chiasm, tracts, radiations, or cortical structures.[67] Early after injury, a child may appear to be functionally blind. Although vision is often assessed by looking at response to visual threat and visual tracking, these responses do not differentiate between peripheral and central impairments. One must assess cranial nerve function to attempt to make that differentiation.

Optic nerve injury is reported to occur in 1.5% of cases, either complete or partial, and results in impaired visual acuity. It is correlated with the site of impact and not necessarily with the overall severity of the brain injury. Usually, optic atrophy is a sign that is seen within 1 month after injury.[67] Chiasmatic injury results in bitemporal visual field impairment of varying degree and is found in 0.3% of TBI cases. It may be identified on MR imaging.[68]

Homonymous hemianopsia is seen with injuries to the optic tracts and is often associated with hemorrhage and hemiparesis. Prism lenses may be of assistance as well as learning compensatory techniques to increase scanning of the full environment.[69] The presence of visual field impairments may be associated with more severe neuropsychological impairment.[70]

Central visual dysfunction may be described as visual processing or visual perceptual problems. Cortical injury is responsible for this type of impairment and may not be confined to the occipital lobes. For example, involvement of temporal lobes may produce visual memory impairment, and involvement of parietal lobes may produce impairment of spatial awareness.[71]

Injury of the third, fourth, and sixth cranial nerves may lead to a variety of visual problems.[72] Diplopia may result from extraocular muscle imbalance and may be present at all times or just in particular gazes. Patching is commonly used to eliminate diplopia but results in monocular vision and related disadvantages.[73] In children under 11 years old, it is important to patch eyes in an alternating manner to avoid difficulty with ambliopia.

Difficulties with convergence may also result in diplopia and are believed to be due to supranuclear impairment. Anatomic correlates of diplopia have not been well described.[72] Accommodation may also be impaired.

Common Cognitive Deficits

Cognitive and communication deficits are of significant importance after TBI and are believed to be the largest cause of disability in this group.[74] A constellation of cognitive sequelae is commonly seen after TBI. These sequelae include difficulties with attention and arousal, memory, and higher executive functions. Injury to children is of particular importance because they are still developing and acquiring new cognitive skills. Impairments in these skills can result in learning problems and have profound effects on their ability to function as adults. Also, one may not see the full consequences of the injury until the children reach the age at which one would expect them to have a particular skill. For example, deficits in abstract reasoning in a child who experienced a TBI at age 4 years would not be evident until later.[18,75]

Impairment of Arousal and Attention

Arousal and attention are common areas of impairment. One of the challenges of early rehabilitation is to maintain arousal or a state of readiness to process sensory information and produce a response.[76] There has been interest in looking at pharmacologic intervention for impairments of arousal and attention, as a result of experimental evidence that neurotransmitters decrease after brain injury. It has been suggested that dopamine, norepinephrine, tricyclic antidepressants, and serotonin may be beneficial for disorders of arousal.[77–80] Although variable success has been seen, those publications are generally case reports and not controlled studies. Because studies of children are lacking, it is difficult to draw conclusions for this age group.

Attention allows the individual to focus on the pertinent sensory stimuli and select which stimulus will elicit a response. It is assessed in indirect ways, usually in timed cognitive tasks.[76] Attentional disorders are among the most common deficits noted after TBI, and disorders may persist long-term in significant injury.[81] Difficulty with maintaining attention may at least partially be responsible for the impairment of memory that is commonly seen after TBI as well. Attention deficit is also a problem in many children without TBI, and hyperactive children seem to be more likely to sustain TBI. In one study of consecutive patients admitted to a pediatric rehabilitation program, 35% had a history of learning disability, attention deficit, or emotional problems before the accident.[40] Similar pharmacologic interventions are used for attention deficits related to TBI or independent from TBI. Stimulant medications include methylphenidate, D-amphetamine, and pemoline. The authors' experience has been that stimulants are most effective when the child has had a history of attention disorder before injury.

Agitation

Another impairment of arousal may actually be a hyperaroused state, or agitation or restlessness. Damage to frontal lobes and subcortical areas may result in agitation,which may be associated with more severe injury.[82] The first line of treatment for agitation should be control of the child's immediate environment, by limiting stimulation, using an enclosed or padded bed or room for safety, and perhaps one-to-one supervision. A number of different medications have been tried to help control agitation, including clonidine, bromocriptine, amantadine, tricyclic antidepressants, and buspirone.[82,83] These medications should be stopped after the period of agitation because their use may produce negative side effects.

Memory Impairment

Memory and learning are often affected, particularly in moderate-to-severe injury. Jaffe and colleagues[37] have shown that injury severity correlated with memory deficits. Academic performance also was correlated to the severity of injury. The area that showed the least improvement over the 1 year studied was academic skills. They postulated that academic progress or learning is affected by multiple variables, including the period of absence from school, difficulty with speed of processing, memory, and residual motor skill impairments. They also noted, as have other clinicians, that on many normed assessments, children with TBI do deceptively well despite their difficulties with academic skills. Lord-Maes and Obrzut[84] agree that typical educational assessment may not elucidate the difficulties that a child with TBI is experiencing and have recommended specialized neuropsychologic assessment. Even with such an assessment, children often do not function at the level one would expect from their test scores. It has been suggested that they are unable to use the skills and fund of knowledge that they have with speed and efficiency.[85] Pharmacologic agents used to treat spasticity or epilepsy may contribute to impairment of memory and attention. For example, benzodiazepines, methyldopa, and phenytoin may adversely affect cognitive abilities.[77] There has also been interest in attempting to improve memory through pharmacologic intervention. It has been postulated that memory impairment relates to a deficit in acetylcholine. Therefore administration of acetylcholine-esterase inhibitors may be of benefit.[77,86] Data are not available concerning the use of these agents in children and adolescents.

Altered Performance IQ

When children with TBI are assessed by measurement of performance intelligence quotient (IQ), pronounced impairment may be seen.[85,87] Max and colleagues[88] found that performance IQ correlated with the severity of injury, even when measured several years later. Likewise, Chadwick and colleagues[89] found differences between their study and control groups in IQ score. They also found that the performance score continued to improve over the first year after injury, but the majority of improvement occurred in the first 4 months. Deficits have been noted particularly for tasks that require speed, including reports of decreased response speed.[87]

Impairment of Communication

Impairment of communication is a common problem. Boyer and Edwards[40] found that two-thirds of their patients had difficulty with communication. One-third had dysarthria. The manifestations of communication impairment can be quite varied. For some individuals, it may involve focal deficits associated with focal injuries, but for the majority of patients with closed, nonpenetrating injuries, there is a typical constellation of sequelae. Studies have demonstrated long-term impairment of language.[40,90] Many individuals with TBI test relatively well in vocabulary but show difficulty with naming, verbal fluency, and expression.[90] Prosody and discourse ability have been reported to be impaired as well.[91] It has been suggested that the language problems seen after TBI have the appearance of a subclinical aphasia.[90] The age at injury may influence the ultimate language outcome, as the young child will have experienced less language development before injury.[92]

Behavioral Sequelae

It is common to see behavioral changes after TBI. Families have reported these to be particularly significant and long-term.[93] Children who sustain TBI during preschool years have an increased risk of later behavioral problems that interfere with school performance.[94]

An often-noted deficit is in impulse control, either verbally or motorically. It is thought that this relates to frontal lobe injury.[88] Disinhibition may be manifested as a wide spectrum of behaviors ranging from poor judgment to rage responses in response to minimal provocation. Adolescents may also exhibit hypersexuality. Multiple methods of intervention may be employed to control behavior, including changes in the environment, behavioral techniques, cognitive therapy, and pharmacologic means.[95] A variety of medications have been used, including haloperidol, propranolol, buspirone, amitriptyline, bromocriptine, carbamazepine, valproate, phenytoin, and lithium.[95–97] As is often the case, these reports are in adults, and there is no published information about their efficacy for children.

Abnormal Emotional Expression

Initially, lack of emotional expression is common. In some cases, parents have been concerned by their child's lack of ability to cry, laugh, or smile. Later, emotional lability is frequent and may persist as a long-term problem.[88] The authors have also noted in some children the apparent inability to recognize the emotional responses of others based on the inability to recognize the auditory and visual cues presented to them by others. It was hypothesized that this may be due to difficulty with processing visual spatial information; however, that was not the case in a study of 12 children with TBI. It was then suggested that there may be specific pathways for processing emotional information.[98]

Impairment of Abstract Reasoning

Frequently after TBI, children and adolescents have an impairment of abstract thinking. This affects many aspects of their lives, including not only the ability to function in school, but also their insight into their own areas of weakness and strength. Often when children are asked how they are different now compared with before the injury, they list physical problems, such as weakness, tremor, or balance, but not cognitive problems, such as memory, attention, or impulse control deficits. Also, it is common to note significant egocentricity. Brain-injured children see themselves at the center of everything. When children with TBI have difficulty making themselves understood, they may perceive it as a function of the other person's ability to hear, not their own inability to express themselves. They also frequently have difficulty in the give and take of social exchange.

Social Isolation

Social isolation is often seen after TBI. There are a number of reasons that contribute to this. In normal social exchanges, the child must focus attention on the relevant information, process it quickly to formulate an appropriate response, and be able to refocus and shift set often. This is difficult for the child with TBI. Also the difficulties noted with recognition of emotional cues from others and the general egocentrism seen after TBI contribute to social isolation. People who experience TBI as adolescents appear to have difficulty forming lasting social relationships.[99]

Medical Conditions Associated with Traumatic Brain Injury

There are a number of medical conditions associated with TBI. These vary greatly and can occur directly as a result of the damage to the brain or be associated with multiple trauma and its stress.

Neuroendocrine Dysfunction

Several different types of neuroendocrine dysfunction can be a direct result of the brain injury. The hormonal deficits may be complete or partial. Compression of the pituitary or hypothalamus by edema, fractures, hemorrhage, increased intracranial pressure, and ischemic necrosis secondary to impaired vascular supply may cause these abnormalities.[100] There has also been MR imaging evidence of hypothalamic atrophy.[101]

Diabetes Insipidus

Disorders of fluid and sodium balance may be seen. Diabetes insipidus is characterized by excessive water loss because of a deficiency of antidiuretic hormone (ADH). ADH is produced in the hypothalamus. Those who exhibit diabetes insipidus may also have other hypothalamic disorders. Individuals with diabetes insipidus experience hypernatremic dehydration, polyuria, and polydipsia.[102] Desmopressin acetate (DDAVP) is a synthetic analogue of ADH and is available in tablet, intranasal, or injectable forms. Monitoring of fluid intake and output, urine specific gravity, and restriction of oral fluid intake along with the use of DDAVP may be indicated. Diabetes insipidus is most frequently a temporary problem but may persist and requires careful follow-up.

Syndrome of Inappropriate Antidiuretic Hormone Secretion

Syndrome of inappropriate ADH secretion (SIADH) may also be seen complicating fluid and electrolyte management after TBI. It is associated with decreased urine output, hyponatremia, and a decreased serum osmolarity. The dilutional hyponatremia can generally be managed by fluid restriction.[21] In cases in which fluid restriction is not possible, demeclocycline has been helpful.[103] Rapid correction of serum sodium can cause pontine myelinolysis.[104]

Cerebral Salt Wasting

Cerebral salt wasting syndrome has been reported to be another cause of hyponatremia. It is thought to occur because of direct neural effect on renal tubular function. In these individuals, their hyponatremia is not dilutional, and they are, in fact, volume-depleted, and therefore fluid restriction would be contraindicated. Signs of dehydration and hypovolemia are the key to differentiating cerebral salt wasting from SIADH.[104]

Precocious Puberty

Precocious puberty occasionally develops in young children who have had severe brain injuries.[105–109] In one series of 33 children who had severe TBIs before the onset of puberty, precious puberty was noted in 7.[110] Initial signs of precocious puberty occurred 2 to 17 months after injury. Girls seemed at greater risk for this complication with 54.5% versus 4.5% female-to-male ratio. In addition to precocious secondary sexual development, the affected children showed accelerated linear growth and advanced bone ages after 2 years. Diabetes insipidus, transient in two, was also present in three of the children with precocious puberty. No other endocrine abnormalities were seen concurrently. In this consecutive series, the clinical severity of brain injury was similar in children with or without precocious puberty. The degree of ventricular dilation appeared worse in children with precocious puberty than those without. Focal hypothalamic injury has been demonstrated by MR imaging in one child with precocious puberty.[106]

Authors of another series of severe TBI in young children saw no clear evidence of precocious puberty.[111] Only 12 of 21 patients were prepubertal at the time of injury. Furthermore, only four girls were injured at vulnerable ages. Therefore, it is likely that the series did not have sufficient numbers of children, especially girls, at risk to observe this complication. Also the children reported in this series had only a single examination and were not followed longitudinally.

The preponderance of girls with precocious puberty in the series by Sockalosky and colleagues[110] is in contrast with the sex distribution observed by Balagura and colleagues[112] in another series of precocious puberty of cerebral origin. Precocious puberty is seen more frequently in girls when all causes are considered together.[113,114] A lower threshold for disruption of the luteinizing hormone–releasing hormone (LH-RH) and an earlier maturation of the hypothalamic-pituitary axis has been hypothesized for the increased incidence of precocious puberty in girls.[110]

The onset of precocious puberty creates significant social and emotional consequences for children and their families, more so when occurring in a child with a previous severe brain injury. In addition to these factors, it often results in shortened adult stature because of premature epiphyseal closure. For these reasons, the authors often consider beginning LH-RH analogue therapy in children who have this complication.

Other Endocrine Problems

Other endocrinologic problems associated with hypothalamic or pituitary damage may be seen as well. In contrast to diabetes insipidus and SIADH, the manifestation of these may be less acute. Deficiencies of growth hormone and gonadotropins are seen more commonly than those of corticotropin and thyrotropin. Tests often indicate abnormalities of both pituitary and hypothalamus.[101] Spontaneous recovery of anterior pituitary function is uncommon.[21] Long-term hormonal therapy is usually required.

Respiratory Dysfunction

Most children who ultimately are transferred to a rehabilitation program after TBI have been acutely intubated as part of the initial management of their injury. If prolonged intubation is required for airway management, these children are likely to have a tracheostomy. One study noted that in TBI, the majority of children who had undergone tracheostomy had been decannulated by 6 months after injury.[115] Typically, one downsizes the tracheostomy tube in preparation for plugging the tube. Eventual decannulation is done if the plugging is tolerated. An otolaryngologist can assist with bedside endoscopy to rule out any complications that may interfere with decannulation. Late complications may be seen from prolonged intubation and may include stenosis of the trachea in glottic or subglottic areas, tracheomalacia, and vocal cord injury or paralysis. Pneumonia may be an early respiratory complication.[21]

Gastrointestinal Concerns

Nutritional Management

Nutritional concerns are important in TBI. In the early stage, the child is in a hypermetabolic state. This has been well documented in adults and appears to be mediated by sympathetic hyperactivity.[116] Limited information available on children also supports this. Early after injury, parenteral means may be used to provide nutrition, but usually rapid change to enteral nutrition is possible.

Tube Feedings. Initially, jejunal tubes are frequently used because of concerns about decreased level of responsiveness, reflux, and aspiration. In addition, there is often delayed gastric emptying early after injury.[21] Rehabilitation settings attempt to simulate the home environment as much as possible. It is often helpful to be able to convert children from continuous to intermittent bolus feedings. This allows for a more normal mealtime and decreases the amount of equipment that must accompany the child.[21] The authors also find it helpful to change from nasogastric or nasojejunal tubes to a percutaneously or surgically placed gastrostomy tube relatively early in the rehabilitation stay. Nasogastric and nasojejunal tubes are associated with an increased risk of sinusitis. The presence of the tube in the posterior pharynx may be a source of irritation for a restless or agitated child and may interfere with attempts to assess and facilitate oral motor function and the reintroduction of oral feeding. Splaingard et al.[115] noted that in children gastrostomy tube placement was at a mean of 29 days after injury.

Gastroesophageal Reflux. Before gastrostomy placement, it is advisable to evaluate the child for possible gastroesophageal reflux by an upper gastrointestinal radiologic study, pH probe study, or milk scan. The presence of reflux in a child at risk for aspiration may necessitate surgical intervention to prevent reflux. Nonsurgical means to treat reflux include pharmacologic intervention to decrease gastric acidity and speed gastric emptying as well as elevating the head of the bed.

Transition to Oral Feeding. Speech and language pathology, occupational therapy, and rehabilitation nursing clinicians are all important team members in the attempt to facilitate transition from tube to oral feeding. All can participate in the oral motor stimulation program and in the assessment of positioning and responsiveness as a component of oral feeding. Speech and language pathology along with radiology participate in videofluoroscopic assessment of swallowing and look at the child's ability to handle various consistencies. When able to progress to oral feeding trial, nursing is in a key position to assess oral intake, monitor quantity, and assist in decreasing tube feeding proportionally.

Risk and Prevention of Gastrointestinal Hemorrhage

Early after TBI, individuals often experience a hyperacidic state, potentially as a result of the physiologic stress as well as the administration of corticosteroids. H_2-receptor blockers are commonly used to decrease the risk of gastrointestinal bleeding.[21]

Bowel Management

It is important to establish routine bowel management programs. Early after injury, children may experience gastrointestinal motility reduction on the basis of the injury itself or because of the side effects of some of the narcotic medications administered to assist in the control of intracranial pressure. Use of suppositories to help stimulate bowel evacuation on a routine basis as well as tube feeding formulas with fiber or adding other sources of fiber may be helpful. Some of the commercially available agents for thickening liquids may contribute to constipation.

Bladder Management

Short-term bladder management is to ensure that fluid intake and output are appropriately balanced. When the child is incontinent, output can be measured by weighing diapers. Monitoring of urine specific gravity can also be of assistance in evaluating any difficulty with fluid and electrolyte balance. Later after injury, bladder management becomes a more cognitively based activity, initially beginning with a timed toileting type of program. If incontinence persists, the individual may have a neurogenic bladder with uninhibited bladder contractions. Usually, postvoiding residual volumes are not elevated.[117] Management with anticholinergics may be helpful for increasing bladder volume.

Central Autonomic Dysfunction

Diagnosis

Central autonomic dysfunction (CAD) is a clinical entity manifested by symptoms such as unexplained elevated temperatures, systemic hypertension, sweating, generalized rigidity, decerebrate posturing, and rapid breathing. This syndrome has been recognized by a number of labels, including diencephalic seizures,[118] autonomic dysfunction syndrome,[119] hypothalamic-midbrain dysregulation syndrome,[120] central fever,[121] and posttraumatic hyperthermia.[122]

The clinical features of CAD vary somewhat from patient to patient. The symptoms begin soon after acquired brain injury, usually during the first week.[123] Almost all patients have more than one symptom of CAD simultaneously.[123] Individual episodes of CAD generally last for several hours. Patients with prenatal brain injuries may have dysthermia for most of their lives. Many children with acquired brain injury had some improvement over time; however, 6 of 20 children with CAD still required medical management of CAD 6 or more months after injury.[123]

Epidemiology and Mechanisms

CAD is commonly observed in persons who have had traumatic and other brain injury. CAD was found in 14% of 220 children with severe acquired brain injuries.[123] CAD in this series was seen more frequently after anoxic than traumatic injury. Unexpected low or high body temperature is also commonly seen in persons who have been institutionalized because of brain damage. Approximately 8% of residents in one report had a history of this problem. All had severe cognitive impairment, and approximately one third had brain damage of prenatal origin.[124]

Regardless of cause, the mechanism of CAD is presumed to involve hypothalamic or brain stem dysfunction. Lesions in these areas have been found in some patients with symptoms of CAD, leading to a hypothesis that CAD results from a diencephalic–brain stem disconnection syndrome or brain stem release phenomena.[120] Injury to axons controlling arginine vasopressin has also been hypothesized.[125]

Prognosis of Children with Central Autonomic Dysfunction

The development of CAD features has rather serious implications with regard to prognosis. In a retrospective review in a series of children with acquired brain injury, the presence of CAD after acquired brain injury was correlated with more protracted periods of unconsciousness and worse cognitive and motor outcomes a year or more after injury.[123] Follow-up computed tomography (CT) scans in these children generally showed ventricular enlargement with brain atrophy.

Management of Central Autonomic Dysfunction

The management of CAD can be challenging. Elevated body temperatures are often the initial manifestations of concern to the clinician. When the hyperthermia is initially detected, an extensive evaluation is needed to rule out a treatable infectious illness. In contrast to fever resulting from infectious causes, the hyperthermia associated with CAD may respond poorly to nonsteroidal antiinflammatory drugs.[119] In children,

the authors find that cooling blankets and sponge baths are usually more effective in lowering body temperature.

Systemic hypertension can be alarming. Propranolol is clinically effective in the management of the hypertension and elevated temperature resulting from CAD after TBI.[121] Posttraumatic autonomic dysfunction may respond to bromocriptine and morphine.[118] Using bromocriptine or chlorpromazine in management of 26 of 31 children with CAD after acquired brain injury, the authors have found that these drugs, which are thought to have central effects, can result in decreased need or elimination of antipyretics and antihypertensive medications.[123] The authors continue bromocriptine or thorazine until the child is no longer showing CAD features while on therapy. There have been no controlled series comparing the efficacy of the various pharmacologic approaches.

Heterotopic Ossification

Patients at Risk

Heterotopic ossification is ectopic bone formation and is reported to occur in 14–23% of pediatric TBI patients.[21] Heterotopic ossification is noted to be more common in children over age 11, in those with more severe injury, and in those who had two or more extremity fractures.[126] Most commonly, hips and knees are the sites of ectopic bone formation.[126,127] Because heterotopic ossification is seen more frequently after severe injury, it is associated with poor outcome.

Diagnosis and Management

Heterotopic ossification is usually diagnosed a month or later after injury and suspected because of pain, decreased range of motion, and sometimes swelling.[127] Deep venous thrombosis is unusual in children but may be seen in association with heterotopic ossification.[128] Treatment includes aggressive passive range of motion, splinting and positioning, and nonsteroidal antiinflammatory agents.[126,127] In adults, disodium etidronate has been used, but has been reported to result in a reversible rachitic syndrome when used in a growing child.[129] Heterotopic ossification rarely results in functional impairment or requires surgical intervention in children and adolescents.[21,126,127]

Posttraumatic Epilepsy

The Controversy Concerning Prophylaxis of Posttraumatic Epilepsy

The incidence of seizures is increased both early and late, after 1–2 weeks, after TBI. A patient who has two or more seizures late after TBI is considered to have posttraumatic epilepsy (PTE). In adults, the occurrence of early posttraumatic seizures is correlated with an increased risk of development of PTE; however, that is not seen in children.[130] The risk of development of PTE is correlated with the severity of the TBI.[130] Neither children nor adults who have had minor TBI have an increased risk of PTE compared with the general population. Late seizures occur in 1.6% and 7.4% of children with moderate or severe injury.[130] Clinicians have long been aware of the increased likelihood of PTE after severe TBI.

When antiepileptic drugs became available, there was an attempt to prevent seizures and PTE using medication proven to be effective in managing epilepsy. It has become tradition to begin antiepileptic therapy, generally using phenytoin, in many institutions. Until recently, however, controlled clinical trials had not been conducted to demonstrate the effectiveness of this practice. A large, double-blind, placebo-controlled study of adults with severe TBI has been concluded using phenytoin. Although early seizures were decreased in the treated group, there was no effect in preventing PTE (the tendency to have late seizures) with phenytoin therapy.[131] In fact, a slightly greater but not statistically significant incidence of PTE was observed in those patients receiving phenytoin. A smaller placebo-controlled clinical trial in children with TBI also has shown no efficacy in prevention of PTE using phenytoin therapy.[132]

When medication was discontinued after 1 year of prophylactic therapy, greater functional improvement in some neuropsychological measures occurred in adults who had been receiving phenytoin than did in those in the placebo group.[131,133] This improvement after drug withdrawal implies that phenytoin not only was ineffective in the prevention of PTE, but also was actually detrimental to patients after TBI. Another smaller double-blind, placebo-controlled study reported that both carbamazepine and phenytoin had negative effects on cognitive performance for those recovering from TBI.[134] Because phenytoin fails to prevent PTE and because of its detrimental effect on patients with TBI, the authors concur with Hernandez and Naritoku[135] that prophylactic antiepileptic medication should not be used.

Nevertheless, many children are on phenytoin at the time of transfer to the rehabilitation service. Most children should be withdrawn from phenytoin as soon as possible. If the child has had no seizures after the TBI, the authors obtain a drug level. If that is in a subtherapeutic range, the drug can be immediately discontinued. If therapeutic levels are seen, the dose can be reduced by approximately 50% for 1 week and then discontinued. With this practice, seizures are rarely encountered on the rehabilitation service. If the child has had seizures in the early posttraumatic period, the authors first obtain an electroencephalogram (EEG). If the EEG shows no epileptiform activity, the authors withdraw the child from phenytoin. When definite epileptiform activity is seen on the EEG, a more cautious approach is indicated, and generally phenytoin or other anticonvulsant therapy is continued.

Management of Posttraumatic Epilepsy

When the child continues to have seizures beyond the early posttraumatic period, antiepileptic therapy should be maintained. Drugs with the least depression of cognitive function should be used in the lowest clinically effective dose. Sedating drugs, such as barbiturates or benzodiazepines, should be avoided whenever possible. Because phenytoin frequently has undesirable cosmetic effects and it is difficult to regulate dosage because of nonlinear kinetics, other medications are preferable. Phenytoin, carbamazepine, and valproic acid appear to have comparable negative effects in patients who have had TBI.[136] The authors most frequently use carbamazepine; however, valproate or one of the newer antiepileptic medications is also useful. Fewer adverse effects are seen when monotherapy is used.

Cerebral Atrophy and Hydrocephalus

Enlargement of the ventricular system is commonly seen after severe TBI in children.[137] Ventricular enlargement can be the result either of decrease in brain volume or of obstruction of cerebrospinal fluid flow. True hydrocephalus is almost always the result of obstruction of cerebrospinal fluid flow or absorption and is accompanied by an increase of cerebrospinal fluid pressure and volume. Decrease in brain volume is the end result of a destructive or degenerative process and is recognized as cerebral atrophy or hydrocephalus ex vacuo. The latter term implies that the ventricular system is enlarged to fill the vacuum resulting from loss of brain volume. Cerebral atrophy (or hydrocephalus ex vacuo) is far more frequently seen after severe brain injury than is true hydrocephalus.

What are the clues in the differential diagnosis of cerebral atrophy as opposed to hydrocephalus? Most importantly, by the time atrophy is developing, the child is beginning to show modest clinical improvement, whereas the child with hydrocephalus may show clinical deterioration. In addition, there are usually hints on the CT or MR imaging brain scans. When atrophy is present, frequently there are additional abnormalities, such as areas of encephalomalacia or enlarged sulci.

Neuroimaging and Electroencephalography

Modern neuroimaging techniques (CT and MR imaging brain scans) have proven to be invaluable in the assessment and management of the acute brain-injured patient. The combination of MR imaging and single-photon emission computed tomography (SPECT) scans in some studies has improved the ability to predict outcome.[138] In the context of the child on the rehabilitation service after the initial stabilization phase, scans are generally obtained to assess if acute lesions have resolved and to help understand and predict future clinical function. The clinician caring for children involved in motor vehicle accidents is often called on to testify as a treating physician in legal proceedings. The objective and easily demonstrated images from CT and MR imaging scans are often helpful in illustrating the physician's testimony. In many cases, scans are useful in communications with parents, who may find it difficult to understand why their child has not shown a more significant recovery. In most cases, a follow-up CT or MR imaging scan is obtained 1–2 months after injury. Information from these scans can contribute to understanding the clinical course and influences physicians' statements to families. For example, a follow-up scan that is only mildly abnormal in a still unconscious child would support the parents' hopes for substantial improvement.

There has been some interest in correlating neuropsychological outcome and imaging findings in children.[139,149] MR imaging has been noted to detect abnormalities not seen on CT imaging. Also, evidence has suggested that frontal lesion size is correlated to severity of cognitive impairment.[140]

EEG has a limited role in the evaluation and management of most children after TBI. It has not been helpful in determining severity of injury and prognosis for improvement and therefore does not have to be obtained on most children with TBI. EEGs should be performed on children who have had seizures within the first 2 weeks after injury before deciding whether or not to stop antiepileptic therapy. Of course the EEG is invaluable in confirming clinically suspected seizures. Occasionally when interictal EEGs are nondiagnostic and the clinical events are of sufficient concern, continuous EEG monitoring is indicated to record a clinical event.

Early Rehabilitation

Rehabilitation involves the prevention of secondary impairment or disability, facilitation of improved function, and education in the use of compensatory techniques. Evaluating and potentially modifying the child's environment is also an important consideration in minimizing handicap. It is imperative that children with TBI be involved with rehabilitation services.

Rehabilitation efforts should begin while the child is in the ICU. Early efforts should be aimed at reducing potential complications of immobility. These include ischemic ulcers, compression neuropathy, and contractures. Complications due to excessive pressure can be prevented by frequent repositioning, special mattresses, and padding bony prominences. Also, stimulation therapy is important during the ICU stay. Stimulation therapy involves presenting a brief structured stimulus for which one anticipates a response. It is a means of frequently assessing the child but does not cause awakening. Sometimes, rehabilitation interventions in the ICU must be limited because stimulation can increase intracranial pressure.[57]

It is also helpful to have a social worker begin to meet with the family while the child is still in the ICU to begin education about brain injury and the rehabilitation process as well as to provide support.[57,141] Some authors have found that initiating rehabilitation services early shortens the overall hospital and rehabilitation stay.[141,142] Early transfer to a rehabilitation setting is indicated as soon as the patient is medically stable.

Inpatient Rehabilitation

Sensory Stimulation

Even before a child is following commands, rehabilitation may be initiated. In addition to providing structured stimulation and assessing responses on a frequent basis, physical and occupational therapy may work with positioning, including specialized equipment, and activities. Head and trunk control are facilitated. Also, localized responses are channeled into more purposeful activity using hand-over-hand techniques. Oral stimulation is started to help with evaluating oral motor function and may facilitate more control and begin the process of evaluating for the attempt to transition to oral feeding.[57]

Computer-assisted Services

Computer-assisted rehabilitation can be used at many times in the rehabilitation continuum. Even when a child is not as yet consistently following commands, computer programs may be useful to elicit auditory or visual attention. As responses increase, various types of switches can be used to assess the understanding of causality. Obviously, with children who are cognitively able, there is a wealth of software available to work on various cognitive areas and provide structure and immediate feedback in reference to performance.[57] The use of computers in rehabilitation activities can continue after discharge from the inpatient service. Although commonly used, there is no certainty whether computer-assisted therapy is more effective than more traditional neurorehabilitative intervention. Computers are only one facet of the overall rehabilitation approach.[143]

Interventions Based on the Cognitive Level

As children become more responsive and interactive, therapy can become more cognitively based, addressing specific areas of identified deficits that have been previously noted. An eclectic therapeutic approach should be used.[144] Classic neurorehabilitative therapy approaches, adaptive equipment, the use of technology, and environmental modification all have the ultimate goal of increasing the child's independence and ability to function and continue to facilitate ongoing development and acquisition of skills.

Psychosocial Services

An acquired brain injury of a child changes the entire family. Roles and responsibilities change, and the degree of disability affects the family's future activities and opportunities.[145] Supportive services are essential not only for the injured child, but also for the entire family. It is also important to assess preinjury family functioning because this factor has been shown to have an impact on long-term outcome, especially with regard to behavioral problems.[146] The injured child participates in supportive counseling in addition to cognitive rehabilitation activities. Counseling is imperative to assist in preparing for community reentry and in the recognition of the differences seen after return to the community as contrasted to the artificial environment of the inpatient rehabilitation unit.

Providing supportive counseling and education for the patient's siblings is also essential. Medical play can be an effective technique for both injured children and their siblings. Siblings may also benefit from peer support.[145]

Parents may be helped by counseling in addition to education about TBI and its consequences. Proper training enables them to become advocates for their children and to help their children deal with the challenges they face because of the injury.[147] These counseling and education needs may be long-term because the parents initially may be in denial concerning the severity of injury and permanence of impairment.[145,148] The injury results in the need to negotiate systems with which parents were previously unfamiliar. These include special education, medical and rehabilitation services, and publicly supported programs.[147] Also, for families of children with severe injury and those who had difficulties before injury, stressors continue long-term, and families need additional attention and resources to assist them in coping with the consequences of their child's injuries.[149]

Another issue that requires attention is the potential impact of a child's TBI on family finances. Osberg and colleagues[150] found that parents of children who required transfer to a rehabilitation unit experienced difficulty with work and finances. Proactive planning, contact with employers, and the exploration of alternative funding sources can be of substantial benefit.

Discharge Planning

Rehabilitation has become a continuum of care, being provided at many different sites and intensities of service. It is important to begin discharge planning early in the rehabilitation hospitalization. The costs of caring for children with TBI are significant. The majority of those costs relate to the acute care hospitalization, but for those with significant injury, up to 47% of the hospital costs are due to inpatient rehabilitation.[7]

Most children are discharged to home after TBI. Determining the appropriate services, assisting the family in obtaining them depending on their third-party payer and network requirements, and coordinating with the public school system are essential elements in this planning process. Working closely with the third-party payer case manager can be helpful in obtaining the appropriate services for optimal transition. Family or other caregiver training is imperative in medical or nursing procedures as well as the management of behavioral problems after TBI.

Community Reintegration

School Services

Traumatic Brain Injury Classification

Children who have experienced TBI are more likely than the general population to require special education services.[151] By law, all children are entitled to a free and appropriate education. TBI affects the child's ability to learn and potentially function in a school setting. The availability of *Traumatic Brain Injury* is helpful as a classification in the school setting because that may qualify students for special education services. States have developed their own individual criteria for eligibility for this classification. Frequently, these criteria are more flexible than for other classifications, affording children with TBI improved access to services.

It is also important to remain flexible with regard to duration of the school day and to accommodate to the need for rest periods or continuing outpatient therapy services. It is also important to remember that children with mild and moderate TBI who may not have required inpatient rehabilitation services may also have cognitive impairments shortly after injury. Those children should have screening to ensure that they receive appropriate supportive services on their return to school.[152,153]

Individual Educational Program Planning and Revision

When a child does require inpatient rehabilitation, early and frequent contacts between the rehabilitation facility and the child's home school are essential to facilitate optimal transition from the rehabilitation setting to home. If the rehabilitation unit has school services available on site, valuable information is obtained about the child's functioning. The availability of the rehabilitation facility teacher assists in contacts with the public school system. In some cases, the school accepts assessments done in the rehabilitation facility as their initial assessments for Individual Education Plan (IEP) formulation. Children may need accommodations or modifications to assist with dealing with any cognitive or physical deficits they may be experiencing.

A critical element in planning for school reentry is to plan for frequent IEP review. For many children with special needs, the IEP is expected to be appropriate for the entire school year. Children with TBI generally return to school while still experiencing improvement of function, and therefore more frequent IEP review and update are indicated.[154,155]

Preparing classmates and teachers for the child's reentry is also an important feature. Basic information about TBI and its sequelae are helpful. Also the child with the TBI may benefit from role playing, which practices responses to peer questions and comments before return to school.

Community Supports

In-Home Services

Flexibility is a key to successful discharge planning. TBI results not only in a variety of impairments of the individual, but also in stressors on the family and changes in family roles. One nearly universal change is the need for increased supervision or care for the child. Extended family systems may be of some assistance in dealing with this, but it is not uncommon for children and families to need additional support. Personal care assistants may be helpful in providing supervision and structure, in addition to physical assistance in caring for the child. In some cases, if third-party payers do not cover this service, state or federally supported programs may be available. Coordination with a social worker knowledgeable in this area is essential for exploring funding options.

Out-of-Home Services

As noted previously, most children are discharged to home after TBI. Other settings may include medical foster placement, group homes, or skilled nursing facility types of placements. Options vary depending on the state of residence and funding available.

Planning for Long-term Needs

As children who have sustained TBI and their families age, certain issues must be considered. For those who are severely injured and require physical assistance or constant supervision, parents eventually will no longer be able to provide physical care. Advance planning is essential with regard to guardianship or conservatorship and the long-term living arrangements for those who remain dependent. Early discussion about these issues with a social worker and legal counsel is important.

Returning to Sports and Recreational Activities

Whether the child was injured during a sports activity or as a result of another cause, a frequent issue that faces the child, family, and physician is if and when sports activities can be safely resumed. It is the authors' practice to advise children who have had severe TBI to cease participation in contact sports, especially football, ice hockey, and soccer. The authors also think that it is ill advised for persons who have survived severe traumatic injury to engage in unusually risky activities such as horse back riding and all-terrain vehicle, motorcycle, or snowmobile operation. In addition, the normal safety precautions that apply to all children should be observed. For example, all children should be using helmets when bicycle riding, and they should be properly restrained in motor vehicles.

It is challenging to advise parents whose child has been injured during a sports activity whether the child should resume play. There are several concerns. First is that the child is expected to return to the same activity during which injury occurred. In certain sports, such as high school football, approximately 20% of players incur a concussion each year.[156] In addition, there are clinical reports of a *second impact syndrome*. Patients with this phenomenon have a fatal outcome when incurring repeated, relatively minor head injuries within a short period of time.[157,158] Some doubt has been raised, however, as to the existence of second impact syndrome as a specific entity.[159]

Frequently the child, parent, and physician are under great pressure to allow reentry into the sports activity. There are guidelines in the sports medicine literature to address this problem.[160,161] The Colorado Medical Society has issued guidelines for the management of concussion in sports that are similar and somewhat easier to follow (Table 13–3).[158] Although there have been no clinical investigations to determine if these guidelines are reasonable and effective, they nevertheless serve to support the clinician's decisions. These guidelines are quite conservative. For example, most children with sports medicine head injury severity ratings of moderate to severe would be considered as mild injury using the ratings given earlier in this

chapter. It has also been suggested that premature return to sports could place the individual at increased risk for additional injury because of the neuropsychological sequelae of minor injury, especially impaired speed of information processing and response speed.[159]

Outcomes

Measurement

Efforts to measure outcomes have been quite varied. Neuropsychological and motor testing may be undertaken to outline specific areas of deficit. More global measures of function have also been used. The Coma/Near Coma (CNC) scale has been designed to evaluate small changes in individuals functioning at levels of minimal responsiveness. It is applicable to children and adults. It can be helpful in allowing for a reproducible assessment of responses and relatively subtle changes over time that may precede more significant improvement in neurologic status.[162] For children who have less severe injury or who are regaining skills, the Functional Independence Measure (FIM) and Functional Independence Measure for Children (WeeFIM) are commonly used measures of global functioning.

The Glasgow Outcome Scale classifies individuals according to the following five categories: death, persistent vegetative state, severe disability, moderate disability, and good recovery.[163] This scale is somewhat general, and some authors have attempted to make modifications to increase the differentiation of outcomes of children.[137] The modified Glasgow outcome rating scale for children is shown in Table 13–4.

Survival

Deaths from brain injury may occur early or late (≥ 1 week) after injury. More than two-thirds of deaths from brain injury occur at the

TABLE 13–3.

Colorado Medical Society Guidelines for the Management of Concussion in Sports*

Grade 1: Confusion without Amnesia or Loss of Consciousness
Remove from contest. Examine immediately and every 5 minutes for development of amnesia or postconcussive symptom at rest and with exertion. Permit return to contest if amnesia does not appear and no symptoms appear for at least 20 minutes.

Grade 2: Confusion with Amnesia but with No Loss of Consciousness
Remove from contest and disallow return. Examine frequently for signs of evolving intracranial pathology. Reexamine the next day. Permit return to practice after 1 full week without symptoms.

Grade 3: Loss of Consciousness
Transport from field to nearest hospital by ambulance (with cervical immobilization if indicated). Perform thorough neurologic evaluation emergently. Admit to hospital if signs of pathology are detected. If findings are normal, instruct family for overnight observation. Permit return to practice only after 2 full weeks without symptoms.

* Prolonged unconsciousness, persistent mental status alterations, worsening postconcussion symptoms, or abnormalities on neurologic examination require urgent neurosurgical consultation or transfer to a trauma center.

scene or en route to the hospital.[164] Children with acquired brain injury who have survived the initial stabilization period and become enrolled in a rehabilitation program generally live for many years. In the authors' experience, death in children with profound brain injuries was seen only in those who remained in vegetative states for longer than 90 days after anoxic or traumatic injury. For example, all children who had even minimal responsiveness, such as a social smile, but no language or purposeful motor activity, survived the follow-up period, which was a median of 8 years.[165] Even children in vegetative states usually live for years. Survival for children in vegetative states is dramatically longer than for adults with similar function. In contrast to studies of adults, in which approximately 50% of adults in vegetative states die within 1 year of injury, one-half of children still in vegetative states at 1 year after injury were still living 7–8 years later.[165,166] Although length of survival for children in vegetative states is definitely greatly shortened in comparison with normal children, others have also noted survival for years, dramatically longer than for adults similarly affected. Splaingard and colleagues[115] observed that 86% of children who required tracheotomies and gastrostomies after acquired traumatic and anoxic injury survived 2 or more years after injury. Another report of people (mostly older children and young adults) with profound mental retardation observed that immobile subjects who required tube feeding had a life expectancy of 4–5 additional years.[167] In a more recent report, children in pediatric skilled nursing facilities who were tube-fed, not rolling, and had no hand or arm use had a 66% 8-year survival.[168] The investigators believed that the survival rates, which were better than those previously reported, were likely the result of intense medical management. These survival rates are comparable to what the authors have observed in children of comparable function who are living at home.

Morbidity and Long-term Impairment

Many factors affect the long-term outcome of survivors. The most important of these factors is the severity of injury; however, the cause of injury and age at the time of injury are also important. The relation of each of these factors with expected outcome is discussed separately.

Related to Injury Severity

Although there is considerable variability from case to case, outcome is primarily related to the severity of injury. Some of the variability

TABLE 13–4. Modified Glasgow Outcome Rating Scale

Cognitive Status
0—Normal, no problems
1—Verbal communicator, requires special educational services
2—Limited language but able to express wants and needs, self-contained classrooms
3—No language but socially responsive, smiles, responds to tone of voice
4—Persistent vegetative state

Motor Status
0—Normal, no problems
1—Functional ambulation, no devices, but not normal, needs supervision for ADL
2—Independent ambulation but with devices and/or adaptations or adaptive equipment for ADL
3—Ambulation with physical assistance and/or assistance with ADL
4— Nonambulatory, needs assistance to transfer, dependent on others for ADL
5—No purposeful movements

ADL, activities of daily living.
Modified from Kriel RL, Krach LE, Sheehan M: Pediatric closed head injury: Outcome following prolonged unconsciousness. Arch Phys Med Rehabil 1988;69:678.

might be accounted for by the particular areas of brain injured. Because damage after TBI tends to occur in similar areas in most patients, it is helpful to the clinician to be able to make generalizations primarily by injury severity.

Mild and Moderate Injury. Children who have had minor traumatic injury may have headaches and subtle cognitive changes, primarily for the initial weeks after injury. These can affect the child when returning to school. The authors commonly advise returning to school for half days until experience has demonstrated that endurance is adequate to permit longer days. The cognitive changes seen after minor injury in children often include difficulty with timed tasks and impaired attention and recent memory. They may also have subtle language dysfunction and impaired prosody of speech. Behavior and personality changes may be seen during the early recovery period. The authors suggest assessing the child using a language and psychological screen a few weeks after injury to see whether short-term intervention would be helpful. Children who have had moderate injuries have similar types of cognitive problems; however, they tend to be more severe, to be frequent, and to persist for longer periods of time.

By 1 year after injury, children who have had minor brain injury rarely have impairment that can be attributed to the accident. There are now well-controlled clinical outcome studies of minor traumatic injury in children.[38,169] These studies have carefully compared children with TBI and age-matched controls 1 year or more after injury using extensive batteries of neuropsychological, achievement, and behavioral testing. Both studies have shown that children with minor traumatic injury are clinically indistinguishable from age-matched controls at 1 year after injury. Real-life function in terms of academic achievement, learning disorders, behavior, and adjustment is similar in children who have had minor injury and in control children.

Similar conclusions have been reached by other investigators. A prospective study at the University of California, Los Angeles, attempted to control for the preinjury level of functioning and used two comparison groups.[170] A retrospective history was obtained at time of injury, and the children were reassessed at 1, 6, and 12 months after injury. There were 137 children in the mildly brain-injured group and 114 in the group without brain injury. A battery of cognitive and behavior scales were used in the assessment. Children with and without brain injury did not differ significantly on any test, and mean scores fell well within the normal range. In addition, no differences were noted in measures derived from school records. Because the rates of behavior problems in the mildly brain-injured group actually declined from preinjury level to those 12 months after injury, it was concluded that the head injury did not produce new behavior problems. It was observed, however, that the brain-injured group had elevated incidence of behavior problems before the accident. Because the incidence of learning and attention deficit disorders is substantial even in uninjured children, the clinician should not conclude that these problems have been the result of a minor brain injury despite the pressure from a legal professional to state otherwise.

Severe Injury.   Numerous studies have shown that children with severe TBI show remarkable ability for partial recovery of function. For example, only 1 of 30 children who were unconscious from 7–90 days failed to become ambulatory with or without equipment by 2 or more years after injury.[171] In that same series, 6 of 30 patients attended college after injury. Thirteen of the group were believed to return to their preinjury function. Bruce and colleagues[172] subsequently reported that 87% of children unconscious longer than 6 hours made a good recovery and were able to lead a full independent life with or without minimal neurologic deficit. Although there is general consensus that substantial improvement occurs after severe TBI in the pediatric population, more recent studies have reported that most patients fail to show complete recovery. In a large pediatric series of

severe TBI, 73% became independent in ambulation and self-care within a year of injury.[36] Only 10% of 344 children had normal neurologic examinations 1 year after injury. Almost half of the group with normal neurologic examinations had severe emotional disturbances requiring professional intervention. Jaffe and colleagues[37] observed that 1 year after injury, children who have had severe TBI still have lower scores on standardized tests of intelligence and memory and lower academic achievement. Children with severe TBI have compromised language competence when reassessed as adults.[173]

Profound Injury.   Children with profound brain injury, unconscious longer than 90 days, obviously have a less favorable prognosis for recovery. In a series of profoundly injured children, only 1 of 36 had normal motor outcome, and no child had a normal cognitive outcome. Two-thirds recovered some language function, and one-quarter recovered independent ambulation with or without assistive devices.[165] Although most recovery is generally observed during the first year after injury, some children show modest late improvement. For example, 7 of 9 children who showed only a social smile 1 year after injury eventually developed limited expressive language.

Related to Cause of Injury

Recovery of function is also strongly related to the cause of injury. For example, children with severe or profound traumatic injury generally have more recovery than do those with anoxic injuries. Seventy-five percent of children with TBI unconscious longer than 90 days eventually regained consciousness, whereas only 25% of those with anoxic injury did so.[165] Survival after profound injury was also substantially longer in the trauma group. Although one-fourth of children become ambulatory and most regain some language function even when unconscious 90 days after traumatic injury, that is not the case for children with anoxic injuries (Figs. 13–1 and 13–2).[165] In a series of 26 children with severe anoxic/ischemic brain injuries, all children who regained language skills or became ambulatory were unconscious fewer than 60 days.[174] Children with severe anoxic injuries almost always have profound rigidity, which markedly impairs their motor function.[165] The effect of causes of injury has been observed by other investigators. For example, in series with children who had received gastrostomies and tracheostomies, 45% of children with traumatic injury achieved functional independence, as contrasted with none of those after anoxia.[115]

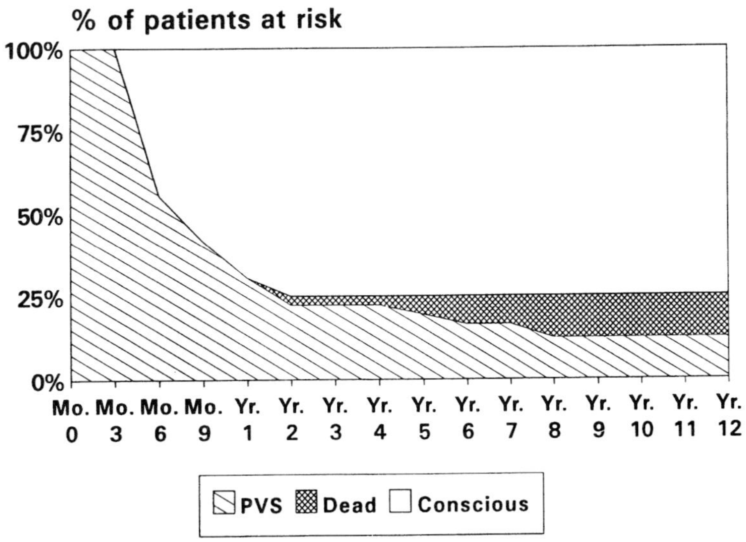

% of patients at risk

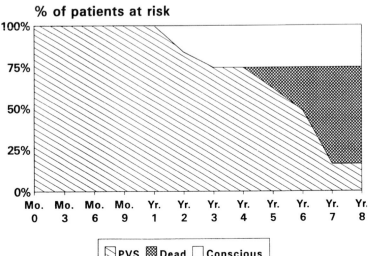

FIGURE 13–1. Survival analysis of 36 children with closed head injuries. (From Kriel RL, Krach LE, Jones-Saete RN: Outcome of children with prolonged unconsciousness and vegetative states. Pediatr Neurol 1993;9:362, with permission.)

Children who have been abused often have worse outcomes. In a consecutive series of 97 children with severe TBI, abused children had significantly worse cognitive and motor outcomes than those injured from other causes.[18] Even in the critical care experience, survival and neurologic outcome are worse for abused children than after other causes of traumatic injury.[175] Frequency of death was 36% versus 12% in the nonabused children; however, these differences did not reach statistical significance. This experience emphasizes that abused children need to be evaluated and observed especially carefully and that there should be expectations for increased utilization of rehabilitation services. It can only be speculated why abused children do worse. Abuse might have the potential for repetitive, nondocumented injury and also tends to occur in younger children who are especially vulnerable to brain injury.

Characteristic motor abnormalities are seen with some causes of acquired brain injury. For example, movement disorders were seen much more frequently after brain injury associated with status epilepticus than with other acquired injury and rigidity after anoxia.[174,176]

Related to Age at Time of Injury

Because children have better survival after brain injury and do well after mild injury, clinicians mistakenly conclude that those with more severe injury also do better than adults. Several clinical reports have observed that young children with diffuse TBI actually have worse recovery than older children or adults.

% of patients at risk

FIGURE 13–2. Survival analysis of 13 children after anoxic brain injury. (From Kriel RL, Krach LE, Jones-Saete RN: Outcome of children with prolonged unconsciousness and vegetative states. Pediatr Neurol 1993;9:362, with permission.)

Some reports emphasized the favorable recovery of children after TBI.[74,177] Eiben and colleagues[74] reported that there was a tendency for a less favorable outcome with increasing age of the child or young adult. Other investigators have found that worse outcomes are more frequently seen in the youngest patients.[18,28,178] Infants have been found to do worse than toddlers, with the percentage of poor recovery 13.4% versus 4.9% when seen at follow-up 3 years after injury.[28] In a series of 97 children unconscious longer than 24 hours, the authors observed that both cognitive and motor outcomes were worse in children under 6 years at age of injury (Table 13–5).[18] Koskiniemi and colleagues[179] also observed that the final outcome was worse in children who were youngest at age of injury and that the watershed of outcome prediction was approximately 4 years of age.

What are the reasons why the youngest children do worse after diffuse brain injury? One explanation is that the causes of traumatic injury differ with age, such as abuse in younger children and bike accidents in teenagers. Another is that the physical characteristics of the young child's skull and brain render it more vulnerable to mechanical injury. Lastly, interruption of neuroanatomic, neurochemical, and neuropsychological developmental sequences should logically have a more catastrophic effect in the younger child.

Although TBI in young children tends to result in the worst cognitive and motor outcomes, injury to adolescents also may have profound impact. In a series of 28 persons severely injured as adolescents, 25 recovered language function and 21 independent ambulation.[99] When seen in follow-up as young adults, significantly fewer of the head-injured patients had graduated from high school and gained employment compared with a reference population. Perhaps most significant in terms of success of interpersonal relations and acceptance was the observation that only one of the head-injured young adults was married compared with 61% of the reference population. Sixty-eight percent of patients reported that social lives and peer relationships had deteriorated after injury. Higher rates of unemployment have been found by others in young adults with sequelae as a result of injury as a child.[180]

Prevention

Because TBI is a frequent cause of significant disability in childhood, efforts should be undertaken to prevent injury. Because motor vehicle accident is the largest cause of TBI in this age group, appropriate restraint of children in the back seat is imperative to prevent injury. Airbag injuries have been reported that occurred when children were not properly restrained.[181] Likewise, the use of protective equipment, such as bicycle helmets, can have a significant impact on decreasing brain injuries, even when accidents involve being struck by motor vehicles.[182] Adults need to model safety-conscious behavior for children in their own appropriate use of seat belts and helmets.

Long-term Follow-up

As is evident by the discussion of potential deficits and the effect of TBI on the child and family, long-term follow-up is an essential part of any comprehensive brain injury rehabilitation program. In children injured at a young age, cognitive deficits may not actually be evident until long after injury. Improvement may continue for a significant period of time. As children and their parents age, alternative programs and living situations may be needed. Rehabilitation involves a continuum of care, and coordination of these services contributes to optimal outcome.

TABLE 5. Outcome Versus Age

Outcome Score	Cognitive Outcome		Motor Outcome	
	< 6 Yr (%)	≥ 6 Yr (%)	< 6 Yr (%)	≥ 6 yr (%)
0	7.4	15.7	7.4	34.3
1	40.7	57.1	33.3	28.6
2	33.3	14.3	22.2	15.7
3	11.1	8.6	7.4	7.1
4	7.4	4.3	18.5	8.6
5	–	–	11.1	5.7
Mean	1.7	1.3	2.3	1.4
t-test	1.86		2.46	
P value	0.03		0.01	

Modified from Kriel RL, Krach LE, Panser LA: Closed head injury: Comparison of children younger and older than 6 years of age. Pediatr Neurol 1989;5:296.

References

1. Annegers JF, Grabow JD, Kurland LT, et al: The incidence, causes, and secular trends of head trauma in Olmsted County, Minnesota, 1935–1974. Neurology 1980;30:912.
2. Thurman DJ, Jeppson L, Burnett CL, et al: Surveillance of traumatic brain injuries in Utah. West J Med 1996;165:192.
3. Kraus JF, Fife D, Cox P, et al: Incidence, severity, and external causes of pediatric brain injury. Am J Dis Child 1986;140:687.
4. Kraus JF, Rock A, Hemyari P: Brain injuries among infants, children, adolescents, and young adults. Am J Dis Child 1990;144:684.

5. Brooks CA, Lindstrom J, McCray J, et al: Cost of medical care for a population-based sample of persons surviving traumatic brain injury. J Head Trauma Rehabil 1995;10:1.
6. Massagli TL, Michaud LJ, Rivara FP: Association between injury indices and outcome after severe traumatic brain injury in children. Arch Phys Med Rehabil 1996;77:125.
7. Jaffe KM, Massagli TL, Martin KM, et al: Pediatric traumatic brain injury: Acute and rehabilitation costs. Arch Phys Med Rehabil 1993;74:681.
8. Michaud LJ, Duhaime A-C, Batshaw ML: Traumatic brain injury in children. Pediatr Clin North Am 1993;40:553.
9. Michaud LJ, Duhaime A-C: Gunshot wounds to the brain in children. J Head Trauma Rehabil 1995;10:25.
10. Vernon-Levett P: Head injuries in children. Crit Care Nurs Clin North Am 1991;3:411.
11. Levi L, Guilburd JN, Linn S, et al: The association between skull fracture, intracranial pathology and outcome in pediatric head injury. Br J Neurosurg 1991;5:517.
12. Berney J, Froidevaux A-C, Favier J: Paediatric head trauma: Influence of age and sex. Childs Nerv Syst 1994;10:517.
13. Aicardi J: Diseases of the Nervous System in Childhood. New York, Cambridge University Press, 1992.
14. Ewing-Cobbs L, Duhaime A-C, Fletcher JM: Inflicted and noninflicted traumatic brain injury in infants and preschoolers. J Head Trauma Rehabil 1995;10:13.
15. Johnston MV, Gerring JP: Head trauma and its sequelae. Pediatr Ann 1992;21:362.
16. Aldrich EF, Eisenberg HM, Saydjari C, et al: Diffuse brain swelling in severely head-injured children. J Neurosurg 1992;76:450.
17. Alderson P, Roberts I: Corticosteroids in acute traumatic brain injury: Systematic review of randomised controlled trials. BMJ 1997;314:1855.
18. Kriel RL, Krach LE, Panser LA: Closed head injury: Comparison of children younger and older than 6 years of age. Pediatr Neurol 1989;5:296.
19. Merten DF, Osborne DRS: Craniocerebral trauma in the child abuse syndrome. Pediatr Ann 1983;12:882.
20. Alexander R, Sato Y, Smith W, et al: Incidence of impact trauma with cranial injuries ascribed to shaking. Am J Dis Child 1990;144:724.
21. McLean DE, Kaitz ES, Keenan CJ, et al: Medical and surgical complications of pediatric brain injury. J Head Trauma Rehabil 1995;10:1.
22. Husson B, Pariente D, Tammam S, et al: The value of MRI in the early diagnosis of growing skull fracture. Pediatr Radiol 1996;26:744.
23. DiScala C, Osberg S, Gans B, et al: Children with traumatic head injury: Morbidity and postacute treatment. Arch Phys Med Rehabil 1991;72:662.
24. Cope DN: The rehabilitation of traumatic brain injury. In Kottke FJ, Lehmann JF (eds): Krusen's Handbook of Physical Medicine and Rehabilitation. Philadelphia, WB Saunders, 1990.
25. Sobus KML, Alexander MA, Harcke HT: Undetected musculoskeletal trauma in children with traumatic brain injury or spinal cord injury. Arch Phys Med Rehabil 1993;74:902.
26. Uomoto JM: Neuropsychological assessment and training in acute brain injury. In Kottke FJ, Lehmann JF (eds): Krusen's Handbook of Physical Medicine and Rehabilitation. Philadelphia, WB Saunders, 1990.
27. Simpson DA, Cockington RA, Hanieh A, et al: Head injuries in infants and young children: The value of the paediatric coma scale. Childs Nerv Syst 1991;7:183.
28. Raimondi AJ, Hirschauer J: Head injury in the infant and toddler: Coma scoring and outcome scale. Childs Brain 1984;11:12.
29. James HE: Neurologic evaluation and support in the child with an acute brain insult. Pediatr Ann 1986; 15:16.
30. Michaud LJ, Rivara FP, Grady MS, et al: Predictors of survival and severity of disability after severe brain injury in children. Neurosurgery 1992;31:254.
31. Papero PH, Snyder HM, Gotschall CS, et al: Relationship of two measures of injury severity to pediatric psychological outcome 1–3 years after acute head injury. J Head Trauma Rehabil 1997;12:51.
32. Ellenberg JH, Levin HS, Saydjari C: Posttraumatic amnesia as a predictor of outcome after severe closed head injury. Arch Neurol 1996;63:782.
33. Ruijs MBM, Keyser A, Gabreels FJM: Assessment of post-traumatic amnesia in young children. Dev Med Child Neurol 1992;34:885.
34. Ewing-Cobbs L, Levin HS, Fletcher JM, et al: The children's orientation and amnesia test: Relationship to severity of acute head injury and to recovery of memory. Neurosurgery 1990;27:683.
35. Iverson GL, Iverson AM, Barton EA: The children's orientation and amnesia test: Educational status is a moderator variable in tracking recovery from TBI. Brain Inj 1994;8:685.
36. Brink JD, Imbus C, Woo-Sam J: Physical recovery after severe closed head trauma in children and adolescents. J Pediatr 1980;97:721.
37. Jaffe KM, Fay GC, Polissar NL, et al: Severity of pediatric traumatic brain injury and neurobehavioral recovery at one year—A cohort study. Arch Phys Med Rehabil 1993;74:587.
38. Fay GC, Jaffe KM, Polissar NL, et al: Mild pediatric traumatic brain injury: A cohort study. Arch Phys Med Rehabil 1993;74:895.
39. McDonald CM, Jaffe KM, Fay GC, et al: Comparison of indices of traumatic brain injury severity as predictors of neurobehavioral outcome in children. Arch Phys Med Rehabil 1994;75:328.
40. Boyer MG, Edwards P: Outcome 1 to 3 years after severe traumatic brain injury in children and adolescents. Br J Accident Surg 1991;22:315.
41. Swaine BR, Sullivan SJ: Longitudinal profile of early motor recovery following severe traumatic brain injury. Brain Inj 1996;10:347.
42. Chaplin D, Deitz J, Jaffe KM: Motor performance in children after traumatic brain injury. Arch Phys Med Rehabil 1993;74:161.
43. Haaland KY, Temkin N, Randahl G, et al: Recovery of simple motor skills after head injury. J Clin Exp Neuropsychol 1994;16:448.
44. Neistadt ME: The effects of different treatment activities on functional fine motor coordination in adults with brain injury. Am J Occup Ther 1994;48:877.
45. Eviatar L, Bergtraum M, Randel RM: Post-traumatic vertigo in children: A diagnostic approach. Pediatr Neurol 1986;2:61.
46. Geurts ACH, Ribbers GM, Knoop JA, et al: Identification of static and dynamic postural instability following traumatic brain injury. Arch Phys Med Rehabil 1996;77:639.
47. Wober C, Oder W, Kollegger H, et al: Posturographic measurement of body sway in survivors of severe closed head injury. Arch Phys Med Rehabil 1993;74: 1151.
48. Newton RA: Balance abilities in individuals with moderate and severe traumatic brain injury. Brain Inj 1995; 9:445.
49. Lehmann JF, Boswell S, Prince R, et al: Quantitative evaluation of sway as an indicator of functional balance in post-traumatic brain injury. Arch Phys Med Rehabil 1990;71:955.

50. Hallet M: Classification and treatment of tremor. JAMA 1991;266:1115.
51. Aisen ML, Holzer M, Rosen M, et al: Glutethimide treatment of disabling action tremor in patients with multiple sclerosis and traumatic brain injury. Arch Neurol 1991;48:513.
52. Krauss JK, Mohadjer M, Braus DF, et al: Dystonia following head trauma: A report of nine patients and review of the literature. Mov Disord 1992;7:263.
53. Lee MS, Rinne JO, Ceballos-Baumann A, et al: Dystonia after head trauma. Neurology 1994:44:1374.
54. Parziale JR, Akelman E, Herz DA: Spasticity: Pathophysiology and management. Orthopedics 1993;16:801.
55. Mayer NH: Functional management of spasticity after head injury. J Neurol Rehabil 1991;5:S1.
56. Katz RT: Management of spasticity. Am J Phys Med Rehabil 1988;67:108.
57. Krach LE: Early rehabilitation interventions for children with traumatic brain injury. In Wild KV (ed): Neurologische Fruhrehabilitation. Munich, W Auckschwerdt Verlag, 1990.
58. Wilson DJ, Childers MK, Cooke DL, et al: Kinematic changes following botulinum toxin injection after traumatic brain injury. Brain Inj 1997;11:157.
59. Milanov DG: Mechanizms of tizanidine action on spasticity. Acta Neurol Scand 1994;89:274.
60. Dall JT, Harmon RL, Quinn CM: Use of clonidine for treatment of spasticity arising from various forms of brain injury: A case series. Brain Inj 1996;10:453.
61. Albright AL, Cervi A, Singletary J: Intrathecal baclofen for spasticity in cerebral palsy. JAMA 1991;265: 1418.
62. Albright AL, Barron WB, Fasick MP, et al: Continuous intrathecal baclofen infusion for spasticity of cerebral origin. JAMA 1993;270:2475.
63. Yousem DM, Geckle RJ, Bilker WB, et al: Posttraumatic olfactory dysfunction: MR and clinical evaluation. Am J Neuroradiol 1996;17:1171.
64. Doty RL, Yousem DM, Pham LT, et al: Olfactory dysfunction in patients with head trauma. Arch Neurol 1997;54:1131.
65. Berry H, Blair RL: Central auditory dysfunction. J Otolaryngol 1977;6:120.
66. Ward PH: The histopathology of auditory and vestibular disorders in head trauma. Ann Otol Rhinol Laryngol 1969;78:227.
67. Tierney DW: Visual dysfunction in closed head injury. J Am Optom Assoc 1988;59:614.
68. Tang RA, Kramer LA, Schiffman J, et al: Chiasmal trauma: Clinical and imaging considerations. Surv Ophthalmol 1994;38:381.
69. Streff JW: Visual rehabilitation of hemianoptic head trauma patients emphasizing ambient pathways. NeuroRehabilitation 1996;6:173.
70. Uzzell BP, Dolinskas CA, Langfitt TW: Visual field defects in relation to head injury severity. Arch Neurol 1988;45:420.
71. Raymond MJ, Bennett TL, Malia KB, et al: Rehabilitation of visual processing deficits following brain injury. NeuroRehabilitation 1996;6:229.
72. Lepore FE: Disorders of ocular motility following head trauma. Arch Neurol 1995;52:924.
73. Politzer TA: Case studies of a new approach using partial and selective occlusion for the clinical treatment of diplopia. NeuroRehabilitation 1996;6:213.
74. Eiben CF, Anderson TP, Lockman L, et al: Functional outcome of closed head injury in children and young adults. Arch Phys Med Rehabil 1984;65:168.
75. Lazar MF, Menaldino S: Cognitive outcome and behavioral adjustment in children following traumatic brain injury: A developmental perspective. J Head Trauma Rehabil 1995:10:55.
76. Whyte J: Attention and arousal: Basic science aspects. Arch Phys Med Rehabil 1992;73:940.
77. Wroblewski BA, Glenn MB: Pharmacological treatment of arousal and cognitive deficits. J Head Trauma Rehabil 1994;9:19.
78. Wolf AP, Gleckman AD: Sinement and brain injury: Functional versus statistical change and suggestions for future research designs. Brain Inj 1995;9:487.
79. Ross ED, Stewart RM: Akinetic mutism from hypothalamic damage: Successful treatment with dopamine agonists. Neurology 1981;31:1435.
80. Reinhard DL, Whyte J, Sandel ME: Improved arousal and initiation following tricyclic antidepressant use in severe brain injury. Arch Phys Med Rehabil 1996; 77:80.
81. Kaufmann PM, Fletcher JM, Levin HW, et al: Attentional disturbance after pediatric closed head injury. J Child Neurol 1993;8:348.
82. Silver BV, Yablon SA: Akathisia resulting from traumatic brain injury. Brain Inj 1996;10;609.
83. Cardenas DD, Alvin McLean J: Psychopharmacologic management of traumatic brain injury. Phys Med Rehabil Clin North Am 1992;3:273.
84. Lord-Maes J, Obrzut JE: Neuropsychological consequences of traumatic brain injury in children and adolescents. J Learn Disabil 1996;29:609.
85. Jaffe KM, Fay GC, Polissar NL, et al: Severity of pediatric traumatic brain injury and early neurobehavioral outcome: A cohort study. Arch Phys Med Rehabil 1992; 73:540.
86. Taverni JP, Seliger G, Lichtman SW: Donepezil mediated memory improvement in traumatic brain injury during post acute rehabilitation. Brain Inj 1998;12:77.
87. Bawden HN, Knights RM, Winogron HW: Speeded performance following head injury in children. J Clin Exp Neuropsychol 1985;7:39.
88. Max JE, Lindgren SD, Knutson C, et al: Child and adolescent traumatic brain injury: Correlates of injury severity. Brain Inj 1998;12:31.
89. Chadwick O, Rutter M, Brown G, et al: A prospective study of children with head injuries: Cognitive sequelae. Psychol Med 1981;11:49.
90. Jordan FM, Murdoch BE: Linguistic status following closed head injury in children: A follow-up study. Brain Inj 1990;4:147.
91. Chapman SB, Levin HS, Matejka J, et al: Discourse ability in children with brain injury: Correlations with psychosocial, linguistic, and cognitive factors. J Head Trauma Rehabil 1995;10:36.
92. Coster WJ, Haley S, Baryza MJ: Functional performance of young children after traumatic brain injury: A 6-month follow-up study. Am J Occup Ther 1994; 48:211.
93. Klonoff H, Clark C, Klonoff PS: Long-term outcome of head injuries: A 23-year follow up study of children with head injuries. J Neurol Neurosurg Psychiatry 1993;56:410.
94. Michaud LJ, Rivara FP, Jaffe KM, et al: Traumatic brain injury as a risk factor for behavioral disorders in children. Arch Phys Med Rehabil 1993;74:368.
95. Cassidy JW: Neuropharmacological management of destructive behavior after traumatic brain injury. J Head Trauma Rehabil 1994;9:43.
96. Bellus SB, Stewart D, Vergo JG, et al: The use of lithium in the treatment of aggressive behaviors with two brain-injured individuals in a state psychiatric hospital. Brain Inj 1996;10:849.
97. Wroblewski BA, Joseph AB, Kupfer J, et al: Effectiveness of valproic acid on destructive and aggressive behaviors in patients with acquired brain injury. Brain Inj 1997;11:37.

98. Parker PJ, Shapiro EG, Kriel RL: Affective recognition in children following head injury. In Wild KV (ed): Spektrum der Neurorehabilitation. Munich, W Zuckschwerdt Verlag, 1993.

99. Kriel RL, Krach LE, Bergland MM, et al: Severe adolescent head injury: Implications for transition into adult life. Pediatr Neurol 1988;4:337.

100. Iglesias P, Gomez-Pan A, Diez J: Spontaneous recovery from post-traumatic hypopituitarism. J Endocrinol Invest 1996;19:320.

101. Grossman WF, Sanfield JA: Hypothalamic atrophy presenting as amenorrhea and sexual infantilism in a female adolescent. J Reprod Med 1994;39:738.

102. Wang LC, Cohen ME, Duffner PK: Etiologies of central diabetes insipidus in children. Pediatr Neurol 1994; 11:273.

103. Anmuth CJ, Ross BW, Alexander MA, et al: Chronic syndrome of inappropriate secretion of antidiuretic hormone in a pediatric patient after traumatic brain injury. Arch Phys Med Rehabil 1993;74:1219.

104. Zafonte RD, Mann NR: Cerebral salt wasting syndrome in brain injury patients: A potential cause of hyponatremia. Arch Phys Med Rehabil 1997;78:540.

105. Sigurjonsdottir TJ: Precocious puberty: A report of 96 cases. Am J Dis Child 1968;115:309.

106. Maxwell M, Karacostas D, Ellenbogen RG, et al: Precocious puberty following head injury. J Neurosurg 1990;73:123.

107. McKiernan J: Precocious puberty and nonaccidental injury. BMJ 1978;14:1059.

108. Shaul PW, Towbin RB: Precocious puberty following severe head trauma. Am J Dis Child 1985;139:467.

109. Blendonohy PM, Philip PA: Precocious puberty in children after traumatic brain injury. Brain Inj 1991;5:63.

110. Sockalosky JJ, Kriel RL, Krach LE, et al: Precocious puberty after traumatic brain injury. J Pediatr 1987;110: 373.

111. Goldman M, Shahar E, Sack J, et al: Assessment of endocrine functions in children following severe head trauma. Pediatr Neurol 1997;17:339.

112. Balagura S, Shulman K, Sobel EH: Precocious puberty of cerebral origin. Surg Neurol 1979;11:315.

113. Rayner PHW: Puberty: Precocious and delayed. BMJ 1976;1:1385.

114. Bierich JR: Sexual precocity. Clin Endocrinol Metab 1975;4:107.

115. Splaingard ML, Gaebler D, Havens P, et al: Brain injury: Functional outcome in children with tracheostomies and gastrostomies. Arch Phys Med Rehabil 1989;70:318.

116. Feldman Z, Contant CF, Pahwa R, et al: The relationship between hormonal mediators and systemic hypermetabolism after severe head injury. J Trauma 1993;34:806.

117. Stover SL: Epidemiology of neurogenic bladder. Phys Med Rehabil Clin North Am 1993;4:211.

118. Bullard DE: Diencephalic seizures: Responsiveness to bromocriptine and morphine. Ann Neurol 1987;21:609.

119. Rossitch E, Bullard DE: The autonomic dysfunction syndrome: Etiology and treatment. Br J Neurosurg 1988;2:471.

120. Pranzatelli MR, Pavlakis SG, Gould R, et al: Hypothalamic-midbrain dysregulation syndrome: Hypertension, hyperthermia, hyperventilation, and decerebration. J Child Neurol 1991;6:115.

121. Meythaler JM, Stinson AM: Fever of central origin in traumatic brain injury controlled with propranolol. Arch Phys Med Rehabil 1994;75:816.

122. Childers MK, Rupright J, Smith DW: Posttraumatic hyperthermia in acute brain injury rehabilitation. Brain Inj 1994;8:335.

123. Krach LE, Kriel RL, Morris WF, et al: Central autonomic dysfunction following acquired brain injury in children. J Neurol Rehabil 1997;11:41.

124. Chaney RH, Olmstead CE: Hypothalamic dysthermia in persons with brain damage. Brain Inj 1994;8:475.

125. Moltz H: Fever: Causes and consequences. Neurosci Biobehav Rev 1993;17:237.

126. Hurvitz EA, Mandac BR, Davidoff G, et al: Risk factors for heterotopic ossification in children and adolescents with severe traumatic brain injury. Arch Phys Med Rehabil 1992;73:459.

127. Citta-Pietrolungo TJ, Alexander MA, Steg NL: Early detection of heterotopic ossification in young patients with traumatic brain injury. Arch Phys Med Rehabil 1992;73:258.

128. Sobus KM, Sherman N, Alexander MA: Coexistence of deep venous thrombosis and heterotopic ossification in the pediatric patient. Arch Phys Med Rehabil 1993;74: 547.

129. Silverman SL, Hurvitz EA, Nelson VS, et al: Rachitic syndrome after disodium etidronate therapy in an adolescent. Arch Phys Med Rehabil 1994;75:118.

130. Annegers JF, Grabow JD, Groover RV, et al: Seizures after head trauma: A population study. Neurology 1980;30:683.

131. Temkin NR, Kikmen SS, Wilensky AJ, et al: A randomized, double-blind study of phenytoin for the prevention of post-traumatic seizures. N Engl J Med 1990; 323:497.

132. Young B, Rapp RP, Norton JA, et al: Failure of prophylactically administered phenytoin to prevent post-traumatic seizures in children. Childs Brain 1983;19:185.

133. Dikmen SS, Temkin NR, Miller B, et al: Neurobehavioral effects of phenytoin prophylaxis of posttraumatic seizures. JAMA 1991;265:1271.

134. Smith KR, Goulding PM, Wilderman D, et al: Neurobehavioral effects of phenytoin and carbamazepine in patients recovering from brain trauma: A comparative study. Arch Neurol 1994;51:653.

135. Hernandez TD, Naritoku DK: Seizures, epilepsy, and functional recovery after traumatic brain injury: A reappraisal. Neurology 1997;48:803.

136. Massagli TL: Neurobehavioral effects of phenytoin, carbamazepine, and valproic acid: Implications for use in traumatic brain injury. Arch Phys Med Rehabil 1991;72:219.

137. Kriel RL, Krach LE, Sheehan M: Pediatric closed head injury: Outcome following prolonged unconsciousness. Arch Phys Med Rehabil 1988;69:678.

138. Newberg AB, Alavi A: Neuroimaging in patients with traumatic brain injury. J Head Trauma Rehabil 1996; 11:65.

139. Levin HS, Amparo EG, Eisenberg HM, et al: Magnetic resonance imaging after closed head injury in children. Neurosurgery 1989;24:223.

140. Levin HS, Culhane KA, Mendelsohn D, et al: Cognition in relation to magnetic resonance imaging in head-injured children and adolescents. Arch Neurol 1993;40:897.

141. Cowley RS, Swanson B, Chapman P, et al: The role of rehabilitation in the intensive care unit. J Head Trauma Rehabil 1994;9:32.

142. Spettell CM, Ellis DW, Ross SE, et al: Time of rehabilitation admission and severity of trauma: Effect on brain injury outcome. Arch Phys Med Rehabil 1991;72:230.

143. Chen SHA, Thomas JD, Glueckauf RL, et al: The effectiveness of computer-assisted cognitive rehabilitation for persons with traumatic brain injury. Brain Inj 1997;11:197.

144. Krach LE: Early rehabilitation of children and adolescents following severe brain injuries. In Wild KV (ed): Spectrum der Neurorehabilitation. Munich, W Zuckschwerdt Verlag, 1993.

145. Waaland PK, Kreutzer JS: Family response to child-hood traumatic brain injury. J Head Trauma Rehabil 1988;3:51.

146. Rivara JM, Jaffe KM, Polissar NL, et al: Family functioning and children's academic performance and behavior problems in the year following traumatic brain injury. Arch Phys Med Rehabil 1994;75:369.

147. Rivara JMB, Jaffe KM, Fay GC, et al: Family functioning and injury severity as predictors of child functioning one year following traumatic brain injury. Arch Phys Med Rehabil 1993;74:1047.

148. Junque C, Bruna O, Mataro M: Information needs of the traumatic brain injury patient's family members regarding the consequences of the injury and associated perception of physical, cognitive, emotional and quality of life changes. Brain Inj 1997;11:251.

149. Rivara JMB, Jaffe KM, Polissar NL, et al: Predictors of family functioning and change 3 years after traumatic brain injury in children. Arch Phys Med Rehabil 1996;77:754.

150. Osberg JS, Brooke MM, Baryza MJ, et al: Impact of childhood brain injury on work and family finances. Brain Inj 1997;11:11.

151. Greenspan AI, Mackenzie EJ: Functional outcome after pediatric head injury. Pediatrics 1994;94:425.

152. Shurtleff HA, Massagli TL, Hays RM, et al: Screen children and adolescents with mild or moderate traumatic brain injury to assist school reentry. J Head Trauma Rehabil 1995;10:64.

153. Ylvisaker M, Feeney T, Mullins K: School reentry following mild traumatic brain injury: A proposed hospital-to-school protocol. J Head Trauma Rehabil 1995;10:42.

154. Frey WF, Savage RC, Ross BJ: The adolescent with traumatic brain injury: Cognitive, psychological and educational issues. Adolesc Med 1994;5:311.

155. Ylvisaker M, Feeney T, Maher-Maxwell N, et al: School reentry following severe traumatic brain injury: Guidelines for educational planning. J Head Trauma Rehabil 1995;10:25.

156. Wilberger JE, Maroon JC: Head injuries in athletes. Clin Sports Med 1989;8:1.

157. Saunders RL, Harbaugh RE: The second impact in catastrophic contact-sports head trauma. JAMA 1984; 252:538.

158. Kelly JP, Nichols JS, Filley CM, et al: Concussion in sports: Guidelines for the prevention of catastrophic outcome. JAMA 1991;266:2867.

159. McCrory PR, Berkovic SF: Second impact syndrome. Neurology 1998;50:677.

160. Cantu RC: Cerebral concussion in sport: Management and prevention. Sports Med 1992;14:64.

161. Fick DS: Management of concussion in collision sports. Postgrad Med 1995;97:53.

162. Rappaport M, Dougherty AM, Kelting DL: Evaluation of coma and vegetative states. Arch Phys Med Rehabil 1992;73:628.

163. Jennett B, Snoek J, Bond MR, et al: Disability after severe head injury: Observations on the use of the Glasgow outcome scale. J Neurol Neurosurg Psychiatry 1981;44:285.

164. Kraus J, Conroy C, Cox P, et al: Survival times and case fatality rates of brain-injured persons. J Neurosurg 1985;63:537.

165. Kriel RL, Krach LE, Jones-Saete C: Outcome of children with prolonged unconsciousness and vegetative states. Pediatr Neurol 1993;9:362.

166. Braakman R, Jennett WB, Minderhoud JM: Prognosis of the posttraumatic vegetative state. Acta Neurochir 1988;95:49.

167. Eyman RK, Grossman HJ, Chaney RH, et al: The life expectancy of profoundly handicapped people with mental retardation. N Engl J Med 1990;323:584.

168. Plioplys AV, Kasnicka I, Lewis S, et al: Survival rates of children with severe neurological disabilities. Ann Neurol 1997;42:501.

169. Bijur PE, Haslum M, Golding J: Cognitive and behavioral sequelae of mild head injury in children. Pediatrics 1990;86:337.

170. Asarnow RF, Satz P, Light R, et al: The UCLA study of mild closed head injury in children and adolescents. In Broman SH, Michel ME (eds): Traumatic Head Injury in Children. New York, Oxford University Press, 1995.

171. Stover S, Ziegler H: Head injury in children and teenagers: Functional recovery correlated with duration of coma. Arch Phys Med Rehabil 1976;57:201.

172. Bruce DA, Schut L, Bruno LA, et al: Outcome following severe head injuries in children. J Neurosurg 1978;48: 679.

173. Jordan FM, Murdoch BE: Severe closed-head injury in childhood: Linguistic outcomes into adulthood. Brain Inj 1994;8:501.

174. Kriel RL, Krach LE, Luxenberg MG, et al: Outcome of severe anoxic/ischemic brain injury in children. Pediatr Neurol 1994;10:207.

175. Goldstein B, Kelly MM, Bruton D, et al: Inflicted versus accidental head injury in critically injured children. Crit Care Med 1993;21:1328.

176. Fowler WE, Kriel RL, Krach LE: Movement disorders after status epilepticus and other brain injuries. Pediatr Neurol 1992;8:281.

177. Jennett B: Head injuries in children. Dev Med Child Neurol 1972;14:137.

178. Lange-Cosack H, Wilder B, Schlesner HJ, et al: Prognosis of brain injuries in young children (one until five years of age). Neuropediatrie 1979;10:105.

179. Koskiniemi M, Kyykka T, Nubo T, et al: Long-term outcome after severe brain injury in preschoolers is worse than expected. Arch Pediatr Adolesc Med 1995;149: 249.

180. Klonoff H, Clark C, Klonoff PS: Outcome of head injuries from childhood to adulthood: A twenty-three year follow-up study. In Broman SH, Michel ME (eds): Traumatic Head Injury in Children. New York, Oxford University Press, 1995.

181. Hollands CM, Winston FK, Stafford PW, et al: Severe head injury caused by airbag deployment. J Trauma 1996;41:920.

182. Thompson DC, Rivard FP, Thompson RS: Effectiveness of bicycle safety helmets in preventing head injuries. JAMA 1996;276:1968.

Chapter 14

Spinal Cord Injuries

Virginia Simson Nelson, MD, MPH

Children and adolescents with spinal cord injury (SCI) must deal with the multisystem involvement imposed by the injury that is compounded by physical and psychological growth and development, which cause complications not seen in the adult patient. Rehabilitation is a process that extends at least until the child is physically and psychosocially an adult. Involvement by a team expert in management of children and adolescents with SCIs should continue throughout this period. This chapter discusses some of the main points to be considered by those who are involved in assisting this rehabilitation process.

Epidemiology

Incidence and Prevalence

Because SCI is not a reportable condition, it is difficult to get an accurate count of the incidence (number of new cases per year) and prevalence (number of people in a given population) of SCIs. From various sources, it is estimated that approximately 10,000 SCIs occur each year in the United States, with 3–5% (300–500) of these occurring in children under age 15 years and 20% (2000) in individuals under age 20. There are approximately 200,000 people living with SCIs in the United States, with approximately 26,000 of these under the age of 25 years.[1] No estimate of the prevalence of pediatric SCI is available. The Major Trauma Outcome Study from 1982 to 1989 found 2.6% of the 114,510 patients had SCI.[2] Forty percent were due to motor vehicle accidents, 20% to falls, and 13.6% to gunshot wounds. Eight percent of patients with SCIs had multiple trauma, with 52% of these having cervical SCIs. Sixty-five percent of those with isolated SCIs had cervical lesions. Hospital mortality was 17% (20% of those with SCI and multiple trauma and 7% of those with isolated SCI). No age breakdown was given in this study.

Demographics: Age, Sex, and Race

Publications[3,4] combined data from the Shriners Hospitals for Children and the Model SCI Care Systems to obtain statistics about SCIs in children. As in adults, boys are four times more likely to have SCIs than girls overall, with this ratio being 1.5:1 in children under 9 years. In children under 3 years, girls have outnumbered boys in some studies. In younger children, there is no statistically significant racial trend, whereas in those over 15 years the percentage of African-Americans was higher than their representation in the general population. These figures are all from specialized hospital data and may not represent those with milder injuries (e.g., incomplete lesions or paraplegia) who are treated in smaller hospitals or those treated in adult settings. There are also SCIs caused by disease, such as tumors, and as medical complications that are not reported. Thus, their incidence and prevalence are not available.

Cause by Age, Sex, Residence, and Month of Year

Younger children more commonly have high cervical lesions, whereas older ones are more likely to have lower cervical lesions, probably because of the relatively large size of the head in younger children. A study by Hadley and colleagues[5] in Arizona reviewed 122 cases of spinal cord and vertebral column trauma in children ages 16 and under. Median age was 15 years in boys and 14 years in girls. SCIs were due to motor vehicle accidents in 39% overall, with motor vehicle accidents the cause in 17% of children under 10 years old, 26% of those 10–14 years old, and 52% in those 15–16 years old. Pedestrian-automobile accidents were the cause in 11% overall, and 33%, 16% and 3% in the three age groups. Falls were the second leading cause under 10 years, with sports the second leading cause at ages 15 and 16. Fifty percent under age 10 had an occiput–C1 injury, with all levels of cervical injuries occurring in 72%, 60%, and 55% in the three age groups. Fifty percent of the subjects were neurologically intact—that is, had vertebral column injury only. Another single institution study by Ruge and colleagues[6] came from Children's Memorial Hospital in Chicago and was composed of 71 children under age 13 years. Forty-three percent were neurologically intact, and 19% had complete lesions. Twenty-one percent had SCI without obvious radiologic abnormality (SCIWORA), with 40% of them neurologically complete lesions. Twenty-two percent under age 4 were male, while 71% aged 4–12 were male. Fifty-six percent under age 4 and 29% aged 4–12 years had C1–2 lesions. Data presented by Vogel[1] in 1997 showed motor vehicle accidents are the leading cause in all ages of children, with violence the second leading cause in those under age 9 years and sports the second leading cause in those aged 9 years and older.

Data from Europe show similar statistics. Turgut and colleagues[7] reported on 82 children with SCI or vertebral column injury treated between 1968 and 1993. Sixty-seven percent were boys. Falls were the most common cause (56%), followed by motor vehicle accidents. Fifty-seven percent of the injuries were cervical. Eighteen percent had complete lesions, and 13% had SCIWORA.

Motor vehicle crashes are the most common cause of SCIs in individuals under 46 years old,[8] with violence the second leading cause under age 9 years and sports the second leading cause in older children. Both violence and sports show a higher incidence in boys, with motor vehicle crashes having a higher incidence in girls. Some studies have shown a difference in causes of SCI in rural versus urban settings, with violence being more common in cities. An increasing proportion of SCIs are caused by violence, with this most marked increase in individuals 16–20 years of age (from 9.7 to 35.9% over the past 20 years).[9] Injuries secondary to sports have been decreasing, probably because of education and improved equipment. There have also been reports of difference in causes at different seasons, with the incidence of SCI being highest in all age groups in the summer. Some causes for SCIs are unique to children, including child abuse, birth injury, and certain preexisting conditions predisposing to SCIs (e.g., Down syndrome and juvenile rheumatoid arthritis).

ASIA Classifications

SCIs are classified by neurologic level and motor and sensory deficits. In children, there is

the additional classification of SCIWORA. In children under age 10 years, SCIWORA is present in 20 to 40% of SCIs.[10] SCIWORA lesions present with normal plain radiographs, but abnormalities may be seen on magnetic resonance (MR) imaging. These lesions are more often complete (American Spinal Injury Association [ASIA] A), with poor prognosis for recovery of function.[9] SCIWORA are thought to be the result of the elasticity of the pediatric spine, which allows transient displacement of structures, injuring the spinal cord, with subsequent self-reduction. This displacement stretches the spinal cord, injuring neural elements, while sparing the vertebral column. Younger children are more likely to have SCIWORA than are older children. Pang[10] combined reports in the literature for a total of 84 children under age 10 years and 178 children 10 years or older. Sixty-three percent of the younger children and 20% of the older children had SCIWORA. Combining numbers from another set of articles, Pang found that 77% of 80 children under age 9 years and 12% of 40 children over 9 years with SCIWORA had *severe* injuries. His exact definition of *severe* is not given, as in one place he talks about *complete injuries*, and in another he talks about *Frankel B and C*.

Dickman and colleagues[11] reported on 26 cases of SCIWORA seen at the Barrow Neurological Institute in Phoenix, Arizona, between 1972 and 1990. These represented 16% of all children seen with SCIs during that time. In young children, SCIWORA occurred in 32% of all injuries with 70% complete lesions. In older children, SCIWORA occurred in 12% of cases and was rarely complete.

The ASIA classification is based on evaluation of motor and sensory function[12] and is a modification of the older Frankel classification system. A neurologic level is assigned based on motor and sensory examination except in the upper cervical (C1–C4), thoracic, and upper lumbar (T2–L1) and sacral (S1–S5) areas where neurologic level is based only on sensation because there are no easily testable motor levels in those areas. Sensory testing consists of four sensory modalities per dermatome: right and left pin prick and right and left light touch. Sensory examination of each side is summed across dermatomes, for a total *pin prick score* and a total *light touch score*. Motor scores are summed for a total motor score as shown in Figure 14–1. Motor level is the level that tests at a 3 with the previous segment testing at 5. For example, if wrist extensors are 3 and the elbow flexors are 5, the motor level is C6. Thus, an individual may be said to have a C5 ASIA A SCI. This means

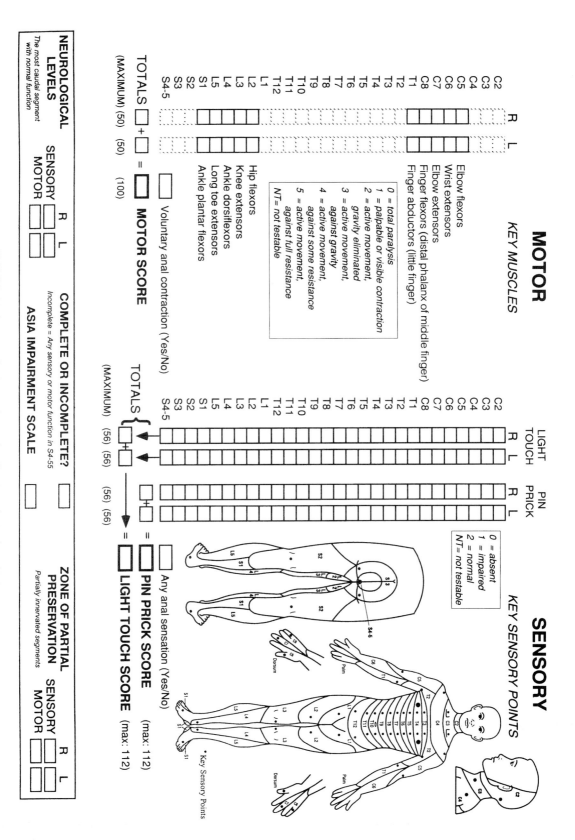

FIGURE 14-1. Standard neurologic classification of spinal cord injury.

ASIA IMPAIRMENT SCALE

☐ **A = Complete:** No motor or sensory function is preserved in the sacral segments S4–S5.

☐ **B = Incomplete:** Sensory but not motor function is preserved below the neurologic level and includes the sacral segments S4–S5.

☐ **C = Incomplete:** Motor function is preserved below the neurologic level, and more than half of key muscles below the neurologic level have a muscle grade less than 3.

☐ **D = Incomplete**: Motor function is preserved below the neurologic level, and at least half of key muscles below the neurologic level have a muscle grade of 3 or more.

☐ **E = Normal:** Motor and sensory function is normal.

CLINICAL SYNDROMES

☐ Central Cord Syndrome
☐ Brown-Séquard Syndrome
☐ Anterior Cord Syndrome
☐ Conus Medullaris Syndrome
☐ Cauda Equina Syndrome

FIGURE 14–2.   ASIA impairment scale.

that the individual has functioning elbow flexors with no motor or sensory function below the level of the C5 dermatome. The ASIA Neurological Classification may be difficult to determine in some children because of their lack of ability to follow directions, either as a result of age or associated brain injury. In children and adolescents who can be tested, the ASIA score provides useful information (Fig. 14–2).

Incomplete SCIs (ASIA B, C, or D) may have a variety of patterns. Central cord syndrome, first described by Schneider and colleagues[13] in 1954, refers to injury predominantly affecting the center of the spinal cord. The clinical picture is one of more involvement of the upper extremities than the lower extremities, with bladder and bowel dysfunction and variable degree of sensory loss below the level of the lesion. There is usually sacral sensory sparing in central cord lesions. This lesion almost always occurs in the cervical region. Brown-Séquard syndrome, first described in 1846, results from hemisection of the spinal cord, usually from penetrating injuries such as stab or gunshot wounds. Pure Brown-Séquard syndrome is characterized by hemiplegia with loss of position and vibratory sense below the level of the lesion on one side with loss of pain and temperature senses one or two levels below the level of the lesion on the other side. Light touch and pressure sensation are usually spared. These findings can be explained anatomically: Light touch and pressure senses have bilateral representation. Pain and temperature sensation are carried in the lateral spinothalamic tract, which ascends one or two levels before crossing and ascending on the contralateral side. Vibratory and position senses are carried in the dorsal columns on the ipsilateral side, and voluntary motor function is carried primarily in the lateral corticospinal tracts on the contralateral side. An easy way to remember this syndrome is that the stronger side has less sensation. Pure Brown-Séquard syndrome is rarely seen because penetrating wounds usually affect more than just one side of the spinal cord.

Anterior cord syndrome is due to a disturbance in blood flow in the anterior spinal artery, resulting in motor deficit and absence of pain and temperature sensations, with relatively preserved position and vibratory senses. This is commonly caused by hypotensive episodes or disturbance of the blood flow to the anterior spinal arteries secondary to lesions of the aorta. Cauda equina syndrome is characterized by flaccid bowel and bladder, saddle anesthesia, and flaccid paralysis of the legs because of injury to the lumbosacral nerve roots within the neural canal. Conus medullaris syndrome is predominantly a sensory syndrome with minimal motor loss and areflexic bowel and bladder and lower limbs. This syndrome is due to injury to the sacral cord. Tumors are a frequent cause of both of these syndromes in children, although they may also occur with severe pelvic trauma.

Data from the Shriner's Hospital SCI Database and the Model SCI System Database indicate that between 50 and 67% of children sustain complete (ASIA A) SCIs.[14] Various incomplete

SCI syndromes each comprise less than 6% of the total, with anterior spinal artery syndrome being the most common at 5.4%.

Prevention

Prevention of injury is always more effective than treatment, and this is especially true in SCI. The hallmark of prevention is safety education beginning in early childhood. Use of safe equipment is the second tenet of prevention, and nowhere has this been more effective than in the use of infant and child auto restraints and of auto lap and shoulder belts. This practice has also caused lap belt injuries, however, including SCIs, which are more common in children than in adults. Other prevention relating to motor vehicles is substance abuse education and laws relating to driving while impaired. Pedestrian safety is promoted almost exclusively through parent and child education. Prevention of sports-related SCIs has improved because of education, rules changes (such as no spearing in football, no checking from behind in hockey), better coaching, and conditioning. Although better equipment such as helmets has decreased the number and severity of brain injuries, data on prevention of SCIs are not available.

The Think First head and SCI prevention program is widely promoted by neurosurgeons and others involved with adolescent trauma programs. An analysis of the impact of this program on the knowledge, attitudes, and behavior of teenagers was done by the Harborview Injury Prevention and Research Center in Seattle, Washington.[15] Their questionnaire survey showed little impact on attitudes, knowledge, or self-reported behavior. An earlier article by Watts and Eyster[16] suggested that the program had a favorable impact on knowledge and attitudes regarding head and SCIs.

Prevention of SCIs resulting from automobile accidents has been investigated by studying the pattern of injuries in motor vehicle accidents. A study of SCIs from motor vehicle accidents in Utah[17] showed 39% of patients were ejected from the vehicle, 70% were involved in a rollover accident, and only 25% were using seat belts. A similar report from Chicago by Sasso and colleagues[18] studied 1352 patients with SCIs in motor vehicle accidents from 1971 to 1993. Only 14% wore seat belts, but the odds of surviving the motor vehicle accident neurologically intact were greater for those who wore seat belts. Neither of these studies focused on the pediatric population, but both suggest the value of seat belt education in preventing SCIs or minimizing the extent of neurologic damage.

A study by DeVivo and Sekar[19] looked at the circumstances surrounding SCIs occurring in swimming pools in patients enrolled in the National Spinal Cord Injury Statistical Center database. Records were reviewed, and a telephone interview was administered. Most injuries occurred in residential pools with no lifeguard present. Alcohol was involved in almost half of the cases. Forty-six percent of the injuries occurred during parties. These data suggest important features to include in a primary prevention program.

A study by Tator and colleagues[20] of spinal injuries (fracture, dislocation, or both) occurring in hockey in Canada between 1982 and 1993 showed an average of 17 major spinal injuries per year, with most of them cervical injuries occurring in players aged 16–20 years playing in supervised games. The authors concluded that the number of severe injuries and those caused by a check from behind were decreasing, even though the total number of injuries was not significantly decreased. Prevention of violence that leads to SCIs in children is beyond the scope of this chapter but is a necessity in today's increasingly violent society.

Treatment of Early Stage of Spinal Cord Injury

Spinal Stabilization

Once it has been determined that the child has an SCI, the spine must be stabilized. The halo external skeletal fixation device was first described in 1968 for use in adults by Nickel and colleagues.[21] It has subsequently been adapted for use in children with modifications required by the unique characteristics of the child's skull, which is thinner. Fixation pins must be carefully placed, with attention paid to both location and depth of insertion.[22] Whether halo traction is used alone or in combination with stabilization in cervical injuries is a surgical decision, with more recent literature and practice being surgical stabilization when the child is medically stable, followed by external immobilization.[23,24] For the child with thoracic or lumbar SCI, immobilization is done with the use of a body cast or thoracolumbosacral orthosis (TLSO) after surgical stabilization.[25] Types of injuries that are managed with external immobilization only include compression fractures and SCIWORA. The length of immobilization varies but is frequently approximately 12 weeks or until there is radiographic evidence of stability and healing as determined by plain radiographs and flexion-extension lateral radiographs.

Use of Steroids

Various studies of the efficacy of the use of methylprednisolone in acute SCI were conducted during the 1980s. The National Acute Spinal Cord Injury Study 2 (NASCIS 2) was published in 1990[26] with the conclusion that patients with acute SCI treated with high-dose methylprednisolone in the first 8 hours after injury had better neurologic outcome than did those treated with naloxone or placebo. This was based on a randomized study of 162 patients, 15% of whom were under age 19 years, with the youngest being 13 years old. The dose of prednisolone was 30 mg/kg initially, followed by 5.4 mg/kg/hr for 23 hours. A more recent article on this topic appeared in the *Journal of the American Medical Association* in 1997.[27] The current recommendation for acute SCIs is administration of methylprednisolone for 24 hours when it is started within 3 hours after injury and administration for 48 hours when started between 3 and 8 hours after injury. Because this recommendation is based on adult data, a recent recommendation is that this regimen should be used in the pediatric population at the discretion of the treating physician.[28]

Respiratory Function

Most children with SCIs have impairment of normal respiratory function because of their injuries, even in the absence of other trauma causing pulmonary problems. The basic muscle groups of respiration are the diaphragm, intercostal muscles, abdominal muscles, and neck accessory muscles. Any SCI that weakens one or more of these muscle groups impairs respiration. The child with weak or absent diaphragm function needs some type of ventilatory support. If the diaphragm is functioning normally, but intercostal and abdominal muscle function is impaired or absent, the child needs assistance with coughing and may need ventilatory support during respiratory illnesses or during sleep. If the child has impairment of abdominal muscles only, assistance with coughing may be the only respiratory support needed.

All children with acute SCIs should be evaluated for respiratory dysfunction. This evaluation should include at least a chest x-ray and measurement of oxygen saturation and end-tidal carbon dioxide or arterial blood gases. If the child is able, vital capacity and maximal inspiratory and expiratory forces should be measured. These measurements should be followed on a daily basis until the child is medically stable. For the child with a history of pulmonary problems, these measurements should also be monitored at routine follow-up. Because the child with an SCI has *bellows failure* and not lung disease, the earliest pulmonary abnormality found will probably be hypercarbia, not hypoxia. By the time there is oxygen desaturation, the child is in or close to respiratory failure. Thus, routine monitoring, if done, should be of carbon dioxide, not just oxygen. A simple way to monitor carbon dioxide is through the measurement of end-tidal carbon dioxide. This noninvasive process is often preferable to measuring blood gases because the child may cry vigorously with pain, thus decreasing the carbon dioxide level markedly and giving a falsely low reading. For the child with an indwelling arterial line, this problem does not occur.

Urinary Function

Most children with acute SCIs have neurogenic bladders. These are generally *spinal shock bladders* initially, or flaccid. As such, they must be drained either periodically (e.g., by the use of clean intermittent cathcterization) or continuously with an indwelling catheter. Because indwelling catheters are often associated with infections, the child should be converted to a clean intermittent catheterization program as soon as there is no medical reason to have continuous monitoring of urinary output. Urodynamic studies of bladder function should be done before hospital discharge to determine whether the child has an upper motor neuron (spastic) or lower motor neuron (flaccid or atonic) bladder. Follow-up of bladder and renal status should be done on a regular basis. The incidence of urinary tract infections varies, although there is no evidence that there is a statistical relationship between the use of clean instead of sterile intermittent catheterization and urinary tract infections.[29]

Gastrointestinal Function

After acute SCI, the gastrointestinal tract usually stops functioning initially. Acute management protocol should require the insertion of a nasogastric tube attached to suction until the ileus is resolved, with parenteral nutrition used until the child is able to take adequate nutrition either orally or via enteral tube feedings. Just as the stomach fails to empty, the bowels also do not work properly because of lack of neural control. A bowel program should be instituted as soon as the child is receiving enteral nutrition. The goal of the bowel program should be continence without impaction. This goal is achieved by normalizing the consistency of the stool through the use of fiber and fluids in the diet and medications, as necessary, and assisting the bowel to evacuate through the use of oral or rectal medications or digital stimulation. Stress ulcers may uncommonly develop in children with acute SCIs. Some physicians advocate the routine use of gastrointestinal medications to reduce stomach acid during the acute stages.

Fluids and Nutrition

Careful attention must be paid to fluid balance and nutrition in the child with an acute SCI. If the child has a concomitant traumatic brain injury, fluids may have to be restricted during the period of brain edema. Once that period has passed, maintenance fluids should be sufficient to assist in maintaining blood pressure, urine output, and hydration of the lungs and gastrointestinal tract. When the child has been changed from an indwelling urinary catheter to intermittent catheterization, there must be a balance between fluids administered and frequency of catheterizations, so that bladder volume does not exceed 400 ml in those who are adult-sized (and proportionately less in smaller children).

To promote healing, the child must receive adequate nutrition. A common standard is to start some form of nutritional support no later than 24 hours after hospital admission. Whether this is parenteral nutrition or via enteral tube or oral is determined by the child's overall medical status. Many children require either tube feedings or parenteral nutrition during most if not all of their acute hospitalization because of their inability or unwillingness to eat an adequate diet. If the child is able to eat orally, calorie and nutrient intake should be carefully monitored, with supplements given via parenteral nutrition or enteral tube.

Immobilization hypercalcemia may occur in children after SCIs and has been reported in 10–23% of individuals with SCI.[3,30] Those at highest risk of developing hypercalcemia are adolescent boys, especially those with quadriplegia and complete lesions. The most common clinical presentation is anorexia, nausea, vomiting, malaise, and behavioral changes. Although this usually occurs after the acute phase, calcium and phosphorus blood levels should be monitored on a regular basis, especially in those at highest risk of developing hypercalcemia, even in the absence of clinical symptoms. Treatment consists of hydration and early mobilization. Hydration should be at least 150% of maintenance needs, usually at least partially by

intravenous route. Furosemide (1 mg/kg per dose) assists in excretion of calcium and the extra fluid but may not be necessary. In patients whose calcium levels do not decline after 7–10 days with hydration and mobilization, consideration should be given to using calcitonin 100 mg subcutaneously once or twice a day. Etidronate disodium may also be used but not in growing children because of the potential development of the rachitic syndrome.[31]

Psychosocial Issues

Psychosocial issues in children who sustain SCIs must be addressed beginning in the early postinjury period. During that time, parents and other family members may have the main adjustment problems. Both the family and the child may go through the classic stages of mourning—denial, anger, depression, and acceptance—although more recent literature discusses individual coping styles as predictors of how patients will cope.[32–34] These stages may be manifest in the child by regressive behaviors and anorexia. Introducing an element of control, even in the acute stage in the intensive care unit, may decrease some of these behaviors.[33] Buffers to adjustment difficulties include family support, premorbid personality style and peer relations, family strengths and coping styles, financial resources, and community support. Risk factors include premorbid depression and personality disorders. Learning disabilities may also affect adjustment and ability to understand procedures and care routines.

Rehabilitation

When a child leaves the acute care setting and enters rehabilitation varies in different institutions. If one thinks of rehabilitation as an ongoing process that starts on the day of injury, the transfer to the rehabilitation unit is merely one of many steps in the process. Rehabilitation of the child with SCI is comparable to rehabilitation of the child with any other acute change in function, usually with less need for cognitive rehabilitation. The entire rehabilitation process should focus on the whole child in the context of his or her family and community and be performed by a rehabilitation team of professionals that focuses only on children. Goals should include maintenance of good health and prevention of secondary complications, while promoting maximal independence possible given the age of the child and type of SCI. Although most rehabilitation occurs during the early postinjury period, rehabilitation must be an ongoing process, especially in children injured at an early age. Thus, a child who is too young to participate in self-care needs to learn this when he or she is older. The ultimate goal is for the child to be either physically independent in his or her daily life or to direct others in those areas where physical independence is not possible. In addition, the child must be encouraged to complete his or her education and prepare for employment as an independent adult.

Mobility

Mobility for the child with an SCI starts with the process of learning to sit up again. This may be facilitated by the use of Ace wraps or support stockings and an abdominal binder to assist in the maintenance of blood pressure. As soon as the child with quadriplegia is able to be upright at least 0.5–1 hour, consideration should be given to providing power mobility, to allow some control over the environment and freedom in movement. Continuing the process of regaining mobility includes relearning to roll in bed; going from supine to sitting and reverse; transferring from sitting to standing or to wheelchair and back; and ambulation or independent wheelchair mobility on all surfaces, including outdoors,

ramps, and curbs. How long the relearning process takes, how complete it can be, and what assistive devices are necessary depends on the child's age and level of injury. See Table 14–1 for recommendations established at a workshop sponsored by the American Academy of Orthopaedic Surgeons and the Shriners Hospitals for Crippled Children.[28]

Activities of Daily Living

By the time children are 5 years old, they are independent in the majority of self-care activities with supervision. Regaining this independence after it has been lost because of an SCI is of utmost importance, especially to adolescents and preadolescents. The first step in this process is allowing some control over the environment in the rehabilitation unit. This may be as simple as a remote control for the television and an accessible nurse call switch or more complex through the use of an environmental control unit accessed via head, mouth, or eye switch. The relearning of self-care skills should follow an orderly pattern but may begin with the activity in which the child is most interested, often self-feeding. Activities that must be relearned include dressing, bathing and hygiene,

TABLE 14–1.   Mobility Guidelines

Level of Injury	Age	Goals	Orthotic Options
C1–4	Bracing available from age 1 year–prepuberty No standing after puberty	Standing	Prone and supine standers (stationary standers)
C4–7	Encourage from ages 1–5 years Available from age 5 years– prepuberty	Static standing and mobility	As above plus parapodiums/swivel walkers/mobile standers
T1–5	Encourage ages 1–10 years after rehabilitation goals are met (increase upper extremity strength/endurance); if surgery is performed, intensive gait training available postoperatively Ages 11–21 years need to meet criteria: 6 parallel bar pushups; 25 wheelchair pushups; transfer level heights; < 20° of hip flexion contracture; < 15° of knee flexion contracture; < 15° of ankle plantarflexion contracture.	Standing and household ambulation	As above plus RGO
T6–12 and L1	Strongly encourage in ages 1–10 years	Household and limited community ambulation	Same as above
L–4	Strongly encourage for all ages	Community ambulation	Above plus HKAFOs, KAFOs, AFOs
L5–S1	Strongly encourage for all ages	Community ambulation	Include AFOs, GRAFOs; strongly encourage for joint protection

AFO, Ankle-foot orthosis; GRAFO, ground reaction ankle-foot orthosis; HKAFO, hip-knee-ankle-foot orthosis; KAFO, knee-ankle-foot orthosis ; RGO, reciprocating gait orthosis.

Adapted from Betz RR, Mulcahey MJ (eds): The Child with a Spinal Cort Injury. Rosemont, IL, American Academy of Orthopaedic Surgeons, 1996;849.

TABLE 14–2. Functional Independence after Spinal Cord Injury

Activities	Level of Injury				
	C1-4	C5	C6	C7	PARAPLEGIA
Feeding	N	A	Y	Y	Y
Dressing UE	N	A	Y	Y	Y
Dressing LE	N	A	A	A	A
Bathing	N	N	N	Y*	Y
Bladder	N	Y*	A	Y	Y
Bowel	N	N	A	Y	Y
Rolling in bed	N	N	Y*	Y	Y
Transfers-level	N	N	Y*	Y	Y
Manual wheelchair	N	Y*	Y	Y	Y
Power wheelchair	Y	Y	Y	X	X
Driving	N	Y*	Y	Y	Y

N, Not independent; Y, Independent; A, Independent with assistive devices; Y*, May be independent, but not expected; X, Not usually needed.

UE, Upper extremities; LE, lower extremities.

feeding, transfers, writing and computer usage, and leisure pursuits. For young children, teaching these activities may be incorporated into play activities. Children with high tetraplegia should be taught how to direct a caregiver to perform the various activities. See Table 14–2 for long-term independence expectations for children with SCI who are old enough and cognitively able to participate in self-care.

Medical Issues

Bladder Function

After the transition from the intensive care unit to rehabilitation, management of the bladder must be converted to a technique that can be done at home. Often, this is also the time that the bladder is changing from flaccid to spastic, with detrusor sphincter dyssynergia. The goals of management are preservation of renal function, prevention of urinary tract infections and stones, continence, and independence. Baseline urologic studies should be done in all children with SCIs. These include urinalysis and culture, renal ultrasound or intravenous pyelogram, and serum blood urea nitrogen (BUN) and creatinine. After the spinal shock has resolved, commonly 6–12 weeks after the SCI, baseline urodynamic studies should be done. These include a cystometrogram and sphincter electromyogram. The cystometrogram provides information on bladder volume and filling and voiding pressures (or leak point pressure). Pressures greater than 40 cm H_2O are known to be related to an increased incidence of upper tract deterioration.[35]

Clean intermittent catheterization or intermittent self-catheterization is the method most commonly used today for bladder drainage after SCI, and numerous studies have shown its efficacy and safety for long-term management of the neurogenic bladder. For those who cannot independently manage intermittent self-catheterization, external sphincterotomy may be considered for continuously draining the bladder but is rarely recommended in children because it destroys any chance for urinary continence when the child is older. It is also rarely recommended in females because of the lack of a satisfactory collecting device for the continuously draining urine. Complications of external sphincterotomy may include penile erosions from the condom catheter collecting device, the need for reoperation, and erectile dysfunction. For females who cannot manage intermittent self-catheterization, consideration may be given to the Mitrofanoff procedure, which brings the bladder stoma to the abdominal wall for easier accessibility for intermittent self-catheterization.[36,37] This is a major surgical procedure and should not be undertaken during the initial rehabilitation period but later after the child has had an opportunity to live at home.

Various medications may be used in the management of the neurogenic bladder. These include antibiotics and anticholinergics. There have been a variety of studies of the usefulness of prophylactic administration of antibiotics or the treatment of asymptomatic bacteriuria. Based on these, the general recommendation is to treat catheter-associated bacteriuria only when it is associated with fever or, on occasion, new incontinence.[35] Anticholinergic medications may be used to reduce bladder pressures and contractility, including oxybutynin (Ditropan), imipramine (Tofranil), and hyoscyamine (Levsin and Cystospaz).

All have the side effect of dry mouth and decreased sweating and may cause blurred vision and constipation. Each should be used with caution in children exposed to high environmental temperatures, and the function of the bowel program should be carefully monitored. Oxybutynin has been used intravesically to relax the bladder directly and avoid systemic side effects. The tablet is crushed, suspended in distilled water, and instilled in the bladder after catheterization. This practice is particularly useful where environmental temperatures are high and children wish to pursue outdoor activities.

Respiratory Function

Although acute pulmonary problems may not be as frequent during rehabilitation as during the initial phase after SCI, close attention should be paid to pulmonary status, especially in children who are younger and less able to communicate and in those with higher levels of tetraplegia or more complete lesions. Clinical symptoms of respiratory problems often develop long before radiologic or laboratory evidence is present. The child should be carefully watched for changes in secretions or cough, shortness of breath, headache, changes in mental status, sleepiness, and snoring. Presence of morning headache should be assumed to be a sign of hypercarbia and promptly investigated. Routine monitoring of pulmonary status during rehabilitation should at the least include daily auscultation, measurement of end-tidal carbon dioxide tension and transcutaneous oxygen saturation, and measurement of vital capacity and maximal inspiratory and expiratory forces in all children with quadriplegia and infants and young children with high paraplegia. Consideration should be given to monitoring oxygen saturation overnight in children with complete quadriplegia because some studies have found that a high percentage of adults with complete quadriplegia have frequent nocturnal desaturations,[38] Prevention of problems may include percussion and postural drainage, assisted cough techniques, respiratory muscle training, pneumococcal immunization and yearly influenza vaccines, adequate nutritional status, and a cardiopulmonary fitness program. An abdominal binder or thoracolumbosacral orthosis may be beneficial by providing support to the abdominal muscles.

Nutrition

Adequate nutrition is necessary to promote healing of injuries and provide energy to participate in the rehabilitation process. For many children, refusal to eat may be present, either because of lack of appetite or because this may be the only activity over which they have any control. Loss of the sense of smell may accompany some injuries, also contributing to anorexia. Nutrition must become a nonnegotiable issue during rehabilitation. If the child is unable or unwilling to eat, short-term use of nasogastric tube feedings should be considered. If the inability to eat continues longer, the placement of a gastrostomy tube should be considered. Once a child has finally begun to eat, care must be taken that he or she not overeat and thus become obese. No nutritional standards are available for children with SCI, but careful monitoring of weight can assist in determining the correct level of calories necessary for growth without promoting obesity.

Bowel Function

With the loss of neural control, the gastrointestinal tract loses voluntary control, and peristalsis slows. Stiens and associates[39] reviewed the anatomy, physiology, and management of the neurogenic bowel.[39] A program to control incontinence while preventing impaction must fit into the child's daily life. Factors to consider are premorbid bowel function, timing, consistency, frequency, and volume of bowel movements. The new bowel regimen should duplicate, as closely as possible, the premorbid patterns. If possible, bowel movements should be timed shortly after a meal to take advantage of the gastrocolic reflex. Factors to be considered in the new program are diet, physical activity, equipment, oral and rectal medications, and scheduling. The diet must contain adequate fluid and fiber to provide sufficient bulk to the stool and keep it moving through the gastrointestinal tract. Certain foods may have a constipating effect (e.g., dairy products or high-fat meals) or cause diarrhea (e.g., caffeine, certain fruits). These need to be balanced to achieve the desired goals. Table 14–3 summarizes many of the medications used for bowel programs for individuals with SCI.

Young children may need only digital stimulation or no special program to evacuate completely. Older children may, likewise, need only digital rectal stimulation to evacuate completely, but, more commonly, one or more medications is necessary.

Skin

Decubitus ulcers are a common complication of pediatric SCI and are caused by pressure, shear, and friction, with moisture being a complicating factor. Ulcers cause a huge burden in terms of time lost from school and other activities, cost, and psychological distress. Prevention is clearly a better solution than any treatment.

TABLE 14–3. Bowel Medications

Medication	Effects	Negative Effects
Bulk-forming Agents		
Psyllium (Metamucil, Fibercon, Citrucel, Perdiem)	Absorbs water to keep stool formed and prevent dry, hard stool	Bloating, flatulence
Stool Softeners		
Docusate (Colace, Surfak)	Allows water to enter stool	Diarrhea, liquid form tastes bitter and is poorly tolerated
Mineral oil	Lubricant	Interferes with absorption of fat-soluble vitamins, causes lipid pneumonia after aspiration
Stimulants		
Senna (Senokot)	Increases intestinal motility, takes 6–12 hours to work	Diarrhea, cramping
Bisacodyl (Dulcolax)	Increases intestinal motility	Diarrhea, cramping (less with rectal suppositories)
Saline Laxatives		
Milk of Magnesia	Draws water into gut to stimulate colonic motility	Diarrhea
Magnesium citrate	Stimulates colonic motility, used for complete bowel evacuation	Large volume, tastes bad, may cause electrolyte imbalance
Saline enemas (Fleet's)	Acts to evacuate distal colon	Cramping, may cause electrolyte disturbance
Hyperosmolar		
Lactulose, sorbitol	Draws fluid into intestine	Diarrhea, cramping, flatulence
Polyethylene glycol (GoLYTELY)	Draws fluid into intestine, used for complete bowel emptying	Cramping, diarrhea
Glycerine suppositories	Irritant	
Prokinetic Agents		
Cisapride (Propulsid)	Affects neurotransmitters to increase gastrointestinal motility, including gastric emptying, antiemetic	Interacts with many drugs, cardiac arrhythmia
Metoclopramide (Reglan)	Promotes gastric emptying	Behavior problems
Rectal Agents		
Therevac mini-enemas	Triggers colonic peristalsis	
Carbon dioxide suppositories (Ceo-Two)	Causes rectal distention	

The basis of prevention is thorough education of the child and family about pressure relief, avoiding moisture, and treatment of ulcers in the earliest stage. Data from the Model SCI Care Systems in 1997 show that 34% of patients developed ulcers while still hospitalized, including 51% of those with complete tetraplegia, 40% of those with complete paraplegia, 30% of those with incomplete tetraplegia, and 19% of those with incomplete paraplegia.[8] Fifteen to twenty percent of those seen for annual examinations developed ulcers per year during the first 5 years after injury. Although these figures may be less in children, ulcers nonetheless are costly.

There are various systems of classification used for pressure ulcers (Tables 14–4 and 14–5).

Large pressure ulcers may not heal with the relief of pressure for long periods of time, and surgery may be necessary. Various types of closures include linear closure and several types of flaps, which are well detailed by Apple and Murray.[42]

TABLE 14–4. Shea Classification of Pressure Ulcers

Grade	Description
1	Red area or ulcer of epidermis or into epidermis
2	Full dermis thickness to subcutaneous fat
3	Fascia and muscle exposed
4	Bone visible
5	Large cavity through a small sinus

Adapted from Bergman SB, Yarkony GM, Stiens SA: Spinal cord injury rehabilitation: 2. Medical complications. Arch Phys Med Rehabil 1997;78:S53.

TABLE 14–5. National Pressure Ulcer Advisory Panel Classification

Grade	Description
I	Nonblanchable erythema
II	Partial skin loss of epidermis, dermis
III	Full-thickness skin loss
IV	Damage through fascia, muscle, or bone

Adapted from Yarkony GM: Pressure ulcers: Classification and overview. In Betz RR, Mulcahey MJ (eds): The Child with a Spinal Cord Injury. Rosemont, IL, American Academy of Orthopedic Surgeons, 1996.

Autonomic Hyperreflexia

Autonomic hyperreflexia (dysreflexia) (AH) is dysfunction of the autonomic nervous system after SCI at or above T6. As a result of noxious stimuli below the level of injury, there is increased sympathetic activity leading to vasoconstriction below the level of injury and hypertension. The central nervous system response is vasodilation above the level of injury with increased vagal tone and bradycardia. Symptoms of AH include pounding headache, sweating above the level of the lesion, red *splotches* on the face and neck, and nasal congestion. Bradycardia may be present. Inciting factors are bladder and bowel distention and rapid change in position from sitting to supine. Urinary tract infection, renal or bladder stones, and suppository or enema insertion may also be inciting factors. AH can present as an acute emergency, more commonly in older adults than in children, who are better able to withstand extreme hypertension.

Treatment of AH consists of relief of inciting factors. The child is immediately placed in the sitting position, and the bladder is emptied. Most episodes of AH resolve with these treatments. If a rectal examination must be done, this may exacerbate the AH and should be done with the use of local anesthetic on the glove. If AH persists, nifedipine should be administered sublingually. An older treatment is nitroglycerine paste which can be wiped off the skin, terminating its action once the hypertension resolves. Prevention of AH consists of effective bowel and bladder management programs.

Hypercalcemia

As discussed previously, hypercalcemia is most likely to occur in adolescent boys in the first 2–3 months after SCI. Serum calcium should be routinely followed throughout the rehabilitation inpatient course, and treatment with fluids, furosemide, and calcitonin as described previously should be instituted.

Deep Venous Thrombosis

Deep venous thrombosis (DVT) and pulmonary embolism are common potentially life-threatening complications in SCI. Although DVT is somewhat less common in prepubertal children, it still does occur. The most common time of occurrence is during the first few weeks after the SCI. Recommendations for prophylaxis against DVT in pubertal children include minidose heparin or low-molecular-weight heparin and calf compression pumps during the rehabilitation hospitalization. Late-occurring DVT most commonly occurs with increased immobilization related to illness or surgery.

Symptoms of DVT include a swollen, warm extremity. If the child has sensation, this may be accompanied by pain. Differential diagnoses include cellulitis, fracture, reflex sympathetic dystrophy, and heterotopic ossification. Diagnosis is confirmed by Doppler ultrasound. If the ultrasound is negative and the index of suspicion for DVT is high, a venogram or MR imaging may be necessary. Plain radiographs should be obtained, especially in prepubertal children and in those whose SCI occurred more than 3 months previously. Once a DVT is confirmed, treatment is bed rest until adequate heparinization is achieved to maintain the partial thromboplastin time 1.5–2.5 times control. The patient is converted to warfarin (Coumadin) for long-term management, with the international normalized ratio maintained at 1.5–2.5 times control values. Treatment should continue for 3–6 months. Complications of heparin and warfarin include bleeding for both and heparin-induced thrombocytopenia. Warfarin may interact with many medications, and the patient and family should be fully educated about this if warfarin is to be continued after hospital discharge.

Temperature Regulation

Children with SCI above T6 frequently have problems with temperature regulation because of the loss of central control of sympathetic and voluntary muscles.[43] They must thus dress according to the environmental temperature. Before investigating the source of hyperthermia or hypothermia, investigation should be made into the temperature of the environment where the child has been. Often undressing the child or putting a blanket over the child is all that is necessary to treat the hyperthermia or hypothermia. For children who reside in areas with cold weather, the use of a mylar Space blanket to maintain body heat is recommended for emergency situations. Occasionally, severe spasticity may cause extreme hyperthermia.[44]

Latex Allergy

Latex allergy is commonly seen in children with myelodysplasia and is now being recognized in children with SCI. A report states the incidence of latex allergy in children with SCI is 6–18%.[1] Children and families should be educated about this potential problem and encouraged to avoid latex when possible.

Spasticity

Approximately 50% of children with SCI have spasticity, which tends to be more common

TABLE 14–6. Common Spasticity Medications

Medication	Site of Action	Side Effects
Baclofen (Lioresal)	Spinal cord–GABA receptor agonist	Sedation, nausea, seizures (especially with rapid withdrawal)
Diazepam (Valium)	Brain	Sedation, potential for substance abuse
Dantrolene (Dantrium)	Muscle	Liver dysfunction, weakness
Tizanidine (Zanaflex)	Spinal cord	Sedation, nausea
Clonidine (Catapres)	Spinal cord	Hypotension (less with transdermal than oral), dry mouth, constipation
Gabapentin (Neurontin)	Central	Gastrointestinal
Botulinum toxin (Botox)	Local muscle	Weakness

GABA, γ-Aminobutyric acid.

in those with incomplete lesions.[45] Management of spasticity has the goals of promoting function and preventing contractures and pain because of the spasticity. Simple measures include ranging, positioning, and the use of orthoses. Some patients and families think that spasticity is reduced with a daily passive standing program. If spasticity still interferes with function, medications may be considered. See Table 14–6 for a summary of common antispasticity medications.

Local spasticity may be treated with splinting or casting or, if severe, with the use of intramuscular botulinum toxin. If spasticity continues to be severe and generalized after physical measures are employed and medications are maximized, surgical management of spasticity should be considered. Selective dorsal rhizotomy has been used in the United States since the mid-1980s. Although usually performed in children with spasticity of cerebral origin, the same technique may be used to reduce spasticity in children with SCIs who are at least 6 months postinjury. A newer surgical technique is the implantation of a pump for continuous administration of baclofen into the intrathecal space.[46] Potential complications seen with intrathecal baclofen include infection, catheter disconnection or blockage, seroma around the pump, cerebrospinal fluid leak, seizures, failure to respond to increasing doses of baclofen, and pump failure. Some deaths have been reported after implantation of a baclofen pump in children with SCI.[47]

Psychosocial Issues

The primary psychosocial issue during rehabilitation is funding for care, equipment, therapies, and environmental modifications after discharge from inpatient rehabilitation. While parents are dealing with these issues, they must also adjust to the new needs of their child and assist their child in adjusting. The child must adjust to the new function of his or her body and learn to reenter home, community, and school. Recreation therapy can be of great help in assisting the child learn to move about in the community, both from the physical and from the psychosocial perspective.

Education and Vocation

While the child is relearning mobility and self-care skills, he or she must also begin to resume school work. Adaptations necessary in the school environment need to be addressed, including architectural barriers, attitudinal barriers, and how to function with different physical skills. The child may need new ways to access computers for school or something as simple as two sets of school books—one for home and one in each classroom—to ease the physical challenges of returning to school. School staff and students need to be educated about SCIs to the extent the child and family wish this to be done. Often it is helpful for several members of the rehabilitation team to visit the school to discuss spinal cord injury and present a videotape of the child engaged in some common activities. If this can be a question-and-answer session for the other students and school staff, many misconceptions can be eliminated and school reentry eased.

Equipment and Environment

For the child who has had an SCI and is nonambulatory, a barrier-free environment is necessary at home, at school, and in the community. Home evaluation by an occupational therapist with recommendations for making the home wheelchair-accessible is necessary as soon as the child's long-term status is known. Minimal needs are ramping to enter the house, wide enough doorways to move about, and some type of access to a bathroom for hygiene and bathing. For some families, accessible housing can be obtained only if they move or the child lives with another member of the extended family.

Wheelchairs

For the child with an SCI, needs related to wheeled mobility must be addressed as soon as possible after the injury and frequently reassessed as the child grows. Even if the child is expected to be a household ambulator, he or she may need a wheelchair for independence in the community. Children with high tetraplegia need powered mobility to be independent in the community, and children as young as 2 years have been shown to have the ability to use power wheelchairs.[48] Electric riding toys are available commercially that can often be adapted for use by children with SCIs. The advantages of these toys are cost and their appearance as a *normal* preschool toy. For the older child who needs powered mobility, a backup manual wheelchair or stroller is also necessary for those times when the power wheelchair is nonoperable or when it cannot be transported.

Most children with tetraplegia and paraplegia should be fitted for a wheelchair by age 3 or 4 years. The chair should fit the child, have the potential to be grown, and accommodate equipment such as orthoses and ventilators. If the child is to be transported by van or school bus in the wheelchair, it should meet local and state transportation standards. It should be a commonly available model with service and parts readily available in the community in which the child lives. See Table 14–7 for a summary of seating systems.

TABLE 14–7.   Seating Systems for Children with Spinal Cord Injury

Medical Considerations	Suggested Equipment Components	Rationale	Comments
Respiratory compromise requiring daytime ventilation	Ventilator Tray	To transport ventilator	The wheelchair must have at least a 16-inch seat width to accommodate ventilator
High tetraplegia	Tilt-in-space power option and/or power recline	Used for pressure relief and prevention of pressure ulcers; avoid transferring out of chair for catheterization for females	A tilt-in-space system maintains a consistent back (hip) angle while tilting the entire seat on its posterior axis; thus, there are no shear forces. The power recline system lowers the seat back, elevates the legs, and moves the hips into an extended position, causing shearing forces. The power recline system may be preferable if perineal care or catheterization is made easier
	Elevating leg rests Arm troughs	Necessary to maintain position of legs and arms when using the tilt-in-space or power recline	
	Head rest and/or Hensinger collar	Necessary for postural alignment to promote functional abilities and to provide support for weak neck muscles	The Whitmyer SOFT head support is recommended as it is cosmetically appealing and allows for many adjustments
Spinal deformities	Lateral supports Molded seat system if severe (> 40°)	Good postural alignment necessary for functional activities and appropriate sensory stimulation	Lateral supports are more easily transferred from seat to seat
Spasticity	Belts, toe and heal loops, lateral supports, molded seating system	Good postural alignment necessary for functional activities and appropriate sensory stimulation	
Hypotonicity	Thoracolumbosacral orthosis Lateral supports, molded seating system	Good postural alignment necessary for functional activities and appropriate sensory stimulation	
Hip instability/ dislocation	Cut out seat for leg length discrepancy > 1 inch Molded seat	To maintain postural alignment to distribute pressure evenly	
Pressure ulcer history	Tilt-in-space or recliner system Air bladder cushion	To provide pressure relief	All children with pressure sores on their buttocks should stay off them until healed

Adapted from Betz RR, Mulcahey MJ (eds): The Child with a Spinal Cord Injury. Rosemont, IL, American Academy of Orthopaedic Surgeons, 1996;845.

TABLE 14–8. Comparison of Orthotic Options at C7, T5 and T12–L1.

	C7	T5	T12–L1
Primary mobility	Wheelchair	Wheelchair and RGO/HKAFO	Wheelchair and RGO/HKAFO
Standers/ parapodium	Full body support Exercise, household, classroom use	Full body support Functional indoor use May pivot walk with parapodium/walker	May be initial means of upright mobility for early standing
RGO	Not generally recommended	Household and classroom ambulator	Short community ambulator
	Limited exercise use on level surfaces only Requires modified walker Requires physical assistance	Limited outdoor use Walker or forearm crutches Assistance required, depending on age	Walker or crutches, depending on age Midthoracic uprights to control lordosis
HKAFO	Not recommended	Same as above for RGO Walker or crutches with swing to/through gait	Same as above for RGO Crutches with swing-through gait
KAFO	Not recommended	Not recommended	Household ambulation Watch for development of lordosis Energy-consuming
AFO	Positioning use only	Positioning use only	Positioning use only
TLSO	Recommended for trunk support and postural alignment	Recommended for trunk support and postural alignment	May be used for postural alignment

RGO, Reciprocating gait orthosis; HKAFO, hip-knee-ankle-foot orthosis; KAFO, knee-ankle-foot orthosis; AFO, ankle-foot orthosis; TLSO, thoracolumbosacral orthosis; GRAFO, ground reaction ankle foot orthosis.
Adapted from Creitz LL, Nelson VS, Haubenstricker L, Backer G: Orthotic Prescriptions. In Betz RR, Mulcahey MJ (eds): The Child with a Spinal Cord Injury. Rosemont, IL, American Academy of Orthopedic Surgeons, 1996;552.

Training in wheeled mobility should begin as soon after the injury as the child can begin sitting up. Training should include smooth level surfaces, carpeted surfaces, ramps, and curbs. For the older child with strong arms, training may also include riding escalators. Safety is an important part of both manual and power wheelchair training, and the child should understand that his or her *driver's license* will be revoked for infractions of safety rules. A final part of training in wheelchair mobility is introduction to wheelchair sports.

Orthotics for Standing and Ambulation

Orthotic management of the child with an SCI must consider the child's developmental level, growth potential, functional status, and cognitive abilities. The goals of walking might include functional independence, maintenance of lower extremity range of motion, promotion of cardiovascular fitness, and perhaps spasticity reduction. The type of orthosis depends on the spinal level and the presence of deformities. See Tables 14–8 and 14–9 for options at various levels of SCI.[49]

TABLE 14–9. Comparison of Orthotic Options at L3 and L5

	L3	L5
Primary mobility	RGO/KAFO and wheelchair	AFO/GRAFO
Standers/ parapodium	May be initial means of upright mobility for early standing	Not applicable
RGO	Independent community ambulator Independent at functional activities May be able to unlock knees	Generally not used at this level Consider using if hip extensors/abductors are weak
HKAFO	Same as above for RGO	Same as above for RGO
KAFO	Same as above for RGO Watch for development of lordosis	May use to control genu valgum or varum Watch for development of lordosis
AFO	Positioning use If strong quadriceps, may be able to use for standing and/or walking	Watch for knee deformity May not need crutches
TLSO	Not required for ambulation	Not required for ambulation

RGO, Reciprocating gait orthosis; HKAFO hip-knee-ankle-foot orthosis; KAFO, knee-ankle-foot orthosis, AFO, ankle-foot orthosis; TLSO, thoracolumbosacral orthosis; GRAFO ground reaction ankle-foot orthosis.
Adapted from Creitz LL, Nelson VS, Haubenstricker L, Backer G: Orthotic Prescriptions. In Betz RR, Mulcahey MJ (eds): The Child with a Spinal Cord Injury. Rosemont, IL, American Academy of Orthopedic Surgeons, 1996;552.

All children with SCI should be encouraged to stand at young ages, with household ambulation encouraged in those with T12–L1 paraplegia and community ambulation encouraged for those with L3 and lower paraplegia. Once children reach puberty, they should be allowed to decide under what conditions to stand and walk. Of primary importance is independent function in age-appropriate activities in the community, not walking to the exclusion of other activities.

Activities of Daily Living and Upper Extremity Function

After SCI, children need to relearn self-care skills. Children with SCI C7 and lower can be expected to be independent in basic self-care by adolescence if they are in a barrier-free environment. Assistive devices, such as tenodesis orthoses, palmar bands, balanced forearm orthoses, forearm-wrist orthoses, and reachers, can all be useful in increasing function.[50] Acceptance of these by children and adolescents is dependent on cosmesis, reliability, and the amount they increase function. If parents do not accept assistive devices, young children will not, although adolescents may. The role of functional electrical stimulation with implanted electrodes is still being debated, but early results are promising for adolescents and adults with C5 and C6 level SCI. Surgical reconstruction to improve upper extremity function has been written about extensively in the adult SCI literature, with more recent articles about its role with children. A careful evaluation of the child's function must be done, and the family and child must be educated about the procedure and what can be achieved with the surgery.

Assistive Technology

An assistive technology device is any item that increases or improves functional capabilities for an individual with a disability. An assistive technology device need not be high technology. Assistive technology service is service that assists the disabled individual in the selection and use of technology, such as a device. Depending on the child's needs, assistive technology may include any of the following devices: augmentative communication, computer, seating and postural support, powered mobility, environmental control unit, recreation equipment, and motor vehicle adaptations. Identifying and using assistive technology is an ongoing, dynamic process for the child with an SCI, especially for those who sustain injury at an early age. Children with SCI should be introduced to assistive technology early in their rehabilitation by a team

knowledgeable in the simplest, least complicated equipment that will increase the child's functional abilities and promote independence.

Special Considerations in High Tetraplegia

Children with high tetraplegia (C1–4 levels) all have some type of partial or complete respiratory dysfunction. Whether they require full-time or part-time mechanical ventilation depends on their level and the completeness of their lesion. Some may be ventilated only at night by face mask, whereas others require tracheostomies and full-time ventilation. Issues unique to this latter group include airway problems, increased risk of pulmonary infection, developmental impact of being assisted by a machine for life support, and impact of a tracheostomy on communication and swallowing. School reintegration is another issue because these children require assistance with their respiratory management, bowel and bladder care, and all usual school activities. Who provides this assistance must be negotiated between the school, parents, and rehabilitation physician.

Respiration and Airway

Various options are available for the home mechanical ventilation of children with high tetraplegia. Ventilation may be invasive (i.e., through a tracheostomy) or noninvasive (via face mask, tank respirator, or cuirass). The important fact to remember is that *the best ventilation is not necessarily the least ventilation*. It is better for the child to be healthy while using respiratory support than to be unhealthy and free of the ventilator. The reader is referred to *The Ventilator-Assisted Child: A Practical Resource Guide*[51] for more details. Table 14–10 summarizes ventilation options.

Communication

Oral communication is a complex process involving oromotor, vocal fold, and respiratory muscles. If a child has a tracheostomy with or without cranial nerve involvement from SCI, oral communication is affected, and the child must learn to communicate in a new manner. Although the primary purpose of the tracheostomy tube is to provide an attachment to the ventilator and an opening for suctioning, the type and size chosen must also allow for an air leak to promote oral communication, if at all possible. The ventilator should be set at a low rate with a long inspiratory time because ventilator users talk on the inspiratory cycle. Consideration

TABLE 14–10. Types of Mechanical Ventilation

	Indications	Limitations	Advantages
BIPAP-Trach	For respiratory support for child who can initiate breath Transition between trach-IPPV and mask-BIPAP Improve functional residual capacity Augment tidal breathing with pressure support Stabilize airways Improve pulmonary hygiene Rest respiratory muscles Intolerance of mask	Not usable for child who has no respiratory effort Trach imposes changes in lifestyle (e.g., swimming) Requires external battery and alarms Inability to trigger in small babies	Direct access to trachea for suctioning Smaller machine than *traditional* ventilator Shorter learning curve than for *traditional* IPPV Leak compensation in children with uncuffed trachs
BIPAP-mask	For respiratory support for child who can initiate breath Transition between trach-IPPV and mask-BIPAP Improve functional residual capacity Augment tidal breathing with pressure support Stabilize airways Improve pulmonary hygiene Rest respiratory muscles	Portable with external battery Skin irritation on face may limit use Not usable with severe oral motor dysfunction No direct trachea access for suctioning Not useable for child who has no respiratory effort Not practical for 24-hour use	No trach (noninvasive) Less costly than IPPV Shorter learning curve Better humidification than passover humidifier and trach
Trach-IPPV	Need for full respiratory support	Trach imposes changes in lifestyle (e.g., swimming)	Ventilator is portable and can be transported on wheelchair
Cuirass	For respiratory support for child who can initiate breath independently, but needs some support Rests respiratory muscles	Must be custom-made for small children and those with chest deformities (e.g., scoliosis) Does not work well with decreased chest compliance No internal battery—electrically powered Difficult to don independently	No trach No face mask
Iron Lung	For respiratory support for child who can initiate breath independently, but needs some support Rests respiratory muscles	Large size does not fit well in most homes Does not work well with decreased lung compliance Cannot use without assistance Positioning is difficult Portable unit (Porta-lung) weighs approximately 100 lbs	Machinery is simple to service No face mask and sometimes no trach May be used with or without trach

BIPAP, Bilevel positive airway pressure; IPPV, intermittent positive-pressure ventilation; trach, tracheostomy.
Adapted from Driver LE, Nelson VS, Warschausky SA (eds): The Ventilator-Assisted Child: A Practical Resource Guide. San Antonio, Communication Skill Builders, 1997.

should also be given to using a one-way speaking valve such as the Passy Muir.[52]

Spinal Orthoses and Abdominal Support

Children with high tetraplegia often need the support of a thoracolumbosacral orthosis (TLSO) or abdominal binder to assist them in maintaining the upright position, to support the diaphragm when they are not using mechanical ventilation, and to prevent hypotension in the upright position. A traditionally molded TLSO often restricts chest and abdominal excursion and may be uncomfortable, especially after meals. For the child with high tetraplegia, the TLSO should be molded with the child on a tilt-table or wedge elevated at approximately 30 degrees. As soon as the molding plaster is dry enough, the cast should be cut along the middle front. If the child has a tracheostomy, he or she should be given several large breaths with an ambu-bag, allowing the chest and cast to expand. Both sides of the cast should be lubricated with petroleum jelly, and several layers of plaster should be placed over this opening. This new cast is larger than the original one, and a TLSO fabricated from it is more comfortable and allows for better ventilation and expansion for eating. The TLSO should be fabricated with a belly hole, which is lined with ¼-inch foam.[53]

Mouthsticks

Mouthsticks are lightweight sticks with specialized tips that can be used to perform various activities, such as keyboarding, switch control, writing, and turning pages. The mouth end may be Y-shaped or custom-molded to fit the child's mouth. The length of the mouthstick varies, according to the size of the child and the activity for which the mouthstick is to be used. Mouthstick activities may be used for therapeutic goals of increasing neck range, strength, and endurance and improving the use of a chin joystick for wheelchair control. All children with high tetraplegia should be introduced to the use of mouthsticks and encouraged to use them for a variety of activities, including writing, painting, playing games, and page turning.

Neck Exercises

Isometric neck exercises should begin as soon as medical clearance has been obtained. Once the child with high tetraplegia has been released from cervical bracing, active range of motion and strengthening exercises should begin, since greater strength and range of motion of the neck make accessing various types of controllers such as joysticks or pneumatic switches easier. The stronger the neck muscles and the more symmetric the pull, the greater the ability of the child to control switches to access assistive technology. Practice with mouthsticks and driving with a chin joystick both assist in strengthening neck muscles.

Wheelchairs

All children with complete high tetraplegia need some type of wheelchair. Those old enough should be strongly considered for power mobility. Their wheelchairs become their portable homes, with ventilator, suction equipment, oxygen if necessary, and all supplies contained on the chair. Most of these children need to have tilt-in-space features to allow for pressure relief and access for catheterizing, suctioning, and so forth. A power wheelchair should have controls that are fully accessible to the child. The ventilator should be mounted as far as possible above the ground to prevent dirt and moisture from entering it. A convenient mounting system is the gimble mount, which allows the ventilator to swivel and stay level as the seating is tilted or reclined. Various control systems can be used, including chin, pneumatic (sip-and-puff), and head-controlled switches. The child should be allowed to practice with various types before a final decision is made. Generally the chin control is the easiest to use because the head control requires more neck strength.

Long-term Follow-up

Effect of Growth on the Child with Spinal Cord Injury

Growing children often encounter complications because of the effects of growth on their body. The most common one is contracture, which is most likely to occur during periods of rapid growth. Other growth-related complications include hip subluxation and scoliosis. In children who sustain SCI before puberty, more than 90% develop scoliosis with two-thirds requiring surgical management.[54] An equal percentage develop hip subluxation or dislocation.[55] Although not directly related to growth, approximately 14% of children with SCI develop pathologic long bone fractures, many with no known cause.[56] Treatment should consist of removable splints or orthoses. Approximately 50% of children with SCI may develop syringomyelia as seen on MR imaging. A common symptom of this is severe spasticity. Routine surveillance of the child with SCI should watch for these complications, with more frequent follow-ups during periods of rapid growth.

Advocacy

As the child and family adjust to life with an SCI, they are confronted with the many barriers to participation in usual activities. Children and their families need to learn advocacy skills to open doors for them to participate in all types of activities. This advocacy training begins during acute rehabilitation. Children and their families can be introduced to peer counseling and educated about laws, advocacy methods, internet resources, and consumer groups. They should be assisted by the rehabilitation team as they re-enter the community and school and resume usual childhood activities.

References

1. Vogel LC: Unique management needs of pediatric spinal cord injury patients: Etiology and pathophysiology. J Spinal Cord Med 1997;20:10.
2. Burney RE, Maio RF, Maynard F, Karunas R: Incidence, characteristics, and outcome of spinal cord injury at trauma centers in North America. Arch Surg 1993;128:596.
3. Vogel LC: Management of medical issues. In Betz RR, Mulcahey MJ (eds): The Child with a Spinal Cord Injury. Rosemont, IL, American Academy of Orthopedic Surgeons, 1996.
4. Vogel LC, DeVivo MJ: Etiology and demographics. In Betz RR, Mulcahey MJ (eds): The Child with a Spinal Cord Injury. Rosemont, IL, American Academy of Orthopedic Surgeons, 1996.

5. Hadley MN, Zabramski JM, Browner CM, et al: Pediatric spinal trauma: Review of 122 cases of spinal cord and vertebral column injuries. J Neurosurg 1988;68:18.

6. Ruge JR, Sinson GP, McLone DG, Cerullo LJ: Pediatric spinal injury: The very young. J Neurosurg, 1988; 68:25.

7. Turgut M, Akpinar G, Akalan N, Ozcan OE: Spinal injuries in the pediatric age group: A review of 82 cases of spinal cord and vertebral column injuries. Eur Spine J 1996;5:148.

8. National Spinal Cord Injury Statistical Center: The 1997 Annual Statistical Report for the Model Spinal Cord Injury Care Systems. Birmingham, AL, National SCI Statistical Center, 1997.

9. Vogel LJ, Mulcahey MJ, Betz RR: The child with a spinal cord injury. Dev Med Child Neurol 1997;38:202.

10. Pang D: Spinal cord injury without radiographic abnormality (SCIWORA) in children. In Betz RR, Mulcahey MJ (eds): The Child with a Spinal Cord Injury. Rosemont, IL, American Academy of Orthopedic Surgeons, 1996.

11. Dickman CA, Zabramski JM, Hadley MN, et al: Pediatric spinal cord injury without radiologic abnormalities: Report of 26 cases and review of the literature. J Spinal Disord 1991;4:296.

12. American Spinal Injury Association/International Medical Society of Paraplegia (ASIA/IMSOP): International Standards for Neurological and Functional Classification of Spinal Cord Injury, Revised. Chicago, American Spinal Injury Association, 1996.

13. Schneider RC, Cherry G, Pantek H: The syndrome of acute central cervical spinal cord injury: With special reference to the mechanisms involved in hyperextension injuries of cervical spine. J Neurosurg 1954;11:546.

14. Cawley MF: Incomplete spinal cord injury. In Betz RR, Mulcahey MJ (eds): The Child with a Spinal Cord Injury. Rosemont, IL, American Academy of Orthopedic Surgeons, 1996.

15. Wright M, Rivara FP, Ferse D: Evaluation of the Think First head and spinal cord injury prevention program. Injury Prevention 1995;1:81.

16. Watts C, Eyster EF: National head and spinal cord injury prevention program of the American Association of Neurological Surgeons and the Congress of Neurological Surgeons. J Neurotrauma 1992;9(Suppl 1): S307.

17. Thurman DH, Burnett CL, Beaudoin DE, et al: Risk factors and mechanisms of occurrence in motor vehicle-related spinal cord injuries: Utah. Accident Analysis and Prevention 1995;27:411.

18. Sasso RC, Meyer PR, Heinemann AW, et al: Seat-belt use and relation to neurologic injury in motor vehicle crashes. J Spinal Disord 1997;10:325.

19. DeVivo MJ, Sekar P: Prevention of spinal cord injuries that occur in swimming pools. Spinal Cord 1997;35:509.

20. Tator CH, Carson JD, Edmonds VE: New spinal injuries in hockey. Clin J Sport Med 1997;7:17.

21. Nickel VL, Perry J, Garrett A, et al: The halo: A spinal skeletal traction fixation device. J Bone Joint Surg 1968;50A:1400.

22. Loder RT: Halo use in children. In Betz RR, Mulcahey MJ (eds): The Child with a Spinal Cord Injury. Rosemont, IL, American Academy of Orthopedic Surgeons, 1996.

23. Ward WT, Doyle JS: Management of upper cervical spine injuries: Occiput to C3. In Betz RR, Mulcahey MJ (eds): The Child with a Spinal Cord Injury. Rosemont, IL, American Academy of Orthopedic Surgeons, 1996.

24. Klassen RH, McGrory BJ: Management of C3-C7 injuries. In Betz RR, Mulcahey MJ (eds): The Child with a Spinal Cord Injury. Rosemont, IL, American Academy of Orthopedic Surgeons, 1996.

25. Dekutoski MB: Management of thoracic, thoracolumbar, lumbar, and sacral fractures in the pediatric population. In Betz RR, Mulcahey MJ (eds): The Child with a Spinal Cord Injury. Rosemont, IL, American Academy of Orthopedic Surgeons, 1996.

26. Bracken MB, Shepard MJ, Collins WF, et al: A randomized controlled trial of methylprednisolone or naloxone in the treatment of acute spinal cord injury. N Engl J Med 1990;322:1405.

27. Bracken MB, Shepard MH, Holford TR, et al: Administration of methylprednisolone for 24 or 48 hours or tirilazad mesylate for 48 hours in the treatment of acute spinal cord injury. JAMA 1997;277:1597.

28. Workshop Statements. In Betz RR, Mulcahey MJ (eds): The Child with a Spinal Cord Injury. Rosemont, IL, American Academy of Orthopedic Surgeons, 1996.

29. Van Hala S, Nelson VS, Hurvitz EA, et al: Bladder management in patients with pediatric onset neurogenic bladders. J Spinal Cord Med 1997;20:410.

30. Maynard FM: Immobilization hypercalcemia following spinal cord injury. Arch Phys Med Rehabil 1986; 67:41.

31. Silverman SL, Hurvitz EA, Nelson VS, Chiodo A: Rachitic syndrome after disodium etidronate therapy in an adolescent. Arch Phys Med Rehabil 1994;75:118.

32. Anderson CJ: Unique management needs of pediatric spinal cord injury patients: Psychosocial issues. J Spinal Cord Med 1997;20:21.

33. Warschausky S, Engel L, Kewman D, Nelson VS: Psychosocial factors in rehabilitation of the child with a spinal cord injury. In Betz RR, Mulcahey MJ (eds): The Child with a Spinal Cord Injury. Rosemont, IL, American Academy of Orthopedic Surgeons, 1996.

34. Buckelew SP, Frank RG, Elliott TR, et al: Adjustment to spinal cord injury: Stage theory revisited. Paraplegia 1991;29:125.

35. Pontari MA, Bauer SB: Urologic issues in spinal cord injury: Assessment, management, outcome, and research needs. In Betz RR, Mulcahey MJ (eds): The Child with a Spinal Cord Injury. Rosemont, IL, American Academy of Orthopedic Surgeons, 1996.

36. Mitrofanoff P: Trans-appendicular continent cystotomy in the management of the neurogenic bladder. Chir Pediatr 1980;21:297.

37. Horowitz M, Kuhr CS, Mitchell ME: The Mitrofanoff catheterizable channel: Patient acceptance. J Urol 1995; 153:771.

38. Flavell H, Marshall R, Thornton AT et al: Hypoxia episodes during sleep in high tetraplegia. Arch Phys Med Rehabil 1992;73:623.

39. Stiens SA, Bergman SB, Goetz LL: Neurogenic bowel dysfunction after spinal cord injury: Clinical evaluation and rehabilitative management. Arch Phys Med Rehabil 1997;78:S86.

40. Bergman SB, Yarkony GM, Stiens SA: Spinal cord injury rehabilitation: 2. Medical complications. Arch Phys Med Rehabil 1997;78:S53.

41. Yarkony GM: Pressure ulcers: Classification and overview. In Betz RR, Mulcahey MJ (eds): The Child with a Spinal Cord Injury. Rosemont, IL, American Academy of Orthopedic Surgeons, 1996.

42. Apple DF, Murray HH: Surgical management of pressure ulcers. In Betz RR, Mulcahey MJ (eds): The Child with a Spinal Cord Injury. Rosemont, IL, American Academy of Orthopedic Surgeons, 1996.

43. Schmidt KD, Chan CW: Thermoregulation and fever in normal persons and in those with spinal cord injuries. Mayo Clin Proc 1992;67:469.

44. Mandac BR, Hurvitz EA, Nelson VS: Hyperthermia associated with baclofen withdrawal and increased spasticity. Arch Phys Med Rehabil 1993;74:96.

45. Vogel LC: Spasticity: Diagnostic work-up and medical management. In Betz RR, Mulcahey MJ (eds): The Child with a Spinal Cord Injury. Rosemont, IL, American Academy of Orthopedic Surgeons, 1996.

46. Meythaler JM, Steers WD, Tuel SM, et al: Continuous intrathecal baclofen in spinal cord spasticity: A prospective study. Am J Phys Med Rehabil 1992;71:321.

47. Armstrong RW, Steinbok P, Farrell K, et al: Continuous intrathecal baclofen treatment of severe spasms in two children with spinal cord injury. Dev Med Child Neurol 1992;34:731.

48. Butler C, Okamoto G, McKay T: Powered mobility for very young children. Devel Med Child Neurol 1983;25:472.

49. Creitz LL, Nelson VS, Haubenstricker L, Backer G: Orthotic prescriptions. In Betz RR, Mulcahey MJ (eds): The Child with a Spinal Cord Injury. Rosemont, IL, American Academy of Orthopedic Surgeons, 1996.

50. Miner LJ, Nelson VS: Upper limb orthoses. In Redford JB, Basmajian JV, Trautman P (eds): Orthotics: Clinical Practice and Rehabilitation Technology. New York, Churchill Livingstone, 1995.

51. Driver LE, Nelson VS, Warschausky SA (eds): The Ventilator-Assisted Child: A Practical Resource Guide. San Antonio, Communication Skill Builders, 1997.

52. Driver LE, Hilker DF: Oral and written communication needs of the ventilator-assisted child. In Driver LE, Nelson VS, Warschausky SA (eds): The Ventilator-Assisted Child: A Practical Resource Guide. San Antonio, Communication Skill Builders, 1997.

53. Backer G, Howell B: Physical therapy goals and intervention for the ventilator-assisted child or adolescent. In Driver LE, Nelson VS, Warschausky SA (eds): The Ventilator-Assisted Child: A Practical Resource Guide. San Antonio, Communication Skill Builders, 1997.

54. Lubicky JP, Betz RR: Spinal deformity in children and adolescents after spinal cord injury. In Betz RR, Mulcahey MJ (eds): The Child with a Spinal Cord Injury. Rosemont, IL, American Academy of Orthopedic Surgeons, 1996.

55. Miller F, Betz RR: Hip joint instability. In Betz RR, Mulcahey MJ (eds): The Child with a Spinal Cord Injury. Rosemont, IL, American Academy of Orthopedic Surgeons, 1996.

56. Betz RR: Unique management needs of pediatric spinal cord injury patients: Orthopedic problems in the child with spinal cord injury. J Spinal Cord Med 1997;20:14.

Chapter 15

Neuromuscular Diseases

Craig M. McDonald, MD

Progressive acquired or hereditary neuro-muscular diseases (NMDs) are disorders caused by an abnormality of any component of the lower motor neuron—anterior horn cell, peripheral nerve, neuromuscular junction (presynaptic or postsynaptic region), or muscle. While some neuromuscular diseases have pathologic abnormalities isolated to one anatomic region of the lower motor neuron, with primary or secondary changes in muscle, other neuromuscular diseases have been recognized as multisystem disorders. For example, myotonic muscular dystrophy may affect skeletal muscle, smooth muscle, myocardium, brain, and ocular structures; Duchenne muscular dystrophy gives rise to abnormalities of skeletal and cardiac muscle, the cardiac conduction system, and brain; Fukuyama congenital muscular dystrophy affects skeletal muscle and brain; and mitochondrial encephalomyopathies may affect the mitochondria of multiple tissues.

Neuromuscular diseases may be acquired (e.g., poliomyelitis, Guillain-Barré syndrome, myasthenia gravis, or polymyositis), but the most common cause is genetic (e.g., spinal muscular atrophy, hereditary motor sensory neuropathy, congenital myasthenia gravis, or Duchenne muscular dystrophy).

Tremendous advances have occurred in the past decade in our understanding of the molecular genetic basis and pathophysiology of neuromuscular diseases affecting children and adults. Traditional approaches to the classification of neuromuscular disorders use clinical history, family history, clinical examination findings, electrodiagnostic findings, and histopathologic analysis of muscle and/or nerve biopsy specimens to provide clinical diagnosis. Molecular genetic advances have led to the discovery of specific genes for over 100 neuromuscular disorders and have provided pathophysiologic explanations for phenotypically divergent disorders such as Duchenne and Becker muscular dystrophy. The wide range of clinical phenotypes of childhood spinal muscular atrophy (from the severe infantile type I form to the mild ambulant type III form) and genetic heterogeneity has been identified within specific syndromes. For example, at least 14 genetically distinct subtypes of hereditary motor sensory neuropathy (HMSN) have been described, some with undetermined gene loci; six genetically distinct subtypes of autosomal recessive limb-girdle muscular dystrophy have been identified; and two genetically distinct subtypes of Bethlem myopathy exist. In fact, the gene loci for approximately 100 distinct neuromuscular disorders and over 40 mitochondrial encephalomyopathies had been identified at the time this chapter was written.

Appropriate rehabilitation management of neuromuscular diseases requires an accurate diagnosis. The clinician must be able to obtain a relevant patient and family history and perform focused general, musculoskeletal, neurologic, and functional physical examinations to direct further diagnostic evaluations. Laboratory studies may now include relevant molecular genetic studies in certain instances; however, specific genetic entities need to be strong diagnostic considerations because these studies may be expensive and have limited sensitivity and specificity. Electromyography (EMG) and nerve conduction studies remain an extension of the physical examination and help to guide further diagnostic studies such as muscle and nerve biopsies or even motor point biopsies applied to the evaluation of congenital myasthenic syndromes. All diagnostic information needs to be interpreted, not in isolation but within the context of relevant historical information, family history, physical examination findings, laboratory data, electrophysiologic findings, and pathologic information, if obtained.

A skilled synthesis of all available information may provide the patient and family with (1) a precise diagnosis or as accurate a diagnosis as medically possible; (2) prognostic information (if available for a specific entity); and (3) anticipatory guidance for the near future. Knowledge of the natural history of specific neuromuscular conditions helps in the ongoing rehabilitative management of progressive impairments, disabilities, and handicaps. This chapter summarizes the diagnostic evaluation, natural history and impairment profiles, and rehabilitation management of childhood neuromuscular diseases.

Diagnostic Evaluation of Neuromuscular Diseases

Neuromuscular Disease History

The common chief presenting complaints from parents or children with suspected neuromuscular disorders may include infantile floppiness or hypotonia, delay in motor milestones, feeding and respiratory difficulties, abnormal gait characteristics, frequent falls, difficulty ascending stairs or arising from the floor, and muscle cramps or stiffness. Teenagers with later-onset disorders may present with chief complaints of strength loss or decreasing endurance, falls, difficulty ascending stairs, exercise intolerance, episodic weakness, muscle cramps, focal wasting of muscle groups, breathing difficulties, or bulbar symptoms such as speech and swallowing difficulties.

Information should be obtained about the recent course of the chief complaint, specifically whether the process is getting worse, staying the same, or getting better. If strength is deteriorating, it is important to ascertain the rate of progression (i.e., whether weakness is increasing over days, weeks, months, or years). It is critical to determine whether the distribution of weakness is predominantly proximal, distal, or generalized. It is also useful to identify factors that worsen or help primary symptoms. A history of muscle twitching may reflect fasciculations. Tremor or balance problems may be due to distal weakness or superimposed cerebellar involvement.

Bulbar involvement may be identified if the individual has difficulty with chewing, swallowing, or speech articulation. Visual complaints (blurriness or diplopia) may indicate the presence of cataracts or possible involvement of extraocular musculature. Distal stocking glove or focal sensory complaints may be consistent with a peripheral neuropathy or focal nerve entrapment. A comprehensive medical and surgical history should be obtained. A history of recent illnesses should be carefully elucidated, including respiratory difficulties, aspiration pneumonias, or recurrent pulmonary infections. In addition, such cardiac symptoms as dizziness, syncope, chest pain, orthopnea, or exertional complaints may indicate superimposed involvement of the myocardium. A review of pulmonary symptoms should be obtained. A history of weight loss may be due to recurrent illnesses, nutritional compromise, swallowing difficulty, or progressive lean tissue atrophy.

A detailed history regarding pregnancy (e.g., quality of fetal movement or pregnancy complications) and perinatal problems (evidence of fetal distress, respiratory difficulties in the recovery room, need for resuscitation or ventilation problems in early infancy, ongoing respiratory difficulties, swallowing/feeding difficulties, and persistent hypotonia) should be obtained. Perinatal respiratory distress in the delivery room may be seen in acute infantile type I spinal muscular atrophy (SMA), myotubular myopathy, congenital hypomyelinating neuropathy, congenital infantile myasthenia, transitory neonatal myasthenia, and severe neurogenic arthrogryposis.

History regarding the child's acquisition of developmental milestones should be ascertained relating to head control, independent sitting, crawling, standing with and without support, walking with and without support, fine motor prehension, bimanual skill acquisition (bringing objects to midline, transfer of objects), and language acquisition. Information regarding gait characteristics (toe walking, excessive lordosis, etc.), running ability, transitions from floor to standing, stair climbing, falls, recreational/athletic performance, pain or muscle cramps and easy fatigue, or lack of endurance, may be important clues to the presence of a neuromuscular disorder. History regarding mental development, type of school, and school performance may be important indicators of superimposed CNS involvement. For the older child, a detailed history regarding the age of onset of symptoms, paralysis progression, distribution of weakness, presence of muscle cramps, fatigue, episodic weakness, presence of atrophy or fasciculations, performance in physical education, current and past ambulatory distances, ability to move from floor to standing, problems climbing stairs, and problems reaching overhead or dressing may all be important functional information.

A history of muscle cramps at rest or with exertion may be associated with a muscular dystrophy, metabolic myopathy, toxic myoglobinuria, inflammatory myositis, or other lower motor neuron disorders.

A thorough anesthetic history should be obtained. Malignant hyperthermia is associated with primary familial malignant hyperthermia, central core congenital myopathy, Duchenne muscular dystrophy (DMD), and Becker muscular dystrophy (BMD). Other NMD conditions occasionally associated with malignant hyperthermia include Fukuyama congenital muscular dystrophy, limb-girdle muscular dystrophy (LGMD), facioscapulohumeral muscular dystrophy (FSH), periodic paralysis, myotonia congenita, mitochondrial myopathy, and the Schwartz-Jampel syndrome.

Family History

Suspicion of a neuromuscular disease warrants the ascertainment of a detailed family history and pedigree chart. Autosomal dominant conditions may have pedigrees of multiple generations affected with equal predilection to males and females. Typically, one-half of offspring within a pedigree are affected. In autosomal recessive conditions, only one generation may be affected with equal proportions of males and females. Proportionally, one-fourth of offspring are clinically affected. Parents in earlier generations may be normal, and the parents of affected children are presumptive heterozygous carriers of the condition. In many instances of autosomal recessive inheritance, no other family members within the nuclear family unit are affected, making the confirmation of inheritance pattern difficult without a molecular genetic marker present or protein abnormality confirmed by immunohistochemistry techniques. In X-linked recessive conditions, males on the maternal side of the family are affected in approximately 50% of instances, and females are carriers in 50% of instances.

Often, it is valuable to examine affected relatives who may be either earlier or later in the course of their neuromuscular disease relative to the affected child. In addition, medical records and diagnostic evaluations of affected family members should be reviewed and the diagnosis confirmed if possible. In some instances, the examination of a parent can help to establish the diagnosis in an affected infant or child, as is frequently the case in myotonic muscular dystrophy (MMD). In this disorder, genetic anticipation with abnormal CTG trinucleotide expansion of unstable DNA results in progressively earlier onset of the disease, with increasing severity, in successive generations.

In the case of dystrophic myopathies, a definitive molecular genetic or pathologic diagnosis established in a sibling or close relative may allow the clinician to establish the diagnosis in a child or adult based on clinical examination, easily obtainable laboratory data, such as creatine

kinase, or molecular genetic testing, thus allowing the avoidance of further invasive testing such as muscle biopsy.

Physical Examination

Physical examination findings help to focus further diagnostic evaluation, using such tools as electrodiagnosis, molecular genetic testing, and histopathologic analysis of biopsy specimens. All diagnostic information must be interpreted within the context of relevant clinical information. In many instances, a precise molecular genetic diagnosis is not medically possible. However, the accurate characterization of an individual patient within the most appropriate neuromuscular clinical syndrome still allows the clinician to provide the patient and family with accurate prognostic information and anticipatory guidance for the future.

Specific aspects of the physical examination relevant to the neuromuscular disease population include simple inspection for the presence of focal or diffuse muscle wasting or focal enlargement of muscles, as with the "pseudohypertrophy" seen in such dystrophic myopathies as Duchenne and Becker muscular dystrophy (Fig. 15–1). The increase in calf circumference in DMD is caused by an increase in fat and

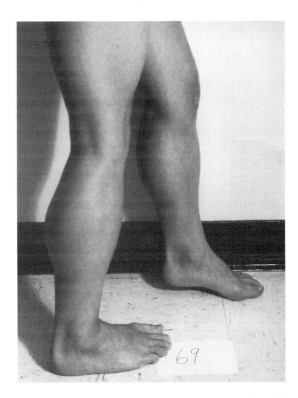

FIGURE 15–1. Calf pseudohypertrophy in a male with Duchenne muscular dystrophy.

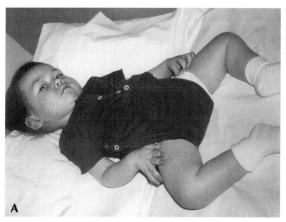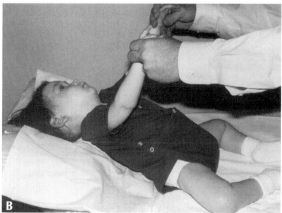

FIGURE 15–2. *A* and *B*, Hypotonia in an 18-month-old with spinal muscular atrophy.

connective tissue, not secondary to true muscle fiber hypertrophy in the gastrocnemius.[1] Over time, the reduced bulk of musculature may be caused by more severe fiber loss in a more active dystrophic process affecting proximal musculature. Other neuromuscular disorders may show calf pseudohypertrophy, such as childhood-type acid maltase deficiency.

Focal atrophy of particular muscle groups may provide diagnostic clues to specific neuromuscular disorders such as SMA, Emery-Dreifuss muscular dystrophy, FSH, and limb-girdle muscular dystrophy. Those with HMSN, particularly those with type II axonal forms, demonstrate distal atrophy or "stork leg appearance" relatively early in the disease course. Palpable nerves in the cubital tunnel, posterior auricular region, or around the fibular head may be indicative of "onion bulbs" seen in hereditary demyelinating neuropathies such as HMSN I subtypes or Dejerine-Sottas disease (HMSN type III).

Muscle fasciculations may be seen as nonspecific findings of a variety of lower motor neuron disorders. Fasciculations are particularly common in such lower motor neuron disorders as SMA. Distal fine tremor may be seen in a large proportion of HMSN patients (30–50%) and in other patients with weakness such as SMA. Polyminimyoclonus, another variant of muscle fasciculations characterized by a fine tremor of the fingers and hands, may be evident in SMA types I and II.

Infants with NMD show infantile hypotonia (Fig. 15–2), the differential for which is large (see Chapter 5).

A thorough general physical examination of cardiac, pulmonary, and gastrointestinal systems should be performed on all patients suspected of having a neuromuscular disease. Hepatomegaly may be seen in metabolic myopathies such as acid maltase deficiency (type 2 glycogenosis) and type 3 and 4 glycogenosis. The skin should be evaluated for characteristic skin rashes and nail bed capillary changes if an inflammatory myopathy such as dermatomyositis is suspected. Craniofacial changes and dental malocclusion are common in congenital myotonic muscular dystrophy, congenital myopathies, congenital muscular dystrophy, and type II SMA. A neurologic examination should include a thorough evaluation of cranial nerve function, muscle tone, muscle strength, sensory and cerebellar function, deep tendon reflexes, and assessment for the presence of percussion and/or grip myotonia (Fig. 15–3) in situations in which a myotonic syndrome is suspected. Musculoskeletal examination will reveal the presence of limb contractures and spinal deformity.

Some neuromuscular disorders, such as congenital myotonic muscular dystrophy, Fukuyama congenital muscular dystrophy, selected

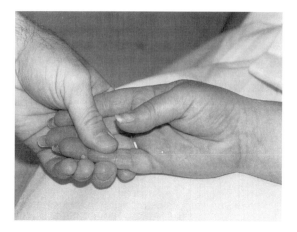

FIGURE 15–3. Percussion myotonia of the thenar eminence.

cases of mitochondrial encephalomyopathies, and a small proportion of Duchenne muscular dystrophy cases, may have significant intellectual impairment.

A thorough functional examination is essential in the diagnostic evaluation of a patient with suspected neuromuscular disease. This includes an evaluation of head control, bed/mat mobility, transitions from supine-to-sit, sit-to-stand, sitting ability without hand support, standing balance, gait, stair climbing, and overhead reach. An evaluation of overhead reach examining the patient from the front and from behind is important in evaluation of shoulder girdle weakness. Careful assessment of scapular winging, scapular stabilization, and scapular rotation is very helpful in the assessment of patients with FSH and limb-girdle syndrome. The scapula is stabilized for overhead abduction by the trapezius, rhomboids, and serratus anterior. Abduction to 180° requires strong supraspinatus and deltoid in addition to strong scapular stabilizers.

Patients with proximal weakness involving the pelvic girdle muscles may rise off the floor using the classic Gowers' sign, through which the patient usually assumes a four-point stance on knees and hands, brings the knees into extension while leaning the upper extremities forward, substitutes for hip extension weakness by pushing off the knees with the upper extremities, and sequentially moves the upper extremities up the thigh until an upright stance with full hip extension is achieved (Fig. 15–4). A Gowers' sign is not specific to any one neuromuscular condition but may be seen in a variety

of neuromuscular diseases, including DMD, LGMD, SMA type III, severe childhood autosomal recessive muscular dystrophy (SCARMD), congenital muscular dystrophy, congenital myopathy, myasthenic syndromes, severe forms of HMSN (e.g., HMSN types III and IV), and other neuromuscular diseases producing proximal weakness. Patients with proximal lower extremity weakness often exhibit a classic myopathic gait pattern (Fig. 15–5). Initially, weakness of the hip extensors produces anterior pelvic tilt and a tendency for the trunk to be positioned anteriorly to the hip joint. Patients compensate for this by maintaining lumbar lordosis, which positions their center of gravity/weight line posterior to the hip joints, thus stabilizing the hip in extension on the anterior capsule of the hip joint. Subsequently, weakness of the knee extensors produces a tendency for patients to experience knee instability and knee buckling with falls. Patients compensate for this by decreasing stance-phase knee flexion and posturing the ankle increasingly over time into plantar flexion. This produces a knee extension moment at foot contact, and the plantar flexion of the ankle during mid-to-late stance phase of gait helps to position the weight line/center of gravity anterior to the knee joint (thus producing a stabilizing knee extension moment). Patients with Duchenne muscular dystrophy progressively demonstrate toe walking with initial floor contact with the foot increasingly moving forward onto the midfoot and finally the forefoot as they reach the transitional phase of ambulation before wheelchair reliance (see Fig. 15–5).

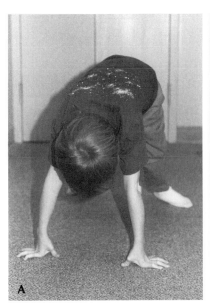 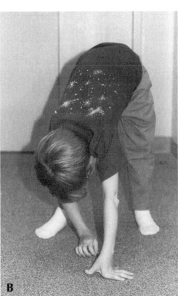 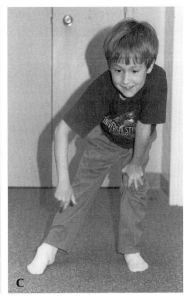

FIGURE 15–4. *A–C,* Gowers' sign in 7-year-old boy with Duchenne muscular dystrophy due to hip extensor weakness.

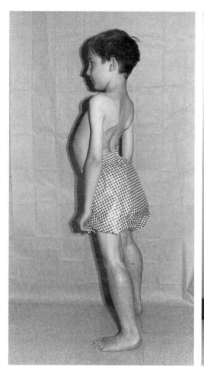 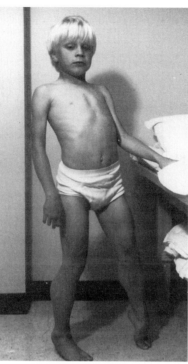

FIGURE 15–5 (Left). "Myopathic" stance in an 8-year-old boy with Duchenne muscular dystrophy. Note the lumbar lordosis compensating for hip extensor weakness and primarily forefoot contact compensating for knee extensor weakness.

FIGURE 15–6 (Right). Trendelenburg or "gluteus medius" gait pattern in a male with Duchenne muscular dystrophy. Note the lateral lean over the stance side due to hip abductor weakness; ankle dorsiflexion weakness necessitates swing phase in circumduction for clearance.

Finally, weakness of the hip abductors produces a tendency toward lateral pelvic tilt and pelvic drop of the swing-phase side. Patients with proximal weakness compensate for this by bending or lurching the trunk laterally over the stance-phase hip joint (Fig. 15–6). This produces the so-called "gluteus medius lurch" or Trendelenburg gait pattern.

Patients with distal weakness affecting the ankle dorsiflexors and ankle everters and less severe proximal weakness (e.g., HMSN, Emery-Dreifuss muscular dystrophy, myotonic muscular dystrophy, FSH, and other conditions) often exhibit a foot slap at floor contact with a steppage gait pattern to facilitate swing-phase clearance of the plantar-flexed ankle. Alternatively, these patients may clear the plantar-flexed ankle using some degree of circumduction at the hip or vaulting on the stance-phase side. Milder distal lower extremity weakness may become clinically evident by testing heel walking and toe walking.

Serum Laboratory Studies

Those neuromuscular diseases with inherent sarcolemmal muscle membrane injury often show significant elevations in transaminases, aldolase, and creatine kinase (CK). The CK enzyme catalyzes the release of high-energy phosphates from creatine phosphate. It occurs mainly in muscle and leaks into the serum in large amounts in any disorder involving muscle fiber injury. The MM fraction is specific to skeletal muscle. The CK value may be significantly elevated in early stages of DMD and BMD, with values up to 50–100 times normal. A normal CK value may help to exclude DMD and BMD. Overlap in CK values occurs between DMD and BMD. Other forms of muscular dystrophy, such as Emery-Dreifuss muscular dystrophy, limbgirdle muscular dystrophy, FSH, and congenital muscular dystrophy, may show moderate elevations in CK. However, in congenital muscular dystrophy, the CK value may be extremely variable, ranging from normal values to a fairly marked elevation. There is no close association between disease severity and CK values. In all dystrophic myopathies, the CK values tend to decrease over time with increasing severity of the disease owing to progressive loss of muscle fiber and irreversible cell death. Thus, a 3-year-old with DMD may have a CK value of 25,000, whereas a 10-year-old with DMD may show a CK value of 2,000. Other conditions with significant elevations in CK may include polymyositis, dermatomyositis, acute rhabdomyolysis, and malignant hyperthermia. In many of the congenital structural myopathies, such as central core disease, nemaline rod myopathy, and fiber-type disproportion syndrome, a serum CK value is likely to be normal or only mildly elevated.

CK levels have ranged from normal to 2–4 times elevated in SMA I and II.[2] SMA III patients have also been found to have normal to slightly elevated CK values[3] with elevations generally to 2–5 times normal. A serum CK level greater than ten times the upper limit of normal generally is an exclusionary criteria for SMA, and, in this setting, work-up for other disorders such as inflammatory or dystrophic myopathies should be pursued. In a child with muscle weakness, a normal CK does not exclude a myopathy or other NMD conditions; however, a severely elevated CK is suggestive of, but not diagnostic of, a dystrophic or inflammatory myopathy. Serial CK measurements in the morning after several days of sedentary activity are still useful in the evaluation of potential female DMD carriers who do not have a detectable gene deletion on molecular genetic studies. Three normal CK values in the females are approximately 90% specific for ruling out carrier status. Even one abnormally elevated CK makes a carrier status a possibility.

Lactate and pyruvate levels are useful in the evaluation of possible metabolic myopathy. The presence of a lactic acidosis may be seen in such mitochondrial encephalomyopathies as Kearns-Sayre syndrome, myoclonic epilepsy and ragged-red fibers (MERRF), and mitochondrial encephalomyopathy with lactic acidosis and stroke-like episodes (MELAS). Whenever clinical evidence suggests a disorder of oxidative metabolism, blood lactate and pyruvate levels should be obtained. Arterial lactate values are a more reliable guide. Lactate elevations under ischemic or exercise stress suggest mitochondrial dysfunction. In a setting of lactic acidemia, the lactate/pyruvate ratio may aid in the differential diagnosis. Children with suspected encephalomyopathy should be evaluated with CSF lactate levels because these values are less subject to flux than are either venous or arterial values. The ischemic forearm test, initially utilized by McArdle, is the most widely used means of assessing muscle in anaerobic metabolism in older, more cooperative patients.[4–6]

Electrodiagnostic Studies

Nerve conduction and electromyography are an extension of the physical examination and a powerful tool for the localization of lesions within the lower motor neuron. In addition, EMG and nerve conduction studies help to guide further studies, such as muscle biopsy, by providing information about the most appropriate muscle site for the biopsy. With spinal muscular atrophy, an electrodiagnostic evaluation allows the clinician to defer muscle biopsy and proceed with molecular genetic studies of the survival motor neuron gene. Electrodiagnostic studies in patients with HMSN help to categorize the neuropathy as either primarily demyelinating or axonal, and such information may help to focus subsequent molecular genetic analyses. In patients with suspected HMSN and positive family histories with molecular genetically confirmed diagnoses, the diagnosis may be further confirmed in the clinic by a simple, reliable, and relatively inexpensive nerve conduction study.

A thorough discussion of the role of electrodiagnosis in neuromuscular disease is provided in Chapter 5.

Molecular Genetic Studies

The application of molecular genetic techniques has resulted in enormous gains in our understanding of the molecular and pathophysiologic basis of many neuromuscular diseases. In addition, molecular genetic studies now aid in the diagnostic evaluation of the dystrophin-deficient muscular dystrophies (DMD, BMD), myotonic muscular dystrophy, predominantly proximal autosomal recessive spinal muscular atrophy, and Charcot-Marie-Tooth disease (hereditary motor and sensory neuropathy). The clinical application of molecular genetic studies is described in the sections on specific neuromuscular conditions.

Muscle Biopsy Evaluation

Muscle Biopsy Technique. The two techniques for obtaining a muscle biopsy specimen include the traditional open biopsy and the needle biopsy.[7,8] Either technique can be performed under local anesthesia; however, most clinicians in the United States use general anesthesia for open biopsies and local anesthesia for needle biopsies. There may be some disruption in the architecture of the tissue with needle biopsy technique, which can affect the evaluation of histologic examination and electron microscopy. Immunocytochemistry analyses, such as Western blot and metabolic studies, do not require strict maintenance of the muscle cellular architecture.

Muscle Biopsy Site Selection. Selection of the muscle is based on distribution of muscle weakness found clinically in addition to electrodiagnostic findings, if obtained. In a dystrophic myopathy, the muscle biopsy should be clinically affected, but not so severely affected that it is largely replaced by fat and connective tissue with minimal residual muscle fiber present for evaluation. The insertional activity on EMG or muscle imaging studies can be helpful in this respect. Sufficient normative information about proportional fiber type and diameter should be available with age-appropriate norms. A diagnosis of congenital myopathy with fiber-type disproportion cannot be made without careful consideration of the normal fiber-type predominance in a given muscle. For example, the vastus lateralis contains two-thirds of type II fibers (with equal proportions of type IIa and type IIb fibers) and one-third of type I fibers. The anterior tibialis, on the other hand, contains a predominance of type I fibers, and the anconeus mostly contains type I fibers. In addition, some muscles, such as the quadriceps and biceps, have longitudinally running fibers that facilitate orientation of the specimen for preparation of cross-sectional slices. The gastrocnemius muscle, on the other hand, may be difficult to orient because fibers run in different plains. Muscles that have undergone recent needle electromyographic evaluation should be avoided as biopsy sites because of the possibility of cellular changes in the muscle fiber secondary to the needle study.

For routine diagnostic studies, the vastus lateralis muscle in the lower extremity and the triceps or biceps in the upper extremity are often preferred. When proximal muscles are severely affected or only distal muscles are involved, the extensor carpi radialis or anterior tibialis muscles are often biopsied.

Histology/Histochemistry

The histopathologic study is likely to provide information about whether the basic disease process is primarily a myopathy or a neurogenic process. In some instances, the diagnosis of specific disorders (such as dystrophic myopathy or inflammatory myopathy) is delineated. In analyses of paraffin sections, basic pathologic reactions of muscle may include fiber necrosis, central nuclei indicative of regeneration, abnormalities of muscle fiber diameter (atrophy, hypertrophy, abnormal variation and fiber size), fiber splitting, vacuolar change, inflammatory infiltrates, and proliferation of connective tissue/fibrosis. A dystrophic myopathy frequently is characterized by the presence of normal fibers, hypertrophied fibers, degenerating fibers, atrophic fibers, regenerating fibers, and connective tissue and fatty infiltration. Neurogenic changes may be characterized by small or large groups of atrophic fibers with or without target fibers and frequently by hypertrophy of the nonatrophic fibers.

A variety of histochemical stains are used to differentiate between fiber types (types I, IIa, IIb, and IIc). Based on the histochemical analyses, information is obtained about (1) pattern of fiber types (e.g., normal predominance, fiber-type predominance, selective fiber type involvement, or reinnervations evidenced by fiber type grouping); (2) analysis of muscle fiber diameters (e.g., fiber hypertrophy or atrophy, increased variability in fiber diameter or denervation atrophy with narrow range of diameters among atrophic and nonatrophic fibers); or (3) alterations in the muscle fiber (e.g., central nuclei, necrosis, splitting or branching, regeneration, or the presence of a variety of other accumulations and fiber alterations, both specific to certain conditions and nonspecific).

Congenital myopathies are a group of structural myopathies whose diagnosis is based on classic histologic characteristics seen on muscle biopsy (e.g., centronuclear or myotubular, central core, nemaline rod, and fiber-type disproportion myopathies).

Immunoblotting and Immunostaining

Immunoblotting of a muscle sample provides information about amounts of specific muscle protein, such as dystrophin or other structural proteins important in maintaining structural integrity of the muscle membrane. Immunoblotting can be performed with as little as 10 mg of frozen tissue. Quantitative dystrophin analysis using Western blot technique can differentiate DMD from BMD and thus help to determine the prognosis in a young symptomatic patient—information not determined by standard molecular genetic analysis of the dystrophin gene. Dystrophin quantity $\leq 3\%$ is consistent with DMD; 3–20% dystrophin is seen in some patients with less severe "outlier" DMD or severe BMD; and either 20–80% dystrophin or normal quantity and reduced or increased molecular weight of dystrophin are consistent with BMD. A normal dystrophin level in a patient with histologic evidence of a dystrophic myopathy is suggestive of a limb-girdle muscular dystrophy (Table 15–1). Immunofluorescent staining of muscle biopsy sections for dystrophin helps to identify symptomatic female DMD carriers and some female BMD carriers.

The progressive loss of muscle fibers evident in muscular dystrophy is now thought to be caused by primary muscle sarcolemmal membrane abnormalities due to inherited structural abnormalities (abnormal molecular weight, deficiency, or absence) of dystrophin or dystrophin-associated transmembrane glycoproteins. Membrane instability leads to membrane injury from mechanical stresses, transient breaches of the membrane, and membrane leakage. Ultimately, after multiple cycles of degeneration and regenerations, irreversible muscle cell death occurs. The muscle fiber is then replaced by connective tissue and fat, and this fibrotic replacement of the muscle may be exceedingly aggressive. This has given rise to the concept of diseases of the dystrophin-glycoprotein complex (Table 15–2). Primary genetic abnormalities lead to abnormalities of intracellular dystrophin, transmembrane sarcoglycans, or transmembrane dystroglycans. Specific abnormalities of muscle cytoskeletal proteins lead to specific dystrophic disease phenotypes, as shown in Table 15–2. An abnormality in the muscle protein merosin, located in the extracellular matrix, gives rise to one of the forms of congenital muscular dystrophy. Immunoblotting and/or immunofluorescent staining of the proteins of the dystrophin-glycoprotein complex now allows many limb-girdle muscular dystrophy patients to be subtyped (see Table 15–1).

Electron Microscopy

Electron microscopy (EM) is used to evaluate ultrastructural changes of muscle fiber organelles/internal components, as well as changes in the muscle fiber. At times, this may provide additional complementary information to the histologic and histochemical assessment of muscle fibers that may be diagnostically relevant. For example, ultrastructural alterations of mitochondria may provide important information and direct additional metabolic studies in the work-up of mitochondrial myopathy. In a congenital structural myasthenic syndrome, ultrastructural alterations at the neuromuscular junction may be detected by EM, either pre- or postsynaptically.

Metabolic Studies

Depending on clinical suspicion and histologic and ultrastructural changes on muscle biopsy, additional metabolic studies may be obtained to evaluate for the presence of metabolic myopathies, including glycogenoses, lipid disorders, or mitochondrial myopathies.

Nerve Biopsy

Nerve biopsies are occasionally useful in the characterization of more severe hereditary motor sensory neuropathies, congenital hypomyelinating neuropathy, and neuroaxonal dystrophy. In addition, perineural immune complex deposition seen in some autoimmune neuropathies and changes consistent with vasculitis also may be useful diagnostically. Otherwise, nerve biopsies rarely add specific information to the diagnostic evaluation of the NMD patient beyond

TABLE 15–1. Limb-Girdle Muscular Dystrophy

Autosomal Recessive	Gene Location	Protein
LGMD 2A	15q15.1–q21.1	Calpain-3
LGMD 2B	2p	?
LGMD 2C	13q12	γ-Sarcoglycan
LGMD 2D	17q12–q21.33	α-Sarcoglycan (adhalin)
LGMD 2E	4q12	β-Sarcoglycan
LGMD 2F	5q33–q34	δ-Sarcoglycan

Autosomal Dominant	Gene Location	Protein
LGMD 1A	5a	?
LGMD 1B	?	?

that information obtained from nerve conduction studies and EMG.

Generally, the sural nerve is used. Because this is a pure sensory nerve, the usefulness of this specimen is limited to those disorders giving rise to demyelinating or axonal changes in sensory fibers. Occasionally, a small portion of the motor nerve can be obtained simultaneously with an anconeus motor point biopsy, in which the motor branch is excised along the entire muscle from origin to insertion.

Specific Neuromuscular Diseases

Dystrophic Myopathies

Duchenne Muscular Dystrophy

Duchenne muscular dystrophy is an X-linked disorder caused by an abnormality at the Xp21 gene loci.[9] The DMD/BMD gene occupies 2.5 million base pairs of DNA on the X chromosome and is about ten times larger than the next largest gene identified to date. The gene contains 79 exons of coding sequence.[10] The primary protein product, called dystrophin, is localized in the plasma membrane of all myogenic cells, certain types of neurons, and in small amounts of other

TABLE 15–2. Diseases of the Dystrophin-Glycoprotein Complex

Protein	Chromosome	Disease
Dystrophin	Xp21.2	DMD, BMD
α-Sarcoglycan	17q12–q21.33	SCARMD/LGMD 2D
β-Sarcoglycan	4q12	LGMD 2E
γ-Sarcoglycan	13q12	SCARMD/LGMD 2C
δ-Sarcoglycan	5q33–q34	LGMD 2F
β-Dystroglycan	3	Unknown
α-Dystroglycan	3	Unknown
Merosin	6q2	Congenital MD
Calpain-3	15q15.1–q21.1	LGMD 2A

cell types.[11,12] Dystrophin deficiency at the plasma membrane of muscle fibers disrupts the membrane cytoskeleton and leads to the secondary loss of other components of the muscle cytoskeleton.[13] The primary consequence of the cytoskeleton abnormalities is membrane instability, leading to membrane injury from mechanical stresses, transient breaches of the membrane, and membrane leakage. Chronic dystrophic myopathy is characterized by aggressive fibrotic replacement of the muscle and eventual failure of regeneration with muscle fiber death and fiber loss.

The incidence of Duchenne muscular dystrophy, based on a number of population studies as well as neonatal screening, has been estimated to be around 1:3,500 male births.[14] As many as one-third of isolated cases may be due to new mutations, which is considerably higher than observed in other X-linked conditions. This high mutation rate may relate to the large size of the gene. The history of hypotonia and delayed motor milestones are often reported in retrospect because the parents are often unaware of any abnormality until the child starts walking. There has been variability reported in the age of onset.[15,17] In 74–80% of instances, the onset has been noted before the age of 4 years.[15,16] The vast majority of cases are identified by 5–6 years of age. The most frequent presenting symptoms have been abnormal gait, frequent falls, and difficulty climbing steps. Parents frequently note the toe walking, which is a compensatory adaptation to knee extensor weakness, and a lordotic posture to the lumbar spine, which is a compensatory change due to hip extensor weakness (see Fig. 15–5).

Occasionally, Duchenne muscular dystrophy is identified presymptomatically in situations in which a markedly elevated CK value is obtained, malignant hyperthermia occurs during general anesthesia for an unrelated surgical indication, or a diagnosis is pursued in a male with an affected older sibling.

Difficulty negotiating steps is an early feature, as is a tendency to fall due to tripping, stumbling on a plantar-flexed ankle, or the knee buckling or giving way because of knee extensor weakness. There is progressive difficulty getting up from the floor with presence of a Gowers' sign (see Fig. 15–4).

Pain and enlargement of muscles, particularly the calves (see Fig. 15–1), are commonly noted. Recently, children aged 8–11 years with Duchenne muscular dystrophy have been noted to exhibit an unusual clinical examination sign that results from selective hypertrophy and wasting in different muscles in the same region.[18] Viewed from behind with arms abducted to 90° and elbows flexed to 90°, DMD patients demonstrate a linear or oval depression (due to wasting) of the posterior axillary fold with hypertrophied or preserved muscles on its two borders (i.e., infraspinatus inferomedially and deltoid superolaterally), as if there were a valley between the two mounts (Fig. 15–7). The tongue is frequently enlarged. Also, an associated wide-arch to the mandible and maxilla with separation of the teeth, presumably secondary to the macroglossia, is a common sign.

Earliest weakness is seen in the neck flexors during preschool years (Fig. 15–8). Weakness is generalized but predominantly proximal early in the disease course. Pelvic girdle weakness precedes shoulder girdle weakness by several years. Ankle dorsiflexors are weaker than ankle plantar flexors, ankle everters are weaker than

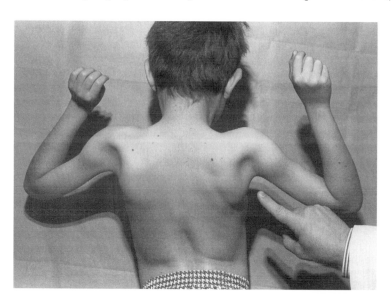

FIGURE 15–7.   Posterior axillary depression sign in Duchenne muscular dystrophy. Note the prominent deltoid superolaterally and infraspinatus inferomedially.

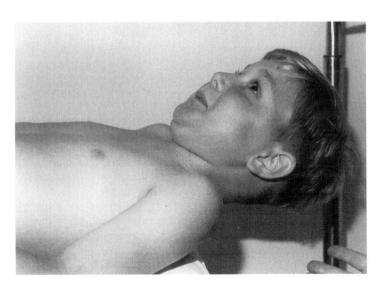

FIGURE 15–8. Weakness of neck flexors in an 8-year-old boy with Duchenne muscular dystrophy makes it difficult for him to bring his chin to the chest when supine and to hold his head up when placed at the end of the examination table.

ankle inverters, knee extensors are weaker than knee flexors, hip extensors are weaker than hip flexors, and hip abductors are weaker than hip adductors.[17]

The weakness progresses steadily, but the rate may be variable during the disease course. Quantitative strength testing shows greater than 40–50% loss of strength by 6 years of age.[17] With manual muscle testing (MMT), DMD subjects exhibit loss of strength in a fairly linear fashion from ages 5–13 years, and measurements obtained several years apart will show fairly steady disease progression. A variable course may be noted when analyzing individuals over a shorter time course.[17] Previous investigators have noted a change in the rate of strength loss at approximately ages 14–15 years.[17,19] This change in the rate of progression does not appear to be associated with achievement of a particular score on the manual muscle test scale but rather consistently occurs in various muscle groups in the early second decade. Thus, the author recommends that natural history control trials evaluating therapies for DMD should be cautious about including subjects transitioning to the teenage years because of the flattening of the MMT strength curve with increasing age.[17,20] Quantitative strength measures have been shown to be more sensitive for demonstrating strength loss than MMT when strength grades were 4–5.[17]

Average age to wheelchair in an untreated DMD population has been 10 years with a range of 7–13 years. Timed motor performance is useful for the prediction of time when ambulation will be lost without provision of long-leg braces. One large natural history study showed that all DMD subjects who took 9 seconds or longer to ambulate 30 feet lost ambulation within 1 year.[17]

Ambulation past the age of 14 years should raise the suspicion of a milder form of muscular dystrophy such as BMD or limb-girdle muscular dystrophy. Ambulation beyond 16 years was previously used as an exclusion criterion for Duchenne muscular dystrophy. Immobilization for any reason may lead to a marked and often precipitous decline in muscle power and ambulatory ability. A fall with resultant fracture leading to immobilization and loss of ambulatory ability is not an uncommon occurrence.

Significant joint contractures have been found in nearly all Duchenne muscular dystrophy children older than age 13 years.[17,21,22] The most common contractures include ankle plantar flexion, knee flexion, hip flexion, iliotibial band, elbow flexion, and wrist flexion contractures.[17] Significant contractures have been shown to be rare in DMD for all joints before age 9 years. There is no association between muscle imbalance around a specific joint (defined as grade 1 or greater difference in flexor and extensor strength) and the frequency or severity of contractures involving the hip, knee, ankle, wrist, and elbow in DMD.[17] Flexion contractures have been shown to be rare in those with ≥ grade 3 extensor strength about a joint, an expected finding because of the definition of a grade 3 muscle on MMT. For those DMD subjects with less than antigravity strength about a joint, there is low correlation between the MMT strength of these specific muscle groups and the severity of joint contracture.[17] The presence of lower extremity contractures in DMD has been shown to be strongly related to onset of wheelchair reliance.[17] Lower extremity contractures are rare while DMD subjects are still upright, but develop soon after they attain a sitting position in a wheelchair for most of the day. The occurrence of elbow flexion contractures also appears to be directly related to prolonged static positioning of the limb, and these contractures develop soon after wheelchair reliance. The relationship between wheelchair reliance and hip and knee flexion contractures has been noted.[17] Mild contractures of the iliotibial bands, hip flexor muscles, and heel cords occur in most DMD patient by 6 years of age.[23] Limitations of knee, elbow, and wrist extension occur about 2 years later;[25] however, these early observed contractures are relatively mild. Given the tremendous replacement of muscle by fibrotic tissue in DMD subjects, it is not surprising that a muscle of less than antigravity extension strength, statically positioned in flexion, develops a flexion contracture (subsequent to wheelchair reliance). The lack of lower extremity weight bearing likely contributes to the rapid acceleration in the severity of these contractures after transition to wheelchair. Ankle plantar flexion contractures are probably not a significant cause of wheelchair reliance, as few subjects exhibit plantar flexion contractures of ≥ 15° before their transition to a wheelchair.[17] Natural history data suggest that weakness is the major cause of loss of ambulation in DMD, not contracture formation.

Reported ultimate prevalence of scoliosis in DMD varies from 33% to 100%.[24] This marked variability is primarily due to retrospective selection for scoliosis, the inclusion or exclusion of functional curves, and dissimilar age groups. The prevalence of scoliosis is strongly related to age. Fifty percent of DMD patients acquire scoliosis between the ages of 12 and 15 years, corresponding to the adolescent growth spurt. Ten percent of older DMD subjects with no treatment of scoliosis show no clinical spinal deformity. This is consistent with Oda's report[25] that 15% of older DMD patients show mild nonprogressive curves (usually 10–30°). The rate of progression of the primary or single untreated lateral curve has been reported to range from 11° to 42° per year, depending on the age span studied. Johnson and Yarnell[26] reported an association between side of curvature, convexity, and hand dominance. McDonald's study,[17] on the other hand, showed no correlation between side of primary convexity and handedness. Oda and colleagues[25] reported that the likelihood of severe progressive spinal deformity could be predicted by type of curve and early pulmonary function measurements. Those with spines lacking significant kyphosis or hyperlordosis and a peak-obtained, absolute forced vital capacity (FVC) greater than 2,000 ml tended not to show severe progressive scoliosis.

No cause-and-effect relationship has been established between onset of wheelchair reliance and occurrence of scoliosis.[17,26,27] Wheelchair reliance and scoliosis have been found to be age-related phenomena. The causal relationship between loss of ambulatory status and scoliosis is doubtful, given the substantial time interval between the two variables in most subjects (scoliosis usually develops after 3–4 years in a wheelchair). Both wheelchair reliance and spinal deformity may be significantly related to other factors (e.g., age, adolescent growth spurt, increase in weakness of trunk musculature, and other unidentified factors) and thus represent coincidental signs of disease progression.

In DMD, absolute FVC volumes increase during the first decade of life and plateau during the early part of the second decade.[17] A linear decline in percent predicted FVC is apparent between 10 and 20 years of age in DMD.[17] Rideau[28] reported FVC to be predictive of the risk of rapid scoliosis progression. In the most severe DMD cases, maximal FVC reached a plateau of less than 1,200 ml. This was associated with loss of ability to walk before age 10 years and severe progressive scoliosis. Moderately severe DMD cases with respiratory compromise reached maximum FVCs between 1,200 ml and 1,700 ml. Spinal deformity was present consistently in these cases but varied in severity. The least severe DMD cases reached plateaus in FVC of greater than 1,700 ml. Similarly, McDonald and colleagues[17] found that those patients with higher peak FVC (> 2,500 ml) had a milder disease progression, losing 4% predicted FVC per year. Those with peak predicted FVC less than 1,700 ml lost 9.6% of predicted FVC per year. Thus, the peak obtained absolute values of FVC usually occurring in the early part of the second decade are an important prognostic indicator of severity of spinal deformity, as well as ultimate severity of restrictive pulmonary compromise due to muscular weakness.

Maximal static airway pressures (both maximal inspiratory pressure and maximal expiratory pressure) are the earliest indicators of restrictive pulmonary compromise in DMD with impaired values noted between 5 and 10 years of age. Vital capacity typically increases concomitant with growth between 5 and 10 years of age with percent predicted FVC remaining relatively stable and close to 100% predicted. DMD patients typically show a linear decline in percent predicted FVC between 10 and 20 years of age. An FVC falling below 40% of predicted may contraindicate surgical spinal arthrodesis, irrespective of scoliotic severity, because of increased perioperative morbidity.[29] Ultimately, respiratory failure in DMD is insidious in its onset and results from a number of factors, including (1) respiratory muscle weakness and fatigue; (2) alteration in respiratory system mechanics; and (3) impairment of the central control of respiration. Noninvasive forms of both positive and negative pressure ventilatory support are increasingly being offered to DMD patients.

The dystrophin protein is present in both the myocardium and the cardiac Purkinje fibers.[30] Abnormalities of the heart may be detected by clinical examination, electrocardiogram (ECG), echocardiography, and Holter monitoring. Cardiac examination is notable for the point of maximal impulse palpable at the left sternal border because of the marked reduction in anteroposterior chest dimension common in DMD. A loud pulmonic component of the second heart sound suggests pulmonary hypertension in patients with restrictive pulmonary compromise. Nearly all patients over the age of 13 years demonstrate abnormalities of the ECG.[17] Q-waves in the lateral leads are the first abnormalities to appear, followed by elevated ST-segments and poor R-wave progression, increased R/S ratio, and finally resting tachycardia and conduction defects. ECG abnormalities have been demonstrated to be predictive for death from cardiomyopathy with the major determinants including R-wave in lead V1 less than 0.6 mV; R-wave in lead V5 less than 1.1 mV; R-wave in lead V6 less than 1.0 mV; abnormal T-waves in leads II, III, AVF, V5, and V6; cardiac conduction disturbances; premature ventricular contraction; and sinus tachycardia.[31] Sinus tachycardia may be due to low stroke volume from the progressive cardiomyopathy, or in some cases may be sudden in onset and labile, suggesting autonomic disturbance or direct involvement of the sinus node by the dystrophic process.[32,33]

Autopsy studies[34] and thallium-201 single photon emission computed tomography (SPECT) imaging have demonstrated left ventricular lateral and posterior wall defects that may explain the lateral Q-waves[35] and the increased R/S ratio in V1 seen on ECG.[36] Localized posterior wall fibrosis was found to be peculiar to DMD and was not found in other types of muscular dystrophy. Pulmonary hypertension leading to right ventricular enlargement also is known to affect prominent R-waves in V1 and has been demonstrated in patients with DMD.[37]

Ventricular ectopy and sudden death are known complications of the cardiomyopathy in DMD, and this association likely explains observed cases of sudden death. Severe ventricular ectopy in DMD has been associated with left ventricular dysfunction[38] and sudden death.[39,40] Yanagisawa and colleagues[40] reported an age-related increase in the prevalence of cardiac arrhythmias detected by ambulatory 24-hour electrocardiographic recordings. They also noted an association between ventricular arrhythmias and sudden death in DMD. Clinically evident cardiomyopathy is usually first noted after age 10 years and is apparent in nearly all patients over age 18 years.[41,42] Development of cardiomyopathy is a predictor of poor prognosis.[43] Echocardiography has been used extensively to follow the development of cardiomyopathy and predict prognosis in patients with DMD. The onset of systolic dysfunction noted by echocardiography is associated with a poor short-term prognosis.[43] The myocardial impairment remains clinically silent until late in the course of the disease, possibly caused by the absence of exertional dyspnea secondary to lack of physical activity. Death has been attributed to congestive heart failure in as many as 40–50% of patients with DMD by some investigators.[44,45] Regular cardiac evaluations with an ECG, echocardiography, and Holter monitoring should be employed in teenagers with preclinical cardiomyopathy.

The dystrophin isoform is present in the brain.[46] Previous studies on intellectual function in children with DMD have generally revealed decreased IQ scores when these children are compared with both control and normative groups.[17] A mean score for the DMD population of 1.0–1.5 SD below population norms has been reported. There has generally been a considerable consistency in the degree of impairment across measures reflecting a rather mild global deficit. Some studies[47–49] have demonstrated relative deficits in verbal IQ. In a longitudinal assessment of cognitive function, McDonald and colleagues[17] found IQ measure in DMD to be stable over time. On neuropsychological testing, a large proportion of DMD subjects fell within the "mildly impaired" or "impaired" range according to normative data.[17] Again, there were no particular areas of strength or weakness identified. These findings likely reflect a mild global deficit rather than focal nervous system impairment.[17]

Substantial anthropometric alterations have been described in DMD. Short stature and slow linear growth with onset shortly after birth have been reported.[50,51] Accurate measurement of linear height is extremely difficult in this population. Arm span measurements may be an alternative measure of linear growth; however, this measurement may also be difficult as elbow flexion contractures of greater than 30° are frequently present in patients older than age 13 years. Forearm segment has been proposed as an alternative measurement in DMD patients with proximal upper extremity contractures, and radius length may be followed for those with wrist and finger contractures. Obesity is a substantial problem in DMD, subsequent to the loss of independent ambulation.[52,53] Weight control during early adolescence has its primary rationale in ease of care, in particular ease of transfers during later adolescence.

Longitudinal weight measurements in DMD confirm significant rates of weight loss in subjects aged 17–21 years.[17,53] This is likely caused by relative nutritional compromise during the later stages when boys with DMD have higher protein and energy intake requirements because of hypercatabolic protein metabolism. Protein and calorie requirements may often be 160% of that predicted for able-bodied populations during the later stages of DMD.[54,55] Restrictive lung disease becomes more problematic during this time, and this may also influence caloric intake and requirements. Self-feeding often becomes impossible during this period because of biceps weakness. In addition, boys with DMD may develop signs and symptoms of upper gastrointestinal dysfunction.[56]

Becker Muscular Dystrophy

Existence of a form of muscular dystrophy with a pattern of muscle weakness similar to that seen in Duchenne muscular dystrophy, X-linked inheritance, but with later onset and a much slower rate of progression, was first described by Becker and Kiener in 1955.[57] The disorder has the same gene location as the DMD gene (Xp21) and is thus allelic. On immunoblotting or immunostaining of muscle biopsy specimens, the presence of altered size or abundance of dystrophin suggests a Becker muscular dystrophy phenotype. Either 20–80% levels of dystrophin or normal quantity and reduced or increased molecular weight of dystrophin are consistent with BMD. Becker muscular dystrophy has a lower incidence than DMD, with prevalence rates ranging from 12–27 per million and a recent estimated overall prevalence of 24 per million.[14,58]

The demonstration of a deletion in the Xp21 gene with cDNA probes is useful in the diagnostic evaluation of dystrophin-deficient myopathies. In the gene deletion test, small blood samples are used as a source of patient DNA, and the dystrophin (DMD, BMD) gene is tested to determine whether it is intact or not. This is done by polymerase chain reaction (PCR) or Southern blotting, and the methods determine whether all segments of the gene are present. If

any segment is missing, the findings indicate the presence of a "deletion mutation." Not all DMD and BMD patients have deletion mutations—many have point mutations that cannot be detected by these methods. Because the gene is so large and complex, it is currently not feasible to routinely test for the other types of smaller mutations. About 55% of DMD patients and 70% of BMD patients show deletion mutations of the gene.[59,60] A positive DNA test result (presence of a deletion) is diagnostic of a dystrophinopathy (Duchenne or Becker dystrophy)—there are no false-positives if the test is done appropriately. Differential diagnosis between DMD and BMD is best done by family history of clinical phenotype. If the patient is still ambulating at 16–20 years of age and has a deletion mutation, then the correct diagnosis is BMD. Some laboratories will report "the reading frame." This information differentiates between a DMD and BMD diagnosis in approximately 90% of deletion-positive cases.[61] Mutations at the Xp21 locus, which maintain the translational reading frame (in-frame mutations), result in an abnormal and partially dysfunctional dystrophin, whereas in Duchenne muscular dystrophy the mutations shift the reading frame (out-of-frame mutations) so that virtually no dystrophin is produced. The reading frame interpretation is most accurate for deletions in the center of the gene (exons 40–60) and is least accurate for deletions in the beginning of the gene (exons 1–20).

Absent dystrophin or levels less than 3% of normal generally are considered diagnostic of Duchenne muscular dystrophy; however, 5% of such patients have BMD phenotypes. In BMD, dystrophin typically has abnormally small molecular weight (< 427 kDa). A minority of patients have dystrophin of larger than normal molecular weight (> 427 kDa), or normal molecular weight. Most BMD patients with larger or smaller molecular weight of dystrophin also have decreased quantities of the protein. All BMD patients with normal molecular weight of dystrophin have decreased quantities, usually less than 30% normal. Smaller-sized dystrophin typically is caused by deletion mutations, and larger-sized dystrophin by duplication mutations. A further refinement is the use of antibodies specific to the carboxy-terminal (C-terminal) region of dystrophin. Using such antibodies, immunohistochemistry reveals that the C-terminal region is almost always absent in DMD but invariably present in BMD.[62] Thus, when this region of the molecule is missing, a more severe phenotype is likely.

Studies have shown significant overlap in the observed age of onset between DMD and BMD.[16] Although determination of the quantity and molecular weight of dystrophin has substantially improved the early differentiation among BMD, outlier DMD, and the more common and rapidly progressive DMD phenotype, Bushby and colleagues[60] found no clear correlation between abundance of dystrophin and clinical course within the BMD group.

A series of Bushby and Gardner-Medwin,[60] which included 67 BMD subjects, supported the presence of two major patterns of progression in BMD—a typical slowly progressive course and a more severe and rapidly progressive course. All of the severe BMD cases showed difficulty climbing stairs by age 20 years, whereas none of the typical BMD cases had difficulty climbing stairs before age 20 years. Abnormal ECGs were seen in 27% of typical BMD subjects and 88% of severe subjects. Bushby and Gardner-Medwin[60] found BMD subjects to have a mean age of onset of 12 years in the typical group and 7.7 years in the severe group. Some patients with BMD present with major muscle cramps as an isolated symptom.[60,63]

The most useful clinical criterion to distinguish BMD from DMD is the continued ability of the patient to walk into late teenage years. Those with BMD will typically remain ambulatory beyond 16 years. Some patients may become wheelchair users in their late teens or early 20s, whereas others may continue walking into their 40s, 50s, or later. Outlier DMD cases generally stop ambulating between 13 and 16 years of age.

As in DMD, preclinical cases are often identified by the finding of a grossly elevated CK value. There is also considerable overlap in CK values between DMD and BMD cases at the time of presentation. Thus, CK values cannot be used to differentiate DMD from BMD.

BMD patients have distribution of weakness similar to those with DMD.[16,65,66] Proximal lower limb muscles are involved earlier in the disease course. Gradual involvement of the pectoral girdle and upper limb musculature occurs 10–20 years from onset of disease. Extensors have been noted to be weaker than flexors.[16,66] The muscle groups that are most severely involved earlier in the course of disease include the hip extensors, knee extensors, and neck flexors.[16,65]

Calf enlargement is a nonspecific finding in BMD, as is the presence of a Gowers' sign. The gait over time is similar to that in other neuromuscular conditions with proximal weakness. Patients often ambulate with a lumbar lordosis, forefoot floor contact, decreased stance-phase knee flexion, and a Trendelenburg or gluteus medius lurch, often described as a waddle.

Early development of contractures does not appear to be a feature of BMD.[16,60,65,66] As with DMD, nonambulatory BMD subjects may develop equinus contractures, knee flexion contractures, and hip flexion contractures. Because of the tremendous replacement of muscle in BMD subjects by fibrotic tissue, it is likely that, as in DMD, a muscle with less than antigravity extension strength, which is statically positioned in flexion, is more likely to develop a flexion contracture subsequent to wheelchair reliance.

Spinal deformity is not nearly as common or severe in BMD, as compared with DMD. Spinal instrumentation is rarely required by BMD patients.[16,60]

Compromised pulmonary function is much less problematic in BMD as opposed to DMD.[16,28,60] The percent predicted forced vital capacity does not appear substantially reduced until the third to fourth decade of life. The percent predicted maximal expiratory pressure appears relatively more reduced at younger ages than the percent predicted maximal inspiratory pressure, a finding seen in DMD and other neuromuscular diseases.[17,67–69] This may be caused by more relative involvement of the intercostal and abdominal musculature with relative sparing of contractile function in the diaphragm in BMD. As in DMD and other neuromuscular diseases, it appears that predicted maximal expiratory pressure (MEP) may be a useful quantitative measure of impairment and perhaps disease progression early in the course of BMD.

The pattern of occasional life-threatening cardiac involvement in otherwise mild and slowly progressive BMD has been reported by many.[60,65,70–73] A significant percentage of BMD cases develop cardiac abnormalities, and the rate of progression of cardiac failure may be on occasion more rapid than the progression of skeletal myopathy.[74–76] In fact, successful cardiac transplantation has been increasingly reported in BMD subjects with cardiac failure.[74,75,77,78] Approximately 75% of BMD patients have been found to exhibit ECG abnormalities.[16,79] The abnormal findings most typically reported include abnormal Q-waves, right ventricular hypertrophy, left ventricular hypertrophy, right bundle-branch block, and nonspecific T-wave abnormalities. Unlike DMD, resting sinus tachycardia has not been a frequent finding. Echocardiography has shown left ventricular dilation in 37%, whereas 63% have subnormal systolic function because of global hypokinesia.[79] Thus, the cardiac compromise may be disproportionately severe, relative to the degree of restrictive lung disease in some BMD subjects. The evidence for significant myocardial involvement in BMD is sufficient to warrant screening of all of these patients at regular intervals using ECG and echocardiography. The slowly progressive nature of this dystrophic myopathy, which is compatible with many years of functional mobility and longevity, makes these patients suitable candidates for cardiac transplantation if end-stage cardiac failure occurs.

Some cases with BMD may present with an isolated cardiomyopathy with no clinical manifestation of skeletal muscle involvement. The diagnosis can be established by demonstration of a deletion in the Xp21 gene or by muscle biopsy. Isolated cases of cardiomyopathy in children, particularly those with family histories indicative of X-linked inheritance, should be screened for BMD with an initial serum CK estimation and molecular genetic studies of the Xp21 gene.

Cognitive testing in BMD subjects has shown large variability in IQ scores and neuropsychological test measures. Mildly reduced intellectual performance has been noted in a subset of BMD patients; however, the degree of impairment is not as severe as that noted in DMD.[16]

Other atypical clinical presentations include a sole complaint of cramps on exercise in individuals with no muscle weakness.[60,63] In addition, patients with focal wasting of the quadriceps, previously diagnosed with quadriceps myopathy, have recently been diagnosed with BMD, based on molecular genetic testing and/or dystrophin analysis on muscle biopsy.[16]

Severe Childhood Autosomal Recessive Muscular Dystrophy (SCARMD)

A heterogenous group of dystrophic myopathies, with childhood onset from 3–12 years, equal male to female prevalence, and a distribution and pattern of weakness similar to DMD but with a slower rate of progression, have been linked to abnormalities of the dystrophin-associated glycoproteins (DAG), in particular, alpha-sarcoglycan (adhalin), a 50-kDa DAG, and gamma-sarcoglycan. The 50-kDa DAG protein has been linked to the 17q12–q21.33 locus,[80] and more recently this type of SCARMD has been referred to as autosomal recessive limb-girdle muscular dystrophy (LGMD) 2D. Other families with SCARMD have been linked to chromosome 13q12,[81] and these individuals with LGMD 2C may show a primary deficiency of gamma-sarcoglycan and a secondary deficiency of alpha-sarcoglycan (see Table 15–1). LGMD 2E patients (chromosome 4q12) show a primary deficiency in beta-sarcoglycan, and LGMD 2F patients (chromosome 5q33–q34) show a primary deficiency of delta-sarcoglycan. Most of the primary sarcoglycan abnormalities lead to secondary deficiencies of alpha-sarcoglycan. Dystrophin analysis is generally normal in these

subjects. It should be noted that all of the DAGs are reduced in DMD patients[82] because the C-terminal portion of dystrophin binds to the dystrophin-associated proteins and maintains their integrity. A less severe autosomal recessive dystrophic myopathy (LGMD 2A) has been linked to chromosome 15q1–q21.1, the gene for the protein calpain-3. Diagnosis of SCARMD or LGMD subtypes is confirmed by muscle biopsy.

Dystrophin analysis is generally normal in subjects with LGMD. Of the seven recessive loci identified to date, four are sarcoglycan genes (see Table 15–1).[23,84] These four proteins make up the sarcoglycan complex, which is thought to interact directly with the 43-kDa DAG and with dystrophin.[85] Dystrophin-associated glycoproteins probably provide connections between the extracellular matrix (the protein merosin) and the intracellular membrane cytoskeleton (attached to dystrophin).[86,87] An abnormality of the dystrophin-glycoprotein complex, resulting from primary deficiencies of one or more of the dystrophin-associated glycoproteins, results in a disruption in the linkage between the intracellular sarcolemmal cytoskeleton and the extracellular matrix. Disruption of the membrane cytoskeleton is common to the pathophysiology of most muscular dystrophies, the dystrophinopathies (see Table 15–2).

SCARMD patients may exhibit calf hypertrophy and a Gowers' sign. Loss of ambulation generally occurs between 10 and 20 years but occasionally after 20 years. In one series,[88] several differences between DMD and SCARMD were noted. The limb extensors were not weaker than limb flexors. In particular, ankle dorsiflexors were similar in strength to ankle plantar flexors, knee extensors showed similar strength compared with knee flexors, and hip extensors and hip flexors showed similar strength values. The severity and rate of progression often varies between and within the families of SCARMD patients. Contractures appear to be much less prevalent and severe in SCARMD compared with DMD. The prevalence of joint contractures in SCARMD subjects was found to be similar to that observed in BMD subjects in one series.[88]

Spinal deformity appears to be much less problematic in SCARMD than in DMD. Less than 50% of SCARMD subjects were found to have curves of mild-to-moderate severity, ranging from 5–30°. The prevalence and severity of spinal deformity in SCARMD appears to be similar to that observed in BMD.

Restrictive pulmonary insufficiency is observed in SCARMD, but it does not appear to be as severe as that seen in DMD. Again, the prevalence of severe restrictive lung disease in

SCARMD is similar to that observed in BMD.[88]

Few studies have systematically evaluated the cardiac manifestations of SCARMD and other limb-girdle dystrophies. In one series,[88] the prevalence of abnormal ECG findings in SCARMD was 62%. ECG abnormalities include evidence of infranodal conduction defects, evidence of left ventricular hypertrophy, increased R/S ratio in V1, and abnormal Q-waves.

Congenital Muscular Dystrophy

The term congenital muscular dystrophy has been widely used for a group of infants presenting with hypotonia, muscle weakness at birth or within the first few months of life, congenital contractures, and a dystrophic pattern on muscle biopsy. The condition tends to remain relatively static, but some subjects may show slow progression, whereas others may gain developmental milestones and achieve the ability to walk.

There are several syndromes of congenital muscular dystrophy with central nervous system abnormality. Fukuyama congenital muscular dystrophy[89-91] is associated with mental retardation, structural brain malformations evident on MR imaging, and a dystrophic myopathy. The gene locus has recently been identified to be at 9q31–33.[92]

Muscle-eye-brain disease[93,94] describes a syndrome comprising congenital muscular dystrophy, mental retardation, and ocular abnormality. Infants present with congenital hypotonia, muscle weakness, elevated CK, myopathic EMG, and dystrophic changes on muscle biopsy. Ophthalmologic findings include severe visual impairment with uncontrolled eye movements associated with severe myopia. Patients often deteriorate around 5 years of age with progressive occurrence of spasticity. CT scans have shown ventricular dilatation and low density of the white matter.

Walker-Warburg syndrome[95] is described as congenital muscular dystrophy with mental retardation and consistent central nervous system abnormalities on imaging (type II lissencephaly, abnormally thick cortex, decreased interdigitations between white matter and cortex, and cerebellar malformation). Ocular abnormalities and cleft lip or palate may also be present.

Cases with more pure congenital muscular dystrophy without CNS involvement have been identified. The main clinical features are muscle weakness and hypotonia, congenital contractures, histologic changes of a dystrophic nature, often with extensive connective tissue or adipose proliferation but no substantial evidence of necrosis or regeneration, normal to moderately elevated CK, normal intellect, and brain imaging that may be either normal or show changes in the white matter on CT or MRI. One form results from merosin deficiency, an extracellular protein important for maintenance of sarcolemmal membrane stability in the muscle fiber.[96] The locus for merosin-deficient congenital muscular dystrophy has been linked to chromosome 6q.[96] A further subtype of congenital muscular dystrophy without CNS involvement and normal merosin has been reported, but the genetic locus has not been established.

Patients with congenital muscular dystrophy often exhibit early contractures, including equinovarus deformities, knee flexion contractures, hip flexion contractures, and tightness of wrist flexors and long finger flexors. The contractures may become more severe over time with prolonged static positioning and lack of adequate passive range of motion and splinting/positioning.

Facioscapulohumeral Muscular Dystrophy

Facioscapulohumeral (FSH) muscular dystrophy is a slowly progressive dystrophic myopathy with predominant involvement of facial and shoulder girdle musculature. The condition is autosomal dominant with linkage to the chromosome 4q35 locus.[97,98] Prevalence has been difficult to ascertain because of undiagnosed mild cases, but has been estimated at 10–20 per million.[14]

Facial weakness is an important clinical feature of FSH muscular dystrophy. The initial weakness affects the facial muscles, especially the orbicularis oculi, zygomaticus, and orbicularis oris. These patients often have difficulty with eye closure but not ptosis. An individual may assume an expressionless appearance and exhibit difficulty whistling, pursing the lips, drinking through a straw, or smiling (Fig. 15–9).

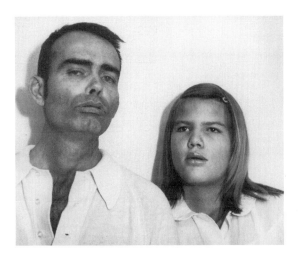

FIGURE 15–9. Facial weakness and expressionless faces in FSH muscular dystrophy. Both father and daughter demonstrate difficulty whistling and pursing their lips.

Even in the early stages, forced closure of the eyelids can be easily overcome by the examiner. Masseter, temporalis, extraocular, and pharyngeal muscles characteristically are spared in FSH muscular dystrophy.

Patients with FSH muscular dystrophy show characteristic patterns of muscle atrophy and scapular displacement. Involvement of the latissimus dorsi, lower trapezius, rhomboids, and serratus anterior results in a characteristic appearance of the shoulders, with the scapula positioned more laterally and superiorly, giving the shoulders a forward-sloped appearance (Fig. 15–10). The upper border of the scapula rises into the trapezius, falsely giving it a hypertrophied appearance. From the posterior view, the medial border of the scapula may exhibit profound posterior and lateral winging. The involvement of the shoulder girdle musculature in FSH muscular dystrophy may be quite asymmetric.

Presentation is commonly in adolescence or early adulthood. Initially, patients show predominant involvement of facial and shoulder-girdle musculature. Scapular stabilizers, shoulder abductors, and shoulder external rotators may be significantly affected, but at times the deltoids

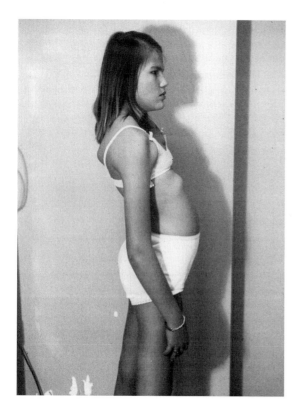

FIGURE 15–10. Posterior and lateral scapular winging, high-riding scapula, and hyperlordosis in FSH muscular dystrophy.

are surprisingly spared if tested with the scapulae stabilized. Both the biceps and triceps may be more affected than the deltoids. Over time, ankle dorsiflexion weakness often becomes significant in addition to pelvic girdle weakness, and some patients exhibit ankle dorsiflexion weakness fairly early in the disease course. Late in the disease course, patients may show marked wrist extension weakness. Some authors have found asymmetric weakness in the dominant upper extremity.[99]

A sensory neural hearing deficit was originally observed in Coats' syndrome (early-onset FSH muscular dystrophy). These individuals have a myopathy that presents in infancy. The disease progression is fairly rapid, with most individuals becoming wheelchair-reliant by the late second or third decade of life. These individuals also have a progressive exudative telangiectasia of the retina. Early recognition and photocoagulation of the abnormal retinal vessels may prevent loss of vision. Several audiometry studies have demonstrated hearing deficits in many later-onset FSH patients in addition to those with Coats' syndrome, suggesting that impaired hearing function is more common than expected in FSH muscular dystrophy.[100–102]

Contractures are relatively uncommon in FSH muscular dystrophy. In the most comprehensive study to date,[99] 22 subjects had range of motion (ROM) testing of major upper and lower extremity joints. Clinically significant loss of ROM (defined as a reduction in ROM greater than 20°) was present in 2 subjects at the wrist and in 1 subject (5%) at the hip, knee, and ankle. This subject had been wheelchair-dependent for 15 years at the time of ROM testing.

Spinal deformity presents as scoliosis or hyperlordosis (Fig. 15–10), alone or in combination. Patients with hyperlordosis, with or without scoliosis, account for 20% of spinal deformities in FSH muscular dystrophy.[99] Rarely, severe and progressive hyperlordosis is associated with FSH muscular dystrophy. FSH patients with scoliosis have mild and nonprogressive curves. Patients with severe hyperlordosis may use their lordotic posturing to compensate for hip extensor weakness.

Mild restrictive lung disease has been reported in nearly one-half of FSH patients.[99] Expiratory musculature appears to be more affected than inspiratory muscles.

The presence of cardiac abnormalities in FSH muscular dystrophy is debated. While diverse ECG abnormalities have been noted, one study showed no abnormalities on ECG, chest radiography, Holter monitoring, and echocardiography.[103] Nuclear scanning with thallium-201 has demonstrated diffuse defects consistent with diffuse fibrosis.[36] Abnormalities in systolic time intervals on echocardiography[104] and elevations in atrial natriuretic peptide are consistent with subclinical cardiomyopathy. Cardiac complications in FSH muscular dystrophy are rare, and patients in general have normal longevity. There is usually no associated intellectual involvement in this dystrophic myopathy.

Changes on muscle biopsy are relatively slight, with the most consistent finding being the presence of isolated small atrophic fibers. Other fibers may be hypertrophied. Serum creatine kinase levels are normal in a substantial proportion of patients. Molecular genetic testing for the FSH muscular dystrophy gene is now available for diagnostic confirmation.

Emery-Dreifuss Muscular Dystrophy

Emery-Dreifuss muscular dystrophy (EMD) is an X-linked recessive progressive dystrophic myopathy with a gene locus identified at Xq28.[105] The muscle protein that is deficient in EMD has been termed emerin. The condition usually presents in adolescence or early adulthood, and many clinical features may be seen in early childhood. Patients may present with a selective scapulohumeral peroneal distribution weakness with striking wasting of the biceps, accentuated by sparing of the deltoids and forearm muscles. Ankle dorsiflexors often are weaker than ankle plantar flexors. Significant atrophy usually is present in the upper arms and legs due to focal wasting of the calf muscles and biceps.

An associated cardiomyopathy usually presents with arrhythmia and may lead to sudden death in early adulthood. The cardiomyopathy may progress to four-chamber dilated cardiomyopathy with complete heart block and ventricular arrhythmias.[106] Atrial arrhythmia usually appears before complete heart block. Reported features include first-degree heart block, followed by Wenckebach phenomenon, complete atrial-ventricular dissociation, and atrial fibrillation or flutter with progressive slowing of the rate.[103,108] Syncope or near-syncope commonly occurs later in the second decade or early in the third decade.[109] Evidence of cardiac arrhythmia, sometimes only present at night, may be detected on 24-hour Holter monitoring. The provision of a cardiac pacemaker to the patient with arrhythmia may be life-saving and considerably improve the life expectancy.

Some cases with EMD may show evidence of nocturnal hypoventilation, as a result of restrictive expansion of the chest in association with the rigid spine, and partly due to involvement of the diaphragm.

The creatine kinase may be moderately elevated, with a value between two and five times the upper limit of normal. Electromyography usually shows a myopathic pattern. Muscle biopsy shows a myopathic process with variation in fiber size, clusters of atrophic fibers, mild proliferation of connective tissue, and some focal necrosis of fibers.

A hallmark of EMD clinically is the early presence of contractures of the elbow flexors with limitation of full elbow extension. Heel cord tightness may be present early in the disorder, concomitant with ankle dorsiflexion and toe walking. Unlike DMD, the toe walking in EMD usually is secondary to ankle dorsiflexion weakness and not a compensatory strategy to stabilize the knee because of proximal limb weakness. Tightness of the cervical and lumbar spinal extensor muscles, resulting in limitation of neck and trunk flexion, with inability to flex the chin to the sternum and to touch the toes, also has been reported in EMD.

A dominantly inherited disorder with a similar phenotype has been reported, but the gene locus is unknown. Some reported cases of "rigid spine syndrome," a form of congenital muscular dystrophy, may be EMD cases in view of the marked predominance of males in this disorder and the associated contractures reported at the elbows and ankles.

Limb-Girdle Syndromes

The term *limb-girdle syndrome* is used to describe varied lower motor neuron disorders presenting in childhood and adulthood and characterized by *predominantly proximal weakness* of the shoulder- and pelvic-girdle muscles. The differential diagnosis of limb-girdle syndromes remains quite large and may include LGMD subtypes, polymyositis, dermatomyositis, congenital myasthenic syndromes, inclusion body myositis, type III spinal muscular atrophy, manifesting carrier of DMD, BMD, FSH, scapuloperoneal myopathy, Emery-Dreifuss muscular dystrophy, congenital myopathies occasionally presenting later in childhood or adulthood (e.g., adult-onset nemaline rod disease, central core disease, centronuclear myopathy, fiber-type disproportion, multi-core disease, sarcotubular myopathy, fingerprint myopathy, reducing-body myopathy), mitochondrial myopathies with limb-girdle weakness, and other metabolic myopathies that may present in adulthood.

Congenital Myopathies

The term *congenital myopathy* is used to describe a group of heterogenous disorders that usually present with infantile hypotonia due to genetic defects causing primary myopathies with the absence of any structural abnormality of the central nervous system or peripheral nerves, and a specific diagnosis of each entity is made on the basis of specific histologic and electron-microscopic changes found on muscle biopsy. While patients may be hypotonic during early infancy, they later develop muscle weakness that is generally nonprogressive and static. The weakness is predominantly proximal, symmetric, and in a limb-girdle distribution.

The serum creatine kinase values are frequently normal, and the EMG may be normal or may show mild, nonspecific changes, usually of a myopathic character (small-amplitude polyphasic potentials). The only congenital myopathy consistently associated with abnormal spontaneous activity on EMG is myotubular (centronuclear) myopathy. In this disorder, the EMG reveals myopathic motor unit action potentials with frequent complex repetitive discharges and diffuse fibrillation potentials. These myopathies may be considered primarily structural in nature; thus patients do not actively lose muscle fibers, as is the case in dystrophic myopathies.

Central Core Myopathy

This is an autosomal dominant disorder with autosomal dominant gene locus at 19q13.1,[110] the same gene locus as the malignant hyperthermia gene. Indeed, these patients have a high incidence of malignant hyperthermia with inhalational anesthetic agents. Histologically, the muscle fibers have amorphous-looking central areas within the muscle that may be devoid of enzyme activity. Electron microscopy shows the virtual absence of mitochondria and sarcoplasmic reticulum in the core region, a marked reduction in the interfibrillary space, and an irregular zig-zag pattern (streaming) of the Z-lines.[111] There is a predominance of high-oxidative low-glycolytic type I fibers and a relative paucity of type II fibers, resulting in a relative deficiency of glycolytic enzymes.

Clinically, patients generally demonstrate mild and relatively nonprogressive muscle weakness, either proximal or generalized, which presents in either early infancy or later. There may be mild facial weakness. Patients often achieve gross motor milestones such as walking rather late, and they continue having difficulty going upstairs. They may show a Gowers' sign. The disorder remains fairly static over the years. There may be frequent occurrence of congenital dislocation of the hip.

Central core myopathy and familial malignant hyperthermia appear to be allelic, as the ryanodine receptor chain implicated in malignant hyperthermia has the same locus.[112]

Nemaline Myopathy

Nemaline myopathy, also referred to as rod-body myopathy, represents a varied group of disorders with different modes of inheritance, but the most typical form is autosomal recessive. Although the rods are easily overlooked on routine hematoxylin-eosin staining and they are rarely demonstrated with the Gomori trichrome stain, they are demonstrated readily on electron microscopy. They are thought to be abnormal depositions of Z-band material of a protein nature and possibly alpha-actinin.

A severe form of the disease may present in the neonatal period with very severe weakness, respiratory insufficiency, and often a fatal outcome. Most cases present with a mild, nonprogressive myopathy with hypotonia and proximal weakness. In more severe cases, swallowing difficulty may be present in the neonatal period. Skeletal abnormalities, such as kyphoscoliosis, pigeon chest, pes cavus feet, high arched palate, and an unusually long face, have been noted. Cardiomyopathy has been described in both severe neonatal and milder forms of the disease.

Autosomal dominant inheritance has been described in a few instances[113] with the gene localized to chromosome 1q21–q23. The locus of the more common autosomal recessive forms has not yet been located.

Myotubular Myopathy (Centronuclear Myopathy)

Patients with non–X-linked myotubular myopathy have muscle biopsies that show a striking resemblance to the myotubes of fetal muscle. Patients typically present with early hypotonia, delay in motor milestones, generalized weakness of both proximal and distal musculature, and ptosis with weakness of the external ocular muscles as well as weakness of the axial musculature. The author has seen severe cardiomyopathy in an adult female with documented autosomal dominant inheritance. Nocturnal hypoventilation has been described.

The gene locus has not been identified to date, but most known non–X-linked forms appear to show autosomal dominant inheritance.

Severe X-linked (Congenital) Myotubular Myopathy

Cases with neonatal onset and severe respiratory insufficiency have been identified with an X-linked recessive mode of inheritance. The gene for this disorder has been located to Xq28.

Muscle biopsy shows characteristic fetal-appearing myotubes.

Patients present with severe generalized hypotonia, associated muscle weakness, swallowing difficulty, and respiratory insufficiency. They often become ventilator-dependent at birth. If they are able to be weaned from the ventilator, subsequent death due to pulmonary complications is not uncommon. Aspiration pneumonias are common. Additional clinical features include congenital contractures, facial weakness, and weakness of the external ocular muscles. Electromyography shows many fibrillations and positive sharp waves.

Mini-core Disease (Multi-core Disease)

This is a relatively rare congenital myopathy with muscle biopsies showing multiple small, randomly distributed areas in the muscle with focal decrease in mitochondrial oxidative enzyme activity and focal myofibrillar degenerative change. Characteristic changes are present on electron microscopy. There is a predominance of type I fiber involvement.

Clinically, patients present with hypotonia, delays in gross motor development, and nonprogressive symmetric weakness of the trunk and proximal limb musculature. There may be mild facial weakness, and there is also associated diaphragmatic weakness, placing patients at risk for nocturnal hypoventilation. Subtle ultrastructural changes allow this condition to be distinguished from central core disease. Inheritance is autosomal recessive; however, the gene location has not yet been established.

Congenital Fiber-type Disproportion

Congenital fiber-type disproportion represents a heterogenous group of conditions most likely with varied genetic defects. The condition was initially delineated by Brooke[114] on the basis of the muscle biopsy picture demonstrating type I fibers, which are smaller than type II fibers by a margin of more than 12% of the diameter of the type II fibers. Congenital muscular dystrophy, myotonic muscular dystrophy, and severe spinal muscular atrophy all may show small type I fibers and should be excluded. The diagnosis of congenital fiber-type disproportion should be made only in the presence of normal-sized or enlarged type II fibers and not in cases in which both type I and type II fibers are small.

Patients typically present with infantile hypotonia and delay in gross motor milestones. The severity has been noted to be quite variable, but it is generally nonprogressive. Patients generally exhibit short stature and low weight, a long narrow face, high-arched palate, and deformities of the feet, including either flat feet or occasionally high-arched feet. Kyphoscoliosis has been reported. Lenard and Goebel[115] documented a case with fairly severe weakness and associated respiratory deficit, necessitating tracheostomy. The author has managed two cases (a mother and son with presumed autosomal dominant inheritance), who both developed nocturnal hypoventilation requiring bilevel positive airway pressure (BIPAP).

Patients with muscle biopsies indicative of congenital fiber-type disproportion and ptosis should be evaluated for a congenital myasthenic syndrome, because the author has seen a number of cases in recent years of congenital structural neuromuscular junction disorders that had associated nonspecific changes on muscle biopsy, which were interpreted to be congenital fiber-type disproportion. This is an important distinction because some of these patients with congenital myasthenia respond to pharmacologic intervention.

The mode of inheritance for congenital fiber-type disproportion is varied with both autosomal recessive and autosomal dominant patterns of inheritance reported. Genetic loci have not been identified to date.

Myotonic Disorders

Myotonic Muscular Dystrophy

Myotonic muscular dystrophy (MMD) is an autosomal dominant multisystem muscular dystrophy with an incidence of 1 per 8,000.[14] The disorder affects skeletal muscle, smooth muscle, myocardium, brain, and ocular structures. Associated findings include baldness and gonadal atrophy (in males), cataracts, and cardiac dysrhythmias. Insulin insensitivity may be present. The gene has been localized to the region of the DM protein kinase (DMPK) gene at 19q13.3.[116,117] Patients demonstrate expansion of an unstable CTG trinucleotide repeat within the region. Molecular genetic testing is now available. Normal individuals generally have < 37 repeats, which are transmitted from generation to generation. MMD patients may have 50 to several thousand CTG repeats with remarkable instability. The age of onset is inversely correlated with the number of CTG repeats.[118–120] Mild, late-onset MMD usually is associated with 50–150 repeats, classic adolescent- or young adult-onset MMD shows 100–1,000 repeats, and congenital MMD shows greater than 1,000 repeats. The expanded CTG repeat domain further expands as it is transmitted to successive generations, providing a molecular basis for genetic anticipation. Both maternal-to-child and paternal-to-child transmission occurs. Repeat size in offspring exceeding 1,000 CTG repeats is generally seen in maternal rather than paternal transmission. Affected fathers seldom transmit alleles larger than 1,000 copies to offspring, owing to a lack of sperm containing such alleles.

Several characteristic facial features of MMD may be noted on inspection (Fig. 15–11). The adult with long-standing MMD often has characteristic facial features. The long, thin face with temporal and masseter muscle wasting is drawn and has been described by some as "lugubrious." Adult males often exhibit frontal balding.

Myotonia, a state of delayed relaxation or sustained contraction of skeletal muscle, is easily identified in school-aged children, adolescents, and adults with MMD. Grip myotonia may be demonstrated by delayed opening of the hand with difficult extension of the fingers following tight grip. Percussion myotonia may be elicited by percussion of thenar eminence with a reflex hammer, giving an adduction and flexion of the thumb with slow return (see Fig. 15–3).

MMD is one of the few dystrophic myopathies with greater distal than proximal weakness. Although neck flexors, shoulder-girdle musculature, and pelvic-girdle musculature may become significantly involved over decades, initial weakness is often most predominant in the ankle dorsiflexors, ankle everters and inverters, and hand muscles.[121] As with other dystrophic myopathies, significant muscle wasting may occur over time. In MMD patients with infantile onset, a congenital clubfoot or talipes equinovarus is a

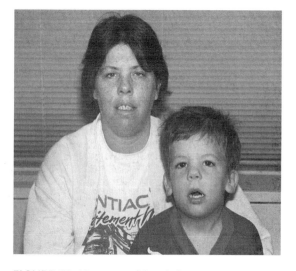

FIGURE 15–11. Typical facial characteristics in myotonic muscular dystrophy (MMD) and congenital MMD. The symptomatic mother has 660 trinucleotide CTG repeats at the DM protein kinase (DMPK) gene locus in chromosome 19q13.3, whereas the child has 1,560 repeats.

fairly common deformity (Fig. 15–12). In patients with noncongenital MMD, contractures at the wrist, ankle, and elbows are relatively uncommon and mild.[121] Patients with congenital-onset MMD may develop spinal deformity requiring surgical spinal arthrodesis.[121]

Cardiac involvement is a common feature of MMD. Abnormalities on ECG and echocardiography are demonstrated in approximately 70–75% of patients.[122] Prolongation of the PR-interval, abnormal axis, and infranodal conduction abnormalities are all suggestive of conduction system disease, which may explain the occurrence of sudden death in less than 5% of MMD patients.[123] Ventricular tachycardia may also contribute to the syncope and sudden death associated with MMD. Some patients have required implantation of cardiac pacemakers. Q-waves have been reported on screening ECGs in MMD patients, and this abnormality may reflect myocardial fibrosis.[122] Any MMD patient with dyspnea, chest pain, syncope, or other cardiac symptoms should receive thorough cardiac evaluation.

Individuals with noncongenital MMD have a high incidence of restrictive lung disease.[121] Involvement of respiratory muscles is a major cause of respiratory distress and mortality in affected infants with MMD. Swallowing difficulties that produce aspiration of material into the trachea and bronchial tree, along with weakened respiratory muscles and a weak cough, have been reported as factors that may result in pulmonary complications in MMD patients. Care should be taken during general anesthesia in MMD because of risk for cardiac arrhythmias and malignant hyperthermia.

Constipation is a fairly common complaint in congenital MMD, owing to smooth muscle involvement. MMD patients should also be screened for diabetes mellitus because insulin insensitivity is not uncommon.

Those with congenital MMD usually show significantly reduced IQ, often in the mentally retarded range.[121,124] In noncongenital MMD, there is evidence for a generally lower intelligence of a mild degree (full-scale IQs have been reported to be in the 86–92 range.[121] There is a wide range of IQ values found in this population, with many subjects scoring in the above-average range. Cognitive functioning also appears to be directly related to the size of the CTG repeat domain expansion at the MMD gene locus.

Myotonia Congenita

Myotonia congenita (Thomsen's disease) is inherited as an autosomal dominant condition. Symptoms may be present from birth, but usually develop later. Myotonia may be manifested as difficulty in releasing objects or by difficulty walking or climbing stairs. It is exacerbated by prolonged rest or inactivity and may be aggravated by cold. Patients may demonstrate grip myotonia, lid lag following upward gaze or squint and diplopia following sustained conjugate movement of the eyes in one direction. The other common feature of myotonia congenita is muscle hypertrophy. Patients may exhibit a "Herculean" appearance.

A recessive form of myotonia congenita (Becker form) also exists with later-onset, more marked myotonia, more striking muscle hypertrophy, and associated muscle weakness. The dominant form seems more prone to aggravation by cold.

Diagnosis is essentially clinical with confirmation by classical myotonic discharges on EMG. Muscle biopsy is essentially normal apart from the presence of hypertrophy of fibers and an absence of type IIb fibers.

Paramyotonia Congenita

Paramyotonia congenita is an autosomal dominant myotonic condition with mild involvement, cold aggravation, hypertrophy of musculature, and more severe involvement of hands and muscles of the face. Myotonic episodes usually subside within a matter of hours.

Schwartz-Jampel Syndrome

Schwartz-Jampel syndrome is an autosomal recessive disorder with myotonia, dwarfism, diffuse bone disease, narrow palpebral fissures, blepharospasm, micrognathia, and flattened facies (Fig. 15–13). Limitation of joint movement may be present along with skeletal abnormalities, including short neck and kyphosis. Muscles are typically hypertrophic and clinically stiff. The symptoms are not progressive.

Electrodiagnostic studies show continuous electrical activity with electrical silence being difficult to obtain. There is relatively little waxing and waning in either amplitude or frequency of complex repetitive discharges. Abnormal sodium channel kinetics in the sarcolemma of muscle has been demonstrated.[125] Some therapeutic benefit has been reported with procainamide[126] and carbamazepine.

Neuromuscular Junction Disorders

Transient Neonatal Myasthenia

Transient neonatal myasthenia occurs in about 10–15% of infants born to myasthenic mothers and is due to transplacental transfer of circulating acetylcholine receptor (AChR) antibodies from the mother to the fetus. Symptoms appear within the first few hours of birth; however, occasionally onset may be delayed for 3–4

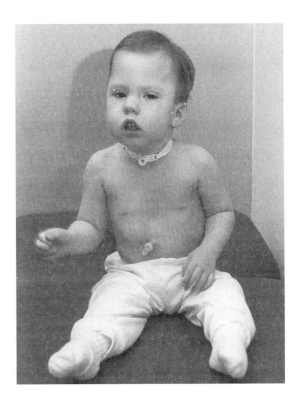

FIGURE 15–12. Congenital myotonic muscular dystrophy with respiratory insufficiency requiring tracheostomy and part-time ventilatory support. Note the temporal wasting and equinovarus foot deformities. The child has over 2,200 CTG repeats at chromosome 19q13.3.

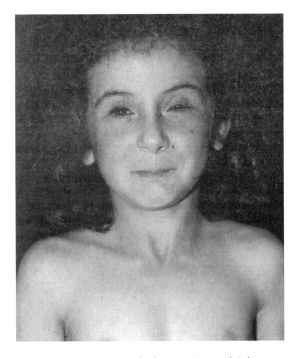

FIGURE 15–13. Facial characteristics of Schwartz-Jampel syndrome in a 7-year-old girl. Note the narrowing palpebral fissures and blepharospasm.

days. Typical clinical characteristics include feeding difficulty, generalized weakness and hypotonia, respiratory difficulties, fetal cry, facial weakness, and, less frequently, ptosis.

The author prefers diagnostic confirmation by evaluating the response to edrophonium or neostigmine with repetitive nerve stimulation studies performed at baseline and subsequent to infusion of the anticholinesterase agent (see Chapter 5). A response decrement with slow rates of stimulation (2–5 Hz) over a train of four to five stimuli may be repaired by edrophonium (Tensilon®) or neostigmine.

Treatment is largely supportive and the condition self-limiting with resolution generally occurring within 2–3 weeks, although occasional cases may persist longer.

Congenital Myasthenic Syndromes

Congenital myasthenia is a term used for a heterogenous group of disorders that are genetically determined rather than autoimmune-mediated. Patients may present in the neonatal period, later in childhood, or even in adult life. Patients often exhibit ptosis, external ophthalmoparesis, facial weakness, general hypotonia, greater proximal than distal muscle weakness, and variable degrees of functional impairment.

Patients show absence of anti-AChR antibodies. At least 12 subtypes have been described, and congenital myasthenia may be classified according to congenital structural presynaptic defects, postsynaptic defects (with or without AChR deficiency), and other miscellaneous syndromes such as AChR deficiency with paucity of secondary synaptic clefts.[127]

Ultrastructural evaluation of the neuromuscular junction with electron microscopy usually is performed on a biopsy of the deltoid or biceps, including the muscle region containing the neuromuscular junction (NMJ) or the "motor point." For in vitro electrophysiologic and immunocytochemical studies of the neuromuscular junction, a short muscle usually is removed from origin to insertion along with its motor branch and NMJ. Muscles obtained have included the anconeus muscle near the elbow, the external intercostal muscle in the fifth or sixth intercostal space near the anterior axillary line, or the peroneus tertius muscle in the lower extremity. Such in vitro electrophysiologic studies allow specific delineation of the congenital myasthenic syndrome into one of the numerous specific subtypes.

Autoimmune Myasthenia Gravis

This disorder is similar to the autoimmune myasthenia gravis observed in adults. The onset is often insidious, but at times patients may present with acute respiratory difficulties. Patients usually present with variable degrees of ophthalmoparesis and ptosis. In addition, they may exhibit facial weakness, swallowing difficulties, speech problems, and weakness of the neck, trunk, and limbs. Proximal muscles are more affected than distal, and the upper limbs are more affected than the lower.

Fluctuation in the disease course with relapse and remission is common. Patients often complain of fatigue and diplopia, as well as progressive difficulty with chewing or swallowing. Patients are often worse with fatigue toward the end of the day. Thymoma, which occurs in about 10% of adult cases, is not a feature of the childhood-onset disease.

Diagnosis may be confirmed by clinical response to an anticholinesterase drug such as edrophonium (Tensilon®). Alternatively, neostigmine, a longer-acting agent, may be used. Repetitive nerve stimulation studies show a characteristic decrement in the compound muscle action potential with slow stimulation rates (2–5 Hz) over a train of 4–5 stimuli. Decrements greater than 12–15% are often noted. Electrophysiologic studies may be more sensitive with proximal muscle groups such as the accessory nerve to the trapezius or study of the facial nerve. Single-fiber EMG is usually impractical in children. Anti-AChR antibodies are detected in the serum in about 85–90% of patients with generalized myasthenia gravis and in about 50% of those with ocular myasthenia.

Management may include treatment with anticholinesterase drugs, such as pyridostigmine, corticosteroids (prednisolone), immunosuppressants (Azathioprine, cyclosporine, or intravenous immunoglobulin), plasma exchange, or thymectomy.

Infantile Botulism

Infants with botulism usually present between 10 days and 6 months with an acute onset of hypotonia, dysphagia, constipation, weak cry, and respiratory insufficiency. The neurologic examination shows diffuse hypotonia and weakness, ptosis, ophthalmoplegia with pupillary dilation, reduced gag reflex, and relative preservation of deep tendon reflexes. The diagnosis may be made by electrodiagnostic studies (see Chapter 5) or by measurement of *Clostridium botulinum* toxin in a rectal aspirate-containing stool.

Noninfantile Acquired Botulism

Older children and adults acquire botulism through poorly cooked, contaminated food with the toxin or through a cutaneous wound that becomes contaminated with soil containing

Clostridium botulinum. The toxin often can be identified in the serum and the food source. Clinical findings include acute onset of constipation, ptosis, diplopia, bulbar weakness, respiratory difficulties, ophthalmoparesis, pupillary dilation, and diminished deep tendon reflexes. Recovery may take months. The diagnosis is generally made from electrodiagnostic studies.

Peripheral Nerve Disorders

Acute Inflammatory Demyelinating Polyradiculoneuropathy (Guillain-Barré Syndrome)

Acute inflammatory demyelinating polyradiculoneuropathy (AIDP) is primarily a demyelinating neuropathy with autoimmune causation. Incidence in children is similar to that seen in adults. Children often have a prodromal respiratory or gastrointestinal infection occurring within 1 month of onset. Common precipitating infections include *Mycoplasma*, cytomegalovirus, Epstein-Barr virus, *Campylobacter jejuni*, and various vaccinations.[127] Weakness generally begins distally in the lower extremity with a progressive ascending paralysis ultimately involving the upper limbs. Pain and sensory symptoms are not uncommon. The most common cranial nerve abnormality is an ipsilateral or bilateral lower motor neuron facial paralysis. Objective sensory loss has been documented in the minority of children.[128] In one series, only 15% required mechanical ventilation.[129] The maximal degree of weakness generally reaches a peak within 2 weeks of onset, and time to maximum recovery was 7 ± 5 months in one series.[130] Complete recovery occurs in most children. Classic criteria for poor recovery in adults (low median compound muscle action potentials [CMAPs] and fibrillation potentials) do not apply to children.[130]

Disturbances of the autonomic nervous system are common in children, including transient disturbances of bowel and bladder, excessive sweating or vasoconstriction, mild hypertension or hypotension, and occasionally cardiac arrhythmias.

Diagnosis is generally confirmed by electrodiagnostic studies (see Chapter 5), and the CSF protein is characteristically elevated in a majority of children.

Treatment has typically included corticosteroids, plasma exchange, or more recently, intravenous immune globulin.[131–134] Recovery is often quite good in children without treatment.[130]

Chronic Inflammatory Demyelinating Polyradiculoneuropathy

Children with chronic inflammatory demyelinating polyradiculoneuropathy (CIDP) often have a presentation similar to AIDP; however, the disorder continues with a chronic or relapsing course. The disorder may begin as early as infancy, but is seen in children and adults. Electrophysiologic studies show focal conduction block, temporal dispersion of CMAPs, prolongation of distal motor latencies, markedly slow conduction velocities, and absent or prolonged H-wave and F-wave latencies. CIDP cases often demonstrate axonal loss on EMG. The CSF protein is elevated in most cases.

The differential diagnosis usually includes HMSN types I and III. The presence of acute relapsing episodes points toward CIDP. Because of the more severe involvement of proximal nerves and nerve roots, a distal sural nerve biopsy may not always show inflammatory changes and demyelination.

Treatment may include corticosteroids (prednisone), plasma exchange, and intravenous immunoglobulin.

Hereditary Motor Sensory Neuropathy

Charcot-Marie-Tooth (CMT) neuropathy, also called hereditary motor sensory neuropathy (HMSN), is a heterogenous group of inherited diseases of peripheral nerves that affects both children and adults and causes significant progressive neuromuscular impairment. It has been estimated that 1 per 2,500 persons has some form of CMT.[14] Type I HMSN denotes individuals with a hypertrophic demyelinating neuropathy (onion bulbs), frequently seen on peripheral nerve biopsy, and reduced nerve conduction velocities, whereas type II HMSN refers to individuals with an axonal neuropathy and normal or slightly reduced nerve conduction velocities. Individuals with type III HMSN (Dejerine-Sottas disease) have a primarily demyelinating peripheral neuropathy with a more severe phenotype. Type IV HMSN refers to autosomal recessive HMSN. Types I, II, and III are now believed to be autosomal dominant conditions with type III HMSN patients exhibiting point mutations with frame shift.

Onset is usually during the first or second decade of life. Both motor and sensory nerve function are affected. The clinical features include distal muscle weakness, impaired sensation, and absent or diminished deep tendon reflexes. Weakness usually is greatest initially in the distal lower extremities and subsequently in the distal upper extremities. Slow progressive weakness, more proximally in the knees, elbows, and pelvic and shoulder girdles, may occur over decades.[68] The various gene locations and known protein abnormalities associated with various forms of CMT (HMSN) are given in Table 15–3.

TABLE 15–3.   Charcot-Marie-Tooth Neuropathy (Hereditary Motor Sensory Neuropathy) and Related Disorders

	Gene Locus	Protein	Inheritance	Gene Abnormality
Charcot-Marie Tooth I (HMSN I)				
CMT IA	17p11.2–12	PMP-22	AD	Duplication/point mutation
CMT IB	1q22–23	P_0	AD	Point mutation
CMT IC	Unknown	Unknown	AD	Unknown
Charcot-Marie Tooth II (HMSN II)				
CMT IIA	1p35–36	Unknown	AD	Unknown
CMT IIB	3q13–22	Unknown	AD	Unknown
CMT IIC	Unknown	Unknown	AD	Unknown
CMT IID	7p14	Unknown	AD	Unknown
Dejerine-Sottas Disease (HMSN III)				
DSDA	17p11.2–12	PMP-22	AD	Point mutation
DSDB	1q22–23	P_0	AD	Point mutation
Charcot-Marie-Tooth IV (HMSN IV)				
CMT IVA	8q	Unknown	AR	Unknown
Charcot-Marie-Tooth X				
CMT X	Xq13.1	Connexin-32	XD	Point mutation
Hereditary Neuropathy with Liability to Pressure Palsies (HNPP)				
HNPP A	17p4.2–12	PMP-22	AD	Deletion/point mutation
HNPP B	Unknown	Unknown	AD	Unknown

XD, X-linked dominant, AD, autosomal dominant, AR, autosomal recessive.

The majority of CMT I pedigrees demonstrate linkage to chromosome 17p11.2–12 and are designated CMT IA.[135] CMT IA duplication results in increased expression of peripheral myelin protein-22 (PMP-22). Defects in the human myelin zero gene (P_0) on chromosome 1q22–q23 lead to CMT IB.[136,137] P_0 is the major protein structural component of peripheral nervous system myelin.

CMT II is a less common disorder than CMT I. Generally, CMT II patients demonstrate later age of onset, less involvement of the small muscles of the hands, and no palpably enlarged nerves. Wasting in the calf and anterior compartment of the leg may give rise to an "inverted champagne bottle" or "stork-leg" appearance. CMT type IIA has been linked to chromosome 1p35–36, type IIB to chromosome 3q13–22, and type IIC to chromosome 7p14.[137,138]

Dejerine-Sottas disease (HMSN III) is a severe hypertrophic demyelinating polyneuropathy with onset in infancy or early childhood. Nerve conduction velocities are greatly slowed, and elevations in CSF protein may be present. Dejerine-Sottas disease may be associated with point mutations in either the P_0 or the PMP-22 gene.[138] Although this disorder was previously believed to be autosomal recessive, many cases are due to de novo point mutations. One form of autosomal recessive CMT (type IVA) maps to the chromosome 8q locus.[139]

Hereditary neuropathy with liability to pressure palsies (HNPP) is an autosomal dominant disorder that produces episodic recurrent nerve entrapments with focal demyelination. Patients may present with peroneal palsies, carpal tunnel syndrome, and other entrapment neuropathies. Peripheral nerve biopsies may demonstrate segmental demyelination and tomaculous or sausage-like formations. A deletion at the PMP-22 gene locus (chromosome 17p11.2–12) causes this autosomal dominant condition.[140]

Patients with an X-linked dominant form of CMT (CMT X) have been described. Male-to-male transmission is not observed, and the disorder generally shows earlier onset and faster rate of progression. The gene locus Xq13 codes for the connexin-32 protein,[141] which is a major component of gap junctions that provide a pathway for the transfer of ions and nutrients around and across the myelin sheath.

DNA testing for the duplication associated with CMT IA is commercially available and should be considered as part of the evaluation of any patient with suspected demyelinating hereditary neuropathy and no molecular genetic diagnosis among relatives. It has been estimated that 70–80% of patients with a clinical diagnosis of CMT I carry the 17p11.2–12 duplication.[138] Other molecular genetic tests are available for CMT IB, CMT X, and HNPP.

Congenital Hypomyelinating Neuropathy

A severe and often fatal newborn disorder often presents with respiratory distress in the delivery room. These infants often have severe generalized hypotonia and associated arthrogryposis. Diagnostically, these infants have absent sensory nerve action potentials (SNAPs) or low-amplitude SNAPs with prolonged distal latencies. Compound muscle action potentials are either absent or low-amplitude with motor conduction velocities ranging from 6–12 m/s.[142] Sural nerve biopsy is the definitive diagnostic procedure. Inheritance may be autosomal recessive, and the disorder is not linked to the PMP-22 gene.[138,142]

Toxic Neuropathies

Toxic polyneuropathies are rare occurrences in children in North America. Toxic exposure to heavy metals and environmental toxins may be more common in other regions of the world. Arsenic polyneuropathy may be axonal or, at times, predominantly demyelinating, simulating Guillain-Barré syndrome or CIDP. The diagnosis is established by obtaining levels of arsenic in blood, urine, hair, and nail samples.

Lead polyneuropathy is most commonly observed in children who have ingested old lead-based paint. Acute exposures more commonly cause lead encephalopathy. Clinical findings may include anorexia, nausea and vomiting, gastrointestinal disturbance, clumsiness, and occasionally seizures, mental status changes, and papilledema. The weakness is predominantly in the lower limbs, but the upper limbs may also be involved. Electrophysiologic studies show a primarily axonal degeneration. A microcytic hypochromic anemia with basophilic stippling of red blood cells establishes the diagnosis. Lead lines may be evident in long-bone films. Lead levels may or may not be elevated in urine and blood, but levels of delta-aminolevulinic acid are usually elevated in the urine.

Mercury poisoning may occur from the ingestion of mercuric salts, exposure to mercury vapor, or use of topical ammonia mercury ointments. Patients present with a generalized encephalopathy, fatigue, and occasionally a skin rash. A predominantly distal motor axonal neuropathy occurs. Deep tendon reflexes may be absent, and the gait is often ataxic. Sensory examination is often normal, although patients may complain of distal paresthesias. Electrophysiologic studies show motor axonal degeneration with normal sensory conduction studies.

Organophosphate poisoning may be due to exposure to insecticides or high-temperature lubricants or softeners used in the plastic industry. Patients present with an encephalopathy manifested by confusion and coma. In acute exposure, cholinergic crisis manifested by sweating, abdominal cramps, diarrhea, and constricted pupils may be present. A predominantly motor polyneuropathy is a late effect. However, the disorder may present as a rapidly progressive polyneuropathy mimicking Guillain-Barré syndrome. Severe paralysis with respiratory failure requiring ventilatory support may occur, and in this situation there may be a superimposed postsynaptic defect in neuromuscular transmission.

Glue-sniffing (N-hexane) neuropathy may be seen in teenaged recreational glue-sniffers. Repeated use may cause symptoms and signs of a predominantly distal motor and sensory polyneuropathy that is predominantly demyelinating. Motor and sensory nerve conduction studies demonstrate moderate slowing.

Chemotherapeutic agents, in particular vincristin, often produce a relatively pure motor axonal polyneuropathy. Severity is dose-dependent. Clinical findings include distal weakness, absent deep tendon reflexes, and at times footdrop. The disorder is often readily apparent by clinical examination, and electrophysiologic studies or nerve biopsy is usually not necessary. The neuropathy usually improves with discontinuation of the medication, although significant electrophysiologic abnormalities (reduced CMAP amplitudes and neuropathic recruitment) may persist.

Metabolic Neuropathies

Uremic neuropathy often occurs in children with end-stage renal disease. If clinical manifestations are present, they consist of a predominantly distal motor and sensory polyneuropathy with "glove-and-stocking" loss of sensation, loss of vibratory sense, and distal weakness, particularly involving peroneal innervated musculature. With successful renal transplantation, clinical findings and electrophysiologic abnormalities normalize.[143] Diabetic polyneuropathy usually is a mixed motor and sensory polyneuropathy with both axonal changes and mild demyelination. The polyneuropathy is less common in children with diabetes mellitus, as compared with adults.[144,145] The severity of the neuropathy may be related to the degree of glucose control.[146]

Motor Neuron Disorders

Predominantly Proximal Spinal Muscular Atrophy

Spinal muscular atrophy (SMA) is a term used to describe a varied group of inherited disorders characterized by weakness and muscle wasting, secondary to degeneration of both anterior horn cells of the spinal cord and brain stem motor nuclei without pyramidal tract involvement. Three subtypes of autosomal recessive,

TABLE 15–4. International SMA Consortium Classification of Autosomal Recessive, Predominantly Proximal Spinal Muscular Atrophy

Type	Onset	Achieved Milestones	Survival
Type I	≤ 6 mo	Never sits without support	Usually less than 2 years
Type II	≤ 18 mo	Sits independently but never stands or walks without aids	Usually greater than 2 years; often to adulthood
Type III	≥ 18 mo	Stands or walks without support	Adulthood

predominantly proximal SMA have been described, all linked to chromosome 5q. A common nomenclature subdivides SMA into types I, II, and III, based on age of onset and age of death, whereas the other approach classifies cases as severe, intermediate, and mild, based on ability to achieve independent sitting, independent standing, and walking. The International SMA Consortium recently attempted to standardize the classification of childhood SMA to provide a rational basis for linkage studies and therapeutic trials (Table 15–4).[147]

SMA type I (severe form) was defined by the International SMA Consortium as follows: onset from birth to 6 months, no achievement of sitting without support, and death usually before age 2 years. In SMA type II (intermediate form), onset is before 18 months; sitting is usually obtained, but standing and ambulation are never obtained; and death occurs after the age of 2 years, usually much later. In SMA type III (mild form), the onset is after the age of 18 months, patients develop the ability to stand and walk, and death is in adulthood. There is considerable variability in severity within each of the three groups, and occasionally some overlap. For example, patients with onset before 6 months may exhibit prolonged survival well past 4 years of age. Patients with onset between 6 and 18 months may ultimately achieve standing and independent ambulation. A modified classification has been proposed by Zares and Rudnik-Shoneborn (Table 15–5).[148]

In 1990, all three forms of SMA were mapped to chromosome 5 (5q13), indicating that allelic variance of the same disease locus accounts for the clinical heterogeneity.[149,150] In 1995, the SMA gene locus was further clarified by the presentation of compelling evidence that at least two distinct genes contribute to the cause of SMA. The survival motor neuron (SMN) gene was shown to be deleted in 93–98% of affected patients with SMA types I, II, and III.[151] The SMN gene deletion test, using PCR techniques to document deletions of exons 7 and 8, can now be used as a confirmatory diagnostic test. In addition, prenatal testing using linkage and deletion data can now be performed. A second gene, the neuronal apoptosis inhibitory protein (NAIP) has been documented to be deleted in 45% of SMA I patients and 18% of SMA II and III patients.[152] A third gene, basal transcription factor 2 (BTF2), may also play a role in the pathogenesis of SMA.[153] It may be that a single gene, such as the SMN gene, may act in concert with other genes to produce the varying phenotypes. Conclusive explanations concerning the observed phenotypic variation in SMA will likely await characterization of the protein products encoded by the SMA-determining genes and determination of the function of these proteins vis-a-vis the maintenance of motor neurons.

Spinal Muscular Atrophy Type I (Werdnig-Hoffman Disease). The majority of cases of SMA type I present within the first 2 months of life with generalized hypotonia and symmetrical weakness. The age of onset of symptoms is less then 4 months in the vast majority of cases. Weak sucking, dysphagia, labored breathing during feeding, frequent aspiration of food or secretions, and weak cry are often noted by history.

Examination shows generalized hypotonia and symmetric weakness involving the lower extremities earlier and to a greater extent than the upper extremities. Proximal muscles are weaker than distal. In the supine position, the lower extremities may be abducted and externally rotated in a "frog-leg" position (see Fig. 15–2). The

TABLE 15–5. University of Bonn (Germany) Spinal Muscular Atrophy Classification

Type	Definition	Mean Age of Onset	Range of Onset	Survival Probability at Age 20 Years
I	Never sat alone	1.9 mo	0–10 mo	0%
II	Sits alone, never walked	8.6 mo	0–18 mo	77%
IIIa	Walks without support; age of onset < 3 yr	17.9 mo	3–30 mo	Normal
IIIb	Walks without support; age of onset 3–30 yr	10.4 yr	3–24 yr	Normal
IV	Age of onset ≥ 30 yr	44.8 yr	33–54 yr	N/A

From Zerres K, Rudnik-Schoneborn S: Natural history in proximal spinal muscular atrophy. Arch Neurol 1995;52:518.

upper extremities tend to be adducted and externally rotated at the shoulders with a semi-flexed elbow. Volitional movements of fingers and hands persist well past the time when the shoulders and elbows cannot be flexed against gravity. The thorax is flattened anteroposteriorly and bell-shaped as a result of intercostal weakness. Pectus excavatum may be variably present. The diaphragm is usually preserved, relative to the intercostal and abdominal musculature. This results in a diaphragmatic breathing pattern during respiration with abdominal protrusion, paradoxical thoracic depression, and intercostal retraction. Neck flexor weakness may result in persistent posterior head lag when the trunk is lifted forward from the supine position. Neck extensor weakness may result in forward head lag when the infant is positioned in the horizontal prone position. With advanced disease, the mouth may remain open as a result of masticatory muscle weakness. Facial weakness may be noted in up to half of the patients. The diagnostic criteria for SMA outlined by the International SMA Consortium[147] list marked facial weakness as an exclusionary criterion for SMA, but this is not an absolute criterion. Tongue fasciculations have been reported in 56–61% of patients,[154,155] so the absence of this finding does not necessarily exclude the disease. In one series,[155] deep tendon reflexes (DTRs) were absent in all four extremities in 74% of cases. Thus, the preservation of DTRs does not exclude the diagnosis of SMA. Appendicular muscle fasciculations and distal tremor are also associated examination findings. Extraocular muscles are spared, as is the myocardium. Hip flexion, knee flexion, and elbow flexion contractures may be observed in some patients along with wrist contractures and ulnar drift of the fingers. Severe arthrogryposis is not typically observed.

Diagnosis is confirmed by a consideration of clinical findings, molecular genetic studies, and, occasionally, electrodiagnostic studies. Muscle biopsy is generally not required to confirm the diagnosis. In a large series from Germany,[148] 197 patients classified as type I (never sits alone) had the following survival probabilities: 32% at age 2, 18% at age 10, and 0% at age 20.

Spinal Muscular Atrophy Type II. Spinal muscular atrophy type II disease onset is usually more insidious than that of SMA type I. The findings of generalized hypotonia, symmetrical weakness, and delayed motor milestones are hallmarks of SMA II. Weakness also involves proximal muscles more than distal muscles, and lower extremity more than upper extremity. A fine tremor of the fingers and hands occurs in a minority of patients. This polyminimyoclonus may be attributed to spontaneous, repetitive rhythmical discharges by the motor neurons that innervate a large territory of muscle. Wasting tends to be more conspicuous in SMA II vs. SMA I. DTRs are depressed and usually absent in the lower extremities. Appendicular or thoracic muscle wall fasciculations may be observed. Tongue fasciculations have been observed in 30–70% of SMA II patients.[147,154–156] Progressive kyphoscoliosis and neuromuscular restrictive lung disease are almost invariably seen in the late first decade of life. Contractures of the hip flexors, tensor fasciae latae, hamstrings, triceps surae, and elbow and finger flexors are quite common. Hypotonic hip dislocations have been noted commonly in SMA II patients. Sensory examination is completely normal, and extraocular muscles and the myocardium are spared. In a large series from Germany[148] of 104 cases classified as SMA II (sits alone, never walks), 98% survived to the age of 10 years and 77% to the age of 20 years. Thus, a longer life span is possible with adequate supportive care.

SMA II is a slowly progressive condition affecting proximal musculature more than distal. The calculated grade of progression for SMA may be a decline of less than one-half manual muscle testing unit per decade.[69] Longitudinal series of 12–39 months' duration have shown essentially stable strength measurements but slow loss of function.[157,158]

Pathologic changes on muscle biopsy have been consistent with hypotrophic change in fetal muscle development. Other changes are consistent with a more active denervating process. Thus, SMA includes a component of myofiber atrophy, comparable to that seen in other denervating diseases, and is not a pure hypotrophic process occurring during early fetal development.

Spinal Muscular Atrophy Type III. In more chronic SMA III, also referred to as Kugelberg-Welander syndrome, weakness usually occurs initially between the ages of 18 months and late teens. Motor milestones may be delayed in infancy. Proximal weakness is observed with the pelvic girdle being more affected than the shoulder girdle.[69] There is an exaggerated lumbar lordosis and anterior pelvic tilt due to hip extensor weakness. There is also a waddling gait pattern with pelvic drop and lateral trunk lean over the stance-phase side, secondary to hip abductor weakness. If ankle plantar flexion strength is sufficient, the patients may show primarily forefoot or toe contact and no heel strike, similar to patients with Duchenne dystrophy.

This is a compensatory measure for knee extensor weakness to maintain a stabilizing knee extension moment at the knee. The patient may exhibit a Gowers' sign when arising from the floor; stair climbing is difficult due to hip flexor weakness. Facial weakness is sometimes noted. Fasciculations are noted in about half of the patients[147] and are more common later in the disease course. Fasciculations in the limb muscles and thoracic wall muscles are common. Calf pseudohypertrophy occasionally has been noted, but wasting of affected musculature is more prominent. Deep tendon reflexes are diminished and often become absent over time. Contractures are generally mild so long as patients remain ambulatory. Scoliosis may be observed in SMA III, but it occurs less frequently and is less severe than scoliosis in SMA II. Although no survival data exist for patients with SMA III, cases have been followed into the eighth decade without mechanical ventilation.[69,148] Ventilatory failure due to neuromuscular restrictive lung disease is a rare event in SMA III, occurring only in adulthood.[69,159]

Zerres and Rudnik-Schoneborn[148] have proposed further subtypes, including SMA IIIa (walks without support; age of onset < 3 years) and SMA IIIb (walks without support; age of onset 3–30 years). In this series, only 44% of SMA IIIa patients remained ambulatory 20 years after onset of weakness, whereas 89% of IIIb patients remained ambulatory after a similar 20-year duration.

Distal Spinal Muscular Atrophy

Distal spinal muscular atrophy, originally described in Asian populations, is a distinct spinal muscular atrophy syndrome with a different inheritance pattern than predominantly proximal SMA.[160] Symptoms often present in the adolescent years with distal weakness of both upper and lower extremities. Patients may have cavus foot deformities and dropfoot and be mistakenly diagnosed with hereditary motor sensory neuropathy. In the upper extremities, the C7, C8, and T1 motor nuclei appear to be predominantly affected. The disorder appears to progress during the second decade of life and becomes relatively static during the adult years. The inheritance pattern is unknown.

Diagnosis of this disorder is usually confirmed by electrodiagnostic studies, which show active denervation in distal musculature greater than proximal musculature and preservation of sensory nerve action potential amplitudes on sensory nerve conduction studies.

Other variants of distal chronic spinal muscular atrophy may present initially with distal lower extremity weakness. The genetics of these variants has not been elucidated.

Progressive Bulbar Paralysis of Childhood (Fazio-Londe Disease)

Fazio-Londe Disease[161] or progressive bulbar paralysis of childhood is a progressive bulbar paralysis that is probably genetically transmitted. The specific genetic characteristics have not been determined yet. Age of onset varies and may be as early as 3 years. Patients may have progressive motor neuron disease with primary involvement of the anterior horn cells in the cervical and upper thoracic cord segments. In addition, there may be widespread degenerative changes in the brain stem. Of cranial nerves, cranial nerve VII is almost always affected. These patients develop dysphagia secondary to cranial nerve XII involvement. The nuclei of cranial nerves III, IV, VI, and X may also be involved; however, clinical impairment of extraocular movement is rare.

Spinocerebellar Degeneration Diseases

Friedreich's Ataxia

Friedreich's ataxia is a spinocerebellar degeneration syndrome with the onset of symptoms before age 20 years. This autosomal recessive condition has been linked to chromosome 9q21. The protein that is abnormal in Friedreich's ataxia has been termed frataxin. Obligate signs and symptoms include progressive ataxic gait, dysarthria, decreased proprioception or vibratory sense (or both), muscle weakness, and absent deep tendon reflexes. Other common signs include cavus foot deformity, cardiomyopathy, upper motor neuron signs, such as a Babinski sign, and scoliosis. The prevalence of scoliosis approaches 100%, but some cases have more severe progressive spinal deformity than others. Those Friedreich's ataxia cases with onset of disease before the age of 10 years generally have more severe progressive scoliosis. Those with the onset of disease during or after puberty have later-onset spinal deformity, which may not require surgical intervention.[24]

Management of Childhood Neuromuscular Diseases

Diseases affecting the lower motor neuron, including those primarily affecting anterior horn cell, peripheral nerve, neuromuscular junction (presynaptic or postsynaptic) or muscle, ultimately lead to progressive loss of functional muscle fiber over time. This loss of functional muscle fiber may lead to progressive weakness, decreased endurance, limb contractures, spinal deformity, body composition changes, decrease in mobility, decreased pulmonary function, and occasionally cardiac impairment if the myocardium is affected. Genetic defects causing CNS structural protein alterations may lead to intellectual impairment. Rehabilitation approaches directed at improving impairment and/or resultant disability may substantially improve the quality of life and community integration of children with neuromuscular diseases. The following discussion emphasizes general principles in the rehabilitation management of childhood neuromuscular disease with several specific conditions used to illustrate key concepts.

Exercise in Neuromuscular Disease

Exercise prescriptions and recommendations in childhood neuromuscular disease need to consider the specific disease condition as well as the developmental and maturational status of the child.

Strengthening Exercise in Rapidly Progressive Disorders

The more rapidly progressive neuromuscular disorders of childhood generally include the dystrophic myopathies. The inherent instability of the sarcolemmal membrane predisposes to membrane injury due to mechanical loads. Theoretically, eccentric or lengthening contractions produce more mechanical stress on muscle fiber than concentric or shortening contractions. Indeed, many of the muscle groups that show the greatest weakness early in the course of Duchenne muscular dystrophy are muscle groups that perform a great deal of eccentric activity, such as the hip extensors, knee extensors, and ankle dorsiflexors. In addition, lower extremity muscles in this population experience more mechanical loads than upper extremity muscle groups, and weakness in the lower extremities generally precedes weakness in the upper extremities. Edwards and colleagues[162] proposed that routine eccentric contractions occurring during gait are a likely source of the pattern of weakness typically seen in myopathies.

There may be increased weakness following strengthening exercise in DMD.[163] There are other instances that have raised concerns regarding overwork weakness in dystrophic myopathies. The dominant upper limb has been found to be weaker in persons with FSH muscular dystrophy than the nondominant, providing circumstantial evidence for overwork weakness.[99,164] A single subject with scapuloperoneal muscular dystrophy had a reversal of rapid strength decline after reducing daily physical activity. Other studies evaluating strengthening intervention in DMD subjects have shown maintenance of strength or even mild improvement in strength over the period of the investigation. However, these studies are limited by use of primarily nonquantitative measures,[165] lack of a control group,[166] and use of the opposite limb as a control without considering the effects of cross-training.[167] Animal work using dystrophic dogs has shown significant increases in creatine kinase values immediately following exercise.[168]

No systemic studies using the DMD population have shown any deleterious effects of resistance exercise. Based on the theoretic susceptibility of the dystrophin-deficient sarcolemmal membrane to mechanical injury and the relative paucity of investigations, it is prudent to recommend a submaximal strengthening program in DMD and other rapidly progressive dystrophic disorders. A great concern is how to incorporate these activities effectively into the daily routine of the child, avoiding use of mundane and tedious regimens that employ progressive resistance exercises. Incorporation of the activity into recreational pursuits and aqua-based therapy is probably the most reasonable approach for the preadolescent child.

Strengthening Exercise in Slowly Progressive Neuromuscular Diseases

Only supervised strengthening programs in this population have been advocated. Recently, a moderate resistance home-exercise program (using a less supervised approach) was devised that demonstrated similar strength gains in both neuromuscular disease patients and normal control subjects without evidence of overwork weakness.[169] Based on this encouraging result, the home program was advanced to high-resistance training in similar subjects without apparent additive beneficial effects; in fact, eccentrically measured elbow flexor strength actually decreased significantly.[170]

Based on the above investigations, the author believes that there is adequate evidence to generally advocate a submaximal strengthening program for persons with slowly progressive NMD. There seems to be no additional benefit to high-resistance, low-repetition training sets, and the risk of actually increasing weakness becomes greater. Improvement in strength will hopefully translate to more functional issues such as improved endurance and mobility.

Aerobic Exercise in Neuromuscular Disease

Aerobic exercise refers to rhythmic, prolonged activity of the level sufficient to provide a beneficial training stimulus to the cardiopulmonary and muscular systems but below the threshold where anaerobic metabolism of fuels is the primary source of energy. The response of normal skeletal muscle to this type of training includes increased capillary density in the muscle to improve substrate transfer, increased skeletal muscle mitochrondrial size and density, higher concentrations of skeletal muscle oxidative enzymes, and improvement in utilization of fat as an energy source for muscular activity. Patients with neuromuscular disease have a diminished capacity for exercise. Children with Duchenne muscular dystrophy have been demonstrated to have low cardiovascular capacity and peripheral oxygen utilization with higher resting heart rate compared with controls.[171] Physical ability and exercise capacity are more likely to be limited by muscle strength than by deterioration of cardiorespiratory function. In a recent study using a home-based aerobic walking program, slowly progressive neuromuscular disease subjects showed modest improvement in aerobic capacity without evidence of overwork weakness or excessive fatigue.[172] It is likely that alternative exercise approaches such as aquabased therapy will need to be used in children with more severe neuromuscular diseases who are nonambulatory and have less than antigravity muscle strength.

Management of Limb Contractures and Deformity

The management of limb contractures in progressive neuromuscular disease and the role of stretching, orthotics, and surgery have recently been comprehensively reviewed.[173] Contracture is defined as the lack of full active or passive ROM due to joint, muscle, or soft tissue limitation. Contractures may be arthrogenic, soft tissue, or myogenic in nature, and a combination of intrinsic structural changes of muscle and extrinsic factors leads to myogenic contractures in selected neuromuscular disease conditions. These factors include the following: (1) degree of fibrosis and fatty tissue infiltration; (2) static positioning and lack of full active and passive ROM; (3) imbalance of agonist and antagonist muscle strength across the joint; (4) lack of upright weight bearing and static positioning in sitting; (5) compensatory postural changes used to stabilize joints biomechanically for upright standing; and (6) functional anatomy of muscles and joints (multijoint muscle groups in which the origin and insertion crosses multiple joints). In general, dystrophic myopathies have a high degree of fibrosis and fatty infiltration, placing these patients at higher risk for contractures. Significant contractures have been identified most commonly in Duchenne muscular dystrophy, Becker muscular dystrophy, Emery-Dreifuss muscular dystrophy, congenital muscular dystrophy, severe childhood autosomal recessive muscular dystrophy, facioscapulohumeral muscular dystrophy, myotonic muscular dystrophy, hereditary motor sensory neuropathy, and spinal muscular atrophy.

Contractures and progressive neuromuscular conditions should be managed with the following concepts in mind:

1. Prevention of contractures requires early diagnosis and initiation of physical medicine approaches such as passive ROM and splinting while contractures are still mild.

2. Contractures are inevitable in some NMD conditions, such as DMD.

3. Advanced contractures become fixed and show little response to stretching programs.

4. A major rationale for controlling contractures of the lower extremity is to minimize the adverse effect of contractures on independent ambulation. However, the major cause of wheelchair reliance in NMD is generally weakness, not contracture formation.

5. Static positioning of both upper and lower extremity joints in patients with weak musculature is the most important cause of contracture formation.

6. Passive stretching for control of lower limb contractures is most successful in ambulatory patients with early mild joint contractures.

7. Upper extremity contractures may not negatively impact the function if they are mild.

8. Joint range of motion should be monitored regularly by physical and occupational therapists using objective goniometric measurement.

Principal therapy modalities must be carried out regularly to prevent or delay the development of lower extremity contractures for those at risk for musculoskeletal deformity. These include (1) regularly prescribed periods of daily standing and walking if the patient is functionally capable of being upright; (2) passive stretching of muscles and joints with a daily home program; (3) positioning of the legs to promote extension and oppose joint flexion when the patient is non–weight-bearing through the lower extremities; and (4) splinting, which is a useful measure for the prevention or delay of ankle contracture.

In the upper extremity, elbow flexion contractures in dystrophic myopathies may occur soon after transition to the wheelchair, secondary to static positioning of the arms and elbow flexion on the armrests of the wheelchair.[17] Other associated deformities in DMD and other dystrophic myopathies include forearm pronator tightness and wrist flexion-ulnar deviation in the later stages of the disease. The regular palm-down position of the hand increases the occurrence of forearm pronator contracture. Mild elbow flexion contractures of ≤ 15° are of no functional consequence to the patient using crutches or a wheelchair. Contractures of the elbows over 30° may interfere with the use of crutches in ambulatory patients with NMD. Severe elbow flexion contractions of > 60° are associated with decreased distal upper extremity function and produce difficulty when dressing.

Passive stretching of the elbow flexors may be combined with passive stretching into forearm supination to help prevent contractures. Prophylactic occupational therapy management of the wrist and hand is recommended in NMD to slow the development of contractures and to maintain fine motor skills. Daily passive stretching of the wrist flexors and intrinsic and extrinsic muscles of the hand and wrist is recommended, as are active range of motion exercises for the wrist and long finger flexors. Nighttime resting splints, which promote wrist extension, metacarpophalangeal extension, and proximal interphalangeal flexion, are recommended. Daytime positioning should emphasize wrist and finger extension, but any splinting should not compromise sensation or function.

Shoulder contractures are less problematic in patients with profound proximal muscle weakness. Combined shoulder internal rotation, adduction contracture, and elbow flexion deformity may interfere with self-feeding. Severe shoulder internal rotation deformities may complicate dressing, produce pain on passive range of motion, and cause pain during sleep.

Bracing/Orthotic and Surgical Management of Limb Deformity

Management of Neuromuscular Diseases with Proximal Weakness

The prototypical disorder in which bracing and surgical management of contractures for prolonged ambulation have been applied is Duchenne muscular dystrophy. In this population, wheelchair reliance is imminent when knee extension strength becomes less than antigravity and time to ambulate 30 feet is greater than 12 seconds.[17] A number of principles should be emphasized for these populations. First, with an appropriate and aggressive home-based therapy program, equinovarus contractures generally are absent or very mild in DMD at the time walking ability ceases.[17] In addition, hip and knee flexion contractures are also absent or extremely mild in ambulatory DMD patients at the time of bracing.[174,175] The wide-based Trendelenburg gait exhibited by these patients with gluteus medius weakness places the hip in an abducted position, leading to iliotibial band contractures. The late phase of ambulation often is associated with more marked joint contractures involving the iliotibial bands and heel cords, because DMD patients spend more time sitting and less time standing. The release of contractures at both the heel cord and iliotibial band generally is necessary to obtain successful knee-ankle-foot orthosis (KAFO).[176–178] Other authors have reported bracing of DMD patients without surgical release of the iliotibial bands.[179–180] Hip and knee flexion contractures generally are not severe enough to interfere with bracing at the time of transition to wheelchair.[17] The iliotibial band contractures may be released with a low Young fasciotomy and a high Ober fasciotomy.

The ankle deformity may be corrected by either tendo Achillis lengthening (TAL) alone or combined with a surgical transfer of the posterior tibialis muscle tendon to the dorsum of the foot. The posterior tibialis tendon transfer corrects the equinovarus deformity but prolongs the time in a cast and recovery time, and it increases the risks of prolonged sitting.

Orthopedic surgical release of these contractures allows the DMD patient to be braced in lightweight polypropylene KAFOs with the sole and ankle set at 90°, drop-lock knee joints, and ischial weight-bearing polypropylene upper thigh component. DMD patients who are braced may or may not require a walker for additional support. At times, DMD patients who have had excellent home stretching programs are placed immediately into KAFO bracing without surgical tenotomies.

While DMD subjects are still ambulating independently without orthotics, they often use their ankle equinus posturing from the gastrocnemius-soleus group to create a knee-extension moment at foot contact, thus stabilizing the knee when the quadriceps muscle is weak. Several authors have cautioned against isolated heel cord tenotomies while DMD patients are still ambulating independently. Overcorrection of the heel cord contracture in a DMD patient may result in immediate loss of the ability to walk without bracing unless the quadriceps are grade 4 or better.[173]

The duration of ambulation in DMD has been successfully prolonged by prompt surgery and bracing, immediately implemented following loss of independent ambulation. The gains in additional walking time have been variable, but generally reported between 2 and 5 years.

Long-term benefits of prolonged walking include decreased severity of heel cord and knee flexion contractures at age 16 years.[181] This may ultimately improve shoe-wearing tolerance and foot positioning on the wheelchair leg rests. Prolonged ambulation by lower extremity bracing in DMD has never been documented to be an independent factor in the prevention of scoliosis. Disadvantages of braced ambulation center on the excessive energy cost of braced ambulation and safety concerns in the event of falls. DMD subjects with KAFO bracing usually need gait training through physical therapy, and they need to be taught fall techniques.

Weakness is the major cause of loss of ambulation in DMD, not contracture formation. Thus, the primary indication of orthopedic surgical tenotomies and posterior tibialis tendon transfers likely is the provision of optimal alignment for KAFO bracing. Little evidence supports the efficacy of early prophylactic lower extremity surgery in DMD for independently producing prolonged ambulation.[17,173,182]

Management of NMD Patients with Distal Lower Extremity Weakness

Ankle dorsiflexors are often clinically weaker than ankle plantar flexors in neuromuscular disease because of selective involvement of the peroneal nerve in many neuropathies and isolated anterior and lateral compartment weakness in several myopathic conditions such as FSH, scapuloperoneal distribution LGMD, DMD, and Emery-Dreifuss muscular dystrophy. Ankle-foot orthotics (AFOs) are often used for patients with distal weakness. AFOs are generally contraindicated in situations in which NMD patients use equinus posturing with forefoot initial contact to maintain a knee extension moment in the setting of quadriceps weakness. Heel cord contractures may need to be surgically lengthened to allow for AFO or KAFO bracing. Cavus feet are common in peripheral neuropathies. Intrinsic muscle weakness of the foot results in hyperextension at the metatarsophalangeal joints and flexion at the interphalangeal joints with resultant claw-toe deformities. This constellation of deformities may cause difficulty in walking, lack of balance, and painful callosities. Treatment of the cavus foot depends on the patient's age, flexibility of the foot, bony deformity, and muscle imbalance. A supple foot may be managed nonoperatively by serial casting in a walking cast, followed by an AFO with a solid ankle in neutral position and a lateral heel wedge if significant hindfoot varus exists. Fixed soft tissue or bony deformity may require orthopedic surgery to produce a plantigrade foot. In skeletally immature children, triple arthrodesis is contraindicated. Triple arthrodesis should be considered only as a salvage procedure for severe heel varus and severe midfoot deformity, with the goal being achievement of hindfoot stability in a skeletally mature patient.

Management of Spinal Deformity

Severe spinal deformity and progressive NMD lead to multiple problems, including poor sitting balance, difficulty with upright sitting and positioning, pain, difficulty in parental or attendant care, and potential exacerbation of underlying restrictive respiratory compromise. Severe scoliosis and pelvic obliquity may, in some instances, completely preclude upright sitting in a wheelchair. The management of spinal deformity and progressive neuromuscular disease has recently been reviewed.[183] Populations at risk for scoliosis include DMD, SCARMD, congenital muscular dystrophy, FSH muscular dystrophy, congenital myotonic muscular dystrophy, spinal muscular atrophy II and III, and Friedreich's ataxia.

Close clinical monitoring is essential for children with NMD at risk for scoliosis. Curves may progress rapidly during the adolescent growth spurt, and children need to be monitored every 3–4 months with clinical assessment and spine radiographs if indicated. In addition, patients who are likely to require surgical arthrodesis at some point should be monitored with pulmonary function tests every 6 months. A forced vital capacity falling below 30–40% of predicted may contraindicate surgery, irrespective of scoliotic severity, because of increased perioperative morbidity. Thus, there is often a critical window of time during which the spinal deformity is evident and likely to continue to progress, and the restrictive lung disease is not of a severity which would contraindicate surgery.

The management of spinal deformity with orthotics is ineffective in DMD and does not change the natural history of the curve. Spinal orthoses are often reported to be uncomfortable and poorly tolerated by DMD patients. Furthermore, vital capacity potentially can be lowered with constrictive orthoses. On the other hand, in neuromuscular diseases with spinal deformity beginning in the first decade of life, such as SMA, congenital muscular dystrophy, congenital myotonic muscular dystrophy, some congenital myopathies, and congenital myasthenic syndromes, spinal bracing is generally used to improve sitting balance in patients who are unable to walk. In addition, spinal orthotics are employed in these younger patients in an attempt to halt curve progression until they are 10–11 years of age, when a single posterior spinal arthrodesis procedure is sufficient. Children younger than 10 years generally require both anterior and posterior spinal arthrodesis because of continued spinal growth, which diminishes after age 11–12 years.

Spinal arthrodesis is the only effective treatment for scoliosis in DMD, SCARMD, congenital muscular dystrophy, congenital myotonic muscular dystrophy, SMA, and Friedreich's ataxia. The decision to pursue posterior spinal instrumentation involves a consideration of the severity of the restrictive lung disease, severity of the cardiomyopathy, severity and flexibility of the spinal deformity, and likelihood that the spinal deformity will continue to progress. Surgical spinal arthrodesis should be deferred to a later date in marginally ambulatory patients with SCARMD, congenital muscular dystrophy, FSH muscular dystrophy, and spinal muscular atrophy type III, because these individuals may use significant lumbar lordosis during gait to compensate for hip extensor weakness.

Provision of Functional Mobility

Generally, antigravity quadriceps is required for community ambulation in childhood neuromuscular disease. Short-distance ambulation may be achieved by some patients with more severe weakness using KAFO bracing with or without a walker. Such orthotic intervention is often provided to children with SMA type III, SCARMD, congenital muscular dystrophy, DMD, and BMD during adulthood. Children with DMD, SMA type II, congenital muscular dystrophy, congenital myopathies, some myasthenic syndromes, and more severe hereditary motor sensory neuropathies use power-mobility devices for functional mobility. Generally, children can be taught to operate a power wheelchair safely when they are at the developmental age of approximately 2 years.[184,185] The initial power wheelchair prescription needs to consider the natural history of the neuromuscular disease condition over the following 5 years because some children will subsequently develop the need for a power recline system and the chair must be able to accommodate such a recline or be retrofit. In more severe disability, the power wheelchair electronics should be sufficiently sophisticated to incorporate alternative drive control systems, environmental control adaptations, and possibly communication systems for patients who are unable to vocalize.

Pulmonary Management

Pulmonary complications are recognized as the leading cause of mortality in childhood neuromuscular disease. Respiratory insufficiency in neuromuscular disease results from a number of factors, including (1) respiratory muscle weakness and fatigue, (2) alteration of respiratory system mechanics, and (3) impairment of a central control of respiration. Progressive muscle weakness and fatigue lead to restrictive lung disease and ultimately to hypoventilation, hypercarbia, and respiratory failure. Increases in elastic load on respiratory muscles occur because of chest wall stiffness, airway secretions, and ineffective cough mechanism. These increases may result in atelectasis and increased airway resistance, and kyphoscoliosis may further alter respiratory mechanics. Defects in central control of respiration may be secondary to hypoxemia and hypercarbia associated with severe restrictive lung disease. Significant nocturnal decreases in partial pressure of oxygen, as well as elevations in arterial partial pressure of CO_2, occur in more severe restrictive lung disease. Hypercapnia or hypoxemia occurring at night may have a role in reducing daytime central respiratory drive. A chronic increase in the bicarbonate pool, generated by respiratory acidosis, may blunt the stimulus to breathe and perpetuate the hypercapnic state. Expiratory muscle weakness may produce ineffective cough and problems with clearance of secretions, and predispose to pulmonary infections.

Respiratory failure may present acutely or insidiously. Respiratory difficulties in the delivery room or early infancy may be seen in acute infantile type I SMA, myotubular myopathy, congenital hypomyelinating neuropathy, congenital infantile myasthenia, congenital myotonic muscular dystrophy, transitory neonatal myasthenia, and severe neurogenic arthrogryposis. In most other childhood neuromuscular diseases, the respiratory insufficiency develops more insidiously, unless an acute decompensation occurs from an event such as an aspiration episode or acute onset of weakness, as seen in Guillain-Barré syndrome, botulism, and myasthenic syndromes. Signs and symptoms of significant respiratory difficulties may include subcostal retractions, accessory respiratory muscle recruitment, nasal flaring, exertional dyspnea or dyspnea at rest, orthopnea, generalized fatigue, and paradoxic breathing patterns. A history of nightmares, morning headaches, and daytime drowsiness may indicate nocturnal hypoventilation with sleep-disordered breathing. Pulmonary function tests have been used to help in the decision-making process regarding the institution of mechanical ventilation. In a study of 53 patients with proximal myopathy, hypercapnia occurred when the maximal inspiratory pressure was less than 30% of predicted and when vital capacity was less than 55% of predicted.[186] Other authors[187,188] have noted lower values for vital capacity measurements in their patients with DMD at the time they require institution of mechanical ventilatory support. Hahn and colleagues[189] have reported the predictive value of maximal static airway pressures in predicting impending respiratory failure. Splaingard et al.[190] reviewed a series of 40 patients with a diverse group of neuromuscular conditions. They noted that all of their patients who required mechanical ventilation had a vital capacity of $\leq 25\%$ with at least one of the following associated findings: (1) $PaCO_2 > 55$ mmHg, (2) recurrent atelectasis or pneumonia, (3) moderate dyspnea at rest, or (4) congestive heart failure.

Noninvasive forms of both positive and negative pressure ventilation are being applied increasingly to children with neuromuscular diseases (Table 15–6). Initially, patients may require ventilatory support for only part of the day. Noninvasive nocturnal ventilation has become a widely accepted clinical practice, providing ventilatory assistance for patients while they are sleeping and allowing them to breathe on their own during the day. Intermittent ventilation may ameliorate symptoms of respiratory failure, reduce hypercarbia, increase oxygenation (even during periods off ventilation), and prolong survival in patients with neuromuscular disease. The long-term use of noninvasive ventilation may be associated with fewer complications than ventilation via a tracheostomy; however, bulbar muscle function should be adequate for safe swallowing.[159] Ventilatory support has allowed prolonged survival and acceptable quality of life in SMA I, SMA II, and DMD.[188,191–193]

TABLE 15–6. Devices Available for Mechanical Ventilation of Patients with Neuromuscular Disease

Negative Pressure Ventilators
Fully-boy ventilator (tank ventilator or iron lung)
Raincoat ventilator ("poncho" or "pneumowrap")
Cuirass ventilator (chest shelf)
Pneumosuit ventilator with leggings

Positive Pressure Ventilators
Via tracheostomy
Noninvasive
  Via full face mask (e.g., BIPAP)
  Via nasal mask (e.g., BIPAP)
  Via mouthpiece with lip seal
  Via intermittent positive pressure breathing (IPPB) using
    mouthpiece adapter

Ventilators Resulting in Passive Movement of the Diaphragm
Pneumobell
Rocking bed

BIPAP, bilevel positive airway pressure.

Improved pulmonary toilet and clearance of secretions can be achieved with assisted cough, deep breathing, incentive spirometry, percussion, and postural drainage, and, in more severe cases, the additional use of interpulmonary percussive ventilation (IPV), given 2–3 times daily.

Nutritional Management

Management of Swallowing Problems

Involvement of palatal and pharyngeal muscles may produce dysphagia. Patients at particular risk include those with SMA, myasthenia gravis, congenital myasthenic syndromes, and congenital myopathies such as myotubular myopathy, oculopharyngeal muscular dystrophy, late-stage Duchenne muscular dystrophy, and late-stage SCARMD. The presence of dysphagia in neuromuscular disease patients has been documented by others.[56,194] The function of the swallowing mechanism is best evaluated with a fluoroscopic videodynamic swallowing evaluation. DMD patients have a high prevalence of dysphagia during the late stages of the disease.[56] DMD patients may also rarely develop acute gastric dilatation secondary to gastric paresis.[195] Bulbar dysfunction and/or respiratory distress may affect feeding in SMA patients. In SMA I, therapeutic modifications may include use of a premature baby nipple with a large opening, use of proper head and jaw position, along with a semireclined trunk position, and use of frequent small feedings to minimize fatigue.[154,196] These larger bolus feeds may distend the stomach and encroach on the diaphragm, thus affecting respiratory status. Improved nourishment in SMA leads to a feeling of well-being and therefore a better quality of life.[196] Poor nutritional status, labored feeding, or symptoms of dysphagia are indications for initiation of supplemental enteral feedings via nasogastric tube or gastrostomy. Gastroesophageal reflux with risk of aspiration may be an indication for placement of a gastrojejunostomy tube.

Energy and Protein Supplementation

Severe deficits in energy and protein intake have been documented in DMD[54,55] during the second decade of life. Substantial weight loss has been documented in DMD to occur between the ages of 17–21 years.[17] Protein and calorie needs in DMD may be approximately 160% of those required for able-bodied adolescents.[54,55] Beneficial effects in weight gain, anthropometric measurements, and nitrogen balance were recently documented for DMD patients, aged 10–20 years, subsequent to a 3-month nutritional supplementation that consisted of an additional 1,000 kcals and 37.2 grams of protein.[197] The positive effects on metabolism observed in this study warrant further investigation.

Branched-chain Ketoacid Supplementation

Based on the observations that muscle protein degradation is accelerated in DMD and that administration of branched-chain ketoacids reduces protein breakdown in fasting obese subjects, Stewart and colleagues[198] conducted a trial of branched-chain ketoacid supplementation. The ketoacids of the branched-chain amino acids leucine, valine, and isoleucine were administered orally as ornithine salts at a dosage of 0.45 gm/kg body weight/day for 4 days in nine boys with DMD, aged 5–9 years. An equivalent amount of protein was removed from the diet during this time. A small but significant reduction in muscle protein degradation was observed as a result of the treatment, and no negative effects were noted. The results warrant further investigation regarding the effects of longer-term branched-chain ketoacid supplementation on muscle protein degradation.

Weight Reduction

DMD patients typically gain excessive weight between 9 and 13 years of age, subsequent to the onset of wheelchair reliance. This increase likely occurs because of a reduction in total daily energy expenditure with increased sedentary existence. Edwards and colleagues[199] demonstrated that weight reduction through a medically supervised decrease in energy intake could be achieved successfully in DMD without compromising skeletal muscle mass. Obesity has also been observed in SMA III patients and has been attributed to a relatively sedentary lifestyle.[196] Increased adiposity has been documented in adults with slowly progressive neuromuscular diseases.[200] Approaches to weight reduction in slowly progressive neuromuscular disease patients have been reviewed recently.[201]

Management of Cardiac Complications

The management of cardiac complications in neuromuscular disease has been reviewed recently.[202] Treatment with angiotensin-converting enzyme inhibitors is probably warranted in DMD when the measured ejection fraction falls below 35%. Digitalis has been demonstrated to be effective in decreasing morbidity from heart failure, but not mortality, and probably is also indicated for the treatment of heart failure observed in DMD patients with cardiomyopathy. Beta blockers also may have a role in DMD. Treatment with coenzyme Q10 remains controversial. Cor pulmonale, confirmed on echocardiography, may

benefit from continuous supplemental oxygen. Patients with known arrhythmias who are at risk for fatal tachyarrhythmias may benefit from antiarrhythmic medication. DMD patients with mitral valve prolapse and mitral regurgitation should be given antibiotic prophylaxis for dental and surgical procedures in accordance with current guidelines.

The management of the cardiomyopathy seen in Becker muscular dystrophy is similar to that seen in DMD; however, in cases of severe end-stage cardiomyopathy, cardiac transplantation should be considered.

Cardiac conduction abnormalities observed in myotonic muscular dystrophy may ultimately require implantation of cardiac pacemakers. In rare instances with cardiomyopathy, treatment may consist of angiotensin-converting enzyme inhibitors, digitalis, and diuretics, based on proven efficacy in cardiomyopathies of other causes.

Emery-Dreifuss muscular dystrophy patients with symptomatic bradycardia or heart block should undergo implantation of a permanent cardiac pacemaker. Atrial standstill, atrial fibrillation, and atrial flutter are all disorders in which blood can pool in the atria, leading to thrombus formation and possible embolic events, including stroke. Anticoagulation with warfarin to an INR of 2–3 has demonstrated a reduction in the incidence of stroke in patients with atrial fibrillation. Prompt referral to a cardiologist should be made for children with cardiac signs or symptoms on screening ECG, echocardiography, or for those with Holter recording abnormalities suggestive of cardiac disease. Late-stage DMD, BMD, and Emery-Dreifuss muscular dystrophy patients should be followed by a cardiologist on a regular basis. Appropriate management of cardiac complications in childhood neuromuscular disease hopefully will increase life expectancy.

Pharmacologic Intervention

The rehabilitation specialist may become involved in the prescription of pharmacologic agents that impact the pathophysiology of various neuromuscular diseases. Evaluation of therapeutic efficacy for pharmacologic agents requires careful objective measurement of strength with quantitative measurements, functional status, and pulmonary function parameters.

Corticosteroids such as prednisone may have an effect on the inflammatory component of the dystrophic myopathy in DMD and slow the progression of the strength loss for a time-limited period of 2–3 years.[203–205] Alternative pulse-dosing regimens may decrease the side effects. Deflazacort is an alternate corticosteroid with a potentially better side-effect profile and efficacy equal to prednisone in DMD. Oxandrolone, an anabolic steroid more potent than testosterone, may be useful in DMD with efficacy similar to prednisone, according to a small pilot study.[206] Results from a study of oxandrolone in DMD in a randomized, double-blind, placebo-controlled trial are forthcoming.

The identification of specific genes and the protein products implicated in the pathogenesis of various neuromuscular disease provides hope that meaningful therapeutic interventions will alter the natural history of many of these neuromuscular diseases. It is likely that traditional rehabilitation approaches will need to be used adjunctively with newer pharmacologic interventions and possibly gene therapy in the management of these conditions.

References

1. Cros D, Harnden P, Pellisier JF, et al: Muscle hypertrophy in Duchenne muscular dystrophy: A pathological and morphometric study. J Neurol 1989;236:43.
2. Eng GD, Binder H, Koch B: Spinal muscular atrophy: Experience in diagnosis and rehabilitation in management of 60 patients. Arch Phys Med Rehabil 1984;65:549.
3. Dorsher PT, Sinaki M, Muller DW, et al: Wohlfart-Kugelberg-Welander syndrome: Serum creatine kinase and functional outcome. Arch Phys Med Rehabil 1991;72:587.
4. Coleman RA, Stajich JM, Pact VW, et al: The ischemic exercise test in normal adults and in patients with weakness and cramps. Muscle Nerve 1986;9:216.
5. Munsat TL: Standardized forearm ischemic exercise test. Neurology 1970;20:1171.
6. Sinkeler SPT, Daanen HAM, Wevers RA, et al: The relation between blood lactate and ammonia in ischemic handgrip exercise. Muscle Nerve 1986;9:216.
7. Dubowitz V: Muscle Disorders in Childhood, 2nd ed. London, WB Saunders, 1995.
8. Mubarak SJ, Chambers HG, Wenger DR: Percutaneous muscle biopsy in the diagnosis of neuromuscular disease. J Pediatr Orthop 1992;12:191.
9. Koenig M, Hoffmann EP, Bertelson CK, et al: Complete cloning of the Duchenne muscular dystrophy (DMD) cDNA and preliminary genomic organization of the DMD gene in mouse and affected individuals. Cell 1987;50:509.
10. Roberts RG, Coffey AJ, Bobrow M, et al: Exon structure of the human dystrophin gene. Genomics 1993;16:536.
11. Hoffman EP, Fischbeck KH, Brown RH, et al: Dystrophin characterization in muscle biopsies from Duchenne and Becker muscular dystrophy patients. N Engl J Med 1988;318:1363.
12. Houzelstein D, Lyons GE, Chamberlain J, et al: Localization of dystrophin gene transcripts during mouse embryogenesis. J Cell Biol 1992;119:811.
13. Ervasti JM, Ohlendieck K, Kahl SD, et al: Deficiency of a glycoprotein component of the dystrophin complex in dystrophic muscle. Nature 1990;345:315.
14. Emery AH: Population frequencies of inherited neuromuscular diseases—A world survey. Neuromuscul Disord 1991;1:19.
15. Dubowitz V: Progressive Muscular Dystrophy in Childhood. MD Thesis, University of Cape Town, 1960.
16. McDonald CM, Abresch RT, Carter GT, et al: Profiles of neuromuscular diseases: Becker's muscular dystrophy. Am J Phys Med Rehabil 1995;74(Suppl 5):S93.
17. McDonald CM, Abresch RT, Carter GT, et al: Profiles of neuromuscular diseases: Duchenne muscular dystrophy. Am J Phys Med Rehabil 1995;74(Suppl 5):S70.
18. Pradhan S: New clinical sign in Duchenne muscular dystrophy. Pediatr Neurol 1994;11:298.
19. Kilmer DMD, Abresch RT, Fowler WM Jr: Serial manual muscle testing in Duchenne muscular dystrophy. Arch Phys Med Rehabil 1993;74:1168.
20. Mendell JR, Province MA, Moxley RT, et al: Clinical investigation of Duchenne muscular dystrophy: A methodology for therapeutic trials based on natural history controls. Arch Neurol 1987;44:808.
21. Brooke MH, Fenichel GM, Griggs RC, et al: Duchenne muscular dystrophy: Patterns of clinical progression and effects of supportive therapy. Neurology 1989;39:745.
22. Johnson ER, Fowler WM Jr, Lieberman JS: Contractures in neuromuscular disease. Arch Phys Med Rehabil 1992;73:807.
23. Brooke MH, Fenichel GM, Griggs RC, et al: Clinical investigation in Duchenne dystrophy. 2. Determination of the "power" of therapeutic trials based on the natural history. Muscle Nerve 1983;6:91.
24. Hart DA, McDonald CM: Spinal deformity in progressive neuromuscular disease: Natural history and management. Phys Med Rehabil Clin North Am 1998;9:213.
25. Oda T, Shimizu N, Yonenobu K, et al: Longitudinal study of spinal deformity in Duchenne muscular dystrophy. J Pediatr Orthop 1993;13:478.
26. Johnson E, Yarnell S: Hand dominance and scoliosis in Duchenne muscular dystrophy. Arch Phys Med Rehabil 1976;57:462.
27. Lord J, Behrman B, Varzos N, et al: Scoliosis associated with Duchenne muscular dystrophy. Arch Phys Med Rehabil 1990;71:13.
28. Rideau Y, Jankowski L, Grellet J: Respiratory function in the muscular dystrophies. Muscle Nerve 1981;4:155.
29. Rideau Y, Glorion B, Delaubier A, et al: The treatment of scoliosis in Duchenne muscular dystrophy. Muscle Nerve 1984;7:281.
30. Bies RD, Friedman D, Roberts R, et al: Expression and localization of dystrophin in human cardiac Purkinje fibers. Circulation 1992;86:147.
31. Akita H, Matsuoka S, Juroda Y: Predictive electrocardiographic score for evaluating prognosis in patients with Duchenne muscular dystrophy. Tokushima J Exp Med 1995;40:55.
32. Miller G, D'Orsogna L, O'Shea JP: Autonomic function and the sinus tachycardia of Duchenne muscular dystrophy. Brain Dev 1989;22:247.
33. Perloff JK: Cardiac rhythm and conduction in Duchenne muscular dystrophy. J Am Coll Cardiol 1984;3:1263.
34. Sanyal SK, Johnson WW, Thapar MK, et al: An ultrastructural basis for the electrocardiographic alteration associated with Duchenne's progressive muscular dystrophy. Circulation 1978;57:1122.
35. Takenaka A, Yokota M, Iwase M, et al: Discrepancy between systolic and diastolic dysfunction of the left ventricle in patients with Duchenne muscular dystrophy. Eur Heart J 1993;14:669.
36. Yamamoto S, Matsushima H, Suzuki A, et al: A comparative study of thallium-201 single photon emission computed tomography and electrocardiography in Duchenne and other types of muscular dystrophy. Am J Cardiol 1988;61836.
37. Yotsukura M, Miyagawa M, Tsuya T, et al: Pulmonary hypertension in progressive muscular dystrophy of the Duchenne type. Jpn Circ J 1988;52:321.
38. Mori H, Utsunomiya T, Ishijima M, et al: The relationship between 24-hour total heart beats or ventricular arrhythmias and cardiopulmonary function in patients with Duchenne muscular dystrophy. Jpn Heart J 1990;31:599.

39. Chenard AA, Becane HM, Tertrain F, et al: Systolic time intervals in Duchenne muscular dystrophy: Evaluation of left ventricular performance. Clin Cardiol 1998;11:407.
40. Yanagisawa A, Miyagawa M, Yotsukura M, et al: The prevalence and prognostic significance of arrhythmias in Duchenne-type muscular dystrophy. Am Heart J 1992;124:1244.
41. Nigro G, Comi LI, Politano L, et al: The incidence and evolution of cardiomyopathy in Duchenne muscular dystrophy. Int J Cardiol 1990;26:277.
42. Nigro G, Comi LI, Politano L, et al: Evaluation of the cardiomyopathy in Becker muscular dystrophy. Muscle Nerve 1995;18:283.
43. Nagai T: Prognostic evaluation of congestive heart failure in patients with Duchenne muscular dystrophy: Retrospective study using non-invasive cardiac function tests. Jpn Circ J 1898;53:406.
44. Gilroy J, Cahalan J, German R, et al: Cardiac and pulmonary complications in Duchenne's progressive muscular dystrophy. Circulation 1963;27:484.
45. Leth A, Wulff K: Myocardiopathy in Duchenne progressive muscular dystrophy. Acta Paediatr Scand 1976;65:28.
46. Nudel L, Zuk D, Zeelan E, et al: DMD gene product is not identical in muscle and brain. Nature 1989;337:76.
47. Dorman C, Hurley AD, D'Avignon J: Language and learning disorders of older boys with Duchenne muscular dystrophy. Dev Med Child Neurol 1988;30:316.
48. Marsh GG, Munsat TL: Evidence of early impairment of verbal intelligence in Duchenne muscular dystrophy. Arch Dis Child 1974;49:118.
49. Sollee ND, Latham EE, Kinndlon DJ, Bresnan MJ: Neuropsychological impairment in Duchenne muscular dystrophy. J Clin Exp Neuropsychol 1985;7:486.
50. Rappaport D, Colleto GM, Vainzof M, et al: Short stature in Duchenne muscular dystrophy. Growth Regul 1991;1:11.
51. Eiholzer U, Boltshauser E, Frey D, et al: Short stature: A common feature in Duchenne muscular dystrophy. Eur J Pediatr 1988;147:602.
52. Scott OM, Hyde SA, Goddard C, Dubowitz V: Quantitation of muscle function in children: A prospective study in Duchenne muscular dystrophy. Muscle Nerve 1982;5:291.
53. Willig TN, Carlier L, Legrand M, et al: Nutritional assessment in Duchenne muscular dystrophy. Dev Med Child Neurol 1993;35:1074.
54. Okada K, Manabe S, Sakamoto S, et al: Protein and energy metabolism in patients with progressive muscular dystrophy. J Nutr Sci Vitaminol (Tokyo) 1992;38:141.
55. Okada K, Manabe S, Sakamoto S, et al: Predictions of energy intake and energy allowance of patients with Duchenne muscular dystrophy and their validity. J Nutr Sci Vitaminol (Tokyo) 1992;38:155.
56. Jaffe KM, McDonald CM, Ingman E, Haas J: Symptoms of upper gastrointestinal dysfunction: Case-control study. Arch Phys Med Rehabil 1990;71:742.
57. Becker PE, Kiener G: Eine neue X-chromosomale Muskeldystrophie. Arch Psychiatr Z Neurol 1955;193:427.
58. Bushby KMD, Thambyayah M, Gardner-Medwin D: Prevalence and incidence of Becker muscular dystrophy. Lancet 1991;337:1022.
59. Comi GP, Prelle A, Bresolin N, et al: Clinical variability in Becker muscular dystrophy: Genetic, biochemical and immunohistochemical correlates. Brain 1994;117:1.
60. Bushby KMD, Gardner-Medwin D, Nicholson LVB, et al: The clinical, genetic and dystrophin characteristics of Becker muscular dystrophy. II. Correlation of phenotype with genetic and protein abnormalities. J Neurol 1993;240:105.
61. Monaco AP, Bertelson CJ, Liechti-Gallati S, et al: An explanation for the phenotypic differences between patients bearing partial deletions of the DMD locus. Genomics 1988;2:90.
62. Arahata K, Beggs AH, Honda H, et al: Preservation of the C-terminus of dystrophin molecule in the skeletal muscle from Becker muscular dystrophy. J Neurol Sci 1992;101:1488.
63. Gospe SM, Lozaro RP, Lava NS, et al: Familial X-linked myalgia and cramps: A nonprogressive myopathy associated with a deletion in the dystrophin gene. Neurology 1989;39:1277.
64. Becker PE: Two new families of benign sex-linked recessive muscular dystrophy. Rev Can Biol 1962;21:551.
65. Bradley WG, Jones MZ, Mussini JM, Fawcett PRW: Becker-type muscular dystrophy. Muscle Nerve 1978;1: 111.
66. Emery AEH, Skinner R: Clinical studies in benign (Becker-type) X-linked muscular dystrophy. Clin Genet 1976;10:189.
67. Smith PFM, Calverley PMA, Edwards RHT, et al: Practical problems in the respiratory care of patients with muscular dystrophy. N Engl J Med 1987;316:1197.
68. Carter GT, Abresch RT, Fowler WM Jr, et al: Profiles of neuromuscular diseases: Hereditary motor and sensory neuropathy, types I and II. Am J Phys Med Rehabil 1995;74(Suppl 5):S140.
69. Carter GT, Abresch RT, Fowler WM Jr, et al: Profiles of neuromuscular diseases: Spinal muscular atrophy. Am J Phys Med Rehabil 1995;74(Suppl 5):S150.
70. Ringel SP, Carroll JE, Schold C: The spectrum of mild X-linked recessive muscular dystrophy. Arch Neurol 1977;34:408.
71. Katlyer BC, Misra S, Somani PN, Chaterji AM: Congestive cardiomyopathy in a family of Becker's X-linked muscular dystrophy. Postgrad Med J 1977;53:12.
72. Yazawa M, Ikeda S, Owa M, et al: A family of Becker's progressive muscular dystrophy with severe cardiomyopathy. Eur Neurol 1987;26:13.
73. Lazzeroni E, Favaro L, Botti G: Dilated cardiomyopathy with regional myocardial hypoperfusion in Becker's muscular dystrophy. Int J Cardiol 1989;22:126.
74. Sakata C, Sunohara N, Nonaka I, et al: A case of Becker muscular dystrophy presenting with cardiac failure as an initial symptom. Rinsho Shinkeigaku 1990;30:210.
75. Quinlivan RM, Dubowitz V: Cardiac transplantation in Becker muscular dystrophy. Neuromuscul Disord 1992;2:165.
76. Yoshida K, Ikeda S, Nakamura A, et al: Molecular analysis of the Duchenne muscular dystrophy gene in patients with Becker muscular dystrophy presenting with dilated cardiomyopathy. Muscle Nerve 1993;16:1161.
77. Casazzo F, Banbilla SG, Salvato A, et al: Cardiac transplantation in Becker muscular dystrophy. J Neurol 1988;235:496.
78. Donofrio D, Challa V, Hackshaw B, et al: Cardiac transplantation in a patient with Becker muscular dystrophy and cardiomyopathy. Arch Neurol 1980;46:705.
79. Steare SE, Benatar A, Dubowitz V: Subclinical cardiomyopathy in Becker muscular dystrophy. Br Heart J 1992;68:304.
80. Roberds SL, Leturcq F, Allamand V, et al: Missense mutations in the adhalin gene linked to autosomal recessive muscular dystrophy. Cell 1994;78:625.
81. Passos-Bueno MR, Oliveira JR, Bakker E, et al: Genetic heterogeneity for Duchenne-like muscular dystrophy (DLMD) based on linkage and 50 DAG analysis. Hum Mol Genet 1993;2:1945.
82. Matsumura K, Tome FMS, Collin H, et al: Deficiency of the 50K dystrophin-associated glycoprotein in severe childhood autosomal recessive muscular dystrophy. Nature 1992;359:320.

83. Duggan DJ, Fanin M, Pegoraro E, et al: Alpha-sarcoglycan (adhalin) deficiency: Complete deficiency patients are 5% of childhood-onset dystrophin-normal muscular dystrophy and most partial deficiency patients do not have gene mutations. J Neurol Sci 1996;140:30.

84. Duggan DJ, Hoffman EP: Autosomal recessive muscular dystrophy and mutations of the sarcoglycan complex. Neuromuscul Disord 1996;6:475.

85. Ozawa E, Yoshida M, Suzaki A, et al: Dystrophin-associated proteins in muscular dystrophy. Hum Mol Genet 1995;4:1711.

86. Campbell KP: Three muscular dystrophies: Loss of cytoskeleton–extracellular matrix linkage. Cell 1995;80:675.

87. Tinsley JM, Blake DJ, Zuelling RA, et al: Increasing complexity of the dystrophin-associated protein complex. Proc Natl Acad Sci USA 1994;91:8307.

88. McDonald CM, Johnson ER, Abresch RT, et al: Profiles of neuromuscular diseases: Limb-girdle syndromes. Am J Phys Med Rehabil 1995;74(Suppl 5):S117.

89. Fukuyama Y, Kawazura M, Haruna H: A peculiar form of congenital progressive muscular dystrophy: Report of 15 cases. Paediatria Universitatis Tokyo 1960;4:5.

90. Nonaka I, Miyoshino S, Miike T, et al: An electron-microscopical study of the muscle in congenital muscular dystrophy. Kumamoto Med J 1972;25:68.

91. Segawa M: Clinical studies of congenital muscular dystrophy: Arthrogrypotic type of congenital muscular dystrophy with mental retardation and facial muscle involvement. Brain Dev 1970;2:439.

92. Toda T, Segawa M, Nomura Y, et al: Localization of a gene for Fukuyama-type congenital muscular dystrophy to chromosome 9q31-33. Nat Genet 1993;5:283.

93. Santavuori P, Leisti J, Kruus S: Muscle, eye and brain disease: A new syndrome. Neuropediatrics 1977;8:S553.

94. Santavuori P, Somer H, Sainio K, et al: Muscle-eye-brain disease and Walker-Warburg syndrome. Am J Med Genet 1990;36:371.

95. Williams RS, Swisher CN, Jennings M, et al: Cerebro-ocular dysgenesis (Walker-Warburg syndrome): Neuropathologic and etiologic analysis. Neurology 1984;34:1531.

96. Tome FMS, Evangelista T, Leclerc A, et al: Congenital muscular dystrophy with merosin deficiency. Life Sci 1994;317:351.

97. Upadhyaya M, Lunt PW, Sarfarazi M, et al: DNA marker applicable to presymptomatic and prenatal diagnosis of facioscapulohumeral disease. Lancet 1990; 336:1320.

98. Wijmenga C, Frants RR, Brouwer OF, et al: The facioscapulohumeral muscular dystrophy gene maps to chromosome 4. Lancet 1990;2:651.

99. Kilmer DD, Abresch RT, McCrory MA, et al: Profiles of neuromuscular diseases: Facioscapulohumeral muscular dystrophy. Am J Phys Med Rehabil 1995;74(Suppl 5):S131.

100. Meyerson MD, Lewis E, Ill K: Facioscapulohumeral muscular dystrophy and accompanying hearing loss. Arch Otolaryngol 1984;110:261.

101. Padberg GW, Brouwer OF, de Keizer RJ, et al: On the significance of retinal vascular disease and hearing loss in facioscapulohumeral muscular dystrophy. Muscle Nerve 1995;2:S73.

102. Verhagen WI, Huygen PL, Padberg GW: The auditory, vestibular and oculomotor system in facioscapulohumeral dystrophy. Acta Otolaryngol 1995;1:140.

103. de Visser M, de Voogt WG, la Riviere GV: The heart in Becker muscular dystrophy, facioscapulohumeral dystrophy, and Bethlem myopathy. Muscle Nerve 1992;15:591.

104. Matsuo S, Oku Y, Oshibuchi R, et al: Systolic time intervals in progressive muscular dystrophy. Jpn Heart J 1979;1:23.

105. Bione S, Maestrini E, Rivella S, et al: Identification of a novel X-linked gene responsible for Emery-Dreifuss muscular dystrophy. Nat Genet 1994;8:323.

106. Emery AEH: Emery-Dreifuss muscular dystrophy and other related disorders. Br Med Bull 1989;45:772.

107. Emery AEH, Dreifuss FE: Unusual type of benign X-linked muscular dystrophy. J Neurol Neurosurg Psychiatry 1966;29:338.

108. Voit T, Krogmann O, Lennard HG, et al: Emery-Dreifuss muscular dystrophy: Disease spectrum and differential diagnosis. Neuropediatrics 1988;19:62.

109. Waters DD, Nutter DO, Hopkins LD, et al: Cardiac features of an unusual X-linked humeroperoneal neuromuscular disease. New Engl J Med 1975;293:1017.

110. Kausch K, Lehmann-Horn F, Janka M, et al: Evidence for linkage of the central core disease locus to the proximal long arm of human chromosome 19. Genomics 1991;10:765.

111. Engel WK, Foster JM, Hughes BP, et al: Central core disease—An investigation of a rare muscle cell abnormality. Brain 1961;84:167.

112. Mulley JC, Kozman HM, Phillips HA, et al: Refined genetic localization for central core disease. Am J Hum Genet 1993;52:398.

113. Laing N, Majda B, Akkari P, et al: Assignment of a gene (NEM1) for autosomal dominant nemaline myopathy to chromosome 1. Am J Hum Genet 1992;50:576.

114. Brooke MH: A neuromuscular disease characterized by fibre-type disproportion. In Kakulas BA (ed): Clinical Studies in Myology. Proceedings of the Second International Congress on Muscle Diseases, Perth, Australia, 1971, Part 2. Amsterdam, Excerpta Medica, ICS, 1973;295.

115. Lenard HG, Goebel HH: Congenital fibre-type disproportion. Neuropediatrics 1975;6:220.

116. Harley HG, Brook JD, Rundle SA, et al: Expansion of an unstable DNA region and phenotypic variation in myotonic dystrophy. Nature 1992;355:545.

117. Ashizawa T, Dubel JR, Dunne PW, et al: Anticipation in myotonic dystrophy: II. Complex relationships between clinical findings and structure of the GCT repeat. Neurology 1992;42:1877.

118. Harley H, Rundle SA, MacMillan JC, et al: Size of the unstable CTG repeat sequence in relation to phenotype and parental transmission in myotonic dystrophy. Am J Hum Genet 1993;52:1164.

119. Hunter A, Tsilfidis C, Mettler G, et al: The correlation of age of onset with CTG trinucleotide repeat amplification in myotonic dystrophy. J Med Genet 1992;29:774.

120. Redman JB, Fenwick RG, Fu Y, et al: Relationship between parental trinucleotide GCT repeat length and severity of myotonic dystrophy in offspring. JAMA 1993;269:1960.

121. Johnson ER, Abresch RT, Carter GT, et al: Profiles of neuromuscular diseases: Myotonic dystrophy. Am J Phys Med Rehabil 1995;74(Suppl 5):S104.

122. Lewis W, Sanjay Y: Management of cardiac complications in neuromuscular disease. Phys Med Rehabil Clin North Am 1998;9:145.

123. Moorman JR, Coleman RE, Packer D, et al: Cardiac involvement in myotonic muscular dystrophy. Medicine 1985;64:371.

124. Tuikka RA, Laaksonen RK, Somer HVK: Cognitive function in myotonic muscular dystrophy: A follow-up study. Eur Neurol 1993;33:436.

125. Lehmann-Horn F, Iaizzo P, Franke C, et al: Schwartz-Jampel syndrome: II. Na+ channel defect causes myotonia. Muscle Nerve 1990;13:528.

126. Spaans F, Wagenmakers A, Saris W, et al: Procainamide therapy, physical performance and energy expenditure in the Schwartz-Jampel syndrome. Neuromuscul Disord 1991;1:371.

127. Engel AG: Myasthenic syndromes. In Engel AG, Franzini-Armstrong C (eds): Myology, 2nd ed. New York, McGraw-Hill, 1994;1798.

128. Jones HR Jr, Bradshaw DY: Guillain-Barré syndrome and plasmapheresis in childhood. Ann Neurol 1991; 29:688.

129. Ouvrier RA, McLeod JG, Pollard JD: Acute inflammatory demyelinating polyradiculoneuropathy. Peripheral Neuropathy in Childhood 1990;10.

130. Bradshaw DY, Jones HR Jr: Guillain-Barré syndrome in children: Clinical course, electrodiagnosis and prognosis. Muscle Nerve 1992;15:500.

131. Epstein MA, Sladky JT: The role of plasmapheresis in childhood Guillain-Barré syndrome. Ann Neurol 1990; 28:65.

132. Lamont PJ, Johnston HM, Berdoukas VA: Plasmapheresis in children with Guillain-Barré syndrome. Neurology 1991;41:1928.

133. Shahar E, Murphy EG, Roifman CM: Benefit of intravenously administered immune serum globulin in patients with Guillain-Barré syndrome. J Pediatr 1990; 116:141.

134. Lavenstein BL, Shin W, Watkin T, Keller S: Four-year follow-up study of use of IVIG in childhood acute inflammatory demyelinating polyneuropathy (GBS). Neurology 1994;44:A169.

135. Chance P, Ashizawa T, Hoffman E, Crawford T: Molecular basis of neuromuscular disease. Phys Med Rehabil Clin North Am 1998;9:49.

136. Kulkens T, Bolhuis PA, Wolterman RA, et al: Deletion of the serine 34 codon from the major peripheral myelin protein P_0 gene in Charcot-Marie-Tooth disease type 1B. Nat Genet 1993;5:35.

137. Saito M, Hayashi Y, Suzuki T, et al: Linkage mapping of the gene for Charcot-Marie-Tooth disease type IIA (CMT IIA) to chromosome 1p and clinical features of CMT IIA. Neurology 1997;49:1630.

138. Ianassecu V: Charcot-Marie-Tooth neuropathies: From clinical description to molecular genetics. Muscle Nerve 1995;18:267.

139. Ben Othmane K, Hentati F, Lennon F, et al: Linkage of a locus (CMT4A) for autosomal recessive Charcot-Marie-Tooth disease to chromosome 8q. Hum Mol Genet 1993;2:1625.

140. Chance PF, Alderson MK, Leppig KA, et al: DNA deletion associated with hereditary neuropathy with liability to pressure palsies. Cell 1993;72:143.

141. Bergoffen J, Scherer SS, Wang S, et al: Connexin mutations in X-linked Charcot-Marie-Tooth disease. Science 1993;262:2039.

142. Warner LE, Mancias P, Butler IJ, et al: Mutations in the early growth response 2 (EGR2) gene are associated with hereditary myelinopathies. Nat Genet 1998;18:382.

143. Bolton CF, Young GB: Neurological Complications of Renal Disease. Boston, Butterworth, 1990;92.

144. Eeg-Oloffson O, Petersen I: Childhood diabetic neuropathy: A clinical neurophysiological study. Acta Paediatr Scand 1966;55:163.

145. Gamstorp I, Shelburne SA Jr, Engleson G, et al: Peripheral neuropathy in juvenile diabetes. Diabetes 1966;15:411.

146. Hoffman WH, Hat ZH, Frank RN: Correlates of delayed motor nerve conduction and retinopathy in juvenile-onset diabetes mellitus. J Pediatr 1983;102:351.

147. Munsat TL, Davies KE: Meeting report: International SMA Consortium Meeting. Neuromuscul Disord 1992; 2:423.

148. Zerres K, Rudnik-Schoneborn S: Natural history in proximal spinal muscular atrophy. Arch Neurol 1995; 52:518.

149. Brzustowicz LM, Lehner T, Castilla LH, et al: Genetic mapping of chronic childhood-onset spinal muscular atrophy to chromosomes 5q11.2–13.3. Nature 1990;334: 540.

150. Gillium TC, Brzustowicz LM, Castilla LH, et al: Genetic homogeneity between acute and chronic forms of spinal atrophy. Nature 1990;345:823.

151. Lefebvre S, Burglen L, Reboullet S, et al: Identification and characterization of a spinal muscular atrophy-determining gene. Cell 1995;80:155.

152. Roy N, Mahadevan MS, McLean M, et al: The gene for neuronal apoptosis inhibitory protein is partially deleted in individuals with spinal muscular atrophy. Cell 1995;80:167.

153. Carter T, Bonnemann C, Wang C, et al: A multicopy transcription-repair gene, BTF2p44, maps to the SMA region and demonstrates SMA-associated deletions. Hum Mol Genet 1997;6:229.

154. Eng GD, Binder H, Koch B: Spinal muscular atrophy: Experience in diagnosis and rehabilitation in management of 60 patients. Arch Phys Med Rehabil 1984; 65:549.

155. Iannoccone ST, Browne RH, Samaha FJ, Buncher CR, for the DCN/SMA Group: Prospective study of spinal muscular atrophy before age 6 years. Pediatr Neurol 1993;9:187.

156. Parano E, Fiumara A, Falsperla R, Pavone L: A clinical study of childhood spinal muscular atrophy in Sicily: A review of 75 cases. Brain Dev 1994:16:104.

157. Russman BS, Iannoccone ST, Buncher CR, et al: Spinal muscular atrophy: New thoughts on the pathogenesis and classification schema. J Child Neurol 1992;7:347.

158. Russman BS, Buncher CR, White M, et al, for the DCN/SMA Group: Function changes in spinal muscular atrophy II and III. Neurology 1996;47:973.

159. Bach JR, Want TG: Noninvasive long-term ventilatory support for individuals with spinal muscular atrophy and functional bulbar musculature. Arch Phys Med Rehabil 1995;76:213.

160. Liu GT, Specht LA: Progressive juvenile sequential spinal muscular atrophy. Pediatr Neurol 1993;9:54.

161. Alexander MP, Emery ES III, Koewrner FC: Progressive bulbar paresis in childhood. Arch Neurol 1976; 33:66.

162. Edwards RHT, Jones DA, Newham DJ, et al: Role of mechanical damage in pathogenesis of proximal myopathy in man. Lancet 1984;8376:548.

163. Bonsett CA: Pseudohypertrophic muscular dystrophy: Distribution of degenerative features as revealed by anatomical study. Neurology 1963;13:728.

164. Johnson EW, Braddom R: Over-work weakness in facioscapulohumeral muscular dystrophy. Arch Phys Med Rehabil 1971;52:333.

165. Vignos PJ Jr, Watkins MP: Effect of exercise in muscular dystrophy. JAMA 1966;197:843.

166. Scott OM, Hyde SA, Goddard C, et al: Effect of exercise in Duchenne muscular dystrophy: Controlled six-month feasibility study of effects of two different regimes of exercises in children with Duchenne dystrophy. Physiotherapy 1981;67:174.

167. DeLateur BKJ, Giaconi RM: Effect on maximal strength of submaximal exercise in Duchenne muscular dystrophy. Am J Phys Med 1979;58:26.

168. Valentine BA, Blue JT, Cooper CJ: The effect of exercise on canine dystrophic muscle. Ann Neurol 1989;26: 588.

169. Aitkens SG, McCrory MA, Kilmer DD, et al: Moderate resistance exercise program: Its effect in slowly progressive neuromuscular disease. Arch Phys Med Rehabil 1993;74:711.

170. Kilmer DD, McCrory MA, Wright NC, et al: The effect of a high-resistance exercise program in slowly progressive neuromuscular disease. Arch Phys Med Rehabil 1994;75:560.

171. Sockolov R, Irwin B, Dressendorfer RH, et al: Exercise performance in 6 to 11 year old boys with Duchenne muscular dystrophy. Arch Phys Med Rehabil 1977;58:195.

172. Wright NC, Kilmer DD, McCrory MA, et al: Aerobic walking in slowly progressive neuromuscular disease: Effect of a 12-week program. Arch Phys Med Rehabil 1996;77:64.

173. McDonald C: Limb contractures in progressive neuromuscular disease and the role of stretching, orthotics and surgery. Phys Med Rehabil Clin North Am 1998;9:187.

174. Scott OM, Hyde SA, Goddard C, et al: Prevention of deformity in Duchenne muscular dystrophy: A prospective study of passive stretching and splintage. Physiotherapy 1981;67:177.

175. Vignos PJ Jr, Archibald KC: Maintenance of ambulation in childhood muscular dystrophy. J Chron Dis 1960;12:273.

176. Eyring EJ, Johnson EW, Burnett C: Surgery in muscular dystrophy. JAMA 1972;222:1067.

177. Siegel IM, Miller JE, Ray RD: Subcutaneous lower limb tenotomy in the treatment of pseudohypertrophic muscular dystrophy. J Bone Joint Surg 1986;50A:1437.

178. Spencer GE, Vignos PJ Jr: Bracing for ambulation in childhood progressive muscular dystrophy. J Bone Joint Surg 1962;44A:234.

179. Heckmatt JZ, Dubowitz V, Hyde SA, et al: Prolongation of walking in Duchenne muscular dystrophy with lightweight orthoses: Review of 57 cases. Dev Med Child Neurol 1985;27:149.

180. Shapiro F, Bresnan MJ: Orthopaedic management of childhood neuromuscular disease. Part III: Disease of muscle. J Bone Joint Surg 1982;64A:1102.

181. Vignos PJ Jr: Management of musculoskeletal complications in neuromuscular disease: Limb contractures and the role of stretching, braces and surgery. Phys Med Rehabil State Art Rev 1988;2:509.

182. Manzur AY, Hyde SA, Rodillo E, et al: A randomized controlled trial of early surgery in Duchenne muscular dystrophy. Neuromuscul Disord 1992;2:379.

183. Hart D, McDonald CM: Spinal deformity in progressive neuromuscular disease. Phys Med Rehabil Clin North Am 1998;9:213.

184. Butler C, Okamoto G, McKay T: Motorized wheelchair driving by disabled children. Arch Phys Med Rehabil 1984;65:95.

185. Butler C, Okamoto G, McKay T: Powered mobility for very young disabled children. Dev Med Child Neurol 1983;25:472.

186. Braun NMT, Aurora NS, Rochester DF: Respiratory muscle and pulmonary function in poliomyositis and other proximal myopathies. Thorax 1983;38:316.

187. Curran FJ: Night ventilation by body respirators for patients in chronic respiratory failure doe to late-stage Duchenne muscular dystrophy. Arch Phys Med Rehabil 1981;62:270.

188. Bach JR: Pulmonary Rehabilitation: The Obstructive and Paralytic Conditions. Philadelphia, Hanley & Belfus, 1995;303.

189. Hahn A, Bach JR, Delauber A, et al: Clinical implications of maximal respiratory pressure determinations for individuals with Duchenne muscular dystrophy. Arch Phys Med Rehabil 1997;78:1.

190. Splaingard ML, Frates RC Jr, Harrison GM, et al: Home positive-pressure ventilation: Twenty years' experience. Chest 1983;84:376.

191. Bach JR, Campagnolo DI, Hoeman S: Life satisfaction of individuals with Duchenne muscular dystrophy using long-term mechanical ventilatory support. Am J Phys Med Rehabil 1991;70:129.

192. Gilgoff IS, Kahlstrom E, MacLaughlin E, Keens TG: Long-term ventilatory support in spinal muscular atrophy. J Pediatr 1989;115:904.

193. Wang TG, Bach JR, Avila C, et al: Survival of individuals with spinal muscular atrophy on ventilatory support. Am J Phys Med Rehabil 1994;73:207.

194. Willig TN, Paulus J, Lacau Saint Guily J, et al: Swallowing problems in neuromuscular disorders. Arch Phys Med Rehabil 1994;75:1175.

195. Benson ES, Jaffe KM, Tarr PI: Acute gastric dilatation in Duchenne muscular dystrophy: A case report and review of the literature. Arch Phys Med Rehabil 1996;77:512.

196. Binder H: New ideas in the rehabilitation of children with spinal muscular atrophy. In Merlini L, Granata C, Dubowitz V (eds): Current Concepts in Childhood Spinal Muscular Atrophy. New York, Springer-Verlag, 1989;117.

197. Goldstein M, Meyer S, Freund HR: Effects of overfeeding children with muscle dystrophies. J Parenter Enter Nutr 1989;13:603.

198. Stewart PM, Walser M, Drachman DB: Branched-chain ketoacids reduce muscle protein degradation in Duchenne muscular dystrophy. Muscle Nerve 1982;5:197.

199. Edwards RH, Round JM, Jackson MJ, et al: Weight reduction in boys with muscular dystrophy. Dev Med Child Neurol 1984;26:384.

200. McCrory MA, Kim HR, Wright NC, et al: Energy expenditure, physical activity, and body composition of ambulatory adults with hereditary neuromuscular disease. Am J Clin Nutr 1998;67:1162.

201. McCrory M, Wright N, Kilmer D: Nutritional aspects of neuromuscular diseases. Phys Med Rehabil Clin North Am 1998;9:127.

202. Lewis W, Yadlapalli S: Management of cardiac complications in neuromuscular disease. Phys Med Rehabil Clin North Am 1998;9:145.

203. Fenichel GM, Florence JM, Pestronk A, et al: Long-term benefit from prednisone therapy in Duchenne muscular dystrophy. Neurology 1991;41:1874.

204. Fenichel GM, Mendell JR, Moxley RT, et al: A comparison of daily and alternate-day prednisone therapy in the treatment of Duchenne muscular dystrophy. Arch Neurol 1991;48:575.

205. Griggs RC, Moxley RT, Mendell JR, et al: Duchenne dystrophy: Randomized, controlled trial of prednisone (18 months) and azathioprine (12 months). Neurology 1993;43:520.

206. Fenichel G, Pestronk A, Florence J, et al: A beneficial effect of oxandrolone in the treatment of Duchenne muscular dystrophy: A pilot study. Neurology 1997;48:1225.

Chapter 16

Pediatric Limb Deficiencies

Deborah Gaebler-Spira, MD
Jack Uellendahl, CPO

Variability in human morphology occurs within the limits of survival and function. Variations such as limb deficiency and limb loss create functional challenges for the child. Children contend with the functional problems within the context of growth and development. Equally important as the child's growth are parents' and siblings' reactions and adaptations. Wilke,[1] well known for his work with the disabled and a bilateral total arm amputee himself, stated that the most important act his parents performed while he was growing up was to have another child. This event illustrated to him that his parents loved who he was sufficiently to risk having another child.

The introduction of appropriately timed medical, rehabilitation, and educational services, including early intervention, physical and occupational therapies, prosthetics, orthopedic consultation, and supportive services, ensures the achievement of optimal function and adaptation. A clinical team is necessary to bring together the professionals who have an impact on the functional outcome of the child and family. Members of the team include the pediatric rehabilitation nurse, social worker, occupational and physical therapists, pediatric physiatrist, pediatric orthopedist, pediatrician, prosthetist, and psychologist.

The American Academy of Orthopedic Surgeons (AAOS) championed an organized approach to juvenile amputee management when Frantz in 1956 created the Committee on Child Prosthetics Program. The goal of this committee was to raise the standards of prosthetic care for children. Before that time, prosthetic components were unavailable in pediatric sizes, and prescriptions were at times delayed until school age. The Child's Prosthetic Committee expanded to include clinic members and has held interdisciplinary conferences since 1972 as the Association of Children's Prosthetics/Orthotic Clinics.[2]

The pediatric physiatrist works in conjunction with many professionals when coordinating the management of children with limb deficiency and amputations. The role of the pediatric physiatrist may vary in each situation and in each clinic.

The physician provides an accurate history and physical examination. Elements in the history that are essential for planning a program include (1) cause of limb loss, (2) surgical history, (3) medical problems related to limb loss, (4) medical problems not related to limb loss (i.e., vision, hearing, learning disabilities), (5) prior and current level of function, (6) medications, (7) developmental stage and educational setting, (8) family support system and current living situation, (9) hobbies and recreational interests, (10) previous exposure to persons with a limb loss, (11) current information regarding prosthetics and limb loss, (12) emotional reactions regarding the limb loss, and (13) the patient's and family's goals for rehabilitation.

A general physical examination with focused assessment of the limb is pertinent. The residual limb or limbs are assessed for length, strength, range of motion, and amount of soft tissue (Fig. 16–1). Careful inspection of the skin for sensation, scarring, and resiliency is important. Motor planning, coordination, behavior, and cognition contribute to the medical examination.

The planning of the rehabilitation program should include (1) clear team member communication; (2) goal setting; (3) prosthetic rationale; (4) outlining a preprosthetic program; (5) prosthetic fabrication; (6) prosthetic training; (7) follow-up program for fit and function; and (8) educational, recreational, and vocational pursuits. Rehabilitation involves education at every opportunity.[3]

The use of a functional outcome tool is helpful for children with prosthetic options. A specific reliable, validated outcome tool called the *Child Amputee Prosthetic Project–Functional*

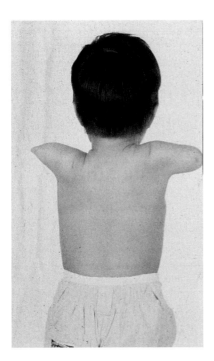

FIGURE 16–1. The physical examination describes the range of motion, strength, and length of the residual limb.

Status Inventory (CAPP-FSI) has been developed.[4] A preschool version has been found to have construct validity.[5] This tool is an inventory of behavioral manifestations of limb deficiency that interfere with a child's typical activities. The CAPP-FSI is specifically designed for the child with limb deficiency.[4] Other functional assessments have been created to address this population, such as the University of New Brunswick's assessment and the Prosthetic Upper Extremity Functional Index (PUFI).[6,7] The advantage of this type of measure rather than the Wee Functional Independence Measure (WeeFIM) or Pediatric Evaluation of Disability Index (PEDI) is the CAPP-FSI sensitivity for the population. In addition to a disability measure, emphasis is placed on the child's quality of life. Measures such as the Child Health Questionnaire or the Modems developed by the American Academy of Orthopedic Surgeons (AAOS) may document quality of life.[8,9] Outcomes of children with disabling conditions should reflect a multidimensional process used by the National Center for Medical Rehabilitation Research. This model includes a profile of the pathophysiologic problem, impairment, functional limitation, disability, and societal limitations.[10]

There are differences in the approach to and management of the lower versus upper limb amputee. The upper limb prosthesis does not replace the sensory function of the hand and is best used

as a mechanical tool.[2] The function of the hand is complex. The hand is used to explore the environment and to manipulate objects within the environment. The hand needs to reach the body and precisely approach an object, grasp, and then release it. Acceptance of the prosthesis is variable. Frequently the exposed skin of a deficient limb is preferable to an encased limb. Stump sensation may even be enhanced to compensate for the loss of prehensile area.[11]

Lower limb prostheses rarely are removed and generally have high acceptance rates. Mobility demands less precision. The primary attributes for a lower limb prosthesis are length and stability. The mechanical principles of gait are predictable and can be incorporated into prosthetic design.

There are two major categories of pediatric patients with limb deficiencies: those who have congenital limb deficiencies and those who have acquired limb deficiencies (i.e., amputations). The two categories of limb deficiency have different characteristics and associated problems. Children with congenital limb deficiency do not have the same experience of loss as the child with amputation. The motivation of the two groups differs. The child with congenital limb deficiency apparently adapts and compensates to do whatever other children do.[2] The child may also have additional congenital anomalies, however, that limit outcome. The child with an acquired amputation has additional challenges of anger and resentment surrounding the events of limb loss.[2] The cause for amputation also affects the overall health of the child.

Congenital Limb Deficiency

The first trimester is the most important for the genesis of limb deficiency. Congenital limb deficiency occurs as a result of failure of formation of part or all of the limb bud. The mesodermal formation of the limb occurs at 26 days' gestation and continues with differentiation until 8 weeks' gestation.[12] The various limb segments develop in a proximal-distal order, so that the arm and forearm appear before the hand and the thigh and leg before the foot.[13]

Maternal diabetes is a risk factor for limb deficiency.[14] Even though alcohol, heroin, cocaine, and smoking have not been found to be related to limb deficiency, all maternal ingestions and first-trimester abnormalities should be documented. The only clearly implicated drug associated with limb deficiency is thalidomide.[15] Uterine abnormalities have been reported in several cases of limb deficiencies theoretically resulting from compression of the fetus.[16]

The International Society for Prosthetics and Orthotics (ISPO) has adopted a definitive system for congenital deficiencies. No longer is it necessary to learn ancient language roots to describe the limb deficiency.[12,13,17,18] Similar to an old language and culture, however, the terminology once used in clinics is difficult to change. Clinical teams often use a fusion of terms.

Seven descriptive terms originally formed the basis of classification of limb anomalies: *amelia*, *phocomelia*, *acheiria*, *adactyly*, and *aphalangia*. The first three are derived from the Greek *melos*, a limb. *Amelia* is absence of a limb, and *hemimelia* is absence of half a limb. *Phocomelia* is based on the Greek word *phoke*, a seal, and refers to the flipperlike appendage attached to the trunk. *Acheiria* and *apodia* derive from Latin for handiwork or close to the same root as surgery, and represent a missing hand or foot. *Adactyly* refers to an absent metacarpal or metatarsal, and *aphalangia* refers to an absent finger or toe.[16]

Many clinics still describe deficiencies by the Frantz classification system. In this system, deficiencies are either terminal, representing the complete loss of the distal extremity, or intercalary, denoting the absence of intermediate parts with preserved proximal and distal parts of the limb (Table 16–1). Those deficits are then divided into horizontal and longitudinal deficits.[16]

The ISPO classification system (Table 16–2) is used in research and academic endeavors because this system facilitates communication and creates a logical, accurate approach. The ISPO classification divides all deformities into transverse or longitudinal. A transverse deficiency has no distal remaining portions, whereas the longitudinal deficiency has distal portions. The transverse level is named after the segment beyond which there is no skeletal portion. Longitudinal deficiencies name the bones that are affected. Any bone not named is present and of normal form. The affected bone is designated as total or partially absent. The approximate fraction of the limb in a transverse deformity is estimated. The longitudinal deficiency has distal portions stated. The number of the digit should be stated in relation to a metacarpal, a metatarsal, and phalanges. Digit numbering proceeds from the radial or tibial side of the limb. Ray refers to the metacarpal or metatarsal and corresponding phalanges.[22]

Congenital Upper Extremity Deficiency

Congenital upper limb deficiency has an incidence of approximately 4.1 per 10,000 live births.[20,21] In most cases, the congenital upper

TABLE 16–1. Examples of Common Deficiencies Named by Three Classification Systems

Original	Frantz	ISPO
Upper extremity amelia	Terminal transverse	Transverse upper arm, total
Fibula hemimelia	Intercalary/normal foot Longitudinal/absent rays Fibular deficiency	Longitudinal fibular deficiency, total or partial
Upper extremity phocomelia	Complete upper-extremity phocomelia	Longitudinal total, humerus, ulna, and radius
	Distal/absent radius ulna Proximal/absent humerus	Carpal, meta-carpal, and phalangeal (total or partial)

limb deficiencies are considered isolated sporadic events with no hereditary implications. The exceptions to this are the deformities that involve hands or feet and, in particular, central ray deficiencies and adactyly involving the first four digits with the fifth intact. These represent a spontaneous mutation with autosomal dominant transmission.[15,21] Craniofacial anomalies are associated with limb deficiencies. Additional neonatal problems may include respiratory difficulty and feeding problems related to the micrognathia and hypoglossia dysgenesis.

TABLE 16–2. ISPO Classification

Upper Limb			Lower Limb
Shoulder Scapula Clavicle	Total Partial		Pelvis Ilium Ischium
Upper arm Humerus	Total Partial Upper Middle Lower Third		Thigh Femur
Forearm Radius Ulna	Total Partial Upper Middle Lower Third		Leg Tibia Fibula
Carpus	Total Partial		Tarsus
Metacarpus	Total Partial Rays 1–5		Metatarsus
Phalanges	Total Partial Fingers/toes 1–5		Phalanges

International Society for Prosthetics and Orthotics: P&O Intl 1991;15:67–69.

TABLE 16–3. Congenital Limb Deficiency

Upper Extremity Syndromes	Associated Problem
TAR	Thrombocytopenia
Fanconi's	Anemia
Holt-Oram	Heart
Baller-Gerold	Craniosynostosis
VACTERL	Vertebral
	Anal atresia
	Cardiac
	Tracheoesophageal fistula
	Renal
	Limb

Inherited Deficiency
Central ray deficiency
Transtibial

TAR, Thrombocytopenia with absence of the radius.

Lengthening of the mandible by distraction callus formation can improve cosmesis and improve medical conditions.[15]

There are five associated syndromes seen with radial deficiency (Table 16–3): (1) TAR syndrome (thrombocytopenia with absence of the radius;[22] (2) Fanconi's syndrome—anemia and leukopenia developing at 5–6 years of age;[23] (3) Holt-Oram syndrome—congenital heart disease, in particular, atrial septal defects and tetralogy of Fallot, as an autosomal dominant trait;[24] (4) Baller-Gerold syndrome—craniosynostosis;[22] (5) VACTERL or VATER multiorgan system involvement (*V*, vertebral; *A*, anal atresia; *C*, cardiac; *TE*, tracheoesophageal atresia; *R*, renal; *L*, limb).[25,26] Not all patients with an absent radius have a syndrome, but all children with an absent radius should undergo a workup or be followed for the associated problems that may affect the child's health and outcome more than the limb deficiency.[15]

Although technology has allowed for early fitting of the upper limb–deficient child with an appropriately sized prosthesis, it is recommended that prosthetic fitting follow the attainment of normal developmental milestones. It has been common for prostheses to be prescribed based more on the limited ability of prosthetic components to meet the age-appropriate needs of a child than on matching prosthetic function with normal development. For example, myoelectric hands of the past were too large and difficult for a 1–2-year-old child to use successfully. Therefore, the experts recommended that these hands not be fitted on children until age 4–5 years. Today it is common for these hands to be fitted successfully on 1-year-olds. The prosthetic technology improved dramatically, as a result of down-sizing and simpler control, to meet the children's needs better.

The most common congenital limb deficiency is the left terminal transradial limb deficiency. For the unilateral transradial level, the first fitting should be performed when the child achieves sitting balance. This usually occurs between 6 and 7 months of age.[27] The goals of prosthetic fitting at this age are to provide a limb that is at the appropriate length for gross two-handed grasp; allow for a limb that encourages normal, symmetric crawling; and develop a wearing pattern for future prosthetic use. The next developmental milestone that indicates that the child is ready for a more sophisticated prosthesis is walking. This usually occurs at about 11–13 months of age.[28] At this time, the child is ready to perform simple grasp and release activities using the prosthesis. It is best to keep the control system as simple as possible at this early age to ensure early success. Other developmental factors to be considered are (1) understanding of holding function, (2) attention span greater than 5 minutes, and (3) willingness to be handled by the occupational therapist to go through training in terminal device opening motion.

A variety of terminal devices may be considered for the first passive prosthesis. Options include hands, hooks of various shapes, mitts, and other nonhand designs (Fig. 16–2). The vast majority of parents prefer a terminal device that looks like a hand. After all, it is only natural to want your child to look like everyone else. For this reason, it is recommended that a passive hand be provided rather than a hook or other nonhand-type device for the initial prosthesis. The two basic passive hand options for infants are the closed, *crawling hand* design and the open hand design. Once the parents become more accepting of their child's limb deficiency, they become more inclined to evaluate prosthetic components based on functional qualities in addition to appearance. The prosthesis is

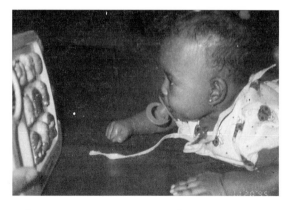

FIGURE 16–2. The passive mit allows upper extremity symmetric weight bearing when prone.

usually self-suspending, using a supracondylar design with or without a suspension sleeve. When the child is developmentally ready for terminal device activation, the options include body-powered hooks or hands as well as myoelectrically controlled hands (Fig. 16–3). Again the majority of parents prefer hands, and the hands that provide optimal function at this age are myoelectrically controlled. At this age, the simplicity of control is of paramount importance. An electric hand that is controlled by one electrode in a voluntary opening control scheme has proved effective and natural. Body-powered devices may not work well for this age group because they lack the requisite force and excursion as well as the cognitive ability to relate shoulder motions to terminal device operation. Again the prosthesis is usually self-suspending, thereby eliminating cumbersome harnessing.

By the time the child is 4–5 years old, he or she is able to operate virtually all types of prosthetic components and control schemes presently available. At this time, the clinical team should be focused on providing prosthetic or other assistive devices that best meet the needs of the particular child rather than focusing on any one fitting method familiar to the clinic. For example, a child might decide after wearing a myoelectric arm since age 1 year that at age 5 it is no longer the best option because of the child's interest in sports. Perhaps a VC hook with interchangeable sport hand is more useful for this child. The clinical team needs to listen to the concerns and needs of the children and parents and prescribe prosthetic components that best accomplish their goals (Fig. 16–4).

Obviously the developmental milestones mentioned previously should guide the fitting schedule of the transhumeral limb-deficient child as well. By comparison to the transradial level, it is advisable to delay the progression only slightly (yet still within normal limits) to achieve optimal results. Because of the nature of a transhumeral prosthesis, it can be more of an encumbrance than the transradial design. This can cause difficulty in rolling over and may impede the infant if fitted too early. Again the terminal device should be activated shortly after the child begins to walk. As mentioned earlier, the terminal devices for the transhumeral level are essentially the

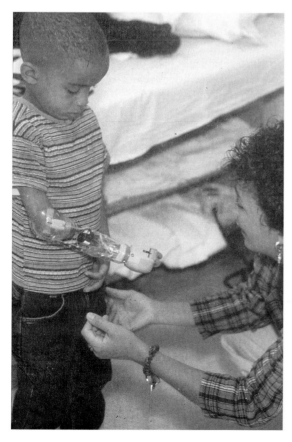

FIGURE 16–3. The therapist evaluates fit and function in a prototype myoelectric prosthesis.

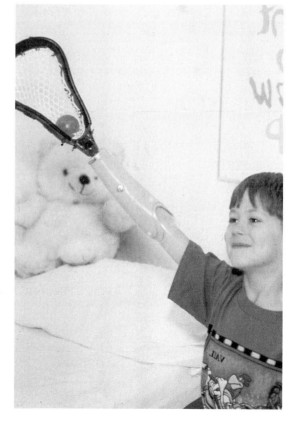

FIGURE 16–4. This boy demonstrates his new prosthesis fitted with a TRS Hi-Fly. The prosthesis is suspended by a silicone socket.

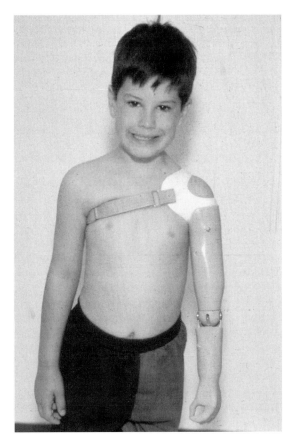

FIGURE 16–5. A myoelectric above-elbow prosthesis for a transhumeral deficiency using a friction elbow.

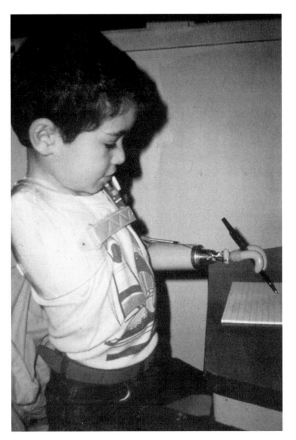

FIGURE 16–6. The child with a transhumeral deficiency chooses a terminal device that improves the control and function needed for childhood tasks.

same as for the transradial, and the same rationale for use applies. The addition of a prosthetic elbow is the key difference. The first prosthesis employs a friction elbow to allow for positioning of the terminal device (Fig. 16–5). It is useful to limit the range of motion at the elbow by producing flexion and extension stops to prevent the elbow from flexing excessively under weight bearing (i.e., during crawling or pushing off of the prosthesis). The initial prosthesis may be suspended either by a harness or by silicone suction suspension. The silicone suction socket has proven effective because it allows free range of motion at the shoulder and provides excellent suspension. As in the case of the transradial deficiency, the transhumeral should be fitted with an activated terminal device once the child begins to walk (Fig. 16–6). Considerations for terminal device selection include appearance, weight, ease of operation, and cost. The myoelectric hand offers reasonable appearance and ease of operation when controlled by a single-site voluntary opening circuit; however, it does make for a heavier prosthesis than a body-powered

hook and is significantly more expensive. Body-powered hooks can be either voluntary opening or voluntary closing. Either design can be used successfully by the transhumeral limb-deficient child once the child is strong enough and has the cognitive ability to understand the operation. This usually is possible at age 2–3 years. When the child is strong enough to operate an active elbow, usually at age 4–5 years, a conventional body-powered elbow may be provided. If the child has insufficient strength or excursion to operate the body-powered elbow, an electric elbow may be considered, although the increased weight may preclude this option.

Even though preservation of the residual limb is a general principle, revision amputation is required in 10% of upper extremity congenital limb deficiencies.[28] Two examples are the radial club hand and the ulnar clubhand. These represent longitudinal deficiencies of the forearm. Treatment is directed at centralization of the hand and reconstructing the thumb.[29]

The Krukenberg procedure (Fig. 16–7) reconstructs the forearm and creates a sensate

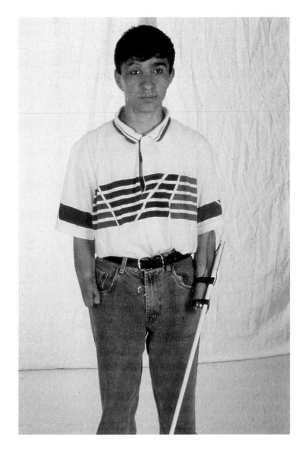

FIGURE 16–7. For the patient with bilateral loss of the hands who is blind, the Krukenberg procedure provides the ability to grasp objects as well as feel them. This man has had a toe transplanted to his right forearm and a left Krukenberg. The left side was fitted with a walking stick attached to an easily removable self-suspending socket.

Given the previous information, the clinical team should offer the child a developmentally appropriate prosthesis when it is reasonable to expect it will improve function. There are no *right* philosophies for the fitting of these complicated cases. The team should recognize that prostheses are to be viewed as tools. Given a tool that is useful, the child will choose to wear it. One that is an encumbrance will be rejected. For the child with bilateral long transradial limbs, passive crawling hands would be an encumbrance. They would cover sensate skin and provide no functional benefit. Later in development, this same child may benefit from activated terminal devices allowing for grasp and release even though the sensation is compromised. In the case of higher-level bilateral deficiencies, it is wise to start as simple as possible, recognizing that each child has a certain level of tolerance for *gadgets*. With the vast array of prosthetic components now available, it would be easy for the well-intentioned clinical team to recommend components that would overwhelm the user. Some of the critical factors in the success of the high-level bilateral prosthesis are prosthetic weight; complexity of control; proprioceptive feedback; wearing comfort components; and, probably less important, motivation and attitude of parents.

prehensile surface for children with absent hands by separating the ulna and radius in the forearm. Because of the cosmetic appearance, the procedure is used rarely with unilateral conditions. Indications for this procedure are absent hands and visual impairment.[30] Another surgical procedure to enhance prehension is the Vilkke, which attaches a toe to the residual limb (Fig. 16–8).[29]

Terminal overgrowth does not occur frequently for the child with congenital limb deficiency but does occur with transhumeral deficiencies. The phocomelic or bilateral total upper extremity transverse deficiency patient rarely requires amputation revision. The terminal digits can activate switches or myoelectric sensors.[28]

Bilateral Upper Limb Deficiency

Because of the wide variety of possible combinations of bilateral limb deficiency, no attempt to propose a fitting time-table is made.

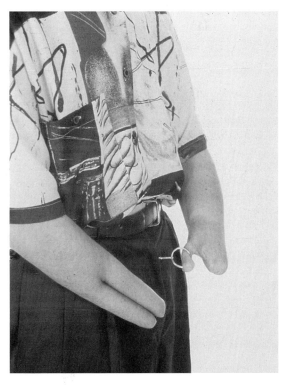

FIGURE 16–8. The transplanted toe provides independence in toileting with a modified pull zipper.

There are a multitude of prosthetic components that may be prescribed for the upper limb-deficient child. This section suggests selection criteria and gives guidance based on clinical experience. Any of the available components may be appropriate for a particular child, and the clinical team needs to listen carefully to the needs and expectations of the child and family when determining appropriate prosthetic components.

Training

In the case of the congenital upper limb-deficient child, the preprosthetic period is mainly focused on the needs of the parents. The clinical team should try to answer all of their questions and educate them about what they can expect in the future regarding the development of their child. The parents should be encouraged to treat the child the same as they would a normally limbed child. Often the parents benefit from being introduced to other parents and children with similar limb deficiencies. It is important during this initial contact for the clinical team

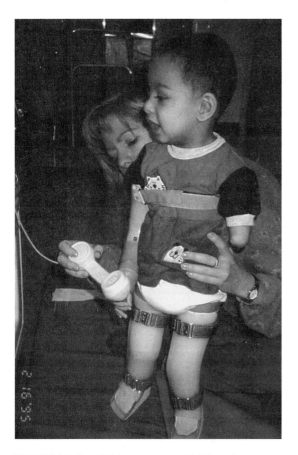

FIGURE 16–9. This boy presents with bilateral transverse upper limb loss at the elbow. The therapist operates the myoelectric hand controlled by a single-site voluntary opening circuit. Not all deficient limbs must be fitted.

to present an honest forecast of the prosthetic plan. Often the only information the parents have is from movies and the media. Their expectations may therefore be unrealistic. The clinical team members must walk a fine line between presenting the prosthetic options in an honest manner without sounding negative or disheartening. After all, prosthetic technology with all of its sophistication is still far from the ideal of replacing a physiologic arm.

Once the child has achieved sitting balance and the prosthetist has provided an initial prosthesis, prosthetic training can begin. The parents should be instructed in the proper donning and doffing, care and maintenance, and proper fitting of the prosthesis. The therapist demonstrates age-appropriate play activities, such as pat-a-cake, peek-a-boo, and cause-and-effect toys such as a busy box and jack-in-the-box. The goal is to increase the child's awareness of the affected side, including the prosthetic device. The child should also be encouraged to use the prosthesis for transitional movements, such as sitting to crawling and leaning on the prosthesis for weight bearing while reaching with the dominant hand. The parent is encouraged to maintain phone contact with the therapist to answer questions regarding follow-through with prosthetic usage. A recheck through the clinic should be scheduled within a month after delivery of the prosthesis and then every 3–4 months.

When the terminal device is activated, the therapist again provides initial instruction to the parents and child. The therapist works with the child and parents using toys that encourage bimanual use, such as Legos, pop beads, and stringing beads (Fig. 16–9). Initially, it is useful to concentrate on activities that require the prosthetic side to hold while the dominant hand manipulates. Simple activities, such as pulling apart a Lego construction, are a good start. Ultimately the goal is to use the prosthesis as an assist for the sound hand. It is unrealistic and thus inappropriate to teach the child to use the prosthesis for dominant hand activities.

Based on clinical experience the best results for functional use of the prosthesis by children in the 1–3-year-old age group are obtained by using a single-site voluntary opening myoelectric control scheme.[31] When training a child in the use of a myoelectric hand using this control scheme, the therapist should encourage activities that cause the hand to open. Because of the placement of the electrode over the forearm extensors, activities that elicit an extensor activity are appropriate. Once the hand is open, the therapist can quickly place a toy in the hand and

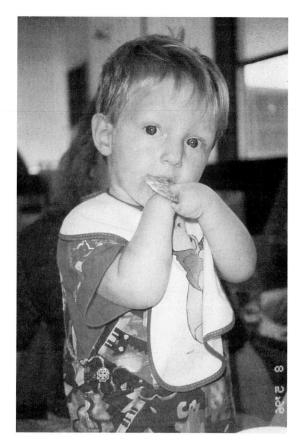

FIGURE 16–10. The child's need to function defines the use of the prosthesis.

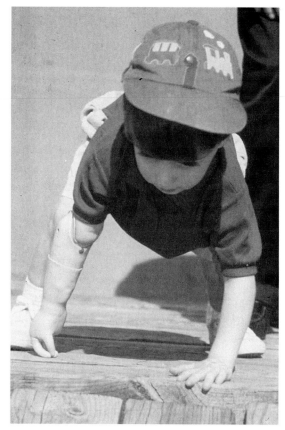

FIGURE 16–11. The child's need to function defines the use of the prosthesis.

encourage the child to release it. By increased repetition, the child learns through cause and effect.

Prosthetic Rejection

Acceptance of a prosthesis is a complex issue with many factors influencing the ultimate outcome. Factors include level of limb loss, presence of other complicating medical conditions, comfort and usefulness of the prosthesis, and acceptance of the limb deficiency by the family. In general, the higher the limb absence, the less likely it is that a child will find a prosthesis useful enough to wear it regularly (i.e., transradial patients tend to wear their prostheses more than transhumeral patients, and transhumeral patients tend to wear their prostheses more than shoulder disarticulation patients (Figs. 16–10 and 16–11).[32]

Case Example

Because the majority of limb-deficient children are missing one arm below the elbow, this case example looks at this level in some more detail. The child who has a wrist disarticulation

or transcarpal limb deficiency presents a challenge because the limb length may be difficult to match, and the end of the physiologic arm can be quite useful left unfitted. The limb is at an appropriate length for opposing the sound side and it has sensation. Fitting a prosthesis covers the sensate skin and might therefore be rejected. Also, these children tend to outgrow their prostheses faster than the transradial group because of the presence of the distal growth center. This is not to say that these children should not be fitted with appropriate prostheses. Some of these children become good wearers and users of their prostheses. They need to be followed closely to keep up with growth, and a consistent wearing pattern has to be fostered for optimal success. Transradial limb–deficient patients are often successful wearers of prostheses. They benefit from the extension of their physiologic limb as well as from the ability to grasp and release objects. At the proximal transradial level, it can be difficult to provide good range of motion at the elbow, and the weight of the prosthesis becomes a more critical factor.

Congenital Lower Limb Deficiency

Transtibial deficiency is more common than transfemoral or transverse deficiency of the thigh (amelia).[33] Fibular longitudinal deficiency, or fibula hemimelia, is the most common congenital lower limb deformity. Bilateral fibular longitudinal deficiency occurs 25% of the time.[34] Unilateral fibular deficiency creates a problem with limb length discrepancy. Ilizarov distraction osteogenesis has expanded the possibilities of equalizing limb length.[35] Efforts to equalize limb lengths by shortening the long side if there is an excess of 7.5 cm are contraindicated because of the loss of total height.[36] In unilateral fibular deficiency, ankle disarticulation provides an end-bearing stump on which the child may walk without a prosthesis.[36] This treatment is indicated with a combination of three-ray foot, tarsal coalition, and short-bowed tibia.

Longitudinal deficiency of the tibia occurs in 1 in 1 million births.[34] The clinical picture includes a varus foot; a short leg; and an unstable knee, ankle, or both. Although various reconstructive surgeries have been attempted, the treatment of choice for tibial longitudinal deficiencies is disarticulation at the knee. For the child with a partial tibial deficiency, the segment length is important. If the tibial segment is short, the surgeon creates a synostosis with the intact fibula and amputation of the foot. This procedure creates a walking surface for the child, which can be stable without a prosthesis. Thirty percent of partial tibial deficiency occurs as an autosomal dominant inherited pattern.[34]

Longitudinal deficiency of the femur or partial proximal femoral focal deficiency (PFFD) describes the congenital defect of the shaft of the femur (Fig. 16–12). PFFD occurs in 1 in 50,000 births.[37,38] Ten to fifteen percent are bilateral. Amstutz and Wilson[39] have defined PFFD as the absence of some quality or characteristic of completeness of the proximal femur, including stunting or shortening of the entire femur. Aitken[30] described four classes related to the presence of a formed acetabulum or absent acetabulum. Type A and B have hip joints and are distinguished from each other by the continuous femoral head cartilage and shaft present in type A. Type C and D have no acetabulum. The difference between type C and D is the presence of the cartilaginous growth plate in type C.[39] Another classification system identifies this defect by the length of the femoral segment remaining.[37] These classification systems allow the pediatric orthopedic surgeon to predict reconstructive surgeries that allow potential growth and height as well as function.[40] The femur is typically short and held in flexion, abduction, and external rotation. The hip is in retroversion. The knee is in valgus, and there is absence of the cruciate ligament. Partial fibular absence and foot deformity are frequent.[33,41]

Treatment depends on whether the deformity is unilateral or bilateral, presence of a hip joint, amount of coxa vara, presence of a pseudarthrosis, and the estimated leg length.[42] If the short side has a fibular deficiency, disarticulation of the ipsilateral ankle equalizes the leg length by allowing an articulated limb on the affected side with an extension prosthesis.[43,44] PFFD presents many challenges for the treatment team. Depending on the clinical picture presented, various surgical as well as prosthetic interventions may be appropriate. Generally, severe forms of PFFD may be converted to provide above-knee function through Syme's amputation and knee fusion. Although still controversial, below-knee function may be simulated through the Van Ness rotation, which involves rotating the foot by 180 degrees so ankle motion can control the prosthesis. Other options include nonstandard prostheses or shoelifts with no surgical conversion.[45]

Frequently congenital lower limb deficiency may present with odd combinations of the absent portions of the extremity and deformities of the remaining segments. The deficiency may include proximal muscles, skin, nails, and parts of the joint. The child with bilateral PFFD may also have upper limb deficiencies, which create challenges for donning and doffing clothes and prosthesis and the use of a prosthesis. Unilateral transverse abnormalities may not pose a risk of deformity.[43]

Fitting Time-Table

The lower limb–deficient child should be fitted with a prosthesis when he or she is ready to pull up to a standing position.[46] This usually occurs between 9 and 10 months.[47] The goals in

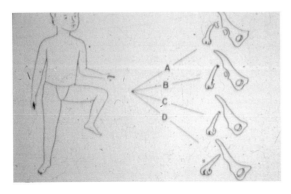

FIGURE 16–12. The classification of proximal femoral focal deficiency.

fitting a prosthesis at this early age are to allow for normal two-legged standing, provide a means for reciprocating gait development, and provide for a normal appearance. The prosthesis should be simple in design, allow for growth adjustment, suspend securely, and be lightweight. At this early age, the transfemoral prosthesis should not use a knee joint because of the complexity of operating a free knee (Figs. 16–13 and 16–14). A knee joint is usually added between ages 3 and 5 years at times with a manual locking option.[48] An extension assist on the knee can be useful to help bring the knee into full extension before loading. Either an endoskeletal or an exoskeletal construction may be employed, each with its own advantages and disadvantages. Endoskeletal construction is good for growth consideration and is generally durable enough in most settings. The foam cover of the endoskeletal design requires more maintenance than an exoskeletal finish. The exoskeletal construction is robust and should be considered for individuals who test the limits of durability.

Components

Traditionally the most common foot prescribed for the child amputee has been the SACH foot. SACH feet have many advantages for this population, including low cost, durable construction, and simple design. In recent years, it has become more popular to fit energy-storing feet on children. Because of the high activity level of many children, these more dynamic feet offer advantages over the SACH foot. As the child grows, the variety of prosthetic feet potentially available increases. All of the usual criteria for foot selection for adult amputees apply to the adolescent amputee population as well.

Selection of the most appropriate prosthetic knee component depends on several factors. These include length and strength of the residual limb, activities of the child, and size of the component. Single-axis knees, with or without a lock, are durable and lightweight. Polycentric knees are particularly good for situations in which the residual limb is long and the knee centers difficult to match. Fluid-controlled knees offer smoother gait and the ability of the knee to adapt to different walking speeds. Fluid-controlled knees are generally reserved until adolescence because of their size and weight. Suspension is a critical design feature of any lower limb prosthesis. The suspension system should be easily adjustable to allow for growth. Suspension sleeves and silicone suction suspension are particularly good because they allow for growth easily and provide excellent suspension.

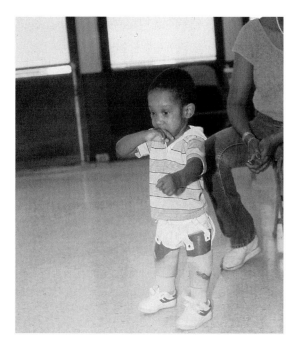

FIGURE 16–13. It is advisable to fit a jointless above-knee prosthesis to the toddler.

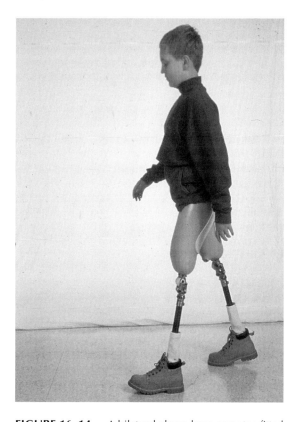

FIGURE 16–14. A bilateral above-knee amputee fitted with suction sockets, polycentric knees, and Flex feet. Because of the high energy consumption required to walk on bilateral above-knee prostheses, the design should be lightweight and as energy-efficient as possible.

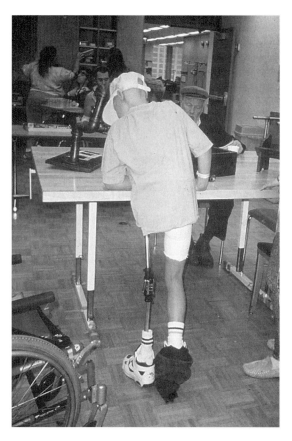

FIGURE 16–15. Weight shifting is taught for dressing skills.

Training

As with the congenital upper limb–deficient child, the preprosthetic period for the lower limb–deficient child is mainly focused on addressing the information needs of the parents. In addition, an assessment of strength, coordination, joint range of motion, skin condition, and sensation should be performed. This information may be useful in determining the timing of initial prosthetic use.

Children tend to do well with lower limb prostheses, often requiring little or no formal gait training. It is important, however, for the treating parties to recognize and understand the normal developmental patterns of gait. For example, toddlers tend to stand and ambulate with a wide-based gait with their lower extremities externally rotated, abducted, and flexed. As their gait matures, these characteristics change to a more narrow-based, upright fashion.[49] The prosthesis should incorporate these features to allow for normal gait development. Because the goal of physical therapy is symmetry of posture and movements during developmental activities, proper alignment and controlled weight shifting

and balance activities are emphasized for children with lower limb prostheses (Fig. 16–15).[48]

The normal child does not establish heel-to-toe gait until about 2 years of age. At about 20 months, the normal child can stand on one foot with help; at 3 years, on one foot momentarily; at 4 years, for several seconds; and at 5 years, for longer periods. The knee of the transfemoral prosthesis is nonarticulated or locked until the child is secure in stiff-legged walking. Prosthetic heel-strike to toe-off gait is not usually attained until the child is about 5 years old or can demonstrate sustained one-legged standing. Efforts to develop a smooth alternating progression should follow. The major causes of gait deviations are growth or worn prosthetic parts.

Frequent follow-up visits should be scheduled for the growing child. The child amputee should be seen every 3–4 months to keep up with growth by adjusting the prosthesis for socket fit and overall length. Prostheses need to be replaced approximately every 15 to 18 months on the growing child.[50]

As children grow, they may completely change their wearing patterns depending on their needs and desires. For example, bilateral above-knee amputees may choose not to wear prostheses when they are young because they feel limited in their mobility. As children mature, cosmesis may become more important to them, and thus prostheses are requested. Therefore, the team should not foster preconceived ideas about prosthetic or assistive device use.[49]

Acquired Amputations

In annual surveys of child amputee clinics, numbers have repeatedly shown that about 40% of the children seen have acquired amputations.[51] In contrast, surveys of prosthetic facilities has revealed that more children with acquired amputations receive prosthetic services than those with congenital limb deficiency. The discrepancy is explained by the fact that complex conditions are still managed by the specialty amputee clinic, whereas the family and child with acquired amputations are comfortable in a community prosthetic setting.[52]

The terminology used for acquired amputations follows the convention for adult limb loss. Upper extremity amputations are shoulder disarticulations, transhumeral (above-elbow amputation), elbow disarticulation, transradial (below-elbow amputation), wrist disarticulation, and partial hand amputations. The types of lower extremity amputations are translumbar (hemicorpectomy), transpelvic (hemipelvectomy), hip disarticulation, transfemoral (above-knee amputation), knee disarticulations (through-knee), transtibial (below-knee amputation), and Symes and partial foot.

Trauma

In the pediatric age group, the most common causes of amputations are trauma and disease.[51] Trauma represents twice as many limb loss causes as those from disease.[53,54] Traumatic injuries include most commonly those resulting from automobile and motorcycle collisions and train accidents. Causes for traumatic injuries depend on the region. In rural areas, farm accidents, lawnmower accidents, and high-tension electric wire injuries occur. For the older child, vehicular accidents, burns, gunshot wounds, and power tools are the most frequent causes of limb loss. Boating accidents can produce amputations by propeller injury. In the 1–4-year-old age range, power tools, such as lawn mowers and household accidents, are frequent.[55]

In more than 90% of acquired amputations, a single limb is involved. In 60% of the cases, the limb involved is the leg. Boys are involved at a rate of 3:2 to girls.[56]

Tumors

Tumors are the most frequent cause of amputations resulting from disease. The highest incidence of malignancy is in the 12–21-year-old age group.[33] Amputation of a limb during adolescence when body image is particularly important may complicate the completion of tasks required during adolescence.[57] Osteogenic sarcomas, Ewing's sarcoma, and, rarely, rhabdomyosarcoma are responsible for the majority of tumors resulting in amputation.[58,59] Definitive surgery for osteosarcoma depends upon the site of the primary tumor and the extent of invasion or metastasis.[60] Surgical removal of the affected bone and the surrounding soft tissue remains the treatment of choice, whether by amputation or limb-salvage procedure. Limb salvage with an endoprosthesis can be offered to 90% of children with osteosarcoma.[61] This procedure, which involves replacing the tumor-ridden bone with a metal endoprosthesis, prohibits contact sports. Additionally the prosthesis needs to be lengthened if growth is incomplete. The surgical procedure of choice attempts to obtain a tumor-free margin of 5–8 cm above the proximal limit of the medullary tumor.[62] Chemotherapy has now proved to be an effective adjunct to surgery. Before 1972, only 15% of afflicted children were disease-free and survived with surgery compared with the 60–70% who now survive with

surgery and the addition of chemotherapy.[63,64] Rehabilitation takes into account the confounding factors of fatigue and the pyschological aspects of combined treatments.

Infections

Infectious emboli from meningococcemia may autoamputate limbs or digits. The process frequently involves all four limbs. Frequently the skin is affected as well as the limb. Over the past few decades, the incidence of invasive meningococcal disease in the United States has remained relatively stable.[65] Strengthening and reconditioning is an important aspect in rehabilitation after prolonged convalescence.

Although the cardinal surgical dictum to conserve all limb length if possible is true for children, disarticulation rather than a transdiaphyseal amputation may be preferred in the growing child.[56] Disarticulation preserves the epiphyseal growth plates and ensures longitudinal growth.[66] Disarticulation also avoids the development of terminal or appositional overgrowth of new bone.

Terminal overgrowth at the transected end of a long bone is the most common complication after amputation in the immature child (Fig. 16–16).[56] It occurs most frequently in the humerus, fibula, tibia, and femur in that order.[66] The appositional growth may be so vigorous that the bone pierces the skin. The treatment of choice is surgical revision. Once surgery is necessary, frequently the problem recurs until skeletal maturity.[56] Stump capping is a surgical option. Bone spurs may form at the periphery of the transected bone. Resection may be necessary. Neuromas rarely need surgical intervention. Adventitious bursa develops in the soft tissue overlying an area of appositional overgrowth. Treatments such as aspiration, steroid

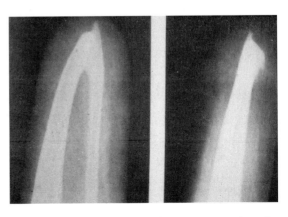

FIGURE 16–16. Overgrowth is common when the midshaft is amputated.

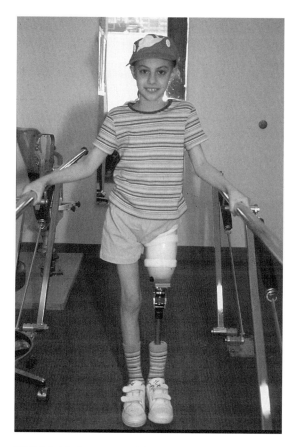

FIGURE 16–17. A variable volume socket is fabricated to accommodate volume changes for the child after tumor resection.

injections, and stump wrapping are usually ineffective.[66] Socket modification and surgical resection permanently correct the condition. Stump scarring that interferes with weight bearing requires prosthetic modifications.

Phantom sensation is the individual's awareness of the missing limb. It is rarely unpleasant. Because phantom sensation is not painful, no treatment is necessary. Several case reports have been written about people with congenital limb loss developing phantom sensations late in life.[67–69] Phantom sensations in children with limb deficiency are explainable if one recognizes the brain as a generator of sensory information.[70] Phantom limb pain rarely occurs in children under age 10 years or during growth but is reported in teenagers. After amputation, the older child may require pain medications for a few weeks.[15]

Fitting Time-Table

The child who acquires an amputation is treated much the same as the congenital limb–deficient child with a few exceptions. A child who undergoes an amputation is likely to require a preparatory prosthesis while the postoperative swelling subsides. The preparatory limb is usually worn for approximately 3 months. In the case of the child who is undergoing chemotherapy treatment, it is useful to use a volume-adjustable socket (Fig. 16–17).

Training

After surgery, the remaining leg must assume the dominant role in all transfer and locomotor activities. Therefore, the sound leg should be evaluated for strength and, if necessary, an appropriate exercise program developed. It is difficult to instruct the young active child in specific exercises and positioning because of limited comprehension and attention span. If specific exercises are indicated, a therapist often needs to be creative with games and use of equipment to get the desired responses, such as using a prone scooter to maintain or work on hip extension.[49] Edema control is accomplished using one of several options, including Ace bandage wrapping, elastic shrinker socks, layers of elastic stockinette, rigid dressing, and removable rigid dressing. It is important that the parent and child understand the proper technique for use of the edema control system. The edema control system should be worn 24 hours a day, being removed only for wound care and hygiene. To avoid increasing the patient's anxiety level, the therapist should not dwell on phantom pain, but the patient should be made aware of the normal postoperative discomfort that is to be expected.[71]

Each child must be assessed as an individual, with consideration given to age, both developmentally and chronologically; physical abilities; interests; and activities. Most children require very little formal physical therapy training. The goal is to develop a normal pattern of gait, including stride length, step length, and velocity whenever possible. Play is the primary motivation for desired movements and activities.[50] Parents should be instructed in how to care for the prosthesis and encouraged to maintain contact with the prosthetist for routine adjustments and follow-up. Often the first sign that an adjustment is needed is noted when the child reduces wearing time or begins to limp.

Outcome

Children with chronic physical handicaps have been found to be at risk for psychological and social adjustment problems.[72] There is a wide variation in a child's adaptation to physical handicap. Some children function quite well, whereas others exhibit adjustment problems. Literature supports a complex interplay of family functioning and temperament in predicting psychological and social adjustment.[73–75] In general, more family cohesion and moral and religious emphasis and organization, in combination with less family conflict, predicted better psychological and social adaptation.[76] In regard to temperament, greater emotionality predicted greater internalizing and externalizing behavior problems and less social competence. By identifying potentially modifiable risk factors, the child and family can be directed to therapies that can improve their overall adaptation.[76,77]

The child's self-perceived physical appearance is related to depressive and anxious symptoms.[75] As a group, classmate, parent, and teacher social support; daily stress; maternal and paternal perceived marital discord; peer acceptance; and athletic competence accounted for 78% of the variance in perceived physical appearance.[75,78]

Perceived social support is another important factor for the child's ability to adjust in a psychologically healthy manner.[77] For the child with limb deficiency, low levels of classroom and classmate social support represent a vulnerability factor.[74] Self-esteem is instrumental in many aspects of the child's life, such as persistence on difficult or challenging tasks, vocational choices, and the child's tendency to take calculated risks. Again the studies illuminate areas where intervention can be directed at improving the child's coping and adjustment strategies. By teaching necessary social skills, including strategies for handling name calling and teasing, professionals validate the child's experiences and prepare the child for interactions that will undoubtedly call attention to the physical deficit.[78,79]

By identifying early the children with vulnerable family dynamics, emotional temperaments, and poor peer interactions, the social and psychological outcome can be modified and psychosocial morbidity reduced. Pediatricians in a general practice setting usually underidentify children with behavioral and emotional problems.[80] A useful screening tool that has been used in epidemiologic studies of behavior and emotional problems, the Child Behavioral Checklist (CBCL), is appropriate to identify objectively those children in need of help.[81] Children are often not perceived by their parents as problematic because of many factors. In addition, the child is unable to identify the underlying social and emotional maladjustment.[82] For these reasons, it behooves professionals not to ignore but to explore the psychological world and behavioral actions of the child.

For children with amputations secondary to tumors, return to school may be difficult. In a study concerning the adjustment after tumor amputation, 67% could not keep up in their classes.[57] In addition to direct intervention for psychological counseling, there are many family support systems available to the families and children with limb deficiency. Many clinics provide opportunity for the interaction and peer support of their population. Frequently the parent-to-parent or child-to-child interactions surpass the effect of professional input for education, information, and resources.[83] Resource guides are available and provide pragmatic information for the child and parents.[84,85]

Functional Substitutions and Function

Children with upper limb deficiency have remarkable aptitudes and flexibility when performing tasks that require two hands. The child with a unilateral terminal transverse radial ulnar limb deficiency accomplishes activities of daily living with the sound intact contralateral hand.[30] For two-handed grasping activities, the elbow joint and residual forearm become the fulcrum for support. The child with asymmetric upper extremity deficiencies functions with the longer residual limb rather than the shorter limb, unless the longer limb has significant problems.[86] The child with bilateral deficiencies of the upper extremity substitutes fine motor tasks with the feet. The feet, which are usually nondexterous, have remarkable potential for fine grasp (Fig. 16–18). Foot function develops in a sequential pattern, which mirrors that of the upper extremity.[87] It is important to teach parents about the loss of surface area corresponding to the absent limb. Children who are active with multiple limb loss have a reduced surface to radiate heat loss, so they may have an increase in sweating and flushing about the head and neck.[15] The younger the child is at the time of amputation, the easier the transformation of hand dominance. In a study of children with amputations secondary to tumors, 75% believed they were independent in and out of the house.[57]

Functional goals for the child with bilateral lower extremity amputations should be optimistic. As long as children have arms with which to balance, they should be expected to walk independently. An adult with transfemoral amputations often needs canes or crutches for walking, whereas the child can walk independently.[33] Weight control is a concern for the child with lower extremity amputations. Dietary instruction should be emphasized early and often. Gait analysis has been performed on adults with amputations.[88] Crutch walking with or without a prosthesis increases energy expenditure during

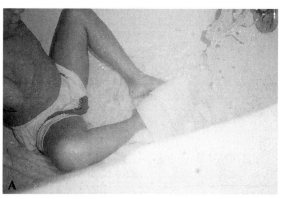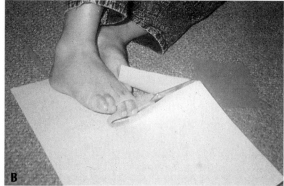

FIGURE 16–18. *A and B,* Foot skills compensate and develop to become functional for activities of daily living and school.

gait. In groups of traumatic amputations, the oxygen costs progressively increase at each higher-level amputation. Amputees preserve their energy expenditure by decreasing their chosen walking speed.[89–91] Children's effort levels have been reported for below-knee amputations between crutch walking, SACH foot, and

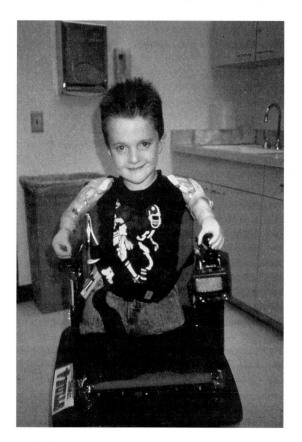

FIGURE 16–19. Independent mobility can be achieved by customizing the power mobility device as well as the prosthesis. This boy has a foreshortened myoelectric prosthesis to drive his chair with a joystick.

the flex foot. Chosen walking speed was higher for the children when using the flex foot, approaching normal. This study involved only five children, so statistical significance could not be determined. A slightly higher oxygen consumption occurred for children using SACH feet.[92]

Children with complex lower extremity limb deficiency, such as tetraphocomelia, benefit from the early introduction of power mobility. Movement provides a sense of independence and competence derived from exploring one's environment. When exploration is restricted, there is a diffuse and long-lasting impact. Motorized wheelchairs traditionally have been used when a child is approximately 5–6 years of age. Innovative seating systems have been developed for the 1–3-year-old child. Salient features include (1) a powered device; (2) proportional control drive with an adjustable joystick used with the head, chin, or lower or upper extremity buds; (3) adjustable positioning seating in an upright frame into which inserts can be attached for growth; (4) compactness, durability, portability, reliability, and safety; and (5) low profile with mounting potential for children to interact on a peer level (Fig. 16–19).[93] In addition to power mobility, other adapted mobility devices are available that are child- and environment-friendly.

Adolescents widen the sphere of mobility to include the community by using public transportation or by driving. The site of the amputation or limb loss determines the degree of difficulty an amputee has driving standard vehicles. In most cases, a person with a partial or full amputation of a limb requires adaptive driving equipment to compensate for the loss of ability to reach and operate driving controls (Fig. 16–20). Most amputees are able to get into and out of a standard-sized sedan independently. Current driving aides are available for the driver who has normal strength and mobility of upper extremities. Control systems used include push-pull control, push–right angle pull control, and push-twist. Each has the acceleration and braking system connected to usable upper extremity function.[94] State licensure for driving and installation of equipment varies. Physicians should be aware of their responsibility in certifying the capabilities of a potential driver. The evaluation for driving potential as well as specific equipment modifications should be discussed and made available for multilimb and complex limb deficiencies.

The child with an isolated limb deficiency or amputation is capable of achieving age-level academic skills. Few studies have been done to define achievement academically. In one study, children with congenital limb deficiency scored above the 50th percentile for their age-matched peers.[95] School placement is almost entirely within the regular school system with an individual education program to address educationally related function.[96] Occupational therapists assist with issues of grasp and fine motor control for paper, computer, and activities of daily living tasks needed in school. Physical therapy is involved with mobility skills such as negotiating the school space and playground. If the limb deficiency does not interfere with hand skills such as writing or mobility skills, an individual education program may not be necessary. In individual cases, the amputee clinic provides input for teachers to assist the child with limb loss in adapting to the classroom. Informational pamphlets have been developed for teachers to prepare able-bodied students for integration of children with physical disabilities into the regular education classroom.[97]

Adapted physical education may be necessary, but frequently regular physical education is sufficient. The philosophy promoted for children with physical disability is that of participation, not observation. Sports and participation in athletic endeavors such as skiing, tennis, and other more mundane exercises improve the self-concept of the child or adult with limb deficiency or amputations. Specialized adaptive prosthetic components that enable unilateral or bilateral handless individual to access sports such as golf, shooting, and ball sports has escalated since the 1980s. The tremendous progress in technology has allowed limb-deficient children to increase their participation and improve competition in athletics (Fig. 16–21). The Carbon Copy II prosthetic foot and Seattle foot are energy-saving designs that permit the athlete a more natural gait.

Little literature exists to define the vocational outcome of the child with limb deficiency.

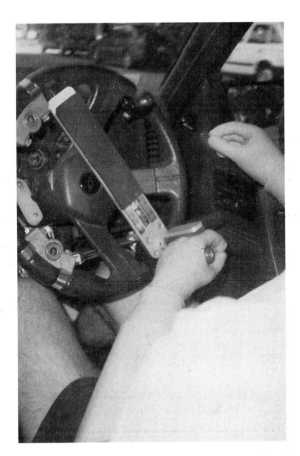

FIGURE 16–20. Adaptations to the steering wheel and myoelectric prosthesis for the bilateral upper extremity amputee create community independence.

Ninety percent of adults with absent radius or transverse radius were employed regardless of surgical intervention.[86] With the passage of the Americans with Disabilities Act, reasonable work accommodations are expected to improve employment opportunities for persons with complex limb deficiency.

Professionals who are involved with the population of children with loss of limb quickly appreciate the possibilities that exist for an individual to compensate and to accomplish as much as the fully limbed individual. Improved materials, improved technology, and greater availability of resources contribute to versatile prosthetic options. Involvement of a child and family with a comprehensive amputee clinic team provides therapeutic choices over the life of the child. Close collaboration of physicians, family, and all professionals is essential for a cohesive and practical rehabilitation program. As in all pediatric conditions, the process of decision making, treatment options, and delivery of care is variable and should be discussed with the child and family. The moving target is always

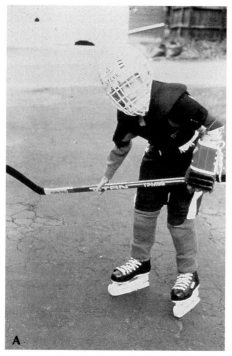

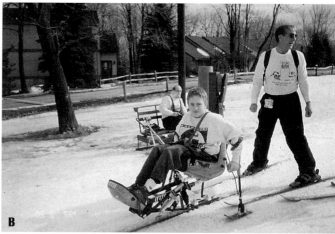

FIGURE 16–21. *A* and *B,* Sports participation by the child with limb deficiencies is possible with equipment substitution.

the growing, developing child, whereas the clinician's aim should be a healthy, happy, well-functioning child, adolescent, and ultimately adult.

References

1. Wilke H: Presidential Guest Speech. Annual Meeting of the Association of Children's Prosthetic/Orthotic Clinics, 1989.
2. Fisk J: Introduction to the child amputee. In Bowker J, Michael J (eds): Atlas of Limb Prosthetics, Surgical, Prosthetic and Rehabilitation Principles. St. Louis, Mosby, 1992.
3. Meier R: Evaluation of and planning for acquired upper-limb amputee rehabilitation. In Atkins D, Meier H (eds): Comprehensive Management of the Upper-Limb Amputee. New York, Springer-Verlag, 1989.
4. Pruitt S, Varni J, Setoguchi Y: Functional status in children with limb deficiency: Development and initial validation of an outcome measure. Arch Phys Med Rehabil 1996;77:1233.
5. Pruitt S, Varni J, Seid M, et al: Functional status in limb deficiency: Development of an outcome measure for preschool children. Arch Phys Med Rehabil 1998;79:405.
6. Stocker D, Biden E, Leckey R: Clinical experiences using the UNB test of prosthetics function. Presented at ACPOC Annual Meeting, Dallas, TX, 1997.
7. Huggins M, Wright H, Hubbard S: The prosthetic upper extremity functional index (the PUFI). Presentation of an Approach to Measurement of a Child's Use of an Upper Extremity Prosthesis. Presented at ACPOC Annual Meeting, Grand Rapids, MI, 1998.
8. American Academy of Orthopaedic Surgeons: Bulletin. Rosemont, IL, 1996;29.
9. Kurtin P, Landgraf JM, Abetz L: Patient-based health status measurement in pediatric dialysis: Expanding the assessment outcome. Am J Kidney Dis 1994;24:376.
10. Granger C, Kelly-Hayes M, Johnston M, et al: Quality and outcome measures for medical rehabilitation. In Braddom RL (ed): Physical Medicine and Rehabilitation. Philadelphia, WB Saunders, 1996.
11. Taylor S, Yuschyshyn H, McIvor J: Stump sensation and prosthetic use in juvenile upper extremity amputees. J Assoc Child Prosthetic-Orthotic Clin 1991;26:24.
12. Burtch R: Nomenclature for congenital skeletal limb deficiencies: A revision of the Frantz and O'Rahilly classification. Artificial Limbs 1996;10:24.
13. Frantz C, O'Rahilly R: Congenital skeletal deficiencies. J Bone Joint Surg 1961;43A:1202.
14. Williamson D: A syndrome of congenital malformations possibly due to maternal diabetes. Dev Med Child Neurol 1970;12:145.
15. Setoguchi Y: Evaluation of the pediatric amputee. In Atkins D, Meier R (eds): Comprehensive Management of the Upper-Limb Amputee. New York, Springer-Verlag, 1989.
16. Graham J Jr, Miller M, Stephen J: Limb reduction anomalies and early in-utero limb compression. J Pediatr 1980;96:1052.
17. Swanson A: Classification for congenital limb malformations. J Hand Surg 1976;1:8.
18. Swanson A, Barsky A, Entin M: Classification of limb malformation on the basis of embryological failures. Surg Clin North Am 1968;48:1169.
19. Day J: The ISO/ISPO classification of congenital limb deficiency. In Bowker J, Michael J (eds): Atlas of Limb Prosthetics. St. Louis, Mosby, 1992.
20. National Center for Health Statistics: Current Estimates From the National Health Interview Survey. Washington, DC, US Department of Health and Human Services, 1990.
21. Goldberg M, Bartoshesky L, O'Toole D: The pediatric amputee: An epidemiologic survey. Orthop Rev 1981;10:40.
22. Carroll R, Louis D: Anomalies associated with radial dysplasia. J Pediatrics 1974;84:409.
23. Silver H, Blair W, Kemp C: Fanconi's syndrome: Multiple congenital anomalies with hypoplastic anemia. Am J Dis Child 1952;83.

24. Holt M, Oram S: Familial heart disease with skeletal malformations. Br Heart J 1960;22:236.
25. Barry J, Auldist A: The Vater association: One end of a spectrum of anomalies. Am J Dis Child 1974;128:769.
26. Lawhon S, MacEwen G, Bunnell W: Orthopedic aspects of the Vater association. J Bone Joint Surg 1986;68A:424.
27. Overby K: Pediatric health supervision. In Rudolph A (ed): Rudolph's Pediatrics, 19th ed. Stamford, CT, Appleton & Lange, 1991.
28. Beasley R: General considerations in managing upper limb amputations. Orthop Clin North Am 1981;12:743.
29. Tooms R: The hand: Amputations. In Crenshaw AH (ed): Campbell's Operative Orthopedics. St. Louis, Mosby, 1980.
30. Aitken G, Pellicore R: Introduction to the child amputee. In Bowker J, Michael J (eds): Atlas of Limb Prosthetics: Surgical and Prosthetic Principles. St. Louis, Mosby, 1992.
31. Meredith J, Uellendahl J, Keagy R: Successful voluntary grasp and release using the cookie crusher myoelectric hand in 2-year-olds. Am J Occup Ther 1993;47:825.
32. Patton J: Developmental approach to pediatric prosthetic evaluation and training. In Atkins D, Meier R (eds): Comprehensive Management of the Upper-Limb Amputee. New York, Springer-Verlag; 1989.
33. Kruger L: Lower limb deficiencies surgical management. In Bowker J, Michael J (eds): Atlas of Limb Prosthetics: Surgical, Prosthetic and Rehabilitation Principles, 2nd ed. St. Louis, Mosby, 1992.
34. McAnelly R, Faulkner V: Lower limb prostheses. In Braddom RL (ed): Physical Medicine and Rehabilitation. Philadelphia, WB Saunders, 1996.
35. Ilizarov G: Possibilities offered by our method for lengthening various segments in upper and lower limbs. Basic Life Sci 1998;48:323.
36. Thomas I, Williams P: The Gruca operations for congenital absence of the fibula. J Bone Joint Surg 1987;69B:587.
37. Gillespie R, Torode I: Classification and management of congenital abnormalities of the femur. J Bone Joint Surg 1983;65B:557.
38. Krajbich I: Proximal femoral focal deficiency. In Kalamachi A (ed): Congenital Lower Limb Deficiencies. New York, Springer-Verlag, 1989.
39. Amstutz H, Wilson P: Dysgenesis of the proximal femur (coxa vara) and its surgical management. J Bone Joint Surg 1962;44A:1.
40. Bryant D, Epps C: Proximal femoral focal deficiency—evaluation and management. Orthopedics 1991;14:775.
41. Kalamchi A, Cowell H, Kim K: Congenital deficiency of the femur. J Pediatr Orthop 1985;5:129.
42. Rossi T, Kruger L: Proximal femoral focal deficiency and its treatment. Orthotics Prosthet 1975;29:37.
43. Mosley C: A straight-line graph for leg length discrepancies. J Bone Joint Surg 1977;59A:174.
44. Von Soal G: Epiphysiodesis combined with amputation. J Bone Joint Surg 1939;21:442.
45. Cummings D, Kapp S: Lower-limb pediatric prosthetics: General considerations and philosophy. J Prosthet Orthot 1992;719.
46. Oglesby D, Tablada C: Prosthetic and orthotic management. In Bowker J, Michael J (eds): Atlas of Limb Prosthetics, 2nd ed. St. Louis, Mosby, 1992.
47. Overby K: Overview of developmental monitoring. In Rudolph A (ed): Rudolph's Pediatrics, 19th ed. Stamford, CT, Appleton & Lange, 1991.
48. Stanger M: Limb deficiencies and amputations. In Campbell S (ed): Physical Therapy for Children. Philadelphia, WB Saunders, 1995.
49. Griffin-Peregrine J: Special considerations for the child amputee. In Karacoloff LA (ed): Lower Extremity Amputation: A Guide to Functional Outcomes in Physical Therapy Management, 2nd ed. Gaithersburg, MD, Aspen, 1992.
50. May B: The child with an amputation. In May B (ed): Amputations and Prosthetics. Philadelphia, FA Davis, 1996.
51. Davies E, Friz B, Clippinger F: Children with amputations. Inter-Clinic Information Bulletin 1969;9:6.
52. Kay H, Fishman S: 1018 Children With Skeletal Limb Deficiencies. New York, New York University Post-Graduate Medical School, Prosthetic and Orthotics, 1967.
53. Cary J: Traumatic amputation in childhood—primary management. Inter-Clinic Information Bulletin 1975;14:1.
54. Lambert C: Etiology. In Aitken G: The Child with an Acquired Amputation. Washington, DC, National Academy of Sciences, 1972.
55. Aitken G: The child with an acquired amputation. Inter-Clin Information Bulletin 1968;7:1.
56. Tooms R: Acquired amputations in children. In Atlas of Limb Prosthetics: Surgical, Prosthetic and Rehabilitation Principles. St. Louis, Mosby, 1981.
57. Tebbi C, Petrilli S, Richards M: Adjustment to amputation among adolescent oncology patients. Am J Pediatr Hematol Oncol 1989;11:276.
58. Mercuri M, Capanna R, Manfrini M, et al: The management of malignant bone tumors in children and adolescents. Management of Malignant Bone Tumors 1991;264:156.
59. Lane J, Kroll M, Rossbach P: New advances and concepts in amputee management after treatment for bone and soft-tissue sarcomas. Clin Orthop 1990;256:22.
60. Rougraff B, Simon M, Kneisl J, et al: Limb salvage compared with amputation for osteosarcoma of the distal end of the femur. J Bone Joint Surg 1994;76A:649.
61. Alman B, DeBari A, Krajbich JI: Massive allografts in the treatment of osteosarcoma and Ewing sarcoma in children and adolescents. J Bone Joint Surg 1995;77A:54.
62. Enneking W, Dunhan W, Gebhardt M, et al: A system for the functional evaluation of reconstructive procedures after surgical treatment of tumors of the musculoskelatal system. Clin Orthop Rel Res 1993;286:241.
63. Link M, Goorin A, Horowitz M, et al: Adjuvant chemotherapy of high-grade osteosarcoma of the extremity. Clin Orthop 1991;270:8.
64. Malawer M, Chou L: Prosthetic survival and clinical results with use of large-segment replacements in the treatment of high-grade bone sarcomas. J Bone Joint Surg 1995;77A:1154.
65. Moore K, Osterholm M: Meningococcal disease and public health practice. JAMA 1998;279:472.
66. Aitken G: Surgical amputation in children. J Bone Joint Surg 1963;45A:1735.
67. Weinstein S, Sersen E: Phantoms in cases of congenital absence of limbs. Neurology 1961;10:905.
68. Poeck K: Phantoms following amputations in early childhood and in congenital absence of limbs. Cortex 1964;1:269.
69. Weinstein S, Sersen E, Vetter R: Phantoms and somatic sensation in cases of congenital aplasia. Cortex 1964;1:276.
70. Melzack R: Phantom limbs, the self and brain (The D.O. Hebb Memorial Lecture). Can Psychol 1989;30:1.
71. Mensch G, Ellis P: Preoperative and postoperative care and the responsibilities of the physical therapist. In Mensch G, Ellis P (ed): Physical Therapy Management of Lower Extremity Amputations. Rockville, MD, 1986.
72. Wallander J, Varni J, Babani L, et al: Children with chronic psychological adjustment. J Pediatr Psychol 1988;13:197.
73. Varni J, Rubenfeld L, Talbot D, et al: Family functioning, temperament and psychologic adaptation in children with congenital or acquired limb deficiencies. Pediatrics 1989;84:323.

74. Varni J, Setoguchi Y, Rubenfeld Rappaport L, et al: Effects of stress, social support and self-esteem on depression in children with limb deficiencies. Arch Phys Med Rehabil 1991;72:1053.

75. Varni J, Setoguchi Y: Self-perceived physical appearance in children and adolescents with congenital/acquired limb deficiencies. J Assoc Child Prosthetic-Orthotic Clin 1991;26:56.

76. Varni J, Setoguchi Y: Psychosocial factors in the management of children with limb deficiencies. Phys Med Rehabil Clin North Am 1991;2:395.

77. Varni J, Setoguchi Y: Perceived physical appearance and adjustment of adolescents with congenital/acquired limb deficiencies: A path-analytic model. J Clin Child Psychol 1996;25:201.

78. Varni J, Rubenfeld L, Talbot D, et al: Stress, social support and depressive symptomatology in children with congenital/acquired limb deficiencies. J Pediatr Psychol 1989;14:515.

79. Costello E, Edelbrock C, Costello A, et al: Psychopathology in pediatric primary care: The new hidden morbidity. Pediatrics 1988;82:415.

80. Jellinek M, Murphy J: Screening for psychosocial disorders in pediatric practice. Am J Dis Child 1988;142:1153.

81. Varni J, Setoguchi Y: Screening for behavioral and emotional problems in children and adolescents with congenital or acquired limb deficiencies. Am J Dis Child 1992;146:103.

82. Weisz J, Weiss B: Studying the "referablilty" of child clinical problems. J Consult Clin Psychol 1991;59:266.

83. O'Donnel P: Structured parent interaction. Inter-Clinic Information Bulletin 1977;16:10.

84. Northwestern University Prosthetics Research Laboratory and Rehabilitation Engineering Research Program: Resource Guide of Prosthetics and Orthotics. 1997.

85. Mooney R: The Handbook: Information for New Upper Extremity Amputees, Their Families and Friends. 1995.

86. Kaniewski B, Coale E, Mochel D, et al: Long-term review of radial defiencies in respect to functional independence. J Assoc Child Prosthetic-Orthotic Clin 1991;26:30.

87. Schmid H: Foot studies in children with severe upper limb deficiencies. Am J Occup Ther 1971;25:160.

88. Gonzalez E, Corcoran P, Reyes R: Energy expenditure in below-knee amputee: Correlation with stump length. Arch Phys Med Rehabil 1974;55:111.

89. Waters R, Lunsford B, Perry J, et al: Energy-speed relation of walking: Standard tables. J Orthop Res 1988;6:215.

90. Waters R, Perry J, Antonelli D, et al: The energy cost of walking of amputees—influence of level of amputation. J Bone Joint Surg 1976;58A:42.

91. Eberhart H, Elftman H, Inman V: Locomotor mechanism of amputee. In Klopsteg P, Wilson P (eds): Human Limbs and Their Substitutes. New York, McGraw-Hill, 1954.

92. Colborne R, Naumann S, Berbrayer D, et al: Biomechanical and metabolic comparison of SACH and Seattle Feet in below-knee amputees. J Assoc Child Prosthetic-Orthotic Clin 1991;26:25.

93. Bleakney D: A powered mobility device for children with tetraphocomelia. J Assoc Child Prosthetic-Orthotic Clin 1990;25:38.

94. Reichenberger A: Assistive driving aids for the disabled. Presented at the Eighth Annual Prosthetics and Orthotic Symposium, Kingsbrook Jewish Medical Center, Brooklyn, New York, 1979.

95. Clarke S, French R: Can congenital amputees achieve academically? Am Corrective Ther J 1978;32:7.

96. Gordon W, Diller-Leonard: The relationship between physical disability and school placement in handicapped children. Proceedings of the 81st Annual Convention of the American Psychological Association, Montreal, Canada, 1993.

97. Popp R: Teaching exceptional children. Learning About Disabilities 1983;15:78.

Chapter 17

Rehabilitation of Burn Injuries

Patricia Taggart, MBA, PT
Robert Haining, MD

Burn injury in children can be a devastating event with lifelong consequences. The management of pediatric burn injury is complex and requires in-depth knowledge of wound care, pain control, normal physiologic parameters, and principles of pediatric rehabilitation.

Epidemiology

Burns are the leading cause of non–motor vehicle deaths in children aged 1–4 years and are the second most common cause of death in children from 4–14 years of age. Scald injuries represent approximately 40–50% of all burns, with the highest incidence seen in the toddler age group.[1,2] In general, increased burn size raises the risk of mortality in children; however, children up to 4 years of age have a higher risk of death independent of burn size.[2,3] The higher mortality rate in younger children may be due to immature immune system and increased fluid requirements, which place them at a higher risk for sepsis and hypovolemic shock after burn injury.[3,4] In children under age 4 years, the male to female ratio is 2:1; this ratio increases to 4:1 in adolescents. Inhalation injury has been cited by investigators as being an important predictor of mortality in burn patients.[5–7]

Scald burns, which may result from spill or immersion, are the single most common cause of pediatric burn injury. In scald spills, the curious toddler pulls hot liquid onto himself or herself, commonly burning the hand, arm, lateral side of the face, neck, and trunk. Immersion scald burns, which occur when a child either climbs or is dipped into a tub of hot water, have been associated with child abuse or neglect.[8] Sixteen percent of all burn injuries are nonaccidental, and approximately half of these are a result of documentable, inflicted abuse.[9]

Flame burns resulting from play with matches, gasoline, firecrackers, and flammable aerosols continue to occur in the 6- to 14-year-old age groups. Educational programs geared toward children in this age group emphasize *stop, drop, and roll* as a method to prevent further ignition of clothing by running.

Household electric current and extension cords are consistently identified as a major cause of electrocution in young children, and risk-taking behavior is the cause for most high-voltage electrocutions in teenagers. Wall outlet–caused injuries represent less than 15% of all pediatric electrical injuries.[10] The majority of the low-voltage injuries occur at home primarily to children under age 12 years. Low-voltage injuries most commonly occur from oral or hand contact with an electrical cord, objects inserted into wall outlets, or direct contact with electrical appliances. High-voltage injuries can be attributed to climbing telephone or power poles, climbing on roofs, playing in abandoned buildings, or subway third rail contact.

Ground fault circuit interrupters (GFCI), instituted in the late 1980s, represent a passive method of preventing electrical injuries. Protective circuits, incorporated into electric wall outlets, detect the loss of current when an individual comes in contact with the current. GFCIs are required in new or reconstructed household bathroom and kitchen outlets, in basements, and in outlets near hot tubs or spas. The use of GFCIs may reduce the number of household electrical burns, but they are not uniformly required by all states.

Physiologic Parameters in Burned Children

Children are different from adults not only in appearance, but also physiologically. Growth dimensions change with increased surface area relative to size. Physiologic parameters of blood pressure, heart rate, respiration, and caloric and fluid requirements change as well. These issues are important not only in acute care, but also in the extended rehabilitation stage.

Infants usually have heart rates greater than 110/min, ranging around 120/min. In response to stress, it is not unusual for the infant's heart rate to be in the 140–160/min range. With variation from the normal levels that would be expected, however, other causes should be looked for. For older adolescents, resting heart rate is more like that of an adult, with the average range falling to 75/min for a 16-year-old boy.

Knowledge of children's response to stress and the changes in the physiologic parameters is mandatory in the care of pediatric burns. Children become dehydrated faster than adults, and proper fluid administration needs to be considered even with small increases in heart rate. Alterations in heart rate also reflect the increased metabolism of children. For these reasons, heart rates should be closely monitored. At times propranolol can be useful to decrease overall metabolic demand.[11] β–Blockers must be used with caution because they mask physiologic responses.

The caloric needs of children with burns are significantly higher than for nonburned children. Normative data for healthy infants and children are listed in Chapter 2. A number of formulas are used in children to calculate caloric need. Improved wound management in burned children suggests that formulas overestimate their caloric needs. It appears from one report that the Galveston formula is closest to actual energy consumption.[12] This is calculated as 1800 kcal/body surface area (m^2) + 1300 kcal/body surface area burned (m^2). Because burned children are catabolic, close attention must be paid to their nutritional needs. The child's nutritional needs may be met orally, enterally, or parenterally. Most common formulas available now supply necessary vitamins; vitamin C at 5–10 × the Recommended Daily Allowance and zinc at 2 × the Recommended Daily Allowance are often supplemented because of their role in wound healing. B vitamins are often needed at twice the Recommended Daily Allowance because of their role as cofactors of metabolism as well.[13] Knowledge of normal fluid and electrolyte needs is important throughout the rehabilitation stay.

Many times the children are reluctant to drink, and adequate hydration must be maintained. Table 17–1 provides a common method of calculating fluids.

Even with optimal nutritional support, children who have suffered moderate-to-severe burns have a reduction in their bone mass and significant growth delays for up to 3 years after the burn. Immobilization may contribute to an acute reduction of bone mass. Increased production of endogenous corticosteroids may lead to reduced bone formation. Hypercalciuria also occurs in the acute period after burns. This may be the result of bone resorption or a high dietary calcium intake. Although the cause remains unclear, a combination of these factors may result in increased susceptibility for fracture.[14]

Function and Structure of the Skin

The skin is a barrier between the body and the environment. It is able to regenerate and repair itself, and because of its elasticity the skin can conform to different postures and shapes of the extremities. The ability to repair and regenerate plays a significant role in the care of burned children. Normally, skin is generated in flat planes, has a smooth appearance, and is soft. When skin is injured, it scars and many times deposits the collagen infrastructure in a disorganized way, giving a whorled and bumpy appearance. The intact skin also acts to keep the underlying structures moist by conserving fluid. It is a major barrier against infection. With skin disruption, the underlying structures are rapidly infected and require local or possibly systemic care.

The skin is composed of the epidermis, dermis, and hypodermis (Fig. 17–1). These layers are superimposed on one another and as a group make up the protective layer. The epidermis is divided into a number of strata. The first three layers adjacent to the dermis (stratum malpighii) are metabolically active. Melanin is produced by melanocytes in the stratum corneum and acts as a protective agent against ultraviolet radiation. Vasculature of the skin allows for blood flow that is much greater than the metabolic demands of the skin itself. Blood flow can exceed up to 10 times the nutritional requirement of the integument and may account for 5% of the cardiac output. This variation in blood flow is important in the thermoregulatory needs of the body. Increasing or decreasing the amount of blood flow elevates or lowers the core temperature. The skin also contains multiple glandular structures, including the sebaceous glands, apocrine glands, and sweat glands. The sweat glands have an important function in thermoregulation. In adults,

TABLE 17–1. Fluid Calculation Method

Body Weight (kg)	Maintenance Fluid Need
≤ 10 kg	100 ml/kg
11–20 kg	1000 ml + 50 ml/kg for each kg above 10 kg
> 20 kg	1500 ml + 20 ml/kg for each kg above 20 kg

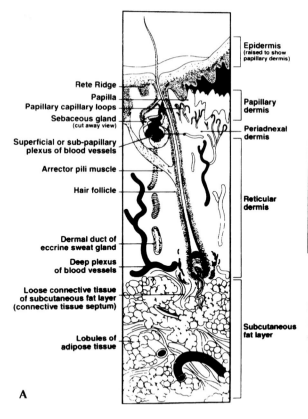

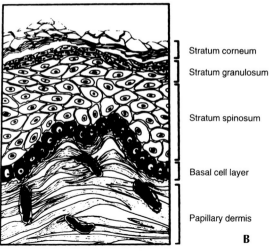

FIGURE 17–1. *A*, Anatomy of the skin. *B*, Epidermal layers and papillary dermis. (From Bennion SD: Structure and function of the skin. In Fitzpatrick JE, Aeling JL (eds): Dermatology Secrets. Philadelphia, Hanley & Belfus, 1996;1–2, with permission.)

sweating can produce up to 10 L/day of fluid.[15] Disruption of this intricate system of protection and thermoregulation imposes many challenges when caring for the burned child.

Burn Classification

Calculation of burn size is relative to total body surface area and varies depending on age. Most clinicians rely on a body diagram and chart to estimate burn size. The modified Lund and Browder[16] chart (Table 17–2) is used most commonly in estimating the extent of burn size in children. This chart is considered more accurate in pediatrics because it relates body proportion to age. The head of a child under 1 year of age is approximately twice as large as an adult's in proportion to the total body surface area.

The rule of 9s (Fig. 17–2) is another frequently used method of estimating burn size. Adult body size is divided into 11 segments of 9% or multiples of 9%. Nine percent of the total body surface area is allocated to the head and neck; 9% to each upper extremity; and 18% each to the anterior trunk, posterior trunk, and each lower extremity. The perineum represents the remaining 1%. The rule of 9s is modified for use with children. Nine percent is taken from the legs and added to the head of a child up to 1 year of

age. For each subsequent year, 1% is returned to the legs until the child is approximately 9 years old, at which time the head is in proportion to that of an adult.

A third method to estimate burn size is the use of the palm of the patient's hand, which represents approximately 1% of total body surface area. This method is useful when estimating small areas of injury.

Classification by Severity

Burns are divided into three classes based on the depth of the injury: (1) superficial, formerly

TABLE 17–2. Child Burn Size Estimation Chart

Burn Area	Age (yr)				
	1	1–4	5–9	10–14	15
Head	19	17	13	11	9
Neck	2	2	2	2	2
Anterior trunk	13	13	13	13	13
Posterior trunk	18	18	18	18	18
Genitalia	1	1	1	1	1
Upper extremity (each)	9	9	9	9	9
Lower extremity (each)	14.5	15.5	17.5	18.5	19.5

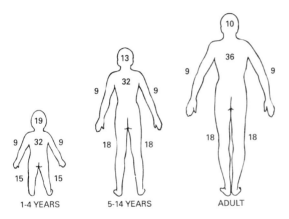

FIGURE 17–2.   The rule of 9s.

known as first degree; (2) partial thickness, formerly known as second degree; and (3) full thickness, formerly known as third degree. The partial thickness category is further subdivided into superficial partial thickness and deep partial thickness. Classification is based on the estimate of remaining epithelial-lined skin appendages that can reepithelialize the wound (Fig. 17–3).[17]

Superficial Thickness Burns

A superficial burn wound can be easily identified and is most commonly associated with sunburn. The area involved is red and slightly moist. The layer of destruction is the epidermis. Blanching is present. This type of wound is painful to touch because nerve endings located in the dermis remain intact. Superficial burns heal by themselves within a relatively short

period of time, 5–7 days with peeling of the injured epidermal cells. There is usually no scarring or pigmentation changes associated with superficial burns.

Partial Thickness Burns

Superficial Partial Thickness Burns

Superficial partial thickness injury generally involves the epidermis and a superficial portion of the dermal layer. These wounds are characterized by erythema and blisters. They are moist and blanch when pressure is applied. Serum leaking from the damaged capillaries is responsible for the wet appearance of partial thickness wounds. Superficial partial thickness wounds are extremely painful because the nerve endings responsible for pain remain intact. Most superficial partial thickness wounds heal by themselves within 7–14 days without scarring. Those that are not healed within 2 weeks may require skin grafting. Some discoloration of the skin may result from this degree of burns.

Deep Partial Thickness Burns

Deep partial thickness burns involve the epidermis and a greater portion of the dermal layer. They are usually red and blanch when pressure is applied because capillary blood flow is intact. Deep partial thickness injuries may be painful if nerve endings remain intact. Partial thickness wounds are also at risk for converting to full thickness injury if tenuous blood supply is lost or if the wound becomes infected. Deep partial thickness wounds usually require skin grafting because without that healing often yields a less

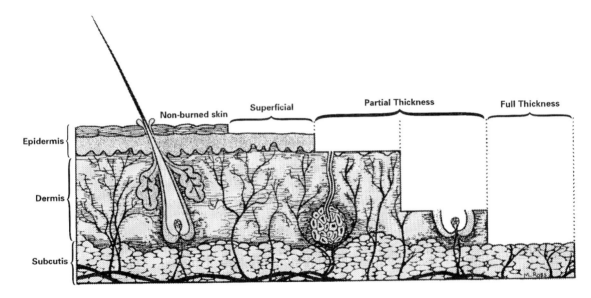

FIGURE 17–3.   Classification of burns by severity.

desirable cosmetic result. The decision to graft is based on the amount of additional burns requiring grafting and donor site availability.

Full Thickness Burns

Full thickness burns involve the epidermis and the dermal layer and may extend into deeper structures, such as fat and muscle. These wounds are dry and leathery in appearance and do not blanch. Because the nerve endings responsible for pain have been destroyed, these wounds are painless. Burns of this depth require skin grafting to heal and often result in scarring.

Criteria for Hospitalization

The American Burn Association established a guideline for hospitalization of a burn patient based on the *5-10-20 rule*.[18] This rule suggests that any patient with burn injury greater than 20% total body surface area should be hospitalized. Special consideration is given to the very young and very old; therefore a burn involving greater than 10% total body surface area in either population suggests hospitalization. Any patient with a full thickness burn greater than 5% requires hospitalization.

Even small burns affecting hands, feet, face, perineum, or joint surfaces and burns resulting from electrical injuries in which deep tissue involvement is suspected should be treated as emergencies and the patient should be hospitalized.[8,19] Any concomitant trauma or medical condition that could compound the effect of the burn injury should be considered as indication for hospitalization (Table 17–3).

Care in Acute Stage

Acute care of the pediatric burn patient begins as soon as the child encounters the emergency medical team in the field or in an emergency department and continues until the inpatient rehabilitation begins. Burns involving greater than 10–15% total body surface area require immediate fluid resuscitation, as do burns associated with smoke inhalation.[19] The ABCs of emergency medicine apply: airway, breathing, and circulation. The team evaluating the child should be ready to evaluate cardiopulmonary status, establish intravenous access, and evaluate the need for insertion of a nasogastric tube and urinary catheter. Once the child has been stabilized, the burn wound should be assessed for severity and depth. Appropriate topical agents and dressings should be applied to the wound. Frequency of dressing changes depends on the topical agent

TABLE 17–3. Indications for Hospitalization

> 20% total body surface area
> 10 % total body surface area in children or elderly
> 5% full thickness injury
Any burns to the eyes, ears, face, hands, feet, genitalia
All inhalation injuries
All electrical burns
All burns complicated by other medical problems
Any burns associated with concomitant trauma

used and the protocol of the facility; this is discussed in detail under wound care.

Factors affecting the acute care management of the pediatric patient include severity of injury, occurrence of life-threatening injury or secondary complications, immediate postburn management, period of time to wound closure, and age and premorbid health of the child.[1] Many burn care facilities have developed clinical guidelines for the care of burned children, often referred to as *critical pathways*. Critical pathways, usually developed based on the severity of the burn diagnosis, provide a road map for interventions used during the inpatient stay. Interventions typically provided during the acute phase by the rehabilitation team include positioning, wound management, range of motion (ROM), and exercise.

Positioning

Proper positioning of the burn patient during the acute phase of care is an essential component of preventing contracture and deformity. Positioning is also useful in controlling edema. Positioning children presents many challenges because of their size, difficulty in keeping them still, and their ability to cooperate. Typically the position of comfort for a burned child is the position that promotes deformity and therefore should be avoided. Positioning can be passive through the use of splints, restraints, or equipment attached to the bed or active through the use of pillows or pads designed to allow the child to change their position. Proper positioning of the burned child is summarized in Table 17–4. Elevation of the hands and feet should be combined with positioning during the first 48–72 hours of the acute phase to avoid edema.

Range of Motion

ROM exercises are performed during the acute phase of burn care on a schedule appropriate to the child's needs. Determination of the frequency of ROM depends on the activity level of the child. Those who are heavily sedated may require only daily ROM if passive positioning can be maintained. Children who are more active

TABLE 17–4. Positioning the Pediatric Burn Patient

Area Involved	Contracture Predisposition	Contracture Preventing Position
Anterior neck	Flexion	Extension, no pillows
Anterior axilla	Shoulder adduction	90° abduction, neutral rotation
Posterior axilla	Shoulder extension	Shoulder flexion
Elbow/forearm	Flexion/pronation	Elbows extended, forearm supination
Wrists	Flexion	15–20° extension
Hands		
MCPs	Hyperextension	70–90° flexion
IPs	Flexion	Full extension
Palmar burn	Finger flexion, thumb opposition	All joints full extension, thumb radially abducted
Chest	Lateral /anterior flexion	Straight, no lateral or anterior flexion
Hips	Flexion, adduction, external rotation	Extension, 10° abduction, neutral rotation
Knees	Flexion	Extension
Ankles	Plantarflexion	90° dorsiflexion

MCPs, Metacarpophalangeals; IPs, interphalangeals.

may require more frequent ROM if the affected body part cannot be maintained in the correct anatomic position. Active exercise should be incorporated into treatment as soon as the child is alert enough to participate.

Inpatient Rehabilitation Phase

As mortality rates for children with large burns continue to decline, the need for therapeutic and rehabilitative intervention becomes increasingly important.[20] The goal of burn rehabilitation is to return the child to the level of function attained before the burn injury. This goal is complicated when the injury occurs in a developing child who has not yet achieved or completed normal developmental milestones. The rehabilitation process, which started during the acute care phase, becomes the primary focus of treatment as the child's wounds progress toward healing. During the rehabilitative phase, evaluation and treatment planning continue and require frequent modification. Children entering into an acute rehabilitation program should undergo complete evaluations by the physiatrist and physical and occupational therapists. A speech pathology evaluation should be considered in cases in which there has been injury to the face, head, or neck; in cases in which the child's injuries required intubation; and in cases in which there is suspicion of anoxia. Rehabilitation

evaluations should include assessment of the wounds, active and passive ROM of all joints, strength, sensation, endurance, gross and fine motor function, posture, activities of daily living, edema and limb circumference, skin quality, and scar formation. Treatment planning should be based on the evaluation stated in terms of functional expectations. The rehabilitation program is a combination of exercises, positioning, and splinting. Static positioning and splinting are usually applied to maintain ROM or to prevent further loss of motion, whereas exercises impart a stretch to healing tissue to preserve or restore movement and improve physiologic and functional status. The initial intent of functional exercises should be directed at promoting a carryover effect of the ROM program.[21] Although exercise programs are based on sound biomechanical and physiologic principles, in the pediatric burn patient, play activities are often the most successful way to induce participation. Treatment should be administered at least twice a day, and exercise should be combined with play and functional activities.

Pain Management

For any child, the perception of pain is the result of many different factors. These include previous experience of pain, ethnic and social behaviors, and personality style. The pain experienced by burn victims can last for months as the patient passes from one aspect of the burn care to the next. Pain experienced, even from intravenous line insertion to debridement, must be appropriately attended to.

Acute Pain Control

During the acute period after a burn, pain control is often based on the use of opiates and even anesthetic agents to provide adequate relief. Because many of these children require controlled ventilation, it is impossible to judge their response to pain other than by physiologic changes of blood pressure and heart rate. It is of utmost importance to give analgesia at a level high enough to ensure that they do not experience pain. Narcotic agents, including fentanyl and morphine, are commonly used by constant infusion. Patient-controlled analgesia has become common and effective in empowering the patient to control pain needs and can be used with young children.

Ketamine can be used as a *dissociative* anesthetic for painful procedures because it has fewer respiratory side effects than the opiates and a short half-life. Transmucosal drug delivery is now becoming more popular as well for short painful procedures. Oral transmucosal fentanyl citrate is now available for children.

Chronic Pain Management

Although children have the most intense pain during the acute phase after a burn, they continue to experience intermittent and at times acute pain during rehabilitation. Pain management must continue to meet the child's needs, but the mechanism and duration of the analgesia change from a predominantly intravenous to an oral route.

The oral bioavailability of morphine is approximately 15–25% of the total dose administered because of first-pass metabolism by the liver. Codeine, oxycodone, and methadone are 60% bioavailable when given orally.[22] Calculating these medications for conversion from parenteral to oral doses should take into account these differences. Methadone can be used effectively to give baseline analgesia and to wean the children from intravenous morphine.

Although opiates should be considered the most important part of acute pain management, nonopiates should be used when possible. As the needs become more chronic, the use of other agents should be instituted to minimize the problems seen with opiates. Nonsteroidal anti-inflammatory medications, such as ibuprofen, can be added to treat the discomfort associated with remobilization and stretching. Other modalities, such as behavioral management and relaxation therapy, should also be used when possible.[23] These techniques are less effective in the very young than in older children. Behavioral distress has been seen to increase with the parents present during medical procedures.[24] Use of anxiolytics, such as lorazepam, should be considered to relieve the child's anxiety during the procedure.

It is not uncommon for children to have neuritic discomfort from the skin healing. Membrane stabilizers, such as carbamazepine or other anticonvulsants, can be useful. Amitriptyline is also effective and can be used in doses much smaller than those used for depression with good effect. The exact mechanism of action, however, is not clearly defined.

Outpatient Pain Management

Once the child is discharged to the outpatient setting, the need for analgesia generally decreases. With necessary ROM exercises and other required activities, however, pain control may need to be considered. Many children are able to tolerate the activities with only acetaminophen.

Other children may need codeine or oxycodone in combination with the acetaminophen to allow them to be compliant. In severe cases in which there is significant deformity, methadone can be used cautiously. Because the pain can also be neuritic in nature, use of carbamazepine or amitriptyline can be continued for a prolonged period without problems.

Wound Management

Burn injury results in damage and disruption to the skin and subcutaneous tissue. The necrotic tissue, commonly referred to as *eschar*, must be removed or damage to capillaries and skin elements results.[25] Debridement is the process of removal of dead material from the wound to promote healing. Burn wounds may be debrided surgically or through gentle, gradual removal of loose necrotic eschar and debris performed by personnel at the bedside or during hydrotherapy.[25] After debridement, the wounds should be washed, patted dry, and covered with an appropriate topical agent. Topical creams and ointments are usually covered with gauze and wrapped in place, particularly if the patient is mobile. The wounds may be covered with topical agents and left open if the patient is immobile (i.e., paralyzed or ventilated). The removal of old bandages and debridement of wounds is often performed using *clean technique*; this method prevents cross-contamination between patients and providers but does not produce or protect a sterile environment. Aseptic, or sterile, technique used to apply topical agents and clean bandages prevents introduction of bacteria to the wound.

Many acceptable methods of wound management are used in burn centers. The frequency of dressing changes generally ranges from every 8 hours to every 24 hours. As wound healing progresses, the dressing regimen and choice of topical agents should be reevaluated for effectiveness.

Topical Agents

Topical antibiotic creams have been the mainstay of burn wound care for the past 20 years and have significantly reduced mortality in burn patients by decreasing the incidence of infection.[25] An ideal topical agent should minimize bacterial growth, encourage reepithelialization, control odor, be easy to apply and remove, be pain-free, cost-effective, and facilitate physical and occupational therapy.[26] The most commonly used topical antibacterial agents are summarized in Table 17–5.

TABLE 17–5. Commonly Used Topical Agents

Agents	Uses	Advantages	Disadvantages	Comments
Silver sulfadiazine 1% cream (Silvadene)	Partial and full thickness burns	Wide spectrum, easy to apply, penetrates and softens eschar, comfortable	Requires regular cleaning, transient leukopenia, sulfa allergy	Most common agent for treating large and deep burns
Mafenide acetate (Sulfamylon)	Partial and full thickness burns, alternative to sulfadiazine	Wide spectrum, effective against *Pseudomonas*, penetrates eschar	Painful on application, sulfa allergy, carbonic anhydrase inhibitor	Also available as solution
Nitrofurazone (Furacin)	Partial and full thickness burns	Wide spectrum, but less effective against *Pseudomonas*, comfortable	Dermatitis, PEG toxicity, less effective against yeast	Available in cream, impregnated gauze, or solution
Bacitracin ointment 50 U/g	Partial and full thickness, general ointment for grafts and donor sites	Effective against gram-positive organisms, useful on faces	Hypersensitivity, ineffective for gram-negative bacteria	Available as solution, good general ointment
Silver nitrate 0.5% solution	Wet dressings for partial and full thickness burns	Wide spectrum, but less effective against *Pseudomonas* and yeast	Painful, stains, solution leaches sodium and chloride	Most commonly used 20–30 years ago, electrolyte imbalance can result from prolonged use
Xeroform gauze	Gauze impregnated with 3% bismuth tribromo-phenate for use on superficial or partial thickness burns	Protects wounds against environmental contamination, mildly deodorizing	May adhere to wound, maceration may occur if multiple layers are used	Inexpensive, when left adherent acts like scab, lifts off as wounds heal
Scarlet red, fine mesh	Gauze impregnated with aniline dye, which enhances epidermal growth	Used on skin grafts and donor sites, or on hypergranulated tissue	May form scab, stains wound	Cheap, easy to use
Enzymes (Travase, Elase, Collagenase Santyl)	Enzymatic debridement of deep partial and full thickness wounds	Speeds eschar removal, prepares wound for graft	May be painful upon application, must be monitored to prevent destruction to surrounding tissue	Controversial agents, frequent infection, may damage normal cells

A number of synthetic burn dressings have been developed. Some of these include Biobrane, Adaptic, Duoderm, Vigilon, Elastogel, Op-Site, Tegaderm, N-terface, and Hydron. Most of these products are occlusive or semiocclusive dressings (i.e., plastic films, hydrocolloids, hydrogels, collagen-impregnated dressings) that claim to provide pain relief, retard evaporative loss, and promote more comfortable movement. These dressings are most commonly used on clean burn wounds, on donor sites, or over skin grafts.

Hydrotherapy

Hydrotherapy is a modality used to wash burn wounds or immerse a patient to cleanse. It is also used to facilitate ROM exercises. The use of immersion to cleanse wounds had created controversy because of the concern that it increases the risk of cross-contamination between patients and from wound to wound within the same patient.[27,28] To decrease or eliminate the risk of cross-contamination, many burn centers use alternative methods to clean wounds, such as the use of spray or shower chairs or tubs and disposable plastic liners on spray tables.

Rehabilitation Principles

Splinting

Splints are a useful adjunct for passive positioning of pediatric burn patients. Children usually present more challenges than adults do in that they have great difficulty staying in a desired position for any length of time. Splints may be used to maintain joint position, correct or prevent deformities, maintain natural body contours, control edema, and complement pressure therapy. The frequency and duration of splint usage are variable depending on the depth and location of the burn and the presence of or potential for joint contracture. Consideration must be given to the anatomic differences present in children, such as thinner, more fragile skin, smaller size, and joint hypermobility.

Splinting is generally initiated at the first indication of developing skin tightness. In large percentage body surface burns involving the neck, axilla, hands, or feet, splinting may be initiated in anticipation of skin tightness as soon as edema subsides. Splinting schedules should be developed to combine passive stretch with active use of the body part. If loss of ROM occurs, the schedule should be adjusted to increase wearing time up to 24 hours daily when not in therapy. In contrast to adults and adolescents, small children do not tend to lose strength or joint mobility when immobilized in splints for extended periods, provided that the splints are removed for regular exercise or activity session.[1]

Small children pose a number of difficulties for splint usage. Because they have less body contour, it may be necessary to fabricate the splint longer to prevent it from sliding. This is especially true when fabricating axillary airplane splints or splints for the lower extremities. Securing splints in place is also difficult; children may remove straps themselves or convince caregivers to remove them. Clever therapists have designed devices that *lock* the splint in place to prevent removal. It may be necessary to cast over a splint with plaster or fiberglass to prevent its removal. Serial casting may also be used in cases in which the use of thermoplastic splinting has failed or when splinting is combined with attempts to place pressure on a body part.

Children wearing splints should have their skin checked regularly to avoid developing pressure areas, decubiti, and nerve compression. Written instructions for donning and doffing splints and wearing schedules should be posted at bedside. Splints should be marked with child's name, date of fabrication, and directional aids (i.e., top, bottom, right side, etc.) to assist staff and family members in correct application.

Range of Motion

Once the child is medically stable, ROM should move from gentle, repetitive action to more aggressive stretching. Because of the fragile nature of children's skin, it may be necessary to combine massage with ROM. Lubrication of the skin makes elongation of tight scar bands and stretching of soft tissue more tolerable to the child. Massage also desensitizes the tissue through tactile stimulation. The clinician should stabilize above and below the joint being ranged to avoid compensation from movement of other body parts. Active or active assisted motion is preferable to passive; however, it may be necessary to combine both to move to the end of the range. The preferred method of tissue elongation to avoid tissue damage is sustained stretch delivered in a slow, prolonged manner to an area of decreased motion or contracture.[21,29] Children should be encouraged to participate in the ROM activities and usually cooperate more fully when given concrete instructions, such as "keep your arm here and count to ten." They also respond well when ROM exercises are combined with play activities or games, for example, basketball. Many children prefer performing ROM exercises in the morning to mobilize joints in preparation for performing functional tasks or activities of daily living.

Activities of Daily Living

Children who have sustained burn injury should be encouraged to participate in activities of daily living as soon as they are medically stable. Activities should be appropriate for age and development and typically include self-feeding, dressing, and assisting in bathing. Assistive devices may be necessary for the child to be independent but should be considered temporary. Play is often considered an activity of daily living for children and should be encouraged whenever possible. Child life specialists invite children to join in play activities, initially at the bedside and later in group or playroom activities.

Exercise: Functional Skills

Children frequently experience loss of strength and motor function as a result of their burn injuries. Immobilization because of skin grafting procedures or mechanical ventilation can have deleterious effects on strength and function. Structured exercise combined with therapeutic, fun activities should begin as soon as the child can actively participate. Exercise programs should emphasize flexibility, strength, and endurance. Allowing the child to choose activities is an important way of giving the child the opportunity to control his or her environment. Activities should be age-appropriate, graded to match the child's level of function, and include fine and gross motor components. Favorite pediatric gross motor activities include ball games and mobility devices such as tricycles, bicycles, and big wheels. Fine motor skills can be attained through the use of puzzles, board games, and crafts.

Ambulation should begin as soon as the child's physical condition allows, often by 48–72 hours after injury, when vital signs are stable and fluid resuscitation is complete.[30] Children with lower extremity burns not requiring skin grafts should be encouraged to ambulate as soon as the wounds are healed and they have successfully completed a lower extremity dependency program. Elastic wraps should be used to control edema and provide circulatory support. The timing of ambulation after lower extremity grafting varies from center to center but most often occurs between the 7th and 14th postoperative days.[21,30] The lower extremities should be supported through the use of elastic wrapping, plaster casts, or Unna's boot.

Modalities

Physical modalities such as fluidotherapy, ultrasound, and paraffin may be helpful additions to scar management. Heat tolerance must be established before the use of such physical agents. Fluidotherapy delivers heat more efficiently than paraffin because high temperatures are better tolerated in a dry environment.[31] Ultrasound may be useful in softening connective tissue in children. Care should be given to avoid overexposure of ephiphyseal plates to ultrasound, avoiding intensities above 3.0 W/cm² when using a stationary transducer for periods of 3 minutes or greater.[32]

Outpatient Phase

Planning for the outpatient phase of burn care begins early during the hospital admission. Information should be gathered regarding the home environment, family support systems available to the child, and services in the home community if the child lives outside the geographic area served by the rehabilitation/burn center. As the child reaches the end of the rehabilitation phase and completion of goals is nearing, implementation of the discharge plan should begin. The patient and family must be well educated about the home care process before discharge.[33] In the outpatient phase, the wound care required is minimal, but ROM needs to be consistently maintained, and the program is geared toward achieving improvements in strength and function. Age-appropriate recreational activities should also be incorporated into the program during the outpatient phase. The patient and family should have a personalized home program, including instructions for wound and skin care, exercise program, activities of daily living, splinting schedule, and pressure program. The child should be monitored for growth during this phase because modifications in pressure garments may be necessary (see scar management).

Reconstructive Phase

The involvement of the rehabilitation team during the reconstructive phase depends on the extent and nature of the reconstruction. Generally the rehabilitation team becomes involved if the area being reconstructed covers a joint or involves the head or neck. In contrast to adults, a growing child is prone to develop recurring contractures until full growth has been achieved, particularly when the burn scars involve the hand or foot or extend over a joint.[34] The reconstruction may require a full rehabilitation program to maximize the effects of surgery.

Burns Requiring Special Consideration

Neck

Neck burns in the pediatric population present challenges to the treatment team. Correct positioning of the child in bed is essential but can be difficult to maintain. While in the acute phase, the child should be positioned with the neck in extension or hyperextension. This can be accomplished by placing a second mattress overlying the first, with the end of the top one slightly above the shoulders. The head then rests on the bottom mattress. Care should be given to avoid allowing the jaw to drop open. The occiput should also be watched for pressure areas if the child remains in supine position for any length of time. The use of thin pressure-relieving devices, such as Spenco pads, under the head is recommended. Pillows should be removed in patients with neck burns to avoid neck flexion.

Thermoplastic splints are useful tools in maintaining neck position. The most commonly used thermoplastic splints for the neck include the anterior neck collar, the wraparound neck collar, and the halo neck splint (Fig. 17–4). Several neck conformers may need to be fabricated to accommodate the different positions of the child's neck when in upright versus recumbent position. The authors have found that appropriately fabricated thermoplastic neck conformers do not inhibit function or play activities in the pediatric burn patient. Other types of splints used to control neck position in children include the soft cervical collar, the watusi collar fabricated from plastic tubes, and commercially available Philadelphia collars.

Axilla

Burns of the axilla are often difficult to treat in the pediatric population. Of all the burn-related contractures, the axilla is most commonly involved.[35] Numerous creative devices have been fabricated to position the shoulder in flexion and abduction. These include special attachments to the bed, such as arm troughs, overhead slings, and pulleys. The most successfully used device in an active patient is the airplane splint (see Fig. 17–4). The airplane splint consists of a piece wrapped around the lateral trunk connected to the arm trough with a bar. The arm trough holds the upper extremity in shoulder flexion and abduction. Care should be taken to support the wrist and hand to avoid edema formation. Straps around the trunk and upper extremity are secured to hold the splint in place. Airplane splints should be monitored and adjusted frequently, especially in children who lack body contour between the waist and hip, as the splints tend to slip downward.

Hands and Feet

The size of the hands and feet in children combined with a tendency toward rapid contracture in partial and full thickness burns makes this an area of special consideration. In hand and foot burns, the development of considerable edema can quickly lead to deformities.[34] During the acute phase, fingers and toes should be wrapped separately to maintain web spaces. Because use is essential to function, deep partial and full thickness burns are frequently treated with early surgical excision and autografting.[36] Splinting is universally used to maintain ROM and preserve function (Figs. 17–5 and 17–6). The method of splinting hand and foot burns depends on the location of the injury (Table 17–6). Hand splints are worn when the child is not engaged in functional activities and commonly worn all night. If both hands are involved, wearing the splints on alternate hands may be suggested to encourage alternate function.

Scar Management

Scarring after a burn is variable in degree for many reasons. Children with darker pigmented skin tend to scar more than those of lighter color. Some children are predisposed to keloid more as the result of genetic factors. Management of these scars is essential to obtain an optimal esthetic result. The use of pressure garments has become standard because the application of constant pressure on the scar flattens it, making it less whorled and thinner. These garments vary in their ability to apply a constant pressure and often require either inserts or overlying thermoplastic splints to apply

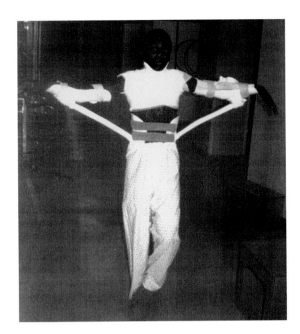

FIGURE 17–4. Neck collar, arm splint—airplane splints.

a firm pressure. It has been reported that the pressures actually applied by these custom-fitted garments can vary a great deal depending

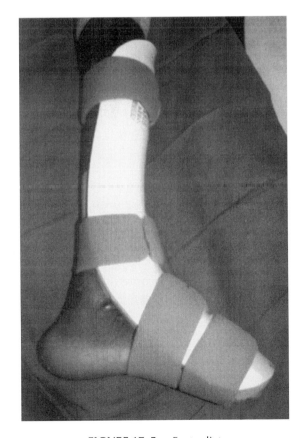

FIGURE 17–5. Foot splint.

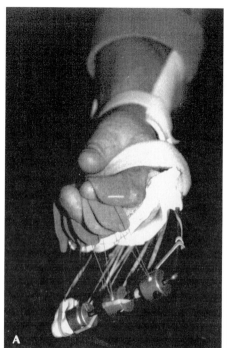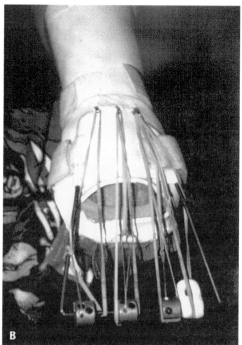

FIGURE 17–6. *A* and *B*, Dynamic hand splint.

on the site of application.[37] As the scar heals, the skin becomes nodular and hypertrophic. The thickness and whorled nature of the scars makes them unsightly. The tissues are initially quite vascular; however, as the scar matures and increases in thickness, the internal portion becomes avascular and fibrotic. The application of the pressure garments and splints appears to minimize fibroblastic activity and allows a more uniform linear deposition of the collagen. To induce capillary occlusion, an even application of 25 and 30 mmHg pressure must be applied. This is more effectively done on the extremities and trunk than over articulations or on the neck. The face is particularly difficult because of the many contours that are relatively mobile. Uvex face masks are used during the day, and cloth masks are applied at night to maintain constant pressure. Although the masks are necessary for an optimal outcome of flattening the

scars, they may cause abnormal facial growth and affect the position of the upper teeth.[38]

The hands and feet can be difficult to fit with pressure garments. Products available to provide pressure to digits include Tubigrip, Coban, and Ace wraps. The use of splints in conjunction with pressure garments can produce optimal results but requires ongoing surveillance to ensure that the splint applied over the garment does not result in excessive pressure (Fig. 17–7).

New Surgical Modalities

The surgical intervention required for burn care varies from center to center. Early excision and grafting of wounds are rather common standards. In scald burns, the excision may be delayed up to 14 days to allow the wound to demarcate, allowing the less involved tissues to heal spontaneously.

Tissue substitutes such as Integra, Aloderm, and Dermagraft-TC are becoming more common in the acute treatment and reconstruction of burns. Substances such as Integra are artificial membranes that allow the underlying tissues to grow into the lesion, allowing for split thickness grafting to be done over a more pliable base. Although it is yet to be seen, this may be useful in improving the appearance of the wound. Aloderm is harvested human dermis, which can be used to fill in defects and minimize wound

TABLE 17–6.   Splinting Hands and Feet

Body Part	Correct Splint Position
Dorsal Hand	MCP flexion 70–90°, IP extension, radial abduction of thumb
Volar hand	MCP/IP full extension, fingers abducted, palmar abduction of thumb
Dorsal foot	Ankle and toes plantarflexion
Sole of foot	Ankle dorsiflexion, toes neutral

MCP, Metacarpophalangeal; IP, interphalangeal.

contraction after grafting. Synthetic occlusive dressings such as Biobrane can be used to cover graft donor sites to improve comfort.[39]

Procedures used more frequently in the care of children include the increased use of tissue expanders and tissue substitutes. The use of tissue expanders can allow for improved esthetic outcome for scalp burns. Even though the complication rate is high, the technique of inserting a balloon under the skin and filling it sequentially allows for skin closure that is adjacent to the area of scar. On the scalp, this can allow the hair to be pulled over to cover the defect.[40]

Psychosocial Concerns

Epidemiologic studies have demonstrated that burn injuries and trauma to children occur more often in families more stressed than the general public.[41] More often these are single-parent families that are economically disadvantaged with a large number of children.[41-43] Emotional disturbance in parents, specifically depression, is associated with higher risk for burn injury in children.[44] A child who sustains burns is more likely to have had emotional or behavioral difficulties preceding the burn injury.[44] The trauma of a burn injury, fear of loss of life, and the threat of disfigurement create numerous psychosocial issues for the burned child and family.

Children, similar to adults, pass through early, intermediate, and long-term stages of recovery.[45,46] There are differences in children's response to hospitalization that vary by age. Infants and toddlers usually experience separation anxiety; school-aged children have difficulties with agitation, anger, and manipulation; and adolescents are sensitive to control issues and react with rebellious noncompliance or regressive withdrawal.[47] Psychological interventions include parental support, providing structure to reduce anxiety and fears, appropriate explanation and demonstration of medical procedures, establishing a *safe area* where no procedures are performed, and providing the child with generous positive reinforcement for participating in medical procedures. Interventions by social workers, child life specialists, psychologists, and psychiatrists are essential in working with the injured child and in helping the team to determine the best approach for handling the child and family.

After discharge, long-term psychological adjustment is usually satisfactory, although young children appear to adjust better than adolescents.[48] There is a greater incidence of adjustment problems in children with visible disfigurement of the hands and face, especially

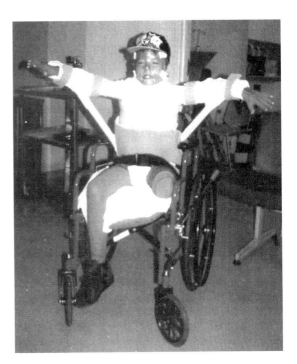

FIGURE 17–7. Neck collar and arm airplane splints with patient sitting in wheel chair.

in adolescents.[49] Resources for psychological counseling or group support should be considered in the pediatric burn injured population, especially in the case of adolescents with visible scars. Burn camps exist throughout the United States and can be a valuable support mechanism for pediatric burn survivors.

School Reintegration

Returning to school after a burn injury presents challenges to the child. Fear and anxiety are common complaints in pediatric burn survivors, and many children expend a great deal of energy in adjusting to their disabilities. The transition back to school can be accomplished through an orientation provided to the school community by trained personnel. Back-to-school programs, either done live or through the use of videotapes, are typically provided by burn center personnel or by selected members of burn foundations. The premise of these programs is that cognitive and affective education of children with burns diminishes their anxiety as well as that of the patient's family, school faculty and staff, and other students.[50] Issues addressed in school reentry programs include what happened to cause the injury, the hospitalization process, scars, splints, pressure garments, and other appliances the student may be wearing. Reentry programs also cover the child's abilities, suggest what friends of the injured child can do, and stress that the burned child may look different on the outside but is the same on the inside.

References

1. Reeves S, Warden G, Staley M: Management of the pediatric burn patient. In Richard R, Staley M (eds): Burn Care and Rehabilitation Principles and Practice. Philadelphia, FA Davis, 1994.
2. Morrow S, Smith D, et al: Etiology and outcome of pediatric burns. J Pediatr Surg 1996;31:329.
3. Erickson EJ, Merrill SW, et al: Differences in mortality from thermal injury between pediatric and adult patients. J Pediatr Surg 1991;26:821.
4. McLaughlin E, McGuire A: The causes, cost and prevention of childhood injuries. Am J Dis Child 1990;144:677.
5. Trudget EE, Shankowsky HA, et al: The role of inhalation injury in burn trauma. Ann Surg 1990;212:720.
6. Herndon D, Langner, et al: Pulmonary injury in burned patients. Surg Clin North Am 1987;67:31.
7. Shirani KZ, Pruitt B, et al: The influence of inhalation injury and pneumonia on burn mortality. Ann Surg 1987;205:82.
8. Hummel R, Greenhalgh D, et al: Outcome and socioeconomic aspects of suspected child abuse. J Burn Care Rehabil 1993;14:121.
9. Feldman K: Child abuse by burning. In Keep, S, Hellfire R (eds): The Battered Child, 3rd ed. Chicago, University of Chicago Press, 1980.
10. Rabban J, Blair J, et al: Mechanisms of pediatric electrical injury: New implications for product safety and injury prevention. Arch Pediatr Adolesc Med 1997;151:696.
11. Baron PW, Barrow R, et al: Prolonged use of propranolol safely decreases cardiac work in burned children. J Burn Care Rehabil 1997;18:223.
12. Holland K, Gillespie R: Estimating energy needs of pediatric patients with burns. J Burn Care Rehabil 1995;16:458.
13. O'Neil CE, Hutsler D, et al: Basic nutritional guidelines for pediatric burn patients. J Burn Care Rehabil 1989;10:278.
14. Klein GL, Herndon DN, et al: Long-term reduction in bone mass after severe burn injury in children. J Pediatr 1995;126:252.
15. Gray's Anatomy, 38th ed. New York, Churchill Livingstone, 1995.
16. Lund C, Browder N: The estimation of areas of burn. Surg Gynecol Obstet 1944;79:352.
17. Miller F, Richard R, et al: Triage and resuscitation of the burned patient. In Richard R, Staley M (eds): Burn Care and Rehabilitation Principles and Practice. Philadelphia, FA Davis, 1994.
18. Resources of optimal care of patients with burn injury. In Resources for Optimal Care of the Injured Patient. American College of Surgeons, Committee on Trauma, 1990.
19. Herndon D, Rutan R, et al: Management of the pediatric patient with burns. J Burn Care Rehabil 1993;14:3.
20. Richard R, Staley M: Burn patient evaluation and treatment Planning. In Richard R, Staley M (eds): Burn Care and Rehabilitation Principles and Practice. Philadelphia, FA Davis, 1994.
21. Kozerefski PM: Exercise and ambulation in the burned patient. In DeGregorio VR (ed): Rehabilitation of the Burned Patient. New York, Churchill Livingstone, 1984.
22. Kealy GP: Pharmacologic management of background pain in burn victims. J Burn Care Rehabil 1995;16:358.
23. Patterson DR: Non-opioid-based approaches to burn pain. J Burn Care Rehabil 1995;16:372.
24. Foertsch CE, O'Hara MW, et al: Parent participation during burn debridement in relation to behavioral distress. J Burn Care Rehabil 1996;17:372.
25. Saffle, J Schnebly W: Burn wound care. In Richard R, Staley M (eds): Burn Care and Rehabilitation Principles and Practice. Philadelphia, FA Davis, 1994.
26. Carr R, et al: Comparative study of occlusive wound dressings on full thickness wounds in domestic pigs. Wounds 1989;1:53.
27. Neville C, Dimick A: The trauma table as an alternative to the Hubbard tank in burn care. J Burn Care Rehabil 1987;8:574.
28. Richard R, et al: Autocontamination of the burn patient by hydrotherapy. Bull Clin Rev Burn Injury 1984;1:40.
29. Braddom R, et al: The physical treatment and rehabilitation of burn patients. In Hummel R (ed): Clinical Burn Therapy. Boston, John Wright-PSG, 1982.
30. Northdurft D, Smith P, et al: Exercise and treatment modalities. In Fissher S, Helm P (eds): Comprehensive Rehabilitation of Burns. Baltimore, Williams & Wilkins, 1984.
31. Borrell R, et al: Comparison of in vivo temperatures produced by hydrotherapy, paraffin wax treatment, and fluidotherapy. Phys Ther 1980;60:1273.
32. Ziskin M, Michlovitz A: Therapeutic ultrasound. In Michlovitz A (ed): Thermal Agents in Rehabilitation. Philadelphia, FA Davis, 1986.
33. Yurko L, Fratianne R: Evaluation of burn discharge teaching. Proc Am Burn Assoc 1988;20:5.
34. Binder H: Rehabilitation of the burned child. In Molnar GE (ed): Pediatric Rehabilitation, 2nd ed. Baltimore, Williams & Wilkins, 1992.
35. Larson D, Huang R, et al: Prevention and treatment of scar contracture. In Artz C, Moncrief A, et al (eds): Burns: A Team Approach. Philadelphia, WB Saunders, 1979.
36. Zamboni W, Cassidy M, et al: Hand burns in children under 5 years of age. Burns 1987;13:476.
37. Mann R, Yeong EK: Do custom-fitted pressure garments provide adequate pressure? J Burn Care Rehabil 1997;18:247.
38. Fricke N, Omnell L, et al: Skeletal and dental disturbances after facial burns and pressure garments. J Burn Car Rehabil 1996;17:338.
39. Housinger TA, Wondrely L: The use of Biobrane for coverage of the pediatric donor site. J Burn Care Rehabil 1993;14:26.
40. De Agustin JC, Morris SF, et al: Tissue expansion in pediatric burn reconstruction. J Burn Care Rehabil 1993;14:43.
41. Blakeney P, Moore M, et al: Parental stress as a cause and effect of pediatric burn injury. J Burn Care Rehabilitation 1993;14:73.
42. Libber S, Stayton D. Childhood burns reconsidered: The child, the family and the burn injury. J Trauma 1984;24:245.
43. Noyes R, Frye S, et al: Stressful life events and burn injuries. J Trauma 1979;19:141.
44. Seligman R, Mac Millan B, et al: The burned child: A neglected area of psychiatry. Am J Psychiatry 1971;128:52.
45. Wilkins T, Campbell J: Psychological concerns in the pediatric burn unit. Burns 1981;7:208.
46. Knudson-Cooper M: Emotional care of the hospitalized burned child. J Burns Crit Care 1982;3:109.
47. Moss B, Everett J, et al: Psychologic support and pain management of the burn patient. In Richard R, Staley M (eds): Burn Care and Rehabilitation Principles and Practice. Philadelphia, FA Davis, 1994.
48. Sawyer M, Minde K, et al: The burned child—scarred for life? Burns 1982;9:205.
49. Bogaerts F, Boecks W: Burns and sexuality. J Burn Care Rehabil 1992;13:39.
50. Blakeney P: School reintegration. J Burn Care Rehabil 1995;26:180.

Chapter 18

Rehabilitation Care for the Child with Joint Disease

Hilary B. Berlin, MD

The rehabilitative care of a child with joint disease must take into account the effect of the disease process on growth and development. The rehabilitation program requires a team approach that includes the child and family. Chronic illness in childhood may have long-lasting consequences related to deformity, growth retardation, loss of function, and social isolation. The goal of rehabilitation is to maintain or restore age-appropriate function and development.

Juvenile Rheumatoid Arthritis

Juvenile rheumatoid arthritis (JRA) is the most common connective tissue disease in children. It is defined by the American Rheumatism Association as the presence of arthritis lasting 6 weeks or longer with onset in children under the age of 16 years. Disease onset is classified in the first six months to be oligoarthritis involving fewer than five joints, polyarthritis with five or more joints involved, or systemic. Exclusion of other diseases is necessary for diagnosis.[1–3] Onset in childhood accounts for about 5% of rheumatoid arthritis cases.[4] The incidence is reported as 13.9 per 100,000 per year with a prevalence of 113.4 per 100,000 children.[5]

Cause

The cause of JRA is unknown. Possible contributing factors include genetic predisposition, immunologic abnormalities, infection, and trauma. There are reported associations of HLA-DR5 with antinuclear antibody (ANA)–positive disease and uveitis[6,7] and of DRw6 with pauciarticular disease.[8] HLA-DR4 is more frequent in rheumatoid factor (RF)–positive adults with rheumatoid arthritis than in RF-positive juvenile-onset arthritis. Immunologic findings include increased number of B cells in the blood, which produce autoantibodies and cytokine activity,

reduced T-cell suppressor activity, and complement activation.[9] The specific role of the immune system in JRA has not been definitively determined.

Infectious cause has been studied with possible agents including *Mycobacterium tuberculosis*, Epstein-Barr virus, and parvovirus B19. Rubella virus has been isolated from the synovial fluid of children with persistent JRA.[10] Epstein-Barr virus–associated suppressor responses are compromised. The pathogenesis of infection causing joint destruction can occur by immune complex deposition, antigen deposition, molecular mimicry leading to an autoimmune response, or arthritogenic toxins.[11]

Pathophysiology

Stimulation of B-cell and T-cell production occurs with infiltration of the synovial tissue. There is inflammation and hypertrophy of the synovial tissue with an increased production of synovial fluid. Joint pressure increases with notable swelling of the joint. Thickening of the synovial membrane occurs, and this may protrude into the joint space. With chronic synovitis and effusion, erosion of the surrounding cartilage and bone can develop. In children, the duration of chronic synovitis is longer before joint destruction occurs than in adults.[12] Enzymes cause destructive changes in the articular cartilage, bone, and other surrounding structures.[13] Joint fluid has increased number of cells.

Clinical Presentation

There are five types of onset in JRA (Table 18–1). Polyarticular-type onset accounts for 35% of children with JRA. Girls are affected more often than boys. More than five joints must be involved in the first 6 months. Asymmetric involvement of large joints occurs. There are two

TABLE 18–1. Juvenile Rheumatoid Arthritis

Onset	Median Age of Onset	Sex	Joints Involved	Serology	HLA	Outcome
Polyarticular			≥ 5			
RF (–)	1–3 yrs	Girls	Large joints; knee, wrist, elbow, ankle often symmetric	Sometimes ANA (+)	—	Variable
RF (+)	12 yrs	Girls	Similar to adult-onset RA	ANA (+)	DR4	Severe arthritis in > 50%
Pauciarticular			≥ 4			
Type I	1–3 yrs	Girls	Large joints; knee, ankle, elbow	ANA (+) RF (–)	DR5 DR6 DR8	Chronic iritis—risk for vision loss, good outcome for arthritis
Type II	10 yrs	Boys	Large joints; hip, sacroiliac	ANA (–) RF (–)	B27	Acute iritis, may progress to spondyloarthropathy
Systemic	Any	Boys and girls	Varied	ANA (–) RF (–)	—	Poor outcome with polyarticular involvement

RF, Rheumatoid factor, ANA, antinuclear antibody.

subgroups: 90% have RF-negative polyarticular arthritis and 10% have RF-positive polyarticular arthritis.

RF-negative polyarthritis comprises 25% of all patients with JRA. Joint stiffness, swelling, loss of mobility, and pain can be present at onset. Joint effusion, synovial thickening, and periarticular edema cause visible swelling. Children may complain of stiffness, but many do not complain of pain with inflamed joints.[10] Popliteal cysts may occur from herniation of thickened synovial tissues and fluid. Onset is symmetric with involvement of the large joints—the knees, ankles, wrists, and elbows. Involvement of metacarpophalangeal joints, interphalangeal joints, and cervical spine occurs as well. Hip involvement is present in half the children and is a cause of late disability from erosion of the femoral head. Extraarticular manifestations include irritability, malaise, mild anemia, and low-grade fever.

RF-positive polyarticular onset occurs in 5% of children with JRA. It is characterized by onset after age 11 years with female predominance. The disease course is similar to adult-onset rheumatoid arthritis. It is reported to be associated with HLA-DR4 in 53–77%[6,14] of cases. Findings include symmetric joint involvement, subcutaneous nodules (Fig. 18–1), and erosive disease. Joints involved include the small joints of the fingers and feet, knees, ankles, wrists, elbows, shoulders, temporomandibular joint, and cervical spine.

The pauciarticular subtype accounts for the largest percentage of children with JRA, approximately 50%. Involvement is limited to five or fewer joints. There are two subgroups—early-onset and late-onset.

The early-onset group are predominantly preschool-aged girls who present before age 4 years. This onset accounts for 30–40% of all children with JRA. Ninety percent are ANA-positive and RF-negative. Most often, large joints, such as the knee, ankle, and elbow, are involved. There is a high risk of iridocyclitis that may be asymptomatic, so these children require routine eye examinations because loss of vision can occur insidiously. There is an association noted in several studies with HLA-DR5, HLA-DR8, and

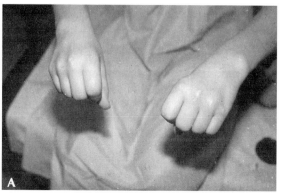
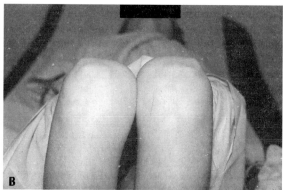

FIGURE 18–1. A and B, Subcutaneous nodules in RF-positive polyarticular-onset juvenile rheumatoid arthritis.

HLA-DR6.[9,15] Eighty percent of these children continue to have fewer than five joints involved with limited disability, but 20% go on to develop polyarticular disease.[12]

The late-onset subgroup occurs in 10–15% of children with JRA and in 9–10-year-old boys. Involved joints are the knees and sacroiliac joints, and enthesitis can be present. There may be tenderness over the iliac crest, patella, calcaneus, or metatarsal heads. These children are at risk for acute iritis. RF and ANA are negative. There is an association with HLA-B27 in 90%. Half of these children later develop ankylosing spondylitis or other seronegative spondyloarthropathy. There are reported cases of a subset of children with oligoarticular-onset JRA who are RF-positive and had early development of erosive disease.[16]

Systemic-onset JRA was first described by Still in 1897[17] and is characterized by the acute onset of high spiking fevers, rash, hepatosplenomegaly, lymphadenopathy, arthritis, fatigue, myalgia, irritability, and pericarditis. The rash is characterized by salmon-colored macular lesions with central pallor over the trunk and affected joints. It can also occur on the palms and soles and is more pronounced with fever. Pericarditis or pleuritis is present in one-third of patients. There is no particular age of onset, with boys and girls affected with equal frequency. Systemic symptoms may precede the arthritis by several months. The joint symptoms may be more notable when fever is present. This onset accounts for 15% of patients with JRA. RF and ANA are negative. The disease course is variable and may progress to severe polyarticular disease with erosions in 25%. These children are at risk for growth retardation and localized growth abnormalities, such as micrognathia and leg length discrepancy. The small joints are most often involved.

Important differences exist in children with JRA compared with adults with rheumatoid arthritis. In JRA, there are five distinct modes of onset. Systemic features are more common in children. Adults have joint destruction earlier, whereas children have synovitis with erosive disease occurring later. Children may have asymptomatic arthritis in which they do not complain of pain but avoid using the involved joint so that muscle atrophy and contracture occur early. The pattern of contracture varies in children compared with adults. Children have large joint involvement more frequently than adults with rheumatoid arthritis. Wrist and hand deviations differ from adults with rheumatoid arthritis. Children tend to have ulnar deviation at the wrist with loss of extension. Radial deviation of the fingers occurs at the metacarpophalangeal joints with finger flexion. Tenosynovitis is more common in children than bursitis. Rheumatoid nodules occur less frequently than in adults. The cervical spine is involved in children more often than in adults. Arthritis in children tends to be ANA-positive, RF-negative, whereas adult rheumatoid arthritis is generally RF-positive. Disturbances of growth and development as well as nutritional parameters must be considered during childhood.

Laboratory Tests

IgM RF is present in up to 20% of children with JRA compared with 80% of adults with rheumatoid arthritis, usually in the subset of adolescent girls with polyarticular presentation. ANA is often positive, especially in children with pauciarticular disease that is RF-positive. A positive ANA does not correlate with disease severity. The erythrocyte sedimentation rate (ESR) can be elevated. Other nonspecific findings are platelet and white blood cell elevation and anemia of chronic disease. Joint fluid is inflammatory with elevated protein, low glucose, low-to-normal complement, and a cell count of 5000–80,000 cells/mm^3. There is little radiographic change early on except for soft tissue swelling. Periarticular bone demineralization is seen radiographically once 50% demineralization is present (Fig. 18–2). Later, subchondral erosions and loss of joint space occur. Magnetic resonance (MR) imaging may reveal increased frequency and severity of joint destruction as well as other changes not seen on radiographs.[18]

Management

The management of children with JRA includes the use of medications, along with rehabilitation, family education, and psychosocial support for the child to function in the age-appropriate environment. A pyramid approach has traditionally been used in adults with rheumatoid arthritis and children with JRA, with nonsteroidal antiinflammatory drugs (NSAIDs) to control the inflammatory process, physical and occupational therapy to prevent deformity and maximize function, and family education and support as the base with additional medications being added (Fig. 18–3). The treatment approach has been reconsidered[19,20] because of concerns of long-lasting effects from the duration and severity of the disease on function and quality of life and from potential harmful side effects of combination NSAID use and slow-acting antirheumatic drugs (SAARDs). It has been suggested that treatment provided once irreversible joint changes are present does not have a significant

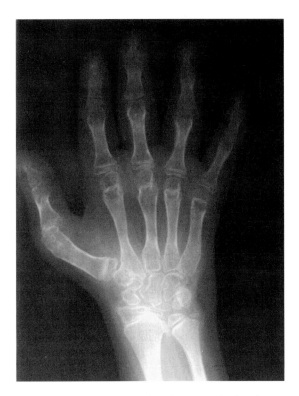

FIGURE 18–2. Radiographic changes in the hand-peri-articular deossification, bony overgrowth at the epiphysis with relative shortening of the distal ulna, erosions at the metacarpal heads.

effect.[13] Current treatment proposals aim toward inducing remission early in the disease course, including the use of intra-articular steroids.

Medications

Medications used in the treatment of JRA are summarized in Table 18–2. Salicylates in the form of aspirin are given for a 6–8 week course. If effective, treatment is continued for 6 months. Side effects are tinnitus, reduced

Experimental
therapy

Immunosuppressive
agents

Steroids

SAARDs

NSAIDs, patient/family education,
family support, rehabilitation, nutrition

FIGURE 18–3. Pyramid approach to management of the child with juvenile rheumatoid arthritis.

platelet function, and gastric irritation. Aspirin is used less frequently because of the occurrence of Reye's syndrome with influenza and varicella infections.

Of the other NSAIDs, naproxen, tolmetin, and ibuprofen are approved for use in children. Naproxen is given in two doses per day, which may be beneficial in the older child when treatment compliance is a concern. It is available in a liquid form. NSAIDs provide pain relief and reduce fever in addition to anti-inflammatory benefits. Ibuprofen has a shorter half-life so the dose is given more frequently. Side effects are similar to salicylates, with gastrointestinal irritation, renal toxicity, hepatic toxicity, and reduced platelet function. NSAIDs can be given with gastrointestinal protective drugs and given with meals to reduce irritation. If no improvement occurs with one medication in 6–8 weeks, a different NSAID is used for another period of 6–8 weeks. More than 50% of children improve with NSAID therapy. Treatment is continued for 1–2 years after suppression of disease activity.

The second line of drug therapy has been termed the *disease-modifying antirheumatic drugs* (DMARDs) or SAARDs. These include gold salts, antimalarials, D-penicillamine, and sulfasalazine. Long-term studies in children and adults do not prove that disease progression is modified.[21] In the traditional approach the DMARDs or SAARDs[22] are used later in the disease course because of the potential toxicity of these agents. These drugs may take several weeks to months to take effect.

Gold salts are given by weekly intramuscular injection. Of children receiving gold salts, 60–70% show improvement.[23] Some studies show less improvement with serious side effects in children with systemic disease.[24] Side effects include skin rash, proteinuria, and bone marrow suppression, so careful laboratory monitoring is necessary. In children with improvement within 6 months, the frequency of dosing is reduced, but it is unclear when treatment should be discontinued. Oral gold (auranofin) has been studied and found to be safe for use in children but with less predictable efficacy[25] than intramuscular administration.

Hydroxychloroquine is the most commonly used antimalarial drug. It is administered orally on a daily basis. Adverse effects are macular degeneration, which is a concern in young children who cannot report vision problems.

D-penicillamine is given orally and induces remission in 60–70% of cases.[26] It can cause bone marrow suppression, rashes, and renal toxicity. Sulfasalazine is a combination of salicylic acid and sulfapyridine. It can be given orally and

TABLE 18–2. Drug Therapy in Juvenile Rheumatoid Arthritis

Drug	Dosage	Usage/Length of Treatment	Side Effects
Aspirin	80–100 mg/kg/d qid up to 25 kg; otherwise 650 mg qid	At least 6–8 wk	Drowsiness, tinnitus, hyperventilation, concern of Reye's syndrome if used during varicella or influenza, reduced platelet function, gastrointestinal irritation
Naproxen	10–20 mg/kg/d bid, suspension available	At least 6–8 wk	Gastrointestinal irritation, cutaneous pseudoporphyria, cutanea tarda
Ibuprofen	35–45 mg/kg/d qid, 45 mg/kg/d if using suspension	At least 6–8 wk	Gastrointestinal, rash, aseptic meningitis
Tolmetin	25–30 mg/kg/d tid		Gastrointestinal irritation
Indomethacin*	1–2 mg/kg/d tid or qid	For fever and pericarditis in systemic JRA	Headache, epigastric pain, difficulty paying attention
Diclofenac*	2–3 mg/kg/d qid		Mild gastrointestinal effects
Piroxicam*	0.3–0.6 mg/kg/d qd	Advantage of once-a-day dosing	
Gold salts	0.75–1 mg/kg/wk, max 50 mg/wk	At least 6 mo use early for polyarthritis	Mucosal ulcers, rash, proteinuria, nephropathy, leukopenia, thrombocytopenia, anemia
Auranofin*	0.1–0.2 mg/kg,d qd or bid, max 9 mg/d		Gastrointestinal, rash
Hydroxychloroquine	5–7 mg/kg/d, max 400 mg/d	8–12 wk	Macular degeneration
D-Penicillamine	3 mg/kg/d, max 250 mg/d 6 g/kg/d, max 500 mg/d 10 g/kg/d, max 750 mg/d	3 mo 3 mo 1–3 yr For polyarthritis; not systemic or pauciarticular	Bone marrow suppression, renal, rash, autoimmune, proteinuria
Sulfasalazine*	40–60 mg/kg/d divided 3–6 doses	6–8 wk	Gastrointestinal, rash, hypersensitivity, renal toxicity, headache
Methotrexate*	0.25 mg/kg/wk orally, increase at 2–4 wk intervals to 1.0 mg/kg/wk; can be given SQ		Avoid use with NSAID because it may potentiate bone marrow suppression, gastrointestinal, hepatotoxicity
Azathioprine*	0.5–2.0 mg/kg/d	Take for 1 yr or more, monitor every 1–2 mo	Gastrointestinal, liver, dose-related leukopenia
Cyclophosphamide*	0.5–1 g/m² IV, monthly		Alopecia, nausea, vomiting, bladder, pulmonary fibrosis, leukopenia, thrombocytopenia
Cyclosporine	3–5 mg/kg/d		Immunosuppression, hypertension, renal insufficiency
Corticosteroids		Most potent anti-inflammatory agent	Growth failure, adrenal suppression, osteopenia, cushingoid appearance, avascular necrosis, weight gain, cataracts, psychosis, myopathy
Prednisone	0.1–1.0 mg/kg/d orally, max 40 mg		
Pulse steroid methyl-prednisolone	10–30 mg/kg/dose; max 1 g		

* Not approved for use in children.

qid, Four times per day; tid, three times per day; bid, two times per day; qd, once a day; NSAID, nonsteroidal anti-inflammatory drug; IV, intravenously; SQ, subcutaneously.

comes in a liquid form. Side effects include gastrointestinal, renal, and central nervous system toxicity; headache; hepatotoxicity; and hypersensitivity reaction. Toxicity may occur more often in children than in adults treated for rheumatoid arthritis.

Immunosuppressive agents have been used in severe systemic or polyarticular disease that has not responded to other means of therapy. There has been hesitation to use these drugs because of the concern that the consequences of treatment may exceed the benefits except in life-threatening stages of illness. Methotrexate can be given orally and is dosed once a week. Toxicity includes bone marrow suppression, hepatotoxicity, and gastrointestinal upset. Laboratory surveillance is necessary. Most data regarding toxicity are in adults with rheumatoid arthritis and children with leukemia on higher doses.[22] Studies[27-29] have found methotrexate effective in achieving remission, but there is concern that flareups may recur once therapy is discontinued.

Cyclosporine blocks the production of interleukin-2 and the proliferation of synovial T cells. Cyclosporine has been used experimentally in children with refractory disease at a dose of 5 mg/kg/day orally and found to reduce the number of joints involved, morning stiffness, fever, and steroid usage.[30] Toxicity may limit usefulness, especially in higher doses, with side effects including renal, liver, and bone marrow toxicity. At low doses, less than 5 mg/kg/day, the most common side effect is gastrointestinal disturbance. The hypertension that limits use in adults, gingival hyperplasia, and hirsutism may not be seen as frequently in children. There may be benefit from combination therapy with methotrexate. Cyclosporine may have disease-modifying as well as anti-inflammatory effects.[31]

Azathioprine has been found to be an effective treatment for children with refractory disease and can reduce the use of steroids. It was not found to change the course of iridocyclitis. The main side effects are gastrointestinal disturbance, hepatotoxicity, and bone marrow suppression.[32]

Systemic corticosteroids are potent anti-inflammatory agents that are used when other options have failed or in severe systemic illness. They reduce symptoms but do not cause remission.[12] Long-term use is limited because of the effects on bone mineralization and growth.

TABLE 18–3. Rehabilitation of the Child with Juvenile Rheumatoid Arthritis

Rest
Splinting
Passive ROM
Active exercises for strengthening
Adaptive equipment
Functional training for ADLs and ambulation
Postsurgical rehabilitation
Nutrition
Counseling family and child

ROM, Range of motion; ADLs, activities of daily living.

Intraarticular steroids can suppress synovitis, and in one study remission was maintained for more than 6 months in 60% of the injected joints.[33] Side effects include subcutaneous atrophy and periarticular calcifications. Radiographic changes consistent with avascular necrosis have been described but may be due to the severe arthritis and not the steroid injection.[33] Topical steroids are used in the treatment of uveitis, and systemic steroids are indicated if inflammation persists.

Intravenous immunoglobulins (IVIG) have been used experimentally in children who failed other treatment, including methotrexate, steroids, and other SAARDs. A study of IVIG use in eight children with systemic-onset JRA showed reduced joint activity and systemic symptoms.[34]

Rehabilitation

Pain and stiffness reduce mobility and limit self-care, activities of daily living (ADLs), and socialization. The goal of rehabilitation (Table 18–3) is to minimize deformity while maintaining as close to a normal lifestyle as possible. Children should be followed early on to maintain joint mobility and flexibility. Rehabilitation also includes patient education.

To plan an individualized treatment program, the evaluation of the patient and family should include information regarding the presence of pain, stiffness, fatigue, systemic manifestations, developmental level, motor and cognitive skills, and restrictions in ADL or mobility. The social situation of the child and family is important to include the caretakers, physical environment and accessibility, availability of transportation, and parental ability to participate in the therapy program.

The physical assessment includes active and passive joint range of motion (ROM), signs of active joint involvement such as swelling, redness, heat, or effusion; presence of pain; muscle bulk and strength; limb length discrepancy (LLD); gait; and ADL. Posture is assessed in sitting and standing with attention to LLD and contracture, which cause asymmetry. Correction may be required to improve gait and stance endurance. Gait is evaluated with and without footwear. There is often a posture of hip (Fig. 18–4) and knee flexion with lumbar lordosis. Internal rotation of the femur may cause genu valgum and tibial external rotation. Loss of knee extension and limitation in hip mobility may be noted. Asymmetric flexion may be caused by an LLD, pelvic obliquity, or scoliosis. The MacBain and Hill[35] functional assessment for children with JRA measures timed ambulation, grip strength, dressing, and undressing.

The treatment program and modalities used depend on the state of the disease process. Therapeutic exercise includes ROM, strengthening, and endurance. Modalities are used in conjunction with exercise.

Pain Relief

It has been reported that young children complain of pain less than adults or may have difficulty localizing pain.[36] The existing pain measurement scale may not account for the cognitive age of the child and thus may not accurately reflect true occurrence of pain. Pain can be assessed using the child visual analogue scale (VAS) or the Varni/Thompson Pediatric Pain Questionnaire, which takes into account the child's cognitive level of development.[37] These measures allow more accurate assessment of pain in children with JRA. Pain is caused by stretching of the capsule, so children tend to limit movement and maintain the joint in flexion to reduce stretch and pain. This practice may hasten the development of flexion contractures. Acetaminophen may provide pain relief, although it does not have anti-inflammatory properties. It can be used in conjunction with NSAIDs. Dosing of medications before therapy may be beneficial. Modalities such as superficial heat and cold can be used on localized areas or by use of a warm bath. The cognitive-behavioral approach includes progressive muscle relaxation, breathing exercises, and guided imagery to reduce perceived pain.[38]

Rest

Rest may be necessary in the management of the child with JRA. Rest can be provided in three forms; bed rest, local joint rest with or without splints, and daily rest periods. Children with systemic-onset JRA may require a period of bed rest for management of myocarditis or pericarditis. Attention to positioning in bed, gentle daily ROM, and use of resting splints are important to prevent flexion contractures. Resting the joint is used more often in the adult population because of the concern that exercise increases joint inflammation.[39] Specific joints can be rested with the use of splinting. For example, splinting of the wrist provides support, rests the joint, and allows function of the fingers. A knee brace can limit knee flexion or control valgus to provide stability while permitting some ROM for ambulation.

In children, the level of fatigue and discomfort may be used as indicators for physical activity. If the child fatigues during the day, rest periods are provided. Rest in the prone position

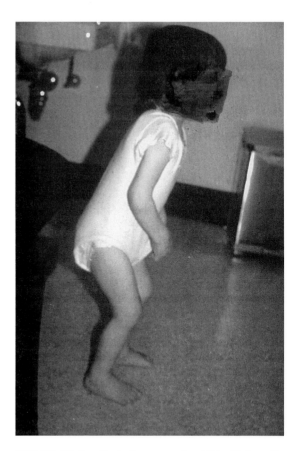

FIGURE 18–4. Typical posture of a child with juvenile rheumatoid arthritis.

allows positioning to reduce hip and knee flexion contracture (Fig. 18–5).[40] Parent and child should be instructed in joint protection to reduce excessive joint stress during activities. Activities that cause impact or excess joint stress, such as running, jumping, and skiing, are discouraged when joint protection is necessary.

Massage

Massage is used to relieve pain, reduce muscle spasm, and mobilize soft tissue. It can be used

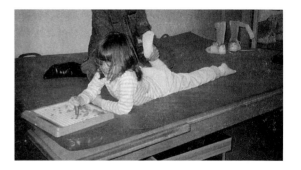

FIGURE 18–5. Resting in the prone position.

in conjunction with heat and cold modalities or prior to stretching and ROM exercises.

Heat

Heat can reduce stiffness, increase the extensibility of tissue, reduce pain, and muscle spasm.[41] Application of heat reduces the sensitivity of the muscle spindle to stretch.[42] Superficial heat can be provided by a warm bath or shower to reduce morning stiffness. Water temperature should be between 90 and 100°F.[43] Play activities for ROM can be performed in the water. Moist heat can be provided to a localized joint and the surrounding muscles to a depth of 1 cm with a hot pack. Paraffin is applied by dipping the involved area, especially the hands, to build up several layers. The area is covered with a towel to retain heat. Once the paraffin is removed, ROM exercises can be done. Fluidotherapy provides superficial dry heat to the hands or feet. Application of superficial heat is thought to reduce joint temperature,[44] but increases in joint temperature can occur with prolonged administration.[45] There is a concern that the application of heat can increase inflammation and accelerate the disease process that leads to cartilage destruction.[46] Ultrasound can provide deep heating but there is concern regarding the effect on the growth plate in children. Sleeping in pajamas, in a sleeping bag, or with warm blankets facilitates a relaxed position because cold induces a flexed position to maintain warmth.[47]

Cold

Cold can provide pain relief, increase the pain threshold, and reduce muscle spasm and swelling by vasoconstriction.[48] It can be used in acute injury to decrease the inflammatory response, pain, and swelling. Cold is applied by cold packs or ice massage. The general preference of children is for use of heat over cold. Cold should be used with caution on insensate areas and is contraindicated in the presence of Raynaud's phenomenon.

Range of Motion

For the child with an involved joint, the position of comfort that increases the joint space is flexion. The presence of pain and related muscle spasm may further induce the flexed position at rest so that flexion contractures occur. Passive ROM to preserve or regain joint mobility is performed daily in a home exercise program with supervision and instruction from the physical and occupational therapist.[49] Excessive flexion increases joint pressure.[50] The pressure rise is higher with greater effusion. Careful ROM

should be continued during the acute phase to prevent contracture, but excessive flexion should be avoided. Once active synovitis is controlled, a more aggressive approach can be taken to improve ROM. Active assisted ROM should be performed with the therapist or parent assisting the child in achieving maximal joint motion. Active ROM exercises can be performed in the bathtub, and play activities such as reaching or throwing can aid in upper extremity ROM.

Strengthening

Isometric strengthening exercises can be performed during acute inflammation or while on bed rest. This requires the cooperation of the child. Older children can perform isometric strengthening exercises while doing other activities, such as sitting in a chair doing homework or while using a computer. Play and recreational activities for ROM and strengthening include throwing a ball, riding a bicycle, and swimming. Exercises with a beach ball can provide range of motion for the elbows and shoulders.[51] Bicycle riding provides lower extremity exercise without weight bearing. The seat height and foot pedals of the bicycle should be set to provide extension at the knee and hip while pedaling. Swimming provides exercise with resistance to joint movement from the water while the buoyancy provides support. Exercising in water provides reduced weight bearing on painful joints.

Activities of Daily Living

ADLs in children refer to age-appropriate self-care skills, play, and school-related activities. Rehabilitation aims at helping the child perform efficiently, compensating for reduced mobility and function, providing assistive devices or environmental modification.[40] Clothing modification to avoid fasteners that are difficult to manage include elastic waistbands, the use of Velcro closures for clothing and footwear, and larger-sized buttons. Specific training can improve dexterity when modifications are not an alternative. To improve independence with feeding, a straw can be used to reduce the need to hold and lift a cup or flex the neck. Other adapted utensils can help to decrease the grip strength necessary for handling them. Bathroom adaptations accommodate limitations in mobility and dexterity. School-related skills can be improved by the use of wrist support, adapted pens to reduce finger grip strength, and computer access. Seating should provide trunk and pelvic symmetry with support if necessary. The feet should be plantigrade, and excess flexion should be avoided at the knee and hip. Desk and table location should be assessed to prevent excess trunk and neck flexion. The child may need to stand or walk around periodically to reduce stiffness.

Physical Fitness

Children with JRA have reduced activity because of pain, limitations in mobility, or disease activity. Children with polyarticular disease were found to be less fit than healthy children.[52] A modified physical education program may be required, especially with cervical spine involvement, to avoid contact sports. General aerobic conditioning programs, such as swimming, walking, dancing, and tai chi, are particularly valuable.

The home exercise program should be incorporated into the child's daily routine and play activities. Goals and time requirement should be realistic to improve compliance. The child should participate where possible in choosing the activities and in performing the exercises. The program is monitored by the physical and occupational therapists.

Splinting

Splinting can be used to reduce inflammation by providing joint rest, position to reduce contracture, support weakened structures, and assist function. Resting splints provide joint alignment and rest. They can be used during the day and removed for ROM exercises or at night. The upper extremity is splinted in a functional position with the wrist in 15–20 degrees of extension; the fingers in some flexion, 25 degrees at the metacarpophalangeal and a few degrees at the proximal interphalangeal; ulnar deviation controlled; and the thumb in opposition (Fig. 18–6). Ring splints (Fig. 18–7) can be applied to individual fingers in the presence of swan-neck or boutonnière deformity. A cervical collar can provide support when there is cervical spine involvement. Knee splints are used at night to maintain extension. A posterior splint should not be applied if contracture is present and there is tibial subluxation.[53] Splinting may be alternated, left side one night and right the next, to allow for use of one extremity so that the child can walk to the bathroom or move in bed or for comfort in sleep.

Dynamic splinting or serial casting is used to improve joint ROM. Continuous stretch is provided by the splint, and the splint is adjusted as improvement occurs. Functional splinting provides support during daily activity. Splints can support the wrist and fingers for ADL. Foot orthoses provide arch support and reduce pain in weight bearing. Splints used for

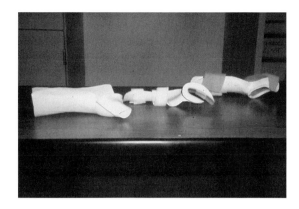

FIGURE 18–6. Hand splints.

functional activities should be lightweight and easy to don.

Adaptive Equipment

Adaptive equipment can be used to improve function and to reduce pain and protect joints. Devices may be poorly accepted in children because they make them *different* from peers and can be burdensome to use. The child should participate in the assessment of useful adaptive devices to improve compliance with use. Dressing sticks and shoe horns with long handles, zipper pulls, and flexible sock cones may improve independence in donning clothing on the lower extremities for the child with limitation in hip or knee flexion. Long-handled hairbrushes and wash mitts can be used for grooming. Elevation of toilet seats and safety bars are necessary if there is limited flexion in the lower extremities. Gait aids can be used to reduce pain on weight bearing and for balance. A cane can be held in the hand opposite the painful lower extremity.[54] If there is elbow or wrist involvement, crutches or a walker with forearm platforms reduces forces on the hands and wrist.[40] Use of a posterior walker encourages upright posture and reduces the tendency toward flexion. Wheelchair

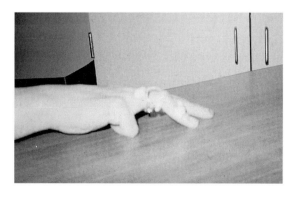

FIGURE 18–7. Finger ring splint.

use is avoided whenever possible to maintain activity and ambulation. When wheelchair use is required for mobility, the child should have a standing program, ambulate when possible, and spend time lying prone to reduce contracture development and to maintain muscle strength.

Surgical Management

Surgical intervention may be necessary to reduce pain and contracture. Soft tissue releases, posterior capsulotomy, and tendon lengthening can correct contracture. Joint replacement is generally delayed until bone growth is complete. Joint replacement can be done in the hands, hips, and knees if there are components to fit the child's size. In the preoperative assessment, other joint involvement that may affect rehabilitation is noted, and a therapy program for the postsurgical period is reviewed. A presurgical rehabilitation program aims at strengthening the muscles required for mobility in the postoperative period and to train ambulation with assistive devices. Difficulty may arise in the postoperative rehabilitation phase in polyarticular involvement. If hip or knee reconstruction requires the use of a walker or crutches, there may be problems because of upper extremity arthritis and contracture. Platform walkers may allow for better distribution of weight-bearing pressure. Loosening occurs in the acetabular component in children as opposed to the femoral component in adults.[55] The life expectancy of the prosthesis may be reduced by loosening from the extent of physical activity in children once pain is reduced and improved ROM allows increased function. Synovectomy can provide relief of pain but does not alter the disease process. The knee is the most common site for synovectomy. There is a possibility of loss of ROM postoperatively, so the arthroscopic approach is preferred.

Specific Joints

Cervical Spine

Cervical spine involvement (Fig. 18–8) occurs more often in children with JRA than in adults with rheumatoid arthritis. Manifestations of cervical spine involvement include restricted ROM, pain, and muscle spasm, which may present as torticollis. Limitation in mobility is seen in extension, rotation, and side-bending. During periods of acute pain with muscle spasm, a soft collar can be used. The collar serves as a reminder to maintain the neck in proper alignment and may provide warmth. Moist superficial heat or cold may reduce pain and muscle spasm. Sleeping with minimal use of pillows is encouraged to maintain a neutral position and reduce the development of flexion contracture. If a pillow is used, it should support cervical lordosis without causing flexion.[56] Subluxation of the atlantoaxial joint can occur when its involvement leads to erosion of the transverse ligament. Excessive flexion can cause neurologic sequelae, which are seen less often in children than adults.[56] If subluxation is present, a firm collar should be worn during automobile travel. Forced ROM at the neck should be avoided, and children should not participate in contact sports that put them at risk for injury. Precautions during intubation for anesthesia include maintaining the neck in a neutral position to avoid hyperextension of the head on a flexed neck.[57]

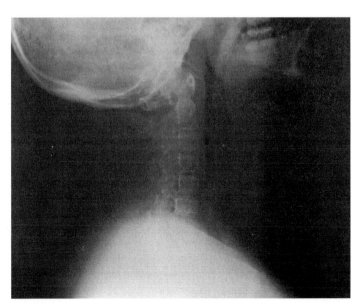

FIGURE 18–8. Cervical spine radiograph with apophyseal joint fusion at C2–C3, C3–C4, C4–C5, C1 on C2 subluxation, and loss of cervical lordosis.

Positioning of books on a stand at eye level and adjustment of desk height, televisions, and computers reduce time spent with the neck in flexion. Children can play or watch television in the prone position to facilitate strengthening of the neck extensors and reduce time spent with the neck flexed. Loss of neck ROM may impair the field of vision so that the child turns the trunk to compensate. This situation can make driving difficult for older adolescents.

Temporomandibular Joint

The temporomandibular joint is involved in up to 50% of the children with JRA.[58] There is an increase in synovial fluid causing increased pressure leading to pain and swelling.[59] The child may complain of pain on chewing and mouth opening. Limited movements can affect the structural development of the mandible.[60] Micrognathia (Fig. 18–9) results from reduced mandibular growth. Unilateral involvement leads to facial asymmetry. Mandibular and facial growth disturbances in symptomatic temporomandibular joint involvement are more common in polyarticular subtypes of JRA.[60] Factors considered in the treatment are the severity of functional deficit and deformity, activity of disease, stage of physical growth, and psychological considerations. The mouth-opening range can be measured and followed during active involvement. Exercises to increase ROM can include chewing gum and biting a large object. Ice packs can be used to reduce muscle spasm, and moist heat can be applied using a hot water–soaked wash cloth.[56] Surgical reconstruction for the mandible is required if growth deficit causes functional problems.

Shoulder

Shoulder involvement is not common at onset of disease, occurring in only 8%. Likelihood of shoulder involvement and severity of loss of mobility increase to 33% with duration of the disease.[61,62] Children lose abduction and internal rotation, in contrast with adults, who lose external rotation.[62–64] Loss of glenohumeral motion is initially compensated for by scapular motion. Loss of shoulder mobility causes difficulty with midline ADLs, such as toileting and grooming. Shoulder position and posture should be maintained when sitting. Exercises such as throwing a ball overhead, painting on an easel, or throwing darts can be performed to maintain shoulder abduction, flexion, and extension and to avoid loss of function in performing midline ADLs. Codman's exercises can be done to eliminate stress on the joint. Gentle stretch along with gentle traction can be used to increase ROM.[56]

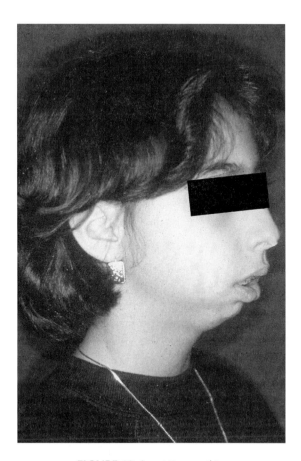

FIGURE 18–9. Micrognathia.

Elbow

At least 90 degrees of flexion range is needed at the elbow for ADL. If elbow flexion contractures occur with loss of supination or pronation, the child compensates with shoulder or trunk motion. These contractures may interfere with eating, grooming, and reaching for objects. The elbow extensors should be strengthened with supination and pronation maintained. Loss of more than 45 degrees of elbow extension limits the ability to use the arms as leverage to rise from a seated position and makes toileting and lower extremity dressing difficult. Dynamic splinting can be applied to increase elbow extension or flexion by providing slow sustained stretch.

Wrist

Wrist involvement is common in children. There is early loss of extension with progression of flexion contracture at the wrist. Children often maintain the wrist in a flexed position during active hand use, which further contributes to flexion contractures. A resting splint is used at night to maintain functional position with the wrist at 15–20 degrees of extension and the fingers in a few degrees of flexion. A splint can be used during the day to support the wrist in extension while allowing the fingers and thumb free motion. Ulnar deviation can also occur and should be controlled with resting splints. Stretching and splinting can be used to prevent contracture development. Strengthening of wrist extension and radial deviation is necessary to reduce contracture in flexion and ulnar deviation. Once contracture develops, serial casting can reduce deformity. Moist heat can be applied to reduce spasm and improve elasticity of tissue; the cast is then applied while the wrist is held in as much extension as possible, with ulnar deviation and subluxation controlled. The cast is removed in 48–72 hours and the process repeated. Stretching can also be provided by commercially available dynamic splinting. If joint ankylosis is inevitable, the hand should be splinted in a neutral position for optimal functional use in self-care.[56]

Hand

Fingers lose both flexion and extension range, causing limitations in functional grasp that may affect ADL and school function. Swan-neck deformity is more commonly seen in adults. It consists of hyperextension at the proximal interphalangeal joint. There may be associated metacarpophalangeal flexion. Boutonnière deformity has flexion at the proximal interphalangeal joint with hyperextension at the distal interphalangeal joint. Concomitant metacarpophalangeal hyperextension may occur. The extensor tendons lengthen and lose the ability to extend the proximal interphalangeal joint. Eventually, there is volar subluxation of the lateral bands. The use of ring splints in metal or plastic can control proximal interphalangeal flexion and extension. Clay can be used for strengthening the fingers during play, and wrist extensors can be strengthened with keyboard use. Activities should incorporate full ROM for the fingers and avoid maintaining flexion with ulnar deviation at the wrist.

Lower Extremities

In the lower extremity, flexion contractures occur at the knee and hip. Knee flexion contracture tends to lead and increase the same at the hips on weight bearing. The child spends more time sitting because ambulation is painful and fatiguing, which encourages further flexion contracture, weakness, and atrophy from deconditioning, disuse, and osteoporosis. Prevention strategies include (1) prone lying 20 minutes per day with the hips and knees extended and the feet off the edge of the bed, (2) ROM exercises to stretch the hip flexors and the hamstrings, (3) strengthening of antagonist muscle groups, (4) encouraging upright posture and ambulation, and (5) resting splints.

Hip

Hip involvement occurs in half of children with polyarticular arthritis. The hips develop flexion contractures with internal rotation and adduction, compared with adults who tend to have external rotation and abduction.[56] There is a compensatory increased lumbar lordosis to maintain the center of gravity. Hip extensor weakness and atrophy, reduced ambulation, and increased time seated contribute to the flexion contracture. Abductor weakness and loss of rotation lead to compensation at the trunk and a higher energy cost in ambulation.[48] The hip flexors can be stretched prone as mentioned or supine with the extremity over the edge of the table or bed. Ambulation in a pool, swimming, and bicycling provide strengthening of the hip extensors. When hip involvement occurs at an early age with reduced weight bearing, it can result in an abnormal femoral neck angle and acetabular development leading to possible lateral subluxation,[48] whereas adults are more likely to develop protrusio acetabuli.[56] Hip development can be assisted or improved by supported standing in a supine or prone stander, which allows upright posture and weight bearing in children who do little standing or ambulation. The child can play or do homework while in the stander. A prone stander allows strengthening of the neck and hip extensors, whereas a supine stander maintains the legs in extension. Hip disease may result in destruction of the femoral head.

Knee

The knee can be maintained in extension with resting splints, or a dynamic splint with an adjustable knee joint can be worn to improve ROM and limit excessive flexion. The knee tends to have a position of flexion with valgus, which can cause difficulty with stairs, jumping, running, and squat-to-stand transitions. The position that minimizes intraarticular pressure is 30 degrees of flexion. The child maintains the leg in flexion as the position of comfort because the intraarticular pressure is reduced.[50,65] Pain-induced hamstring spasm adds to the knee flexion. Eventually, there is quadriceps atrophy with reduction in active extension strength, capsular fibrosis, and contracture.[56] Causes for the valgus tendency may include exaggeration of the normal tendency because of muscle weakness, hamstring spasm pulling the tibia laterally, overgrowth of the medial femoral condyle, external tibial torsion, internal rotation at hip, and vastus medialis atrophy allowing more valgus at the end of extension.[48] Quadriceps strength can be maintained with isometric exercise if ROM is too painful, otherwise with active knee extension exercises. Activities such as kicking, bicycling, and walking can provide strengthening. A knee brace can limit flexion and valgus while permitting extension within the range and allow adjustment as the ROM improves. Caution must be exercised in avoiding forced extension of the knee when contracture is present because this can exacerbate posterior tibial subluxation.[53] When the brace is removed, active exercises to strengthen the quadriceps should be performed. Soft tissue releases may be required for fixed contractures when the joint space is maintained.[53] Joint replacement surgery is generally delayed until skeletal maturity is achieved. If a valgus deformity at the knee is not amenable to conservative treatment, osteotomy can correct alignment.

Ankle and Foot

Involvement of the metatarsophalangeal joint causes reduced pushoff resulting in a flat-foot gait. Molded foot orthoses can be used to reduce pain in weight bearing over the heel and metatarsal heads. Metatarsal pads inserted into shoes reduce weight bearing over the metatarsal heads. Spasm of the long toe flexors and toe extension to reduce weight bearing occur when the metatarsophalangeal joints are involved and cause the clawtoe deformity with hyperextension at the metatarsophalangeal and flexion at the interphalangeal. Varus at the hindfoot causes weight bearing over the lateral foot border. Valgus deformity can contribute to the knee valgus. A UCLB (University of California, Biomechanics Laboratory) type of orthosis can prevent or control varus and valgus deformity. When pain at the heels is present on weight bearing, the child walks on the toes, and plantar flexion contracture results. A posterior leaf spring or hinged-type ankle-foot orthosis can be worn to reduce the loss of dorsiflexion range and to control varus and valgus. Night resting splints are used to prevent plantar flexion contractures, or dynamic posterior leaf spring type of orthosis can be used to improve dorsiflexion range. Ankle rotation exercises, balancing exercises, and raising the heel on a step can strengthen the ankle muscles.[48] Footwear should provide support and comfort. The fit should be adequate to accommodate any deformity present. High heels should be avoided if there is concern about developing plantar flexion contractures. A lift can be added to the shoe to accommodate LLDs.

JRA is a chronic disease characterized by remissions and exacerbations. Even with remission, there can be long-lasting problems related to contractures, LLDs, growth retardation, bone deformity, and osteopenia. This can lead to further disability such as gait deviations and scoliosis as the child grows.

Bone Mineralization

Children with JRA are at risk for developing osteopenia because of failure to achieve adequate skeletal bone mass.[66] Bone mineral density was found to be low in almost 30% of children with JRA who had not been treated with steroids.[67] The low bone mineral density was associated with severity of joint involvement and disease activity. Risk factors include lack of physical activity, inadequate vitamin D and calcium, low body weight, limited sun exposure, and systemic glucocorticoids. Calcium supplementation to increase bone density should be considered for children at risk.[68]

Leg Length Discrepancy

It is important to distinguish true LLD from apparent LLD. Inflammation causing bone overgrowth at the distal femur can cause a true LLD, which later leads to pelvic asymmetry and scoliosis. The increased blood flow can also lead to early epiphyseal closure and overall limb shortening (Fig. 18–10). If the epiphyseal plate is involved, local growth can be reduced causing shortening of an extremity, a small hand or foot, and micrognathia. Long-term steroid use can reduce overall growth of the child. Atrophy occurs in the muscles surrounding the involved joints (Fig. 18–11). Flexion of the longer knee and

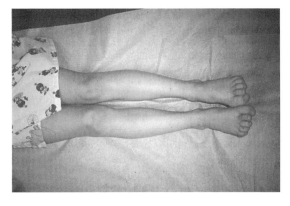

FIGURE 18–10. Asymmetric growth of the lower extremity.

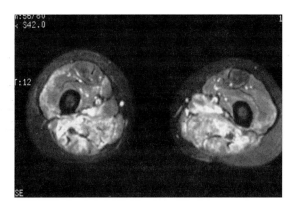

FIGURE 18–11.   MRI showing lower extremity atrophy.

hip to reduce relative leg length causes further contracture. Asymmetric hip flexion contracture is a cause of apparent LLD. Lateral subluxation of the femoral head can also produce apparent LLD. Epiphysiodesis may be needed to reduce growth in the other extremity if the discrepancy is large. In children, LLD should be compensated to ¼ inch.[40] Up to a ¼-inch lift can be accommodated inside the shoe.

Nutrition and Growth

Children with early onset, polyarticular involvement, and systemic disease can have growth retardation during periods of active disease. This growth retardation can be aggravated by the use of corticosteroids.

Outcomes

Functional capacity in JRA is classified using the functional status from the American College

TABLE 18–4.   American College of Rheumatology Revised Criteria for Classification of Functional Status in Rheumatoid Arthritis*

Class I	Completely able to perform usual activities of daily living (self-care, vocational, avocational)
Class II	Able to perform usual self-care and vocational activities but limited in avocational activities
Class III	Able to perform usual self-care activities but limited in vocational and avocational activities
Class IV	Limited in ability to perform usual self-care, vocational, and avocational activities

* Usual self-care activities include dressing, feeding, bathing, grooming, and toileting. Avocational (recreational or leisure) and vocational (work, school, homemaking) activities are patient-desired and age-, and sex-specific.

From Hochberg MC, Rowland WC, Dwosh I, et al: American College of Rheumatology 1991 revised criteria for the classification of global functional status in rheumatoid arthritis. Arthritis Rheum 1992;35:498, with permission.

of Rheumatology (Table 18–4).[69,70] Functional outcomes of children with JRA have been summarized with 31% of the patients having severe functional limitations in class III or IV.[18] This does not take into account length of illness before treatment began or the bias resulting from follow-up of patients with more severe disease. It was reported that the number of patients with severe functional limitation increased with length of follow-up.[71] This classification of functional capacity allows for a wide range of disability within functional class II. Use of this classification may not provide appropriate information to measure outcomes of treatment interventions. The diagnostic criteria also have an influence on outcome studies. Up to 4% of children initially diagnosed with JRA may eventually develop a juvenile-onset seronegative spondyloarthropathy but are included in epidemiologic and outcome data in short-term follow-up for JRA.

A core set of variables was identified to improve the standardization of outcomes as was previously done in adults with rheumatoid arthritis.[72,73] The outcome variables include physician assessment of disease activity, parent or patient assessment of well-being, functional ability, number of joints with active arthritis or with limited ROM, and ESR.[72]

Most outcome studies in children with JRA focus on the effect of intervention on function related to disease activity without emphasis on quality of life.[72] Measurement tools for physical function in children with JRA include the Juvenile Arthritis Functional Assessment Report (JAFAR),[74] the Childhood Health Assessment Questionnaire (CHAQ),[75] and the Juvenile Arthritis Self-report Index. A study proposed that the Juvenile Arthritis Quality of Life Questionnaire (JACQ)[76] include an assessment of quality of life as well as function. Preliminary data suggest good validity and sensitivity of the JACQ.

Seventy-nine percent of children with JRA enter adulthood without severe disability. Remission occurs in up to two-thirds of children, whereas adults usually have progression. Most children are able to attend school or work.[77] The presence of JRA has an impact on school attendance, activities, and participation in physical education programs. PL94-142, the Education for All Handicapped Children Act of 1975, and PL101-476, the Individuals with Disabilities Education Act (IDEA) of 1990, were enacted to meet educational and related service needs of children with disabilities. Physical and occupational therapy services can be arranged as part of the school day. Several studies reported difficulties or reduced participation when the physical education program was not adapted to fit the needs of children with JRA.[78–81] School modifications may include providing transportation, reducing distances of ambulation between classrooms and activities, providing a barrier-free environment, prescribing appropriate seating and positioning, providing adaptive writing equipment, and providing an adapted physical education program. Home tutoring may be necessary during prolonged absence from school.

From preschool through adolescence, children are learning and improving skills. Deficits in mobility, interaction, and socialization affect this development. Exploration of the environment for toddlers is reduced without age-appropriate mobility. Chronic illness causes dependence on family, noncompliance with therapy, absence from school because of medical issues, and altered interaction in the school environment. Frequent assessments of function are necessary as disease fluctuates, and ability to perform self-care, ADL, and mobility fluctuates as well. Body image and appearance are important issues, especially as children enter adolescence.

Poor outcome is related to delay in appropriate treatment; later age at disease onset; longer duration of disease, as remission is unlikely after more than 7 years; RF-positive status; unremitting course; multiple small joint involvement; early appearance of erosion; and hip involvement.[79,82] Disease course may have more prognostic value than disease type at onset, because one-third of children may change subgroup.[79,83] Children with oligoarthritis have the greatest risk of disability from iritis but do well in terms of functional outcome even when contractures occur.[82] Children develop less joint erosion than adults, although further long-term follow-up in cases lasting into adulthood is needed.[73] Death has been reported to occur in 2–4% of children. The death rate in North America is thought to be below 1%.[82,84]

Juvenile-onset Spondyloarthropathy

The juvenile-onset spondyloarthropathies are HLA-B27–associated clinical syndromes in children under age 16 with findings related to arthritis, enthesitis, and tenosynovitis involving joints in the lower extremities, the spine, and the sacroiliac joint. RF and ANA are negative.[85] Conditions include Reiter's syndrome, ankylosing spondylitis, psoriatic arthritis, reactive arthritis, and the arthropathy with Crohn's disease and ulcerative colitis. Most juvenile-onset spondyloarthropathies are undifferentiated at onset. Some children have findings consistent with criteria for juvenile-onset spondyloarthropathy but do not have sacroiliac joint involvement. This is termed *seronegative enthesopathy and arthropathy syndrome* (SEA) and is defined by age of onset before 17 years old, seronegativity, enthesitis most often at the heel or knee, and pauciarticular arthritis usually of the lower extremities.[86] Seventy percent of children with SEA go on to develop definite ankylosing spondylitis or other spondyloarthropathy, especially those with HLA-B27.[87] Juvenile-onset spondyloarthropathies are generally more common in boys than girls.

Ankylosing Spondylitis

The incidence of ankylosing spondylitis is between 1.44 and 2.1 per 100,000 in Canada and 2.0 per 100,000 in the United States. It occurs in children usually older than 8 years old and is more frequent in boys, with a sex ratio ranging from 6:1–2.6:1.[88] Ninety percent of the white patients with ankylosing spondylitis are HLA-B27 positive as compared with 9% of the general population. There is a high concordance rate in monozygotic twins, suggesting a strong genetic susceptibility.[89] The cause is unknown. No bacterial agent has been isolated.

Children with juvenile-onset ankylosing spondylitis present with symptoms often fitting criteria for JRA, especially the pauciarticular type II.[3,85] Tarsal involvement and enthesopathy at onset are more common in ankylosing spondylitis than in JRA. Later, less than half the children with ankylosing spondylitis have upper extremity involvement compared with children with JRA. Axial symptoms (spine and sacroiliac joint) and radiographic sacroiliitis develop in children with ankylosing spondylitis. Children with JRA do not develop radiographic sacroiliitis. Loss of mobility and low back pain occur as the disease persists. Although few joints are involved initially with the onset similar to pauciarticular JRA, eventually more than five joints become involved.[85]

Adults present with decreased spine mobility, back pain, and stiffness related to axial involvement, whereas only 15–24% of children have these findings at onset.[85] Children are more likely to have peripheral joint involvement, as many as 82%, with lower extremity and hip joints most often involved, although the shoulder, costoclavicular, and sternoclavicular joints can be affected as well. Enthesitis, pain at the insertion of tendon to bone, occurs more commonly in children at onset than it does in adults. On physical examination, local tenderness of the enthesis can be present at the patella, tibial tuberosity, and attachment of the Achilles tendon on the calcaneus. Arthritis is asymmetric. Pain may occur at the sacroiliac joint with loss of lumbar lordosis, spine hyperextension, and thoracic kyphosis. There is flattening of the back on forward flexion. Limited chest expansion occurs. Up to 27% have an associated uveitis.[90] Radiographic findings of bilateral sacroiliac joint involvement are necessary for the definitive diagnosis. These findings may not be present for several years after onset, often delaying the diagnosis. Other radiographic findings include osteopenia, joint space narrowing, and ankylosis.

Treatment aims at reducing inflammation and pain, preventing deformity, and maintaining optimal function. Antiinflammatory medications are tolmetin sodium, naproxen, and indomethacin. Sulfasalazine is also used. Glucocorticoid injection may be beneficial for enthesitis. Direct injection into the tendon must be avoided. Ophthalmic steroids are used to treat acute uveitis.

Physical therapy objectives are to maintain ROM of the spine and peripheral joints and erect posture with proper alignment. Exercises focus on preventing hip flexion contractures while strengthening hip extensors and quadriceps. Chest expansion should be assessed, and deep breathing exercises are performed to prevent respiratory complications. Trunk extension is encouraged with swimming. Lateral bending and trunk flexion exercises are also provided to maintain ROM. Shoe inserts relieve weight bearing on the heel and metatarsophalangeal joints to reduce pain.

Hip disease is an indicator for poor outcome. Children tend to have more lasting peripheral joint involvement than adults.[91,92] Surgical correction of foot deformity or hip flexion contractures is often necessary.

Reiter's Syndrome

Reiter's syndrome is more frequent in boys over age 8 years and is characterized by conjunctivitis, urethritis, and symmetric arthritis. The cause may be postinfectious or a reactive arthritis because it occurs after infection with *Chlamydia trachomatis, Chlamydia pneumoniae, Salmonella, Shigella flexneri,* and *Yersinia enterocolitica.* It is not common in children. There is an association with HLA-B27. Oligoarthritis of the knee or ankle is most common but temporomandibular and cervical spine involvement occurs as does enthesopathy. Arthritis is usually the presenting complaint, but low-grade fever may be present. Laboratory findings include an elevated ESR, normal or elevated joint fluid complement,[93] and elevated white blood cell count. Radiographic findings

include erosion at the Achilles tendon insertion and sacroiliac joint changes. The course may be episodic, and some cases develop a chronic destructive arthritis. Rehabilitation goals are to encourage trunk extension, to maintain erect posture in sitting and standing, and to provide breathing exercises for chest expansion.

Arthritis Associated with Inflammatory Bowel Disease

Arthritis occurs in 10–20% of children with ulcerative colitis and Crohn's disease. There is no sex predilection. The arthritis is usually pauciarticular, and spondylitis can be present. Other manifestations of inflammatory bowel disease include erythema nodosum and growth failure. Treatment consists of management of the bowel disease, NSAIDs, and physical therapy.

Psoriatic Arthritis

Psoriatic arthritis is an inflammatory arthritis in children under the age of 16 years associated with psoriasis either preceding the onset or within 15 years.[94] Girls predominate slightly with a peak age of onset of arthritis at 7–11 years and psoriasis at 9–13 years.[90] Fifty percent present with monoarticular arthritis. Most cases progress to involve more than five joints in an asymmetric pattern.[95,96] Commonly involved joints are the knees, ankles, hips, and wrist. The small joints of the feet and hands may be involved. Dactylitis results from inflammation of the flexor tendon sheath causing sausagelike swelling of the digits. Forty percent of cases present with psoriasis, and 10% present with both arthritis and psoriasis.[90] Psoriasis occurs with nail pitting and hyperkeratosis. Anterior uveitis occurs and is indistinguishable from that seen in JRA. Laboratory findings include an elevated ESR. Although RF is negative, the ANA can be positive. Synovial fluid contains mostly polymorphonuclear cells.

Medical treatment starts with NSAIDs— either aspirin, tolmetin, or naproxen. Physical and occupational therapy are necessary to maintain joint ROM and function. If no prompt response occurs, slow-acting antirheumatic drugs, such as gold, indomethacin, or prednisone, are added. Intra-articular steroid injections are used for persistent synovitis. Psoriasis is treated with topical agents. Eighty percent of the cases initially with pauciarticular presentation go on to have involvement of more than five joints.[95] Growth failure can occur because of epiphyseal involvement. A positive ANA may be associated with poor functional outcome.[95]

Systemic Lupus Erythematosus

Systemic lupus erythematosus (SLE) is a multisystem autoimmune disease with episodic inflammation and vasculitis associated with a positive ANA. Immune complex deposition is widespread. The cause is unclear, but possible causes include immune, genetic, environmental, and infectious factors. Exacerbations may be related to intercurrent viral infections. The incidence is 0.53[97] to 0.6[98] per 100,000 population. Twenty percent of the cases begin in childhood. Female-to-male ratio is 4.5:1 but varies depending on age, with a lower ratio in prepubertal children.[99] Children are more likely than adults to present with systemic disease. Clinical findings include malaise; fatigue; weight loss; anorexia; butterfly rash; and joint symptoms such as morning stiffness, joint pain, limited ROM, and swelling. The 11 diagnostic criteria of the American College of Rheumatology are listed in Table 18–5. The presence of four criteria has a 90% sensitivity and a 98% specificity.[100] Laboratory findings include a positive ANA in almost all cases, anti-DNA antibody, other autoantibodies, low complement, anemia, and leukopenia.

One-third of children have an erythematous rash in a butterfly distribution over the bridge of the nose and cheeks. The rash may be precipitated by sunlight. Most children develop a transient arthritis, which is migrating involving the extremities. Joint deformity and erosion on radiographs are not common. Pain may be out of proportion to joint findings on examination. Tenosynovitis of the hands may be present. Proximal muscle weakness may accompany the acute illness or can be from myositis or steroid-induced myopathy. Long-term steroid use can put the child with SLE at risk for avascular necrosis of the femoral head. Raynaud's phenomenon can be present and often suggests the presence of a mixed connective tissue disorder. Cardiac manifestations are pericarditis and endocarditis.

The renal and central nervous system are associated with morbidity and mortality in children with SLE. Central nervous system findings occur in up to one third of cases. Seizures and psychosis are most common, although memory deficits, headache, and behavior changes may also be present. Nephritis is present in 75% of cases and is the main factor in determining outcome in children. The frequency and severity of nephritis in children is greater than that in adults.[101]

The management of children with SLE is symptomatic. Physical activity should be maintained when possible, nutritional considerations should be addressed, excessive sunlight should be avoided, and psychosocial support should be

TABLE 18–5. Diagnostic Criteria in Systemic Lupus Erythematosus*

Malar rash	Pleuritis or pericarditis
Discoid lupus rash	Cytopenia
Photosensitivity	Positive immunoserology
Oral or nasal muco-	LE cells
cutaneous ulceration	Antinative DNA antibodies
Nonerosive arthritis	Anti-Sm antibodies
Nephritis	False-positive test for syphilis
Encephalopathy	Positive antinuclear antibody

* Four or more of the 11 criteria are required for clinical diagnosis.
LE, Lupus erythematosus.
Adapted from Tan EM, Cohen AS, Fries JF, et al: The 1982 revised criteria for the classification of systemic lupus erythematosus. Arthritis Rheum 1982;25:1271.

provided. NSAIDs are used for arthritis and other musculoskeletal symptoms. Systemic steroids are required by most children usually as low-dose prednisone. Fever, dermatitis, arthritis, and serositis usually resolve promptly with low-dose steroids, whereas the serologic findings require several weeks of therapy. Hydroxychloroquine is used for skin manifestations or to lower steroid dosage. Antihypertensives are used when required. High-dose steroids, immunosuppressive agents, and IVIG may be necessary for more severe disease manifestations. Intravenous cyclophosphamide may be used in cases of severe nephritis.

Ten-year survival of greater than 80% has been reported,[102] although it is not as high in lower socioeconomic populations. Adult outcome studies suggest that prognosis is related to urinary protein excretion, serum creatinine, and anemia as well as race and socioeconomic factors.[103] A limited number of outcome studies in children did not find age, race, or sex to be factors in prognosis. Hematuria, proteinuria, persistent hypertension, pulmonary hypertension, chronic active disease, and biopsy-proven diffuse proliferative glomerulonephritis are associated with a poor outcome.

Dermatomyositis

Dermatomyositis is a multisystemic inflammatory disease affecting mainly the muscle and skin. A 20-year study in Pennsylvania found 12% of patients with onset before age 17 years. The incidence is 0.22–0.55 per 100,000 population. The peak age of onset is between ages 5 and 9 years with the ratio of girls to boys increasing with age.[104] The cause is unknown.[105] There is a possible association with coxsackie B virus[106] and *Toxoplasma gondii*.[107] There may be an immune-mediated process related to a genetic predisposition because there is an association with HLA-B8 in 72% and DR3.[108] Muscle biopsy findings demonstrate lymphocyte infiltration with mainly CD4+ cells primarily around the blood vessels, whereas adults have mainly cytotoxic T cells.[109] This infiltration results in formation of thrombi and muscle infarction. It can occur in the blood vessels of dermal connective tissue, gastrointestinal tract, and nerves.

The clinical picture presents as progressive symmetric weakness mainly in the proximal muscles of the extremities and trunk and skin rash. The weakness is more pronounced in the lower extremities. Children have difficulty arising from the floor, running, and climbing stairs. Upper extremity involvement causes difficulty with ADL, such as combing hair. Arthralgias may be present. The skin findings consist of a violaceous rash over the upper eyelids, periorbital edema, or an erythematous rash in a butterfly distribution. There can be involvement of respiratory muscles, pharyngeal muscles, and palatine muscles causing dysphagia and putting the child at risk for aspiration. Extraocular muscles and facial muscles are generally not involved. Vasculitis can involve the gastrointestinal tract. Myocarditis is present in some cases. In half the cases, the presentation is of acute onset. Calcium deposits occur in up to 70% of cases and can lead to further contracture, pain, atrophy, and skin ulceration (Fig. 18–12). Calcinosis is commonly found at the knees and elbows.

The diagnosis is made by the clinical presentation with supporting laboratory data. Deep tendon reflexes may be preserved until late in the disease course. Muscle enzymes, creatine phosphokinase (CPK), aspartate aminotransferase (ASAT), and alanine aminotransferase (ALAT), are elevated. ANA can be elevated, and the ESR is often normal. Electromyography reveals low-amplitude, short-duration polyphasic motor units with early recruitment, positive sharp waves, fibrillations, and complex repetitive discharge. Nerve conduction velocities are normal.[110] Electromyography should exclude one extremity so as not to interfere with muscle biopsy interpretation. Muscle biopsy is consistent with an inflammatory myopathy. Focal degeneration and regeneration, fibrosis, and variation in fiber size are found.

Management

Weakness of respiratory muscles may lead to ventilatory failure requiring mechanical ventilation. Vital capacity and lung function should be followed. Weakness of the posterior pharyngeal muscles involved in swallowing leads to concerns for dysphagia and aspiration. Diet may be

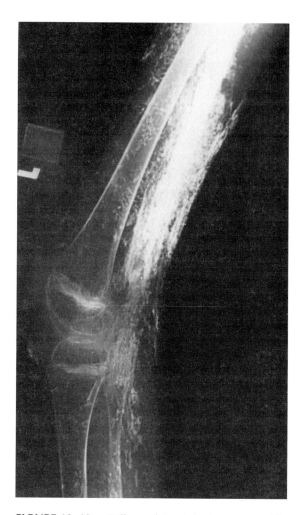

FIGURE 18–12.   Diffuse calcinosis in dermatomyositis.

changed to semisolid, or tube feedings may be required.

Corticosteroid is the main drug therapy used in the treatment of dermatomyositis. High-dose corticosteroids (2 mg/kg/day) are used initially to reduce inflammation. Once there is clinical improvement, alternate-day therapy may be used, and the dosage is tapered. Immunosuppressive agents such as methotrexate are added if there is an inadequate response to prednisone or if the side effects are intolerable.

Physical therapy is initiated in the acute phase to prevent contracture and consists of passive range of motion (PROM) and splinting. Unnecessary immobilization should be avoided. Once inflammation subsides, therapy goals are to strengthen muscles and improve endurance. Skin care is necessary to prevent ulceration or infection. Hydrotherapy may be useful in reducing muscle pain and allowing for ROM exercises when weakness is present.[111] Assessment of ADL is done by the occupational therapist.

TABLE 18–6.	Types of Scleroderma
Morphea	Systemic sclerosis
Localized	Diffuse cutaneous sclerosis
Generalized	Limited cutaneous sclerosis
Guttate morphea	Mixed connective tissue disease
Linear scleroderma	CREST syndrome
En coup de sabre	

CREST, Calcinosis, Raynaud's phenomenon, esophageal dysfunction, sclerodactyly, telangiectasia.

Calcinosis may further limit joint mobility and cause skin breakdown. Discrete calcinosis can be excised surgically.

Most children have a single episode with good functional outcome, whereas 20% develop a more chronic course.[111] Prognosis is related to the degree of vasculitis. Long-term disability is related to persistent contracture, calcinosis, and complications of prolonged steroid use.

Scleroderma

Systemic sclerosis is uncommon in children, and the disease usually presents with linear or focal cutaneous involvement. The cause is unclear with possible immunologic, metabolic, and vascular mechanisms.[82] Girls are affected more often than boys with fibrosis of involved tissue. The average age of onset is between 8 and 10 years with a duration of 7–9 years. Systemic sclerosis is less common than cutaneous involvement. Children account for nearly half of cases of linear scleroderma.[82] The types of scleroderma are listed in Table 18–6.

Cutaneous involvement usually occurs in the form of morphea or linear scleroderma. Morphea are circumscribed areas of hardened skin that may be local or generalized. In guttate morphea, small lesions occur with minimal sclerosis. Morphea tends to be self-limiting over 2–3 years.[112] Linear scleroderma presents with atrophic, erythematous areas, which later become fibrotic with binding of the skin to underlying tissues. Underlying subcutaneous tissue, muscle, and bone are involved. Children may complain of pain associated with the skin changes. Soft tissue atrophy with resorption of soft tissue and bone can occur unilaterally leaving facial or other areas of asymmetry. Scleroderma en coup de sabre (Fig. 18–13) is a unilateral linear involvement of the face and scalp, often with loss of hair on the involved area and asymmetric facial development. Some children develop joint involvement with synovitis involving the lower extremity more often than the upper extremity.[113] Linear scleroderma may be associated with a positive RF, positive ANA, and an elevated ESR.[112]

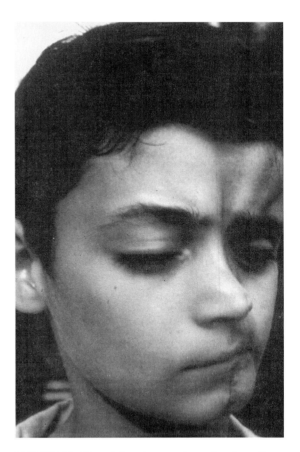

FIGURE 18–13. Scleroderma—Coup de sabre. (From the Clinical Slide Collection on the Rheumatic Diseases. © 1991, 1995, 1997 by the American College of Rheumatology, with permission.)

The systemic form is not common in children and is characterized by Raynaud's phenomenon; symmetric cutaneous involvement; cutaneous ulcers; synovitis; and involvement of the heart, lungs, gastrointestinal tract, and kidneys. Children may present with stiffness, loss of joint function, and skin tightness. Gastrointestinal involvement includes dysphagia and malabsorption. Pulmonary and renal complications are causes of death in childhood.[112] Autoantibodies are frequently positive, including ANA and endothelial antibodies.

The CREST syndrome comprises calcinosis, Raynaud's phenomenon, esophageal dysmotility, sclerodactyly, and telangiectases. It was previously known as acrosclerosis. It is unclear whether it is a separate entity from systemic sclerosis.[82]

There is no specific treatment for scleroderma (Table 18–7). Hypertension is managed medically. Topical steroids can be used for localized skin lesions, but systemic steroids may exacerbate hypertension. Systemic steroids are used to

TABLE 18–7.   Drug Therapy in Scleroderma

Drug	Use
Corticosteroid	
Topical	Localized skin disease
Systemic	Progressive linear disease
D-Penicillamine	Localized skin disease
Methotrexate	Inconclusive
Nifedipine	Raynaud's phenomenon
Captopril	Hypertension

reduce inflammation in progressive linear scleroderma or the early stages of systemic disease. D-penicillamine softens skin lesions but does not improve underlying muscle and bone loss.

Physical therapy is necessary to maintain ROM and prevent contracture because of cutaneous involvement. An exercise program provides soft tissue massage and ROM exercises to maximize mobility around the joints. Moist heat is used before stretching exercises if the child can tolerate the heat. A daily home exercise program includes facial exercises to maintain mouth opening. Raynaud's phenomenon is managed by avoiding cold, biofeedback, and drugs such as nifedipine. Night splinting can aid in reducing or delaying contracture development, and pressure relief can be provided for areas of skin ulceration or bony prominences. Serial casting can correct contracture of the knee, ankle, and wrist.[113] Esophageal dysmotility, if symptomatic, requires management to reduce reflux. Management includes raising the head of the bed; not lying down directly after meals; eating smaller, more frequent meals; techniques to improve swallowing; and the use of antacids.[111]

TABLE 18–8.   Diagnostic Criteria for Mixed Connective Tissue Disease

Raynaud's phenomenon or swollen hands
Anti-ENA and anti-RNP positive
Mixed findings of two connective tissue disorders

SLE	Scleroderma	PM/DM
Lymphadenopathy	Fibrosis	Elevated CPK
Malar rash	Restrictive lung	Myogenic EMG
Polyarthritis	disease	Muscle weakness
Pericarditis or	Esophageal	
pleuritis	hypomotility	
Leukopenia		
Thrombocytopenia		

ENA, Extractable nuclear antigen; RNP, ribonucleoprotein, SLE, systemic lupus erythematosus; PM/DM, polymyositis/dermatomyositis; CPK, creatine phosphokinase; EMG, electromyogram.

Adapted from Kasukawa R, Tojo T, Miyawaki S, et al: Preliminary diagnostic criteria for classification of mixed connective tissue disease. In Kasukawa R, Sharp CG (eds): Mixed Connective Tissue Disease and Antinuclear Antibodies. Amsterdam, Excerpta Medica, 1987;41.

Scarring and fibrosis can limit growth and cause contractures. Long-term management may include surgical reconstruction with support of osseous structures if necessary in cases of severe facial involvement. This surgery should not be done until the disease is inactive and dental maturity is achieved. Tenotomies are useful in treating contractures of the hip flexors and Achilles tendon. Epiphysiodesis of the contralateral limb reduces LLD when there is a concern that lengthening the involved atrophic extremity may worsen contracture or lead to subluxation.[113]

Mixed Connective Tissue Disorder

Mixed connective tissue disease combines features of SLE, JRA, dermatomyositis, and scleroderma. It is usually seen in girls older than age 6 years. The Kasukawa et al.[114] criteria (Table 18–8) are used in children[115] as well as adults. Four of the major diagnostic criteria are necessary for a definitive diagnosis of mixed connective tissue disorder. Clinical findings include arthritis, Raynaud's phenomenon, hand swelling, scleroderma skin changes, rashes of SLE or dermatomyositis, cardiac involvement, hepatosplenomegaly, and thrombocytopenia. Esophageal dysmotility is usually asymptomatic. Bony erosion or joint destruction occurs more often in children than adults.[115] Laboratory findings are antibodies to nuclear ribonucleoprotein and extractable nuclear antigens.[116] Symptomatic treatment includes the use of corticosteroids and NSAIDs. The SLE and dermatomyositis symptoms respond well to corticosteroids. Outcome is varied depending on the disease course.

Infectious Arthritis

Lyme Disease

Lyme disease is caused by the spirochete *Borrelia burgdorferi*, which is transmitted by the deer tick *Ixodes dammini*. The occurrence of arthritis in 12 children was noted in Lyme, Connecticut.[117] The incidence is 5.2 per 100,000 population.[118] In the initial phase of Lyme disease, symptoms such as fever, fatigue, headache, arthralgias, myalgia, and stiff neck occur. Erythema migrans is a characteristic red macule or papule that expands to a large round lesion with central clearing caused by local spread of the spirochete in the skin (Fig. 18–14). It appears 1 to 30 days after the tick bite. These findings usually disappear within 4 weeks of onset. The late phase can last from months to years

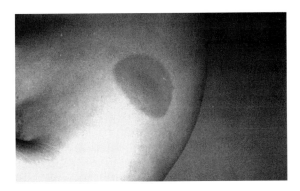

FIGURE 18–14.   Erythema migrans in Lyme disease.

TABLE 18–9.   Antiobiotic Treatment of Lyme Disease

Drug	Dosage	Length of Treatment	Age
Early Disease			
Doxycycline	100 mg bid	14–21 d	> 9 yr
Amoxicillin	30–50 mg/kg/d tid, max 1–2 g/d	14–21 d	
Erythromycin	30 mg/kg/d tid	14–21 d	For penicillin-allergic children, < 9 yr
Late Disease			
Ceftraxone	100 mg/d	14–21 d for CNS involvement	
	50 mg/d	14–21 d for involvement other than CNS	

bid, Two times per day; tid, three times per day.

and is characterized by arthritis, cardiac disease, and neurologic disease. Cardiac manifestations of heart block occur in 5–10% of children. Chronic neurologic manifestations, which occur in 15% of cases, include meningitis, radiculitis, and cranial neuritis. Bell's palsy may be seen more frequently in children than adults. In the classic form, there are intermittent episodes of unilateral arthritis with the knee involved most frequently (88%).[119,120] Other large joints may also be involved, including the hip, shoulder, elbow, wrist, and ankle. Children may also present with an acute onset of unilateral arthritis of the knee or hip, which may be similar to a septic arthritis or toxic synovitis. In some cases, a chronic arthritis develops that resembles pauciarticular JRA.

The pathologic findings are similar to those seen in rheumatoid arthritis, including synovial hyperplasia, mononuclear infiltrates, and vascular proliferation. Diagnosis is confirmed by antibody detection. Serology may be positive for 6–9 months after treatment and resolution of symptoms.[121] Up to 30% have ANA,[122] whereas RF is negative.

Lyme disease is treated with antibiotics for 21 days (Table 18–9). The treatment for early Lyme arthritis is a 30-day course of oral antibiotics. Late disease is treated with intravenous antibiotics. Arthritis may persist up to 6 months, so an observation period of 2 months is recommended before starting another course of antibiotics.[123] When joint fluid is negative for *Borrelia* after the second course of antibiotics, NSAIDs or intra-articular steroids are used. In 85% of children, the arthritis resolves before the end of the initial treatment period, but a chronic inflammatory phase develops in 10%.

Rheumatic Fever

Rheumatic fever occurs in children older than 4 years with boys and girls being affected

equally. Arthritis associated with rheumatic fever presents with pain, swelling, warmth, and limited joint motion in the large joints of the extremities. The most commonly involved joints are the knees, elbows, ankles, and wrists. The arthritis is transient, migrating, and responds rapidly to aspirin. There is periarticular swelling with effusion, but erosion is not seen. Rarely a periarticular fibrosis occurs resulting in a Jaccoud deformity at the metacarpophalangeal joint. The associated findings are carditis, fever, rash, chorea, and nodules. The chorea can be the only presenting symptom of rheumatic fever. It may last from several weeks to years. Diagnosis is clinical by the Jones criteria (Table 18–10). There often is a history of a prior streptococcal infection. Management includes anti-inflammatory medications such as salicylates, corticosteroids

TABLE 18–10.   Jones Criteria for the Diagnosis of Rheumatic Fever*

Major	Minor	Preceding Group A Streptococcal Infection
Carditis	Fever	Throat culture
Polyarthritis	Arthralgia	Rapid streptococcal antigen
Chorea	Elevated ESR or CRP	Elevated streptococcal antibody
Erythema marginatum	Prolonged PR interval	
Subcutaneous nodules		

* Two of the major criteria or one major with two minor are required for diagnosis with evidence of preceding streptococcal infection.

ESR, Erythrocyte sedimentation rate; CRP, C-reactive protein.

Adapted from Dajani AS, Ayoub E, Bierman FZ, et al: Guidelines for the diagnosis of rheumatic fever: Jones criteria, updated 1992. JAMA 1992;268:2069.

for carditis, and physical therapy to maintain joint ROM and mobility. Arthritis does not result in long-term morbidity, but prognosis is related to the extent of cardiac involvement.

Septic Arthritis

Septic arthritis occurs most often in children younger than age 2 years with boys being affected more often than girls.[124] Joint involvement arises by hematogenous spread, by direct extension from local tissues, or as a reactive arthritis. Viral arthritis is more common in older children and adults. Parvovirus B19 affects predominantly girls with symmetric arthritis of the large joints with the knee being involved more often than the hip. The arthritis can be of long duration and may be relapsing. An association was found with HLA-DR4 with those developing arthritis with parvovirus B19 infection.[125] In rubella, a polyarticular, pauciarticular, or monoarticular arthritis can be seen a week after the rash.[126] The arthritis is characterized by pain and morning stiffness in the hands and knees, which usually resolves within 2 weeks. Hepatitis B, Epstein-Barr, and varicella infection are also associated with arthritis. Transient synovitis occurs mainly in boys ages 3–10 years who present with pain in the hip or referred pain in the thigh or knee. It may be preceded by respiratory infection. Laboratory values, including white blood cell count and ESR, and radiographic findings may indicate effusion. There may be a reduced uptake bone scan. Aspiration of synovial fluid is indicated to rule out a septic arthritis and to relieve pain. Transient synovitis is treated with NSAIDs and resting the joint.

Bacterial septic arthritis accounts for 6.5% of arthritis in children.[127] Children have fever and joint pain with loss of mobility in the knees, hips, ankles, and elbows. Monoarticular involvement is most common, but multiple joints may be involved. Osteomyelitis may develop. Septic arthritis of the hip occurs in infants, and premature infants may be at risk because of instrumentation. The leg is positioned in abduction, flexion, and external rotation. Irritability and fever are present. An ambulatory child refuses to bear weight on the extremity. Arthritis associated with syphilis is rare in children and adolescents. Neisseria gonorrhoeae should be considered in adolescents with oligoarthritis, fever, and rash. The most common pathogens are Haemophilus influenzae and Staphylococcus aureus. Joint fluid reveals marked elevation of white blood cells, elevated protein, and low-to-normal glucose. Radiographic findings progress from soft tissue swelling to juxta-articular osteoporosis, narrowing of the joint space, and erosion. Treatment consists of appropriate antibiotic therapy, joint aspiration to relieve pressure, and physical therapy.

Reactive Arthritis

Sterile arthritis in large and small joints can be found after infection with S. aureus. Yersinia enterocolitica infection has been followed by persistence of the organism in the joint fluid with pauciarticular involvement of the knee. Salmonella, Shigella, and Campylobacter have also been associated with arthritis, which is usually transient, involving only a few joints. Some children may develop a chronic arthritis. In arthritis after Salmonella infection, joint fluid should be sterile in reactive arthritis because septic arthritis and osteomyelitis can also occur. Reactive arthritis after Yersinia and Campylobacter has been associated with HLA-B27.

Hemophilia

The hemophilias are the most common congenital coagulation disorders in children. Eighty percent are caused by a deficiency of factor VIII. The disease severity depends on the level of factor in the serum. There is a family history in 80% of the cases. Severe disease is defined as less than 1% factor activity; in moderate disease, activity is greater than 1%. Mild hemophilia occurs when factor levels are greater than 5% of normal, and hemorrhage usually occurs with related trauma or surgery.[128] Large hematomas that occur after minor trauma are often first seen when the child begins to walk. Prolonged bleeding is seen with lacerations. Subsynovial intramural hemorrhage occurs and ruptures into the joint cavity. With repeated hemarthroses, synovial hypertrophy develops with hemosiderin deposition in the synovial lining. Inflammatory tissue produces proteolytic enzymes, which break down cartilage. Later joint deformity occurs as the synovium is replaced by fibrous tissue. Synovial hypertrophy can stimulate epiphyseal plates, leading to growth disturbances. Bony erosions develop. Pain and swelling limit joint mobility leading to contractures.[129] The adjacent muscles atrophy, and osteopenia develops from disuse. Eighty percent of hemarthroses occur in the knee, elbow, and ankle. Shoulder, hip, wrist, finger, toe, and cervical spine involvement is less frequent. Children present with acute pain, joint fullness, swelling, and loss of ROM.

In the upper extremity, shoulder hemarthrosis is accompanied by pain and difficulty finding a position of comfort because of the unsupported position of the arm. Chronic synovitis at the elbow can cause accelerated growth of the radial head limiting movement. Hemarthrosis in the hand usually occurs after trauma. In the lower extremity hip joint involvement can lead to findings similar to Legg-Calvé-Perthes disease.[120] Knee involvement is common and may be related to the weight bearing and joint stresses. Accelerated growth at the distal femoral epiphysis can cause LLD, varus or valgus angulation, and tibial subluxation in addition to flexion contracture. Ankle involvement usually causes plantar flexion contracture, which may be exaggerated in the presence of knee flexion contracture to accommodate an LLD.

Early radiographic changes are in the soft tissue. Hemarthrosis can lead to bony overgrowth when it occurs before epiphyseal fusion. A defect in the intrinsic clotting pathway is indicated by a prolonged partial thromboplastin time with normal platelet count and prothrombin time.

Treatment consists of preventing or minimizing trauma, controlling hemarthrosis, correcting the coagulation problem, and maintaining or restoring function. Factor replacement therapy is given at the earliest sign of hemorrhage. Prophylactic treatment is used in some centers before the development of joint damage with the goal of reducing morbidity and disability.[131,132] Factor VIII replacement had in the past been provided from large plasma pools that were virally inactivated. Recombinant factor VIII and IX concentrates are now available so that the transmission of hepatitis and human immunodeficiency virus (HIV) is eliminated.[133] Arginine vasopressin can be used in mild cases to increase the production of endogenous factor VIII. Antibodies to factor concentrate may develop. Thirty percent of hemophiliacs are currently infected with HIV. The number was 50% in the 1980s, but since 1985 viral transmission has been virtually eliminated by self-exclusion of donors, donor screening for HIV, and viral inactivation of concentrates.[128] Hepatitis B and hepatitis C are transmissible by factor concentrate. Infants with hemophilia are currently immunized for hepatitis B.

The initial management of acute hemarthrosis is early factor replacement therapy. Acute hemarthrosis requires joint immobilization for 48 hours to prevent further bleeding. Once pain and swelling decrease, passive ROM exercises are provided to prevent fibrosis and contracture.[134] Pain management includes analgesics, anti-inflammatory medications, and aspiration of blood from the joint if the overlying skin is tense. Attention must be given to positioning because the painful acute joint is kept in flexion. Joint function may be regained within 12–24 hours with early factor replacement but may take up to 2 weeks when more blood has to be resorbed.[128] Contracture most often occurs in ankle plantar flexion, and hip, knee, and elbow flexion. Contracture may be treated with ROM, casting, and traction. Strengthening of specific muscle groups to provide joint stability is prescribed, and a general conditioning program for strength and endurance is necessary. With established contracture, physical therapy aims at maintaining function and mobility. Exercises can be done in water to reduce stress on the joint while providing support and resistance. Lightweight bracing can be used to support and protect joints. Serial casting and dynamic bracing can be used to reduce deformity. Preventive management includes padding of infant cribs and playpens. Toddlers should be closely supervised to prevent falls and trauma. In older children, exercise participation is recommended for fitness and reducing hemorrhage but sports participation remains controversial. Buzzard[135] reviewed the literature on sports participation for children with hemophilia between 1960 and 1990. It is generally recommended that children with hemophilia avoid contact sports, such as football, hockey, and wrestling, and other activities with a high risk of trauma, such as skiing, whereas activities such as swimming, tennis, hiking, walking, and golf are encouraged. For the child with hemophilia participating in organized sports, injury prevention and early management of injury are important. Exercise should be preceded by a period of stretching to maintain flexibility and provide muscle warm-up. Joint stability requires adequate muscle strength. Appropriate protective gear is necessary as it is for all children participating in sports activities. Replacement therapy may be recommended for children participating in sports activities. The participation of an individual child in a specific sport should also take into account the severity of disease and the child's desire to participate.

Bleeding into muscles and soft tissue can result in pain and contracture. This bleeding occurs most often in the large flexors, the gastrocnemius, and elbow flexors. Fibrous tissue replaces the injured muscle as the blood is reabsorbed. Iliopsoas involvement causes pain on hip extension with preservation of rotation. Hip flexion contracture can develop as can femoral neuropathy from compression of the femoral

TABLE 18–11. Diagnostic Criteria
in Kawasaki Disease

Fever lasting > 5 days
Mucocutaneous changes of the oral cavity
 Strawberry tongue
 Red, peeling lips
 Pharyngeal erythema
Conjunctival injection
Peripheral extremity
 Edema of the hands and feet
 Erythema of the palms or soles
 Desquamation
Rash
Cervical lymphadenopathy

nerve. Bleeding in the gastrocnemius can lead to an ankle plantar flexion contracture. Compartment syndrome may develop in the volar aspect of the forearm and can cause a lasting flexion deformity of the wrist.[128] In most cases, nerve function is recovered, but residual weakness can remain leading to contracture because of muscle imbalance. Nerve stimulation and physical therapy may retard atrophy during the recovery period.

Chronic arthropathy with synovitis can be treated with short courses of NSAIDs such as ibuprofen to reduce pain and inflammation when the precaution of the antiplatelet effect is kept in mind. Surgical procedures are performed with factor replacement and use of minimal incision. Synovectomy is indicated for persistent hemarthrosis with ongoing synovitis despite conservative therapy. It reduces hemarthrosis by removal of the hypertrophic vascular synovium but does not prevent the progression of arthropathy. Loss of ROM can occur even with postoperative physical therapy. Arthroscopic synovectomy has been found to be effective and results in better preservation of ROM.[136,137] Osteotomy can correct varus or valgus deformity. Joint replacement is used in end-stage arthropathy. There is a need for revisions especially when the replacement is performed in a young child. Loosening may occur more often in these patients than in adults.

Kawasaki Disease

Kawasaki disease is a systemic vasculitis that affects young children with an annual incidence of 6 to 7.6 per 100,000 population.[138] Eighty percent of affected children are under age 4 years. It is more common in boys. The cause is unknown, with infectious and immune causes suggested. Clinical manifestations that are seen in the acute phase are summarized in Table 18–11. The acute febrile phase lasts 8–15 days. The child may refuse to walk because of

painful edema, erythema, and desquamation of the feet. Arthritis can develop in the acute phase involving the small joints of the hands and the large weight-bearing joints. It is generally self-limited. Arthrocentesis may be required when large effusions are present. Cardiac manifestations include myocarditis and coronary artery aneurysm, which occur in 20% of cases. Risk factors that increase the development of aneurysm to 50% include age under 18 months, male sex, Japanese origin, and early myocarditis.[139] In the subacute phase the fever resolves, and thrombocytosis develops. During the subacute and convalescent phases, the child is at risk for coronary artery thrombosis and should be followed by echocardiogram. Laboratory findings include elevated acute phase reactants and ESR, with a rise in platelet count after the first week.

Treatment includes aspirin and IVIG. Initially, high-dose aspirin at 80–100 mg/kg/day in four divided doses is used to reduce inflammation and later continued at a dose of 5 mg/kg/day in one dose for the antiplatelet effects. IVIG is given within 10 days of onset to reduce the size and severity of coronary artery aneurysm.

Sickle Cell Disease

Joint involvement may occur in children with sickle cell disease. Septic arthritis is caused by *S. aureus*, *Escherichia coli*, *Enterobacter*, and *Salmonella*.[140] Multiple joints may be involved. More commonly, noninflammatory joint effusions of the knees, ankles, or elbows occur with fever, leukocytosis, and evidence of crisis.[141] Chronic synovitis has been reported with resulting erosive destruction of the wrists, metacarpal heads, and calcanei.[142]

For children with chronic debilitating illnesses, psychological support is needed. Children are often separated from their peers when their physical and medical condition limits participation in sports and physical education programs. Children with chronic disease have a higher rate of absenteeism and lower scores on achievement tests than their peers. Fatigue, inattention, and distractibility play a role in school achievement.[143] Family support and education with instruction for school staff are key factors in providing optimal function and development.

References

1. Brewer EJ Jr, Bass JC, Cassidy JT, et al: Criteria for the classification of juvenile rheumatoid arthritis. Bull Rheum Dis 1972;23:712.
2. Brewer EJ Jr, Bass JC, Baum J, et al: Current proposed revision of JRA criteria. Arthritis Rheum 1977;20(Suppl): 195.

3. Cassidy JT, Levinson JE, Bass JC, et al: A study of classification criteria for a diagnosis of juvenile rheumatoid arthritis. Arthritis Rheum 1986;29:274.

4. Schaller JG, Hanson V (conference chairmen): Proceedings of the First American Rheumatism Association Conference of the Rheumatic Diseases of Childhood. Arthritis Rheum 1977;20(Suppl 2):145.

5. Towner SR, Michet CJ Jr, O'Fallon WM, et al: The epidemiology of juvenile rheumatoid arthritis in Rochester, Minnesota. Arthritis Rheum 1983;26:1208.

6. Howard JF, Sigsbee A, Glass DN: HLA genetics and inherited predisposition to JRA. J Rheumatol 1985;12:7.

7. Glass D, Litvin D, Wallace K, et al: Early-onset pauciarticular juvenile rheumatoid arthritis associated with human leukocyte antigen-DRw5, iritis, and antinuclear antibody. J Clin Invest 1980;66:426.

8. Reekers P, Schretlen ED, van de Putte LB: Increase of HLA-"DRw6" in patients with juvenile chronic arthritis. Tissue Antigens 1983;22:283.

9. Lipnick RL, Tsokos GC, Magilavy DB: Immune abnormalities in the pathogenesis of juvenile rheumatoid arthritis. Rheum Dis Clin North Am 1991;17:843.

10. Chantler JK, Tingle AJ, Petty RE: Persistent rubella virus infection associated with chronic arthritis in children. N Engl J Med 1985;313:1117.

11. Inman RD: The infectious etiology of rheumatoid arthritis. Rheum Dis Clin North Am 1991;17:859.

12. Schaller JG: Juvenile rheumatoid arthritis. In Nelson WE (ed): Nelson Textbook of Pediatrics. Philadelphia, WB Saunders, 1996.

13. Harris ED Jr: Rheumatoid arthritis: Pathophysiology and implications for therapy. N Engl J Med 1990;322:1277.

14. Clemens LE, Albert E, Ansell BM: HLA studies in IGM rheumatoid factor-positive arthritis of childhood. Ann Rheum Dis 1983;42:431.

15. Stastny P, Fink CW: Different HLA-D associations in adult and juvenile rheumatoid arthritis. J Clin Invest 1979;63:124.

16. Sailer M, Cabral D, Petty RE, et al: Rheumatoid factor positive, oligoarticular onset juvenile rheumatoid arthritis. J Rheumatol 1997;24:586.

17. Still GF: On a form of chronic joint disease in children. Med Chir Trans 1897;80:47. [Reprinted in Arch Dis Child 1941;16:156.]

18. Levinson JE, Wallace CA: Dismantling the pyramid. J Rheumatol 1992;19(Suppl 33):6.

19. Roth SH: Rethinking rheumatic disease therapy. J Rheumatol 1989;16:1408.

20. Malleson PN, Petty RE: Remodeling the pyramid—A pediatric perspective. J Rheumatol 1990;17:7.

21. Grondin C, Malleson P, Petty RE: Slow acting antirheumatic drugs in chronic arthritis of childhood. Semin Arthritis Rheum 1988;18:38.

22. Athreya BH, Cassidy JT: Current status of the medical treatment of children with juvenile rheumatoid arthritis. Rheum Dis Clin North Am 1991;17:871.

23. Brewer EJ, Giannini EH, Barkley E: Gold therapy in the management of juvenile rheumatoid arthritis. Arthritis Rheum 1980;23:404.

24. Manners PJ, Ansell BM: Slow-acting antirheumatic drug use in systemic onset juvenile chronic arthritis. Pediatrics 1986;77:99.

25. Giannini EH, Brewer EJ, Kuzmina N, et al: Auranofin in the treatment of juvenile rheumatoid arthritis. Arthritis Rheum 1990;33:466.

26. Ansell BM, Hall MA: Penicillamine in chronic arthritis in childhood. J Rheumatol 1981;8(Suppl 7):112.

27. Giannini EH, Brewer EJ, for the Pediatric Rheumatology Collaborative Study Group: Methotrexate (MTX) in the treatment of recalcitrant JRA—Results of the double-blind, placebo (P) controlled randomized trial. Arthritis Rheum 1989;32:s82.

28. Wallace CA, Archie-Bleyer W, Sherry D, et al: Toxicity and serum levels of methotrexate in children with juvenile rheumatoid arthritis. Arthritis Rheum 1989;32:677.

29. Wallace CA, Sherry DD, Salmonson K: Treatment of juvenile rheumatoid arthritis with higher dose methotrexate. Arthritis Rheum 1990; 33:S39.

30. Reiff A, Rawlings DJ, Shaham B, et al: Preliminary evidence for cyclosporin A as an alternative in the treatment of recalcitrant juvenile rheumatoid arthritis and juvenile dermatomyositis. J Rheumatol 1997;24:2436.

31. Forre O: Radiologic evidence of disease modification in rheumatoid arthritis patients treated with cyclosporine: Results of a 48 week multicenter study comparing low-dose cyclosporin with placebo. Norwegian Arthritis Study Group. Arthritis Rheum 1994;37:1506.

32. Savolainen HA, Kautianen H, Isomaki H, et al: Azathioprine in patients with juvenile chronic arthritis: A long-term follow-up study. J Rheumatol 1997; 24:2444.

33. Allen RC, Gross KR, Laxer RM, et al: Intra-articular triamcinolone hexacetonide in the management of chronic arthritis in children. Arthritis Rheum 1986;29:997.

34. Silverman ED, Laxer RM, Greenwald M, et al: Intravenous gamma globulin therapy in systemic juvenile rheumatoid arthritis. Arthritis Rheum 1990;33:1015.

35. MacBain KP, Hill RH: A functional assessment for juvenile rheumatoid arthritis. Am J Occup Ther 1973; 26:326.

36. Scott PJ, Ansell BM, Huskisson EC: Measurement of pain in juvenile chronic arthritis. Ann Rheum Dis 1977;36:186.

37. Varni JW, Thompson KL, Hanson V: The Varni/Thompson Pediatric Pain Questionnaire: I. Chronic musculoskeletal pain in juvenile rheumatoid arthritis. Pain 1987;28:27.

38. Walco GA, Varni JW, Ilowite NT: Cognitive-behavioral pain management in children with juvenile rheumatoid arthritis. Pediatrics 1992;89:1075.

39. Smith RD, Polley H: Rest therapy for rheumatoid arthritis. Mayo Clin Proc 1978;53:141.

40. Scull SA, Dow MB, Athreya BH: Physical and occupational therapy for children with rheumatic diseases. Pediatr Clin 1986;33:1053.

41. Lehman JF, Masock AJ, Warren CG, et al: Effect of therapeutic temperatures on tendon extensibility. Arch Phys Med Rehabil 1970;51:481.

42. Lehman JF, DeLateur BJ: Diathermy and superficial heat, laser, and cold therapy. In Kottke FJ, Lehmann JF (eds): Krusen's Handbook of Physical Medicine and Rehabilitation. Philadelphia, WB Saunders, 1990.

43. Donovan WH: Physical measures in treatment of JRA. Arthritis Rheum 1977;20(Suppl):553.

44. Horvath SM, Hollander JL: Intra-articular temperature as a measure of joint reaction. J Clin Invest 1949; 28:469.

45. Oosterveld FG, Rasker JJ: Effects of local heat and cold treatment on surface and articular temperature of arthritic knees. Arthritis Rheum 1994;37:1578.

46. Harris ED Jr, McCroskery PA: Influence of temperature and fibril stability on degradation of cartilage collagen by rheumatoid synovial collagenase. N Engl J Med 1974;290:1.

47. Brewer EJ: Reduction of morning stiffness and pain using a sleeping bag. Pediatrics 1975; 56:621.

48. Emery HM, Bowyer SL: Physical modalities of therapy in pediatric rheumatic diseases. Rheum Disease Clin North Am 1991;17:1001.

49. Giescecke LL, Athreya BH, Doughty RA: Home Care Guide on Juvenile Rheumatoid Arthritis (for parents). Atlantic City, NJ, Children's Seashore House, 1985.

50. Jayson M, Dixon SJ: Intra-articular pressure in RA of the knee: III. Pressure changes during joint use. Ann Rheum Dis 1970;29:401.

51. Swezey RL: Exercises with a beach ball for increasing range of joint motion. Arch Phys Med Rehabil 1967; 48:253.

52. Klepper S, Darbee J, Effgen S, et al: Physical fitness levels in children with polyarticular juvenile rheumatoid arthritis. Arthritis Care Res 1992;5:93.

53. Ansell B: Pediatric rehabilitative rheumatology. In Hicks JE, Nicholas JJ, Swezey RL (eds): Handbook of Rehabilitative Rheumatology. Atlanta, American Rheumatism Association, 1988.

54. Lehmann JF, DeLateur BJ: Gait analysis—Diagnosis and management. In Kottke FJ, Lehmann JF (eds): Krusen's Handbook of Physical Medicine and Rehabilitation. Philadelphia, WB Saunders, 1990.

55. Herring JA: Destructive arthritis of the hip in juvenile rheumatoid arthritis. J Pediatr Orthop 1984;4:259.

56. Melvin JL: Arthritis in children and adolescents. In Melvin JL (ed): Rheumatic Disease in the Adult and Child: Occupational Therapy and Rehabilitation. Philadelphia, FA Davis, 1989.

57. Matti MV, Sharrock NE: Anesthesia on the rheumatoid patient. Rheum Dis Clin North Am 1998;24:19.

58. Mayro RE, DeLozier JB, Whitaker LA: Facial reconstruction consideration in Rheumatic disease. Rheum Dis Clin North Am 1991;17:943.

59. Ronning O, Valiaho ML, Laaksonen AL: The involvement of the temporomandibular joint in juvenile rheumatoid arthritis. Scand J Rheumatol 1974;3:89.

60. Mericle M, Wilson VK, Moore TL, et al: Effects of polyarticular and pauciarticular onset juvenile rheumatoid arthritis on facial and mandibular growth. J Rheumatol 1996;23:159.

61. Ansell BB: Joint manifestations in children with juvenile chronic polyarthritis. Arthritis Rheum 1977;20:204.

62. Libby AK, Sherry DD, Dudgeon BJ: Shoulder limitation in juvenile rheumatoid arthritis. Arch Phys Med Rehabil 1991;72:382.

63. Brewer EJ Jr: Juvenile rheumatoid arthritis, manifestations of disease. Maj Prob Clin Pediatr 1977;6:1.

64. Ennevarra K: Painful shoulder joint in rheumatoid arthritis: A clinical and radiological study of 200 cases, with special reference to arthrography of the glenohumeral joint. Acta Rheumatol Scand 1967;11(Suppl):1.

65. Eyrin EJ, Murray WR: The effect of joint position on the pressure of intra-articular effusion. J Bone Joint Surg 1964;46A:1235.

66. Cassidy JT, Hillman LS: Abnormalities in skeletal growth in children with JRA. Rheum Clin North Am 1997;23:3.

67. Henderson CJ, Cawkwell GD, Specker BL, et al: Predictors of total body bone mineral density in non-corticosteroid-treated prepubertal children with juvenile rheumatoid arthritis. Arthritis Rheum 1997,40:1967.

68. Johnston C, Miller J, Slemenda C, et al: Calcium supplementation and increases in bone mineral density in children. N Engl J Med 1992;327:82.

69. Steinbrocker O, Traeger CH, Batterman RC: Therapeutic criteria in rheumatoid arthritis. JAMA 1949; 140:659.

70. Hochberg MC, Chang RW, Dwosh I, et al: The American College of Rheumatology 1991 revised criteria for the classification of global functional status in rheumatoid arthritis. Arthritis Rheum 1992;35:498.

71. Laaksonen AL: A prognostic study of juvenile rheumatoid arthritis. Acta Paediatr Scand 1966;166(Suppl):9.

72. Giannini EH, Rupert N, Ravelli A, et al: Preliminary definition of improvement in juvenile arthritis. Arthritis Rheum 1997;40:1202.

73. Felson DT, Anderson JJ, Boers M, et al: American College of Rheumatology preliminary definition of improvement in rheumatoid arthritis. Arthritis Rheum 1995;38:727.

74. Lovell DJ, Howe S, Shear E, et al: Development of a disability measurement tool for juvenile rheumatoid arthritis—The Juvenile Arthritis Functional Assessment Scale. Arthritis Rheum 1989;32:1390.

75. Singh G, Athreya B, Fries J, et al: Measurement of functional status in juvenile rheumatoid arthritis [abstract]. Arthritis Rheum 1990;33:S15.

76. Duffy CM, Arsenault L, Watanabe Duffy KN, et al: The Juvenile Arthritis Quality of Life questionnaire—Development of a new responsive index for juvenile rheumatoid arthritis and juvenile spondyloarthritides. J Rheumatol 1997;24:738.

77. Ansell BM, Wood PH: Prognosis in juvenile chronic arthritis. Clin Rheum Dis 1976;2:397.

78. Whitehouse R, Shope JT, Sullivan DB, et al: Children with juvenile rheumatoid arthritis at school: Functional problems, participation in physical education. Clin Pediatr 1989;28:509.

79. Gare BA, Fasth A: The natural history of juvenile chronic arthritis: A population-based cohort study: II. Outcome. J Rheumatol 1995;22:308.

80. Lovell DJ, Athreya B, Emery HM, et al: School attendance and patterns, special services and needs in pediatric patients with rheumatic diseases: Results of a multicenter study. Arthritis Care Res 1990;3:196.

81. Flato B, Aasland A, Vinje O, et al: Outcome and predictive factors in juvenile rheumatoid arthritis and juvenile spondyloarthropathy. J Rheumatol 1998;25: 366.

82. Cassidy JT, Petty RE (eds): Textbook of Pediatric Rheumatology. Philadelphia, WB Saunders, 1995.

83. Gare BA, Fasth A: The natural history of juvenile chronic arthritis: A population based cohort study: I. Onset and disease process. J Rheumatol 1995;22: 295.

84. Wallace CA, Levinson JE: Juvenile rheumatoid arthritis: Outcome and treatment for the 1990's. Rheum Dis Clin North Am 1991;17:891.

85. Burgos-Vargas R: The early recognition of juvenile-onset ankylosing spondylitis and its differentiation from juvenile rheumatoid arthritis. Arthritis Rheum 1995;38:835.

86. Rosenberg AM, Petty RE: A syndrome of seronegative enthesopathy and arthropathy in children. Arthritis Rheum 1982;25:1041.

87. Burgos-Vargas R, Clark P: Axial involvement in the seronegative enthesopathy and arthropathy syndrome and its progression to ankylosing spondylitis. J Rheumatol 1989;16:192.

88. Gomez KS, Raza K, Jones SD, et al: Juvenile onset ankylosing spondylitis—more girls than we thought? J Rheumatol 1997;24:736.

89. Brown MA, Kennedy LG, MacGregor AJ, et al: Susceptibility to ankylosing spondylitis in twins. Arthritis Rheum 1997;40:1823.

90. Burgos-Vargas R, Pacheco-Tena C, Vazquez-Mellado J: Juvenile-onset spondyloarthropathies. Rheum Dis Clin North Am 1997;23:569.

91. Garcia-Horteo O, Maldonado-Cocca JA, Suarez-Almazor ME, et al: Ankylosing spondylitis of juvenile onset: Comparison with adult onset disease. Scand J Rheumatol 1983;12:246.

92. Marks SH, Barnett M, Calin A: A case-control study of juvenile- and adult-onset ankylosing spondylitis. J Rheumatol 1982;9:739.

93. Singsen BH, Bernstein BH, Koster-King KG, et al: Reiter's syndrome in childhood. Arthritis Rheum 1977; 20(Suppl):402.
94. Lambert JR, Ansell BM, Stephenson E, et al: Psoriatic arthritis in childhood. Clin Rheum Dis 1976;2:339.
95. Shore A, Ansell BM: Juvenile psoriatic arthritis-an analysis of 60 cases. J Pediatr 1982;100:529.
96. Southwood TR, Petty RE, Malleson PN, et al: Psoriatic arthritis in children. Arthritis Rheum 1989;32:1014.
97. Hochberg M: The incidence of systemic lupus erythematosus in Baltimore, Maryland, 1970–1977. Arthritis Rheum 1985;28:80.
98. Fessel WJ: Epidemiology of systemic lupus erythematosus. Rheum Dis Clin North Am 1988;14:15.
99. Cassidy JT, Sullivan DB, Petty RE, et al: Lupus nephritis and encephalopathy: Prognosis in 58 children. Arthritis Rheum 1977;20(Suppl):315.
100. Tan EM, Cohen AS, Fries JF, et al: The 1982 revised criteria for the classification of systemic lupus erythematosus. Arthritis Rheum 1982;25:1271.
101. Meislin AG, Rosenfield NF: Systemic lupus erythematosus in childhood. Analysis of 42 cases with comparative data on 200 adult cases followed concurrently. Pediatrics 1968;42:37.
102. McCurdy DK, Lehman TJA, Bernstein B, et al: Lupus nephritis: Prognostic factors in children. Pediatrics 1992;89:240.
103. Studenski S, Allen NB, Caldwell DS, et al: Survival in systemic lupus erythematosus: A multivariate analysis of demographic factors. Arthritis Rheum 1987;30:1326.
104. Oddis CV, Conte CG, Steen VD, et al: Incidence of polymyositis-dermatomyositis: A 20-year study of hospital diagnosed cases in Allegheny County, PA 1963–1982. J Rheumatol 1990;17:1329.
105. Pachman LM, Hayford JR, Hochberg MC, et al: New-onset juvenile dermatomyositis. Arthritis Rheum 1997; 40:1526.
106. Christensen ML, Pachman LM, Schneiderman R, et al: Prevalence of coxsackie B virus antibodies in patients with juvenile dermatomyositis. Arthritis Rheum 1986; 29:1365.
107. Schroter HM, Sarnet HB, Matheson DS, et al: Juvenile dermatomyositis induced by toxoplasmosis. J Child Neurol 1987;2:101.
108. Pachman LM, Maryjowski MC: Juvenile dermatomyositis and polymyositis. Clin Rheum Dis 1984;10:95.
109. Cambridge G: What is the role of the immune system in juvenile dermatomyositis. In Woo P, White P, Ansell BM (eds): Paediatric Rheumatology Update. Oxford, Oxford University Press, 1990.
110. Kimura J: Myopathies. In Kimura J (ed): Electrodiagnosis in Diseases of Nerve and Muscle: Principles and Practice. Philadelphia, FA Davis, 1989.
111. Barnes L: Physical therapy management of juvenile arthritis. In Banwell BF, Gall V (eds): Physical Therapy Management of Arthritis. New York, Churchill Livingstone, 1988.
112. Ansell BM, Falcini F, Woo P: Scleroderma in childhood. Clin Dermatol 1994;12:299.
113. Buckley SL, Skinner S, Preston J, et al: Focal scleroderma in children: An orthopaedic perspective. J Pediatr Orthop 1993;13:784.
114. Kasukawa R, Tojo T, Miyawaki S, et al: Preliminary diagnostic criteria for classification of mixed connective tissue disease. In Kasukawa R, Sharp CG (eds): Mixed Connective Tissue Disease and Antinuclear Antibodies. Amsterdam, Excerpta Medica, 1987.
115. Tiddens HAWM, van der Net JJ, de Graeff-Meeder ER, et al: Juvenile-onset mixed connective tissue disease: Longitudinal follow-up. J Pediatr 1993;122:191.
116. Sharp GE, Irving W, Tan E, et al: Mixed connective tissue disease: An apparently distinct rheumatic disease syndrome associated with a specific antibody to an extractable nuclear antigen (ENA). Am J Med 1972;52:148.
117. Steere AC, Malawista SE, Snydman DR, et al: Lyme arthritis: An epidemic of oligoarthritis in children and adults in three Connecticut communities. Arthritis Rheum 1977;20:7.
118. Lyme disease–United States, 1994. MMWR 1995;44:459.
119. Steere AC, Schoen RT, Taylor E: The clinical evolution of Lyme arthritis. Ann Intern Med 1987;107:725.
120. Rose CD, Fawcett PT, Gibney K, et al: Pediatric Lyme arthritis: A longitudinal study of clinical spectrum and outcome. Pediatr Orthop 1994;14:238.
121. Rose CD, Fawcett PT, Gibney KM, et al: Residual serologic reactivity in children with resolved Lyme arthritis. J Rheumatol 1995;23:367.
122. Oski J, Metsola J, Reunamen M, et al: Subacute osteomyelitis caused by Borrelia burgdorferi. Clin Infect Dis 1994;19:891.
123. Athreya BH, Rose CD: Lyme disease. Curr Probl Pediatr 1996;26:189.
124. Wilson NIL, DiPaola M: Acute septic arthritis in infancy and childhood: 10 years' experience. J Bone Joint Surg 1986;68B:584.
125. Klouda PT, Corbin SA, Bradley BA, et al: HLA and acute arthritis following human parvovirus infection. Tissue Antigens 1986;28:318.
126. Mangi RJ: Viral arthritis: The great masquerader. Bull Rheum Dis 1994;43:5.
127. Kunnamo I, Kallio P, Pelkonen P, et al: Clinical signs and laboratory tests in the differential diagnosis of arthritis in children. Am J Dis Child 1987;141:34.
128. Upchurch KS, Brettler DB: Arthritis as a manifestation of other systemic diseases. In Kelly WN, Harris ED, Ruddy S, et al (eds): Textbook of Rheumatology. Philadelphia, WB Saunders, 1997.
129. Atkins RM, Henderson NJ, Duthie RB: Joint contractures in the hemophilias. Clin Orthop 1987;219:97.
130. Pettersson H, Wingstrand H, Thambert C, et al: Legg-Calvé-Perthes disease in hemophilia: Incidence and etiologic considerations. J Pediatr Orthop 1990;10:28.
131. Berntorp E: Methods of haemophilia care delivery: Regular prophylaxis versus episodic treatment. Haemophilia 1995;1(Suppl 1):3.
132. Nilsson IM, Berntorp E, Lofquist T, et al: Twenty five years' experience of prophylactic treatment in severe haemophilia A and B. J Intern Med 1992;232:25.
133. Schwartz RS, Agilgaard CF, Aledort LM, et al: Human recombinant DNA derived antihemophilic factor (factor VIII) in the treatment of hemophilia A. N Engl J Med 1989;320:166.
134. Kock B, Luban NLC, Galioto FM Jr, et al: Changes in coagulation parameters with exercise in patients with classic hemophilia. Am J Hematol 1984;16:271.
135. Buzzard BM: Sports and hemophilia. Clin Orthop 1996;328:25.
136. Klein KS, Aland CM, Kin HC, et al: Long-term follow-up of arthroscopic synovectomy for chronic hemophilic synovitis. Arthroscopy 1987;3:231.
137. Wiedel JD: Arthroscopic synovectomy of the knee in hemophilia. Clin Orthop 1996;328:46.
138. Taubert KA, Rowley AH, Shulman ST: Nationwide survey of Kawasaki disease and acute rheumatic fever. J Pediatr 1991;119:279.
139. Shulman ST, McAuley JB, Pachman LM, et al: Risk of coronary abnormalities due to Kawasaki disease in urban area with small Asian population. Am J Dis Child 1987;141:420.

140. Schumacher HR: Hemoglobinopathies and arthritis. In Kelley WN, Harris ED, Ruddy S, et al (eds): Textbook of Rheumatology. Philadelphia, WB Saunders, 1997.

141. Schumacher HR, Andrews R, McLaughlin G: Arthropathy in sickle cell disease. Ann Intern Med 1973;178: 203.

142. Rothschild BM, Sebes JI: Calcaneal abnormalities and erosive bone disease associated with sickle cell anemia. Am J Med 1981;71:427.

143. Stoff E, Bacon MC, White PH: The effects of fatigue, distractibility, and absenteeism on school achievement in children with rheumatic diseases. Arthritis Care Res 1990;2:49.

Chapter 19

Musculoskeletal Conditions and Trauma in Children

Kevin P. Murphy, MD
Beverly M. Steele, DNSc, RN, CS-FNP

Development of the Bony Skeleton

The skeletal system develops from mesoderm and neural crest cells.[1] Somites form from paraxial mesoderm and differentiate into sclerotomes and dermomyotomes. Sclerotome cells eventually form the vertebrae and ribs. Dermatomes, cells from the dermomyotome, form either the dermis or the primitive muscle cells called *myotomes*.

Limbs and respective girdles, the appendicular skeleton, are derived from cells of the lateral plate mesoderm. Limb buds appear in utero approximately day 26 for the upper extremities and day 28 for the lower extremities.[1] Each limb bud consists of a mass of mesenchyme covered by ectoderm. Despite its simple structure, the mammalian limb bud contains enough intrinsic information to guide its formation, because if transplanted to another region of the body or cultured in vitro, recognizable limb forms develop.[2] The many models for development of the skeletal system are beyond the scope of this chapter. The reader is referred to the appropriate references.[3,4] Vertebrae arise from the fusion of several cartilaginous primordia. The centrum is derived from the sclerotomal portions of paired somites or paraxial mesoderm and serves as the bony floor of the spinal cord, including vertebral body. Neural arches arise independently on either side of the centrum fusing to form a protective roof over the spinal cord. Thirty percent of the spine is ossified at birth. From age 2 years, the neural arches begin to fuse with each other from the lumbar to the cervical region. From about age 7 years, the arches fuse to the centrum from cervical to lumbar regions. The normal adult cervical spine is completely formed by approximately the age of 8 years. Failure of fusion of the dorsal neural arches results in the common anomaly of spina bifida occulta.[5] Failure of fusion and segmentation of these vertebral tissues results in multiple common anomalies of the vertebral column, including hemivertebra and epiphyseal bars.[6] During puberty, secondary ossification centers appear for the tips of the spinous and transverse processes, in addition to epiphyseal plates for the vertebral body forming circumferential bony rings or vertebral ring apophyses. The ring apophyses are the only open vertebral growth center after the age of 10 years. Fusion to the vertebral body usually occurs between the ages of 18 and 25 years. Neurogenic elements or ectoderm generally determines the bony development or mesoderm. This relationship is not seen in reverse. The child with a myelomeningocele generally has an associated bony deficit. Children with spina bifida occulta or hemivertebra or other bony anomalies often do not have corresponding neurologic deficiencies. All parts of the appendicular skeleton begin as cartilaginous components, which convert to true bone by endochondral ossification during embryogenesis generally in a proximal-to-distal sequence.[2,7] By 12 weeks, primary ossification centers are present in nearly all bones of the limbs.[1] The clavicles begin to ossify before any other bones in the body. Virtually all primary ossification centers are present by birth. The part of bone ossified from a primary center is called the *diaphysis* (Fig. 19–1).

The secondary ossification centers of the bones first appear at the distal end of the femur and the proximal end of the tibia approximately 34–38 weeks after fertilization. Most secondary centers of ossification appear after birth. The part of bone ossified from a secondary center is called the *epiphysis* (see Fig. 19–1). The portion of developing bone between the epiphysis and the diaphysis is the metaphysis. Bone age is a good index of general maturation. Determination of

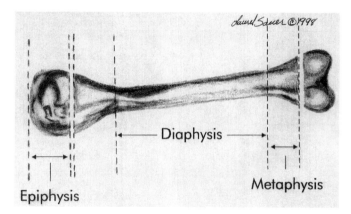

FIGURE 19–1. Diaphysis, metaphysis, and epiphysis of a typical long bone.

the number, size, and fusion of the epiphyseal centers from radiographs is a commonly used method.[8,9] Fusion of the epiphyseal centers happens 1–2 years earlier in females than in males.

Figures 19–2 and 19–3 show the primary and secondary ossification centers in both the upper and the lower extremities along with appearances and closures. Figure 19–4 shows the relative

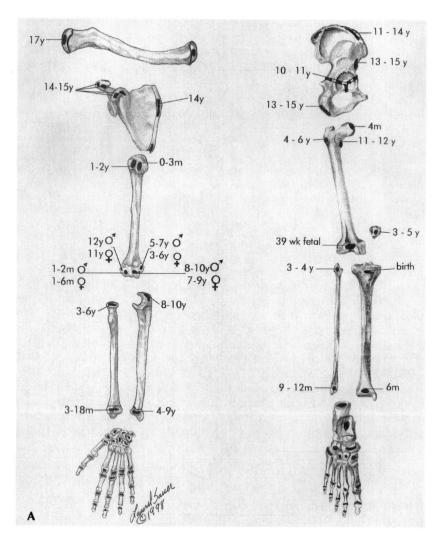

FIGURE 19–2. *A,* Schematic of ages of onset of secondary ossification of major long bones in the arm and the leg.

(Figure continued on following page.)

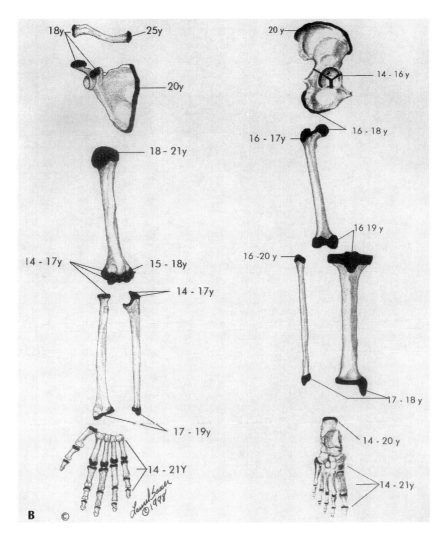

FIGURE 19–2 *(Continued).* *B,* Schematic of ages of physeal closure (physiologic epiphysiodesis) in the major long bones of the arm and the leg.

contributions of individual growth regions to the overall length of an individual bone and composite extremity in both the arm and the leg.

Interruption of any stage of development may result in congenital limb deficiencies of many kinds. Clubfoot, or talipes equinovarus, and other conditions with multifactorial inheritance patterns have also been attributed to persistent mechanical pressures in the uterus, particularly in cases of oligohydramnios.[10] Intrauterine molding may result in some startling postural abnormalities at birth that respond quickly to simple therapy in the first few weeks. Laxity of the musculoskeletal system in neonates provides an opportunity for correction of these deformities by conservative means, such as splinting, not possible weeks later.[11,12] Knowledge of the normal growth and development of the musculoskeletal system and associated deficiencies allows a firm

foundation for the understanding of both congenital and acquired conditions requiring care in the developmental years.

Conditions of the Upper Extremity

Minor limb deficiencies are relatively common in the upper extremities. Syndactyly occurs in 1 in 2200 births,[5] either as cutaneous with simple webbing of the fingers or osseous with fusion of the bones when the digital rays fail to separate during the 8th postconceptual week. It is most frequent between the third and fourth fingers and between the second and third toes and is inherited as a simple dominant or simple recessive trait. Shortness of the digits, brachydactyly, and supernumerary digits, polydactyly, are also seen, the latter being more common. Although minor, many of these abnormalities serve as indicators

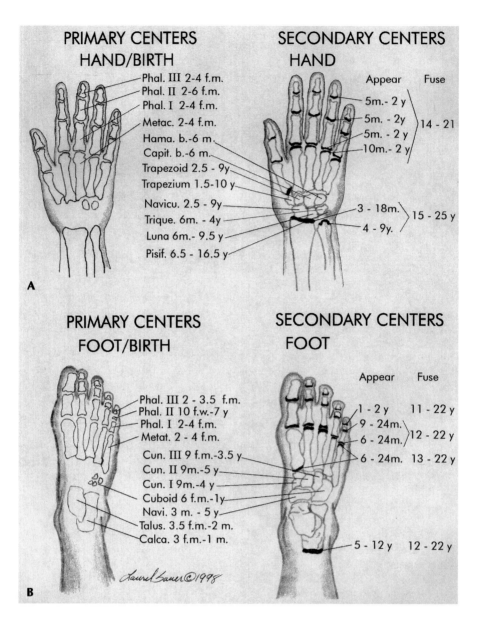

FIGURE 19–3. *A,* Time schedule for appearance of primary and secondary ossification centers and fusion of secondary centers with shafts in the hands. *B,* Time schedule for appearance of primary and secondary ossification centers and fusion of secondary centers with shafts in the feet.

of more serious patterns of malformation.[13] Malformations of the radius are more common than those of the ulna and are associated with numerous syndromes.[7,14] In children with limb anomalies, a multisystemic review is generally indicated because abnormalities in other systems are often present. Simple and multifactorial inheritance patterns may all be causative, in addition to teratogenic effects such as maternal exposure to viral infections and chemical dependency such as alcohol.[15,16]

Multiple ossification centers around a particular joint, such as the shoulder, may result in

malformation. Anomalies of the scapula include a bipartite coracoid, duplication of the acromion process, and dysplasia of the glenoid and scapular clefts.[17] Failure of the scapula to descend from its cervical region overlying the first through fifth ribs results in Sprengel's deformity.[17,18] Congenital dislocation of the radial head unaccompanied by other congenital abnormalities of the elbow or forearm is rare, as fewer than 100 cases have been reported.[7] The direction of displacement of the radial head may be anterior or posterolateral. When the diagnosis is made in the newborn or young infant, closed

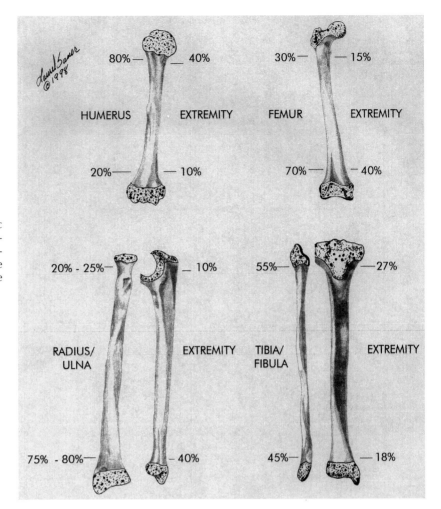

FIGURE 19–4. Schematic of relative contributions of individual growth regions to overall length of an individual bone and composite extremity in the arm *(left)* and the leg *(right)*.

reduction may be attempted. The posteriorly dislocated radial head is reduced by supination of the forearm and extension of the elbow, whereas the anteriorly dislocated radial head is reduced by flexion of the elbow. Reduction is maintained in an above-elbow cast for 4–6 weeks. Closed reduction is often unsuccessful, and an open surgical procedure is required. In the older child, it is impossible to reduce the radial head. The dislocation is left alone until late adolescence, when, if symptoms warrant, the radial head is excised. Congenital conditions persisting into adulthood need to be cared for appropriately because additional biomechanical injuries and overuse syndromes may occur if neglected.

Overuse syndromes are generally conditions caused by unresolved submaximal stress in previously normal tissues. They involve microtrauma resulting from chronic repetitive insults to the musculoskeletal system. With focus on single sports early in life, these injuries have become more prevalent in the pediatric athlete.[19,20] Growth cartilage appears to be more

susceptible to stress and overuse than adult cartilage.[21,22] Growth cartilage is present at three different sites: the physes, the joint surface, and the major muscle-tendon insertions or apophyses. Little League elbow comprises a group of pathologic entities in and about the elbow joint in young developing pitchers. The injury may include medial epicondylar fragmentation and avulsion, osteochondritis of the capitulum or radial head, and delayed closure of growth plates around the elbow. The mechanism of injury appears to be repetitive valgus strain applied to the elbow by throwing.[23–25] Stress injuries to the distal radial and ulnar physes are commonly found in gymnasts.[26–28] X-rays demonstrate widened epiphyses, cystic changes, and beaking of the distal metaphyses. Some risk of distal radial and ulnar growth arrest exists.

Osteochondritis dissecans is a condition resulting in partial or complete separation of a segment of normal hyaline cartilage from its supporting bone. Depending on the separation, cartilaginous or osteochondral intraarticular fragments may form. Mechanical symptoms may arise within the elbow, such as catching and locking. Although it has been more than 100 years since Konig[29] coined the term osteochondritis dissecans, there is still little agreement about the cause. Five theories commonly suggested are ischemia, genetic predisposition, abnormal ossification, trauma, and cyclical strain.

The elbow is the most commonly injured joint in children. Acquired dislocations account for 6–8% of elbow injuries[30,31] and are most frequent in children under the age of 10 years.[32] Typically the injury involves the nondominant extremity with a fall onto the outstretched hand.[33] Nursemaid's elbow consists of radial head subluxation from a sharp upward pull on the extended pronated arm in preschoolers. A generalized ligamentous laxity of children with large cartilaginous components of the distal humerus and proximal ulna, in addition to osseous instability with numerous secondary ossification centers and apophyses, all contribute to the tendency for the pediatric elbow to dislocate. Posterior or posterolateral dislocations account for 80–90% of the injury[34,35] and can be reduced through numerous conservative techniques.[32,33,36] In general, the child refuses to use the arm until reduction is achieved, as discussed previously. Fractures always need to be considered seriously before any reduction, particularly of the coronoid process. Anterior dislocations are less common and usually caused by a direct blow to the posterior olecranon with the elbow flexed.

Shoulder injuries are relatively uncommon in the overall picture of injuries to the pediatric musculoskeletal system.[37] When they occur, they include separation of the acromioclavicular joint from direct trauma, osteolysis of the distal clavicle mostly in weightlifters, and cervical clavicular injuries in the young thrower.[38] Injuries to the rotator cuff are not as common in the young as they are in the older athlete.[38]

Conservative treatment for musculoskeletal injury in children includes rest, ice, compression, and elevation (RICE), in addition to nonsteroidal anti-inflammatory drugs (NSAIDs) (Telectin, naproxen [Naprosyn], ibuprofen [Children's Motrin and Children's Advil]). Appropriate equipment, coaching, recreation environments, and training often prevent these conditions. Surgical referrals need to be considered in all cases.

Tumors may mimic various pain syndromes throughout the body. Primary bone tumors particularly common to the upper extremities include Ewing's sarcoma of the scapula, osteogenic sarcoma of the proximal humerus, and osteoblastomas and chondroblastomas common in the diaphyses and epiphyses of long bones.[7] Osteogenic sarcoma occurs most often during the adolescent growth spurt with a slight preference for boys. Metastasis to the lungs remains the most likely cause of death. Classic radiographs consist of mixed lytic and sclerotic lesions near the metaphysis with a cortical invasion, periosteal elevation, and soft tissue extensions or spicules radiating outward producing a *sunburst* appearance. With Ewing's sarcoma, tumor growth may be so rapid that the center becomes necrotic and osteomyelitis is diagnosed. Because the outlook in childhood cancer continues to change so rapidly and there is such a high level of complexity to the diagnosis and treatment options, referral to a regional oncology center is necessary when neoplasm is diagnosed.

Conditions of the Spine

In about 5% of humans, there are minor variations in the number or proportions of vertebrae.[2] The Klippel-Feil syndrome, sometimes called *brevicollis*, is characterized by a short neck, low hairline, and restricted neck movement.[39] In most cases, the number of cervical vertebrae is decreased. There may be a lack of segmentation of several elements in the cervical spine with smaller cervical nerve roots and intervertebral foramina. Often, there are no other malformations, but some association with additional congenital anomalies exists.[13]

Cleft vertebral column, rachischisis, refers to vertebral abnormalities that primarily affect the axial structures of the spine or axial dysraphic disorders. In infants with rachischisis, the neural folds fail to fuse either because of faulty induction by the underlying notochord or because of the action of teratogenic agents on the neural epithelial cells in the neural folds.[1] The vertebral defects can be quite minor or affect the majority of the spinal column in a startling manner. Congenital abnormalities at the craniovertebral junction are present in about 1% of neonates. Symptoms from these abnormalities may not arise until adult life. Examples of these malformations include (1) basilar invagination or superior displacement of the bone around the foramen magnum, (2) assimilation of the atlas or nonsegmentation at the junction of the atlas and occipital bone, and (3) Arnold-Chiari malformations. Atlantoaxial dislocations may be present in addition to a separate dens or odontoid process because of failure of the centers in the dens to fuse with the centrum of the axis. In children with Down syndrome, atlantoaxial instability may be identified in up to 13%,[40–42] but only 1–2% have symptomatic instability that requires surgery. X-ray examination of the cervical spine in children with Down syndrome should be obtained at about the age of 3 years and before such children enter competitive sports such as the Special Olympics. Repeat x-rays should be taken after the cervical spine has been completely formed, at around the age of 8 years, and then every decade thereafter across the life span as recommended by the American Association of Down's Syndrome. Significant instability is defined as greater than 5 mm of distance between the posterior border of the C-1 arch and the anterior surface of the dens.[43]

Between the vertebrae, the notochord expands to form the gelatinous center of the intervertebral disc called the *nucleus pulposus*.[1,2] This nucleus is later surrounded by circularly arranged fibers from sclerotome-derived mesodermal cells called the *annulus fibrosus*. The nucleus pulposus and the annulus fibrosus together constitute the intervertebral disc. The intervertebral disc is vascular in children up through the age of 7 years. Around the age of 7, the disc begins to develop some of the endarteries common to the adolescent and adult. From the age of approximately 13 years, all endarteries are thought to be formed, and thus the disc has become completely avascular. It may well be that the more vascular nature of the disc is a major reason why discitis occurs almost solely in children.[44-47] Discitis is a rare condition occurring in less than 1% of children. It is commonly divided into septic and aseptic types. Positive cultures are generally more common in younger children, with *Staphylococcus aureus* by far the most common finding. A more slow, indolent form of discitis may develop in a child from brucellosis or tuberculosis. A skin test for tuberculosis may be helpful. Trauma might cause release from the disc tissue enzymes such as phospholipase A_2, known to be a potent inflammatory stimulator, which could, in theory, cause inflammation. Viral causes are also thought to be present and likely make up a substantial component of the aseptic variety. High fever, toxemia, elevated white blood cell counts, positive blood cultures, and bone scan in a child under the age of 3 years who refuses to sit or stand is a common history. The diagnosis must be considered in a child with just mild illness who has abdominal pain or refuses to walk for unclear reasons.

A magnetic resonance (MR) imaging scan shows involvement of the disc space and vertebral bodies (Fig. 19–5). The two most serious diseases in the differential diagnosis include vertebral osteomyelitis, rare in children, and spinal tumors. Biopsy of the disc space may be necessary. Vancomycin may be the treatment of

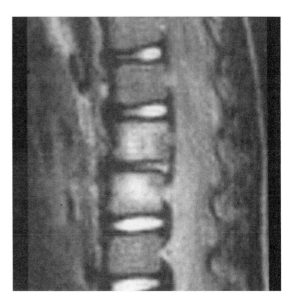

FIGURE 19–5.   Magnetic resonance imaging scan in a 3-year-old child with discitis. Vertebral involvement is present both above and below the dehydrated disc.

choice or other staphylococcal antimicrobials, but only after any attempts for culture or biopsy have been completed. Immobilization of the child may or may not be helpful. Hematogenous spread is the most common cause of vertebral osteomyelitis, with *S. aureus* the most common organism. Vertebral osteomyelitis generally involves the more anterior aspects of the spine and may be associated with paravertebral *collections*. Tuberculous spondylitis, or Pott's disease, remains common worldwide and is still seen in some more neglected areas of the United States.[48]

Progressive scoliosis can be divided into congenital, idiopathic, and neuromuscular types. Idiopathic scoliosis accounts for approximately 80% of patients with structural scoliosis.[7] It is subdivided according to the age of onset with three fairly well-defined periods: infantile, from birth to 3 years of age; juvenile, from 4 years of age until the onset of puberty; and adolescent, at or about the onset of puberty and before the closure of the physes. Idiopathic scoliosis is generally more common in girls, particularly later-onset curvatures with a tendency for left thoracolumbar convexities. Familial tendencies are present, with idiopathic scoliosis occurring, according to some studies, in 1.4–5% of relatives.[49] An autosomal dominant inheritance pattern with a variable penetrance is suspected. School screening has resulted in earlier diagnosis for many children, facilitating timely conservative treatments. Inspection for scoliosis should be part of all routine physical examinations.

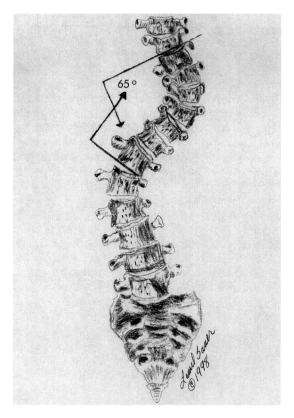

FIGURE 19–6. The Cobb method of measuring the curvature in scoliosis. The angle measured is formed by perpendicular lines drawn through the superior border of the upper vertebra and the inferior border of the lowest vertebra of a given curve.

Posture should be evaluated for shoulder asymmetry, pelvic obliquity, elevation of iliac crests, and exaggerated flank creases. Shift of the trunk can be noted by dropping a plumb line from the prominence of the C7 spinous process and noting whether it deviates laterally at the gluteal cleft. The vertebral body always rotates into the convexity, creating a posterior rib bulge or prominence of the paraspinal muscles on the convex side and an anterior rib prominence on the concave side. Asymmetry of the breasts may also be seen. Forward bending is best to evaluate thoracic asymmetry, along with side-bending assessments, to determine more flexibility or rigidity to the curvatures. A flexible curve that corrects with postural adjustments and sidebending is generally more amenable to bracing than its more rigid counterparts. A thorough neurologic evaluation should occur in addition to checking the bones for leg length discrepancy and hip and knee contractures, and inspecting the skin for café-au-lait spots or hairy patches that may overlie spinal anomalies such as diastematomyelia.

Cobb angles are generally used to measure the degree of spinal curvatures (Fig. 19–6).[50] The curve with the greater number of degrees is the major curve and is designated *left* or *right* according to the side of the convexity. The apex of the curvature is the vertebral body with the fulcrum of maximal angulation. The angles of trunk rotation can be measured with scoliometers on forward bending. An angle of trunk rotation greater than 5 degrees generally indicates a more serious structural curvature, which requires consideration for surgical referral. Compensatory curvatures are by definition not fixed in rotation. Bracing is the usual treatment for curvatures between approximately 20 and 45 degrees in compliant patients. The contact pads are placed just inferior to the apex of the curvature, pressing upward in a superior lateral direction using three points of fixation. On the concave side of the curvature, the distal point of fixation is often the pelvic girdle, and the axillary wall is proximal.[51,52] Bracing is done only during growth and without compromise of respiration or feeding. Both the primary and the secondary curves are braced with emphasis on the primary. To be effective, the orthosis needs to be worn at least 16 hours a day or more until satisfactory correction has been achieved. Curvatures less than 20 degrees are often observed, and if progression is suspected, radiographs are obtained every 6 months. X-rays may include supine and sitting or standing views with anteroposterior and lateral projections, with and without the thoracolumbosacral orthosis (TLSO). Because curvatures of 50 degrees or more are at a high risk for progression, surgical intervention is considered. Significant curvatures may progress during adulthood and increase approximately 1 degree per year. Scoliosis is generally not associated with back pain. When a painful scoliosis is present, other causes need to be considered, such as high-grade spondylolisthesis, neurofibromas, or other spinal tumors.

Congenital scoliosis may be associated with cardiac abnormalities in 10% of cases, with renal in 25% of cases, as well as gastrointestinal anomalies.[53] Family history is positive in 5–10% of siblings and offspring. With more rapid progressions, an MR imaging scan of the spine is indicated to rule out tethering, syrinx, or other intraspinal anomalies. On radiographs, the apex of the curvature is generally where the pathology is located. Epiphyseal bars, failures of separation, are generally more serious and surgically challenging than hemivertebrae, failures of formation. Combinations of hemivertebrae and epiphyseal bars may be the most difficult, particularly when located at junctional areas (i.e., cervicothoracic, thoracolumbar, or lumbosacral). The identification of any congenital vertebral anomaly with progressive curvature requires immediate surgical referral.

Neuromuscular spinal deformity is particularly common in Friedreich ataxia (up to 80% of individuals), spinal muscular atrophy (up to 65% of individuals), Duchenne muscular dystrophy (up to 90% of individuals), cerebral palsy with spastic quadriplegia (up to 70% of individuals), and myelodysplasia (up to 60% of individuals).

Bracing has less to offer in neuromuscular and congenital scoliosis compared with the more idiopathic varieties. Exercise helps to maintain flexibility through spinal segments and maintain strength and respiratory capacities in general. Swimming is helpful, particularly if significant kyphosis is present. TLSO is the usual bracing intervention with curves that have apices at T8 or below. Milwaukee braces are used particularly for kyphotic curvatures with apices above T8.

Progression of scoliosis may occur despite proper bracing and conservative care requiring appropriate surgical referral. Pulmonary function tests are obtained before any surgery and generally must be at least 40% or greater of predicted value for intervention (forced vital capacity and forced expiratory volume in 1 second). Surgical fusions can be anterior or posterior and may include the sacrum. Generally, fusion of the sacrum is avoided in ambulatory individuals for fear of reducing the lumbosacral lordosis and causing gait deterioration. In nonambulators, fusion to the pelvis is more common, particularly in the presence of pelvic obliquity. The individual generally loses 0.07 cm per vertebral segment per year in growth over fused segments. Luque rods with segmental instrumentation, sublaminar hooks, are often the treatment of choice.[54] Posterior spinal fusions are into hard bone and thus generally more secure. Anterior fusions are into softer bone and generally involve taking down the diaphragm with more of a cardiopulmonary challenge to the patient. The reasons for performing an anterior fusion include correction of the spine into more kyphosis with anterior load sharing and a more circumferential fusion. Anterior fusions are associated with the superior mesenteric artery syndrome,[55] and all have sympathectomies. Surgical fusions of the spine are generally delayed until the age of 10 years or more in an attempt to achieve maximal spinal growth. Crankshaft phenomenon[7] may occur with posterior fusions only in children under the age of 10 years who have excessive anterior vertebral body growth over the more superior fused vertebrae. Spinal growth is complete when the iliac apophyses or Risser's lines have been added to the crests of the ilium and the vertebral ring apophyses have fused at an average age of 16.5 years in girls and 17.5 years in boys. Risser's lines[56] appear around the onset of puberty and are graded from 1 to 5 depending on their excursion across the iliac crest. Beginning at the anterosuperior iliac spine and extending backward to the posterior iliac spine, a Risser stage 1 is 25% excursion; stage 2, 50% excursion; stage 3, 75% excursion; and stage 4, complete excursion. A Risser stage 5 occurs when the iliac apophysis fuses to the body of the ilium.

The TLSO and Milwaukee brace[57] are used for other conditions of the spine, such as severe Scheuermann's disease. Scheuermann's disease,[58] or kyphosis, is distinguished from postural roundback by its more rigid structural characteristics. It occurs in 0.5–8% of the population, with an increased prevalence in males. When three or more consecutive vertebrae are wedged more than 5 degrees, radiographic criteria for Scheuermann's disease are met.[59] The radiographic picture includes irregular vertebral end plates, protrusion of disc material into the spongiosum of the vertebral body, Schmorl's nodes, narrowed disc spaces, and anterior wedging of the vertebral bodies. The cause of Scheuermann's disease is unknown but thought by some to fall within the spectrum of repetitive microtrauma and fatigue failure of the immature thoracic vertebral bodies. *Atypical Scheuermann's disease*,[60,61] or thoracolumbar apophysitis, is named because it does not meet the usual radiographic criteria for Scheuermann's disease established by Sorenson.[62] This phenomenon is usually seen at the thoracolumbar junction and may be the pediatric equivalent of an adult compression fracture. There is a 2:1 male-to-female predominance. The peak age of incidence is between 15 and 17 years. When Scheuermann's disease is associated with pain in the presence of one or more irregular vertebral bodies, physical exercise is prohibited. Sometimes the TLSO or Boston brace is required for 3 months to achieve pain control. Conservative care including traditional RICE approach, a gentle flexibility program, and nonsteroidal anti-inflammatory agents may help.

Intervertebral disc injuries in children are uncommon in the young athlete.[44,63–65] In contrast to the selective motor and sensory deficits often observed in adults with disc herniation, athletes under 20 years of age have pain and tenderness localized generally to the midline and to a lesser extent over the course of the sciatic nerve.[66] Current data show that herniated discs account for fewer than 10% of young athletes with low back pain.[67] Spondylolysis has never been found in the newborn. Its occurrence increases between the ages of 5.5 and 6.5 years to a rate of 5%, close to the frequency of 5.8% in the white adult population.[60] Most authors now believe that spondylolysis and prespondylitic stress reactions are overuse injuries.[68–70] The lesion is a pars interarticularis stress fracture treated with bracing and hamstring stretching until healed and asymptomatic. Single-photon emission computed tomography (SPECT) bone scans may be particularly helpful in identifying these lesions and eventual healing, which can take up to 9 months.[71] Spondylolisthesis or slipping forward of the vertebral body may occur during childhood with a prepubertal peak incidence and promoted by hyperlordosis. Grading of spondylolisthesis is according to the classification developed by Meyerding.[71,72] The superior border of the inferior vertebra is divided into four equal quadrants with slips in each quadrant accounting for one grade. Surgical treatment is necessary in the presence of neurologic signs or forward slipping of the vertebral body beyond 50% of its width. Other apophyseal injuries in the spine include the slipped vertebral apophysis or end plate fracture.[73,74]

This condition may mimic a herniated lumbar disc and is often associated with heavy lifting. Commonly the inferior apophysis of L4 is displaced into the vertebral canal along with some attached disc material. Radiographs reveal a small bony fragment pulled off the inferior edge of the vertebral end plate. A computed tomography (CT) scan or MR imaging reveals an extradural mass. Surgical excision provides excellent relief of symptoms. Strains of the lower back are less common in children in view of the open iliac apophyses. Children with iliac apophysitis usually have belt-line pain along the muscular attachments to the superior iliac crest.[63] Lumbar interspinous process bursitis or kissing spines also need consideration in the young patient, especially those participating in gymnastics or other activities involving hyperextension of the thoracolumbar spine.[63]

Congenital cervical stenosis is an additional concern and may account for some of the transient quadriplegia found in older children.[75,76] The diagnosis is made by measuring the anteroposterior diameter of the vertebral body and canal at the level in question. If the canal-to-body ratio is less than 0.8, stenosis is present.[77]

Neoplasms of the spine fall into two groups based on location and the vertebral segment. Osteoid osteoma and osteoblastoma occur in the posterior elements, whereas aneurysmal bone cysts, giant cell tumor, Ewing's sarcoma, eosinophilic granuloma, and osteogenic sarcoma usually occur in the vertebral body.[7,68] Lymphoma also has been reported to cause back pain in the young.[68,78] Remnants of the notochord may persist and give rise to a chordoma. This slow-growing neoplasm occurs most frequently in the base of the skull and in the lumbosacral region. When a neoplasm is diagnosed, referral to a cancer center for proper therapeutic intervention should be arranged.

Conditions of the Lower Extremity

Congenital dysplasia and joint dislocations of the lower extremity may occur at the hip and less often at the knee and patellofemoral joints. Congenital dislocation of the knee is rare,[79,80] with an incidence of 0.7 per 1000 cases in one report. The knee is hyperextended, with the tibia anterior to the femur. Closed reduction with casting in flexion is the initial treatment, followed by surgical reduction if unsuccessful. Congenital dislocation of the patella is also rare and not usually diagnosed in infancy. The condition may be unilateral or bilateral, and there is a familial tendency.[81] The diagnosis should be suspected in the infant presenting with fixed flexion deformity of the knee and excessive lateral rotation of the tibia. The patella does not ossify until 3 years, when the diagnosis is more readily made.[82,83] Closed manipulation to reduce the dislocation is not feasible, and the treatment is open surgical realignment. Congenital absence of the patella is quite rare, is often bilateral, and tends to be associated with talipes equinovarus and congenital dislocation of the hip. Occasionally, it is an isolated lesion.[84] Multipartite patellae arise from two or more centers of ossification, with a fragment sometimes attaching to the main body of the patella by fibrocartilage. These conditions may be bilateral, with the accessory patellae located superolaterally most of the time.[85,86] They can present in the older child and athlete with anterior knee pain and patellofemoral-type symptoms. Multipartite patellae often may be an incidental radiographic finding.[87–89]

Congenital dysplasia of the hip comprises a wide spectrum of conditions ranging from simple hip instability with capsular laxity to complete displacement of the femoral head out of an anomalous acetabular socket. The term *dysplasia* denotes developmental abnormality, whereas congenital dislocation of the hip is considered a progressive deformation of a previously normal hip outside of the acetabulum. It is important to differentiate between two main groups of congenital dislocation of the hip: teratologic and typical. Teratologic dislocation is characterized by associations with other severe malformations, such as arthrogryposis and myelomeningocele. It develops early in utero with severe soft tissue contractures and marked displacement. Typical congenital dislocation of the hip occurs in an otherwise normal infant and may take place in utero, perinatally, or postnatally.[7] Developmental hip dysplasia is relatively common, with a preponderance for a first-born white girl.[90] In the infant with developmental hip dysplasia, subluxation or dislocation usually occurs after birth, often in the first 2 weeks of life. The incidence is higher in breech deliveries. Associations with ligamentous laxity and rearing practices have also been identified (e.g., swaddling the infant with hips in extension). If a congruent reduction is accomplished before the age of 4 years, 95% of hips develop normally.[91] Treatment is usually immediate with a Pavlik harness or other alternative orthoses so that normal remodeling is achieved, it is hoped, before walking. Delays in treatment are associated with recurrence as well as avascular necrosis of the femoral head.

Ultrasonography has become the primary imaging technique of the neonatal hip because the capital femoral epiphyses do not ossify until 3–6 months of age.[92,93] The diagnosis is made by clinical examination, when a palpable clunk is felt while the infant's hip is gently brought into flexion and abduction, thus causing reduction, so-called Ortolani's sign,[94,95] or when the hip is moved slowly into adduction causing dislocation, Barlow's sign.[94,96] As subluxation progresses, asymmetry of the thighs increases with limitation of abduction becoming more apparent. Galeazzi's sign may be present, demonstrating apparent femoral shortening with asymmetric knee levels with the infant supine, heels together, and hips and knees fully flexed. After walking is achieved, Trendelenburg gait is present. The lateral waddle is more evident in bilateral cases. Radiographic changes include an increase in the acetabular index, a break in Shenton's line, and displacement of the femoral head, which may not yet be ossified (Fig. 19–7).[97]

Open reduction of the hip is used when conservative and closed methods fail or there is inability to maintain a stable reduction, which becomes more likely with age.[98] Surgeries may involve various types of acetabular osteotomies to improve lateral coverage of the proximal femur or femoral procedures with various osteotomies redirecting the capital epiphysis into the centrum of the acetabulum.[99] Avascular necrosis, although uncommon, may occur after

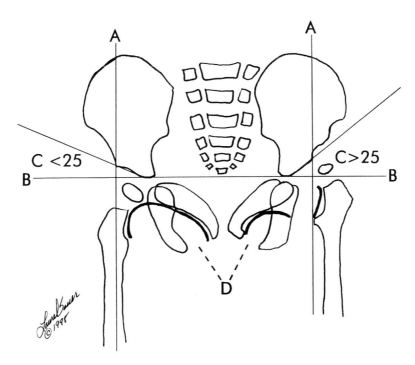

FIGURE 19–7. Radiographic evaluation in developmental hip dislocation. *A,* Perkin's vertical line—perpendicular dropped from the lateral acetabular margin. *B,* Hilgenreiner's line, through the Y cartilages. The femoral head should lie in the lower medial quadrant formed by the intersection of the two lines. *C,* Acetabular index—the angle formed by a line through the acetabular roof and Hilgenreiner's line; normal below 25 degrees. *D,* Shenton's line—the arc appears broken in the presence of dislocation. The abnormal hip appears on the right.

any treatment.[100] If ossification of the femoral head is not seen by the age of 1 year, avascular necrosis is suspected.[90,91] Failure to achieve reduction beyond age 6 years results in a permanently subluxed hip with marked gait deviation and susceptibility to osteoarthritis and pain over time. Spica casts applied after surgery need appropriate infantile care for hygiene and toileting, positioning, and mobility devices, such as scooters, carts, and accessible toys. The importance of early diagnosis and treatment of congenital hip dysplasia or dislocation cannot be overemphasized: the results are generally good with orthopedic intervention and disastrous if neglected.

Clubfoot, talipes equinus, is a common term used to describe several kinds of ankle or foot deformities present at birth. The foot is generally in equinus with forefoot and hindfoot varus and severe adduction. The incidence of clubfoot is approximately 1 in 400 live births.[10] A child born to a parent with clubfoot deformity has 1 chance in 10 of inheriting the condition. Some clubfoot disorders are transient or apparent in nature and result simply from intrauterine crowding. Other conditions may occur in association with myelodysplasia, arthrogryposis, and particularly hip dislocation. Casting in the first few weeks of life often is effective when done in a sequential manner from forefoot to hindfoot and avoiding a rocker-bottom deformity, a vertical talus, or calcaneal equinus. Different surgical procedures are available if the foot is too rigid for manual correction, all approximating various types of posterior medial release.[101,102] Supramalleolar orthoses are effective for maintaining full positioning after surgery and casting. Thereafter, range of motion should be maintained by passive exercise and therapeutic play, particularly into dorsiflexion and eversion. Persistent deformity often results in unstable ankles, lateral sprains, and difficulty with weight bearing and other gross mobility tasks.

A common cause of acquired hip pain in children is acute transient synovitis (ATS). ATS is a self-limited inflammatory condition of unknown cause that generally has an excellent clinical outcome, but often causes considerable anxiety among physicians and family members.[103] The condition may develop any time from toddler age onward, with peak age between 3 and 6 years, and is slightly more common in boys. At least half of the children with ATS have or recently have had an upper respiratory illness, including pharyngitis or otitis media. Trauma of a mild nature is frequently present. ATS is the most common cause of acute hip pain in children,[104,105] reported in up to 0.9% of pediatric

hospital admissions and in as many as 3% of all children. Common presentations include unilateral hip or groin pain with referral pattern to the knee. Radiographs are frequently reported as normal when compared with the opposite side but may show some slight intracapsular effusion. Ultrasonography is especially helpful in detecting effusion and may correlate with MR imaging and a positive radionuclear bone scan. ATS remains a diagnosis made after other entities are excluded. A transient ischemia may occur during the acute synovitis with some rare reports of progression to Legg-Calvé-Perthes disease. Aseptic arthritis also needs to be ruled out. The fundamental treatment consists of rest and age-appropriate NSAIDs. Full unrestricted activity should be avoided until the hip is completely pain-free and there is no evidence of limping.

Legg-Calvé-Perthes disorder is a condition of the femoral head characterized by ischemic necrosis, collapse, and subsequent repair.[106] The condition usually presents between the ages of 4 and 10 years with a peak incidence at 5–7 years. There is a definite male preponderance with 4:1 ratio. Both hips are involved in at least 20% of cases, although rarely simultaneously.[37,107] In the general population, the incidence has been reported to range from 1/1200 to 1/12,000.[103] Delay in skeletal maturation based on bone age has been documented in the early stages of the disease. The definite cause is unknown, but a temporary interruption of the vascular supply to the developing femoral head leading to avascular necrosis has been implicated. The typical presentation is intermittent, mildly symptomatic limping with pain in the groin radiating distally to the knee. Limitations in internal rotation, extension, and abduction of the affected hip are similar to conditions with synovitis. Children presenting with knee pain always require a thorough examination of the hip. Leg length discrepancy may be present and associated with the antalgic gait pattern.

There are four stages of the disease on anteroposterior and frog leg lateral radiographs. Synovitis is the first stage, lasting up to 3 weeks with effusions noted on x-rays. Necrosis of the ossification center with increased density of the capital femoral epiphysis is noted within 1 month to 1 year. The crescent sign occurs early and results from a subchondral fracture, which allows separation of the joint cartilage from the rest of the femoral head. Regeneration or fragmentation occurs within 3 months to 2 years of onset, showing areas of increased and decreased density, flattening of the femoral head or coxa plana, metaphyseal cysts, or subluxation. The final residual or healing stage may show some restoration of sphericity or coxa magna often leading to late degenerative arthritis. Coxa magna is generally caused from overgrowth of the greater trochanteric apophysis into the acetabulum with abutting against the lateral wall of the ilium. This condition contributes further to limited abduction and the Trendelenburg gait. Bone scanning and MR imaging may provide the diagnosis before radiographs. Laboratory tests, including erythrocyte sedimentation rate, C-reactive protein, and white blood cell counts, are often normal unless concurrent illness is present.

Controversy exists about whether treatment of any type affects the natural history of the disorder. The short-term goal is reduction of pain and stiffness of the hip. The disease process is self-limited and may last for 2–4 years. NSAIDs are effective in reducing synovitis. Restriction of activity helps relieve pain, which at times may include non–weight bearing with crutches. Abduction orthoses and casting may at some point be necessary. The important principle of treatment is femoral head containment within a spherical acetabulum so that, at least theoretically, reossification is also spherical. Surgery, including proximal femoral varus osteotomy, may eliminate longer-term bracing and allow earlier resumption of activities in some children. The prognosis of this disease is better with earlier detection, under 8 years, and with less than 50% of femoral head involvement.[107,108] Involvement of the lateral portion of the femoral head carries a poor prognosis, particularly when it affects 40% of the structural part. Return to high-impact athletics is restricted until a pain-free status is found during clinical examination and radiographs show healing. Osteoarthritis later in life is often seen with 50% of untreated patients showing severe changes by the age of 50 years.[109] Other causes of avascular necrosis always need to be considered, including sickle cell anemia, femoral neck fracture, Gaucher's disease, slipped epiphysis, congenital hip dislocations, rheumatoid arthritis and other collagen disorders, and steroid therapy. Bilateral involvement may be confused with multiple epiphyseal dysplasia differentiated by doing a skeletal survey.

A slipped capital femoral epiphysis (SCFE) usually involves posteroinferior displacement of the epiphysis on the proximal femoral metaphysis. More accurately, the epiphysis remains in normal position within the acetabulum, while the remainder of the proximal femur displaces in a superior and anterolateral direction because of weakness in the proximal physis. Radiographic findings include widening of the epiphyseal line with a rare fracture of the proximal femoral metaphysis in the preslip stage and swelling of the joint capsule. Trethowan's sign, a line drawn along the superior surface of the neck passing above the epiphysis rather than through it, indicates initial minimal slippage.[103,107] A peak incidence of SCFE corresponds to the age of accelerated growth and the start of adolescence for girls at 11.5 years and for boys at 13.0 years.[110,111] SCFE is at least twice as common in boys than girls and may be bilateral in up to 25% of cases, 5% of which occur simultaneously.[111] Affected children are often large and overweight, and some association with endocrine factors, such as hypothyroidism, hypopituitarism, hypogonadism, and excessive growth hormone, has been reported.

The cause of SCFE is the application of stress to the proximal femur in an amount exceeding the mechanical integrity of the proximal physis. The two most common features of presentation are pain and altered gait. The pain may come on acutely but more commonly builds over a number of months. As usual with hip pathology in children, pain occurs in the groin region and radiates to the knee and medial thigh. It is aggravated by walking and other high-impact activities. External rotation of the leg may be present with a Trendelenburg gait in the limping child. Physical examination demonstrates a loss of internal rotation, diminished flexion, shortening of the leg, and atrophy of the thigh if symptoms have been long-standing. Mild slips show displacement of the epiphysis up to one-third the width of the metaphysis, moderate slips up to two-thirds, and severe slips greater than two-thirds displacement. The displacement is usually best quantified on lateral radiographs. When SCFE is suspected, ambulation should not be allowed until the child is seen by an orthopedic surgeon.

Surgery is the preferred treatment, preventing further epiphyseal displacement by stabilizing the epiphysis with screws or pins. Cortical bone grafts also are used, crossing from the metaphyses to the epiphyses and resulting in epiphysiodeses. Generally the epiphysis is left in its displaced position because avascular necrosis is a 10–25% risk if manipulation is attempted. After successful physeal closure, it is common for the proximal femur to remodel, rounding angular metaphyseal surfaces anteriorly and forming bone posteriorly.[112] Chondrolysis or acute cartilage necrosis may occur postoperatively in more severe cases, more commonly in African-Americans and girls.[113] If chondrolysis is present, most individuals go on to develop narrowing of the joint space with some ankylosis, degenerative arthrosis, and pain. Weight bearing is generally avoided for at least 6 weeks after surgery, followed by active assistive exercises and strengthening to restore flexion, abduction, and internal rotation. Full identification of this condition while only minimal displacement is present and immediate surgery generally allow rapid mobilization and return to full activity with no sequelae.

Traumatic hip dislocations in children are relatively rare and, when they occur, are usually posterior.[107,114] The mechanism is usually traumatic with a direct blow to the knee with hip and knee flexed, as occurs with a fall during ground impact or dashboard contact injury in a car accident. Some dislocations have occurred during *mini-rugby*, in which players kneeling on the ground have had someone fall on top of them. Avascular necrosis may occur in up to 10% of cases. Sciatic nerve palsy is rare but needs to be ruled out. Posterior hip dislocation is an emergency that requires immediate referral to an orthopedic specialist.

Overuse injuries around the pelvis and hips are common and may be seen along the iliac crest; ischial tuberosities; and anterior, superior, or inferior iliac spine. Sometimes, late diagnosis of an avulsion of the ischial tuberosity is mistaken for an osteosarcoma. An avulsion may occur with a hamstring tear in a child sprinting during sporting activities or other recreational pursuits. Bones grow faster than muscles in children, and with associated growth spurts and limited stretching and warm-up activities, apophyseal avulsions are more common. Treatment of overuse syndromes generally involves conservative modalities and rest, followed by strengthening and stretching of muscle imbalances and gradual return to activity as tolerated. The snapping hip syndrome in children is an entity most commonly associated with iliotibial band irritation of the greater trochanteric bursa on hip flexion, extension, and internal rotation.[115] Osteitis pubis is more common in adults but may occasionally be seen in older teenagers with high mileage running.[116]

The most frequently injured area in childhood and adolescent athletics is the knee.[58,117] The collateral ligaments of the knee, especially the medial collateral ligament, are frequently injured in sports.[118] An isolated injury to the medial collateral ligament usually may be treated successfully without surgery. Although less common, there appears to be an increased incidence of anterior cruciate ligament injuries among children during sports.[118] Often these injuries are associated with avulsion of the anterior tibial spine. Anterior cruciate ligament

reconstructions in children, when performed, need to consider early closure of the distal femoral or proximal tibial physes or other growth disturbances with grafts that might cross the growth plate.[119,120] Autogenous patellar tendon grafting appears to be the surgical choice. The incidence of acute meniscal injuries in children younger than 15 years ranges from 5–9% of sports-related injuries.[121] A meniscal tear in a child under the age of 10 is unusual. Surgery is used only if conservative measures fail. The choice is repair of the meniscus rather than resection because of the increased potential in children for cartilaginous healing.

The lateral discoid meniscus was first described in an anatomic specimen around 1889 by Young.[122] A discoid meniscus should be considered in the differential diagnosis of internal knee derangement in any child. A palpable click, joint line tenderness, restricted range of motion, and occasionally joint effusion may be present. The frequency of discoid meniscus varies worldwide from 3–5% in Anglo-Saxons[123–126] to 20% in Japanese.[127]

Osteochrondritis diseccans, when it occurs in younger people, is most common in the lateral side of the medial femoral condyle with painful exercise and locking sometimes caused by loose bodies. Apophysitides are relatively common at the knee, foot, and ankle, all secondary to traction, overuse, and microtrauma. Apophysitis at the inferior pole of the patella, Sinding-Larsen-Johansson syndrome; at the tibial tuberosity, Osgood-Schlatter disease; and at the posterior calcaneus, Sever's disease, are common examples.[128,129] These conditions generally occur around 10–15 years of age, a few years earlier in girls, and are generally treated conservatively with the RICE protocol. Heel cups may be helpful with Sever's disease, in addition to different types of knee strapping and, at times, short periods of casting or splinting with Osgood-Schlatter disease. Pain-free strengthening of weight-bearing soft tissues, possibly using more closed kinetic chain techniques, may be best. Additional conditions of the patella include chondromalacia[130–132] and acute and recurrent dislocations.[118] Chondromalacia is a term used to describe anterior knee pain of undetermined cause in the younger athlete, associated with softening of the articular cartilage beneath the patellar surface. The pain is frequently worse with squatting and climbing stairs and is associated with a high-riding patellae or malalignment. Patellar dislocations are usually lateral and associated with genu valgum, external tibial torsion, and general ligamentous laxity. The subluxation is usually reducible. Exercises to strengthen the quadriceps, particularly the vastus medialis, and use of patellar tracking braces may be helpful.

Osteochondrosis refers to idiopathic disorders of endochondral ossification that include both chondrogenesis and osteogenesis.[133] Examples include Freiberg's disease, which involves collapse of the articular surface in subchondral bone, usually of the second metatarsal,[134,135] and Köhler's disease, which involves irregular ossification of the tarsonavicular joint with localized pain and increased density.[134,135] Freiberg's disease is more common in girls between the ages of 12 and 15 years, whereas Köhler's disease occurs in younger individuals, aged 2–9 years, and is frequently reversible with conservative care including orthoses and casting.

Flatfeet or pes planus may be flexible or rigid.[136] Flexible pes planus is usually asymptomatic, at least in earlier years, and is the most common type found in children. Inexpensive scaphoid pads or medial inserts may help to create more plantigrade weight bearing in the child, but they do not correct the deformity. Extreme cases, such as in children with hypotonia, may require surgery after the age of 5 years in the form of calcaneal lengthening once the bony cortices are more solid. Untreated progression may occur with compensatory hallux valgus, planovalgus, and secondary bunion and toe deformities. Pes planovalgus is associated with more active or shortened peroneal musculature progressing over time with the development of pain, particularly in later years. Rigid pes planus is a congenital deformity associated with other anomalies in 50% of cases. It is caused by failure of the tarsal bones to separate, leaving a bony cartilaginous or fibrous bridge or coalition between two or more tarsal bones.[136] Tarsal coalition is present in approximately 1% of the population and is bilateral in 50–60% of patients.[137,138] The more common coalitions are talocalcaneal (48%) and calcaneonavicular (43%). Talocalcaneal coalitions tend to become symptomatic earlier, between 8 and 12 years, whereas calcaneonavicular coalitions are more likely to be symptomatic between 12 and 16 years.[137,138] Symptoms are insidious with occasional acute arch, ankle, or midfoot pain. Patients are predisposed to ankle sprain secondary to the limited subtalar motion, and stress to the subtalar and transverse tarsal joints frequently causes pain. CT scans are diagnostic, and initial treatment is conservative with short leg casting or molded orthoses and rest.[139,140] If conservative care fails, surgical intervention is usually necessary. With all symptomatic pes planus, accessory navicular bones need to be considered.[141] Rigid cavus feet

may be associated with metatarsalgia, clawing, and intrinsic muscle atrophy. The atrophy may be caused by an underlying neurologic condition, such as Charcot-Marie-Tooth disease, spinal dysraphism, Friedreich's ataxia, or spinal tumor. Shock absorber inserts or custom orthoses may be helpful.

With any of these lower extremity conditions, gait abnormalities may be present. Although frequently benign, variant gait pattern can be the source of great parental concern. The child's whole posture needs to be looked at carefully, particularly from the waist downward, because malalignment of any lower extremity joint may stem from another.

Figure 19–8 shows anteversion of the femoral head and neck on the femoral diaphysis in addition to coxa valga and coxa vara. The normal angle of the femoral neck and shaft at birth is approximately 160 degrees and decreases to approximately 140 degrees at 5 years and 120 degrees in adulthood. At birth, the normal anterior femoral neck angle relative to the transcondylar line of the distal femur is approximately 40 degrees. This angle declines to approximately 25 degrees by age 5 years and 15 degrees in adulthood.[142,143] An increase in the anteversion angle is frequently associated with in-toeing and increased internal rotation best assessed with the child lying prone. In-toeing may persist into adulthood but often improves with time in the physically normal child. Exercises to strengthen external rotators of the hip and physical and verbal cues to out-toe and compensate may at times offer limited benefit. Severe in-toeing not correcting over time, associated with falls and significantly limited external rotation, can be corrected surgically. Surgery is deferred at least beyond the age of 6 years and frequently closer to 10 years, when there is less chance of postoperative derotation of the surgically corrected torsion. Surgery should not be taken lightly, and good indication should be present along with well-educated parents and child to justify the risk.

Excessive hip external rotation with minimal internal rotation, often tested with the child lying prone with hips extended, is associated with femoral retroversion (opposite of anteversion). This condition is more common in children with low tone and increased joint laxity, such as those with Down syndrome and Ehlers-Danlos syndrome. Gait is with excessive out-toeing, and familial traits may be present. There may be concurrent secondary genu valgum and flexible pes planus.

Tibial torsion, both internal and external, may occur as compensation for the femoral version

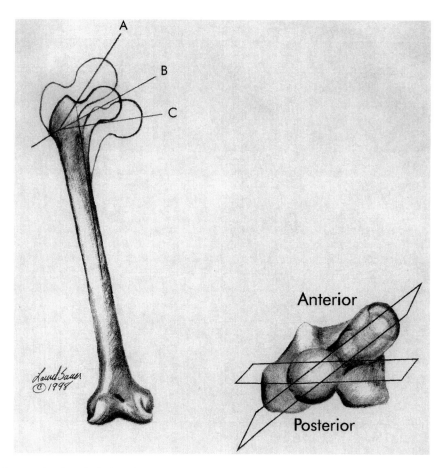

FIGURE 19–8. Angle of neck shaft and anteversion of the femur. *A,* Increased, coxa valga. *B,* Normal. *C,* Decreased, coxa vara. The smaller diagram shows a top view relating a plane from left to right through the greater trochanter and femoral head referenced to the transcondylar femoral axis distally.

or by themselves causing in-toeing and out-toeing. The transmalleolar axis may be palpated in prone and knee-flexed positions. The lateral malleolus is approximately 5–10 degrees posterior to the medial one in the toddler and increases to approximately 15 degrees by adolescence.[144] Denis Browne bars have been prescribed frequently for more severe torsions of the femoral and tibial bones in children under the age of 3 years, when the bones are softer, but their efficacy is questionable.[7]

Angular deformities of the femoral-tibial alignment are also a source of frequent concern for parents and families. At birth, the infant has a bowlegged posture with a genu varum of 10–15 degrees.[145,146] The bowing gradually straightens so that the femorotibial alignment is neutral or 0 degrees by 12–18 months of age. Continued growth results in a peak valgus angulation of 12–15 degrees by the age of 3–4 years. Subsequent growth reduces the genu valgum to normal adult values of approximately 5–7 degrees by the age of 12 years. At any age, there

is a fairly wide standard deviation of normal. Measurements between the medial femoral condyles or intermalleolar distance help to quantitate the deformity.[147] The most common cause of genu varum in children is physiologic bowlegs. Children with this condition have genu varum that persists after the age of 18 months, usually resolving before the age of 3 years. X-rays show symmetric growth plate anatomy and medial bowing that involves the proximal tibia as well as the distal femur. Measurement of the metaphyseal-diaphyseal angle is helpful in the differential diagnosis.[148,149] The differential diagnosis includes infantile tibia vara or Blount's disease, hypophosphatemic rickets, metaphyseal chondrodysplasia, focal fibrocartilaginous dysplasia, and trauma to the epiphyses. Blount's disease occurs in children with no apparent abnormality at birth, with a typical history of genu varum worsening with gait before the age of 2 years. The less frequent juvenile onset may occur between 4 and 10 years and the adolescent form over 11 years. The condition is more frequent in African-Americans and girls and is seen with obesity and in children walking at an early age.[150] Blount's disease is believed to result from abnormal compression of the medial aspect of the proximal tibial physis, causing retardation of growth from that area or increased growth laterally of the proximal tibia or fibula.[150,151] Proximal valgus osteotomies may be required for severe persistent angular deformity after the age of 3 years. Surgical complications can include compartment syndrome with persistent neurovascular compromise. Increased fragmentation, declination, and beaking of the medial proximal epiphyses generally indicate the need for surgery. Hypophosphatemic rickets follows the sex-linked dominant inheritance pattern with a low serum phosphate level. As with all of these conditions, growth is frequently short of stature, generally below the 25th percentile, and may be associated with leg length discrepancies.

Genu valgum or knock-knees is a concern in children who are developing peak valgus alignment around the age of 3–4 years. Almost 99% of the time, this valgus is benign in nature, correcting toward adult values by early adolescence. X-rays show symmetric growth plates with no particular abnormalities. Observation is the treatment of choice in these individuals. Children who have genu valgum with a femoral-tibial angle greater than 20 degrees require follow-up, but generally the problem resolves spontaneously. If abnormal genu valgum persists into the teens, correction by hemiepiphysiodesis, or stapling of the medial physis, may be effective.[145] The advantage of stapling the physis is that staples can be removed before excessive overcorrection occurs.

Leg length discrepancy of less than 1.5 cm is usually just observed. Shoe lifts are helpful for differences up to 3 cm. Appropriate shoe lifts should result in horizontal alignment of the iliac crest or sacral base in the standing position. There are two basic types of leg length discrepancies—true and apparent. True leg length discrepancy is present when bilateral leg length measurements between the greater trochanter and the medial malleolus demonstrate a shortening on one side. Apparent leg length discrepancies are present when bony lengths are the same, but joint alignment or pelvic-femoral asymmetry is present (e.g., adductor spasticity, pelvic obliquity). Radiographic measurement is the most reliable, with the CT scanogram the standard. The Greulich-Pyle norms for skeletal maturation of the hand and the charts of Green Anderson are used for prediction of future growth and the timing of surgery when stapling

or epiphysiodesis of the longer side is considered for true discrepancies between 3 and 6 cm. Discrepancies beyond 6 cm are best treated by limb lengthening through such methods as Wagner or Ilizarov procedures.[7] Prosthetic consideration should be given with any severe limb shortening because it may provide a more functional and cosmetic outlook in future years.

Arthrogryposis multiplex congenita refers to a symptom complex characterized by multiple joint contractures that are present at birth. It is not a single disease, and there are multiple causes. Limited understanding of the entity has made interpretation of the results of treatment difficult.[152] The clinical genetic literature has delineated as many as 150 entities under this term.[153] Neurologists frequently see the newborns with a focus for diagnosing possible neuromuscular disorders or myopathies. Arthrogryposis can be divided into more lethal and nonlethal types. In the more lethal types with limited infantile survival, the great majority of causes are believed to be neurologic, including dysgenesis of the central nervous system, brain stem, and spinal cord, and in about 5–7% myopathic.[154,155] A simpler way of classifying arthrogryposis is by (1) intrinsic causes, abnormalities of the embryo itself, and (2) extrinsic causes, abnormalities of the uterine environment, such as oligohydramnios, or structural abnormalities such as bicornuate uterus causing diminution of movement in an otherwise normally developing embryo. Children who survive infantile arthrogryposis often have upper and lower extremity involvement in typical patterns. Common deformities of the upper extremities include adduction, internal rotation contractures of the shoulders, fixed flexion or extension contractures of the elbows, either wrist flexion and ulnar deviation or extension and radial deviation, and thumb-in-palm deformities. In the lower extremities, flexion, abduction, and external rotation hip contractures with unilateral or bilateral dislocation; fixed extension or flexion contractures of the knees; and severe rigid bilateral clubfeet may be present. Perinatal fractures are common and believed to be secondary to hypotonia and rigid joints.[156]

In the most severe rigid clubfeet, not correctable with casting and conservative care, talectomy may be necessary or talar enucleation in association with the posterior medial releases. An ankle-foot orthosis is generally needed to maintain correction, especially if the patient cannot actively dorsiflex or evert the foot beyond neutral after surgery. Extension wedge osteotomies of the distal femur may be necessary to correct flexion contractures of the knee. There is always a well-recognized risk of neurovascular damage with operative correction of knee flexion contractures needing careful consideration to avoid overstretching of the neurovascular bundle. Shortening osteotomies completed at the same time as the extension wedge osteotomy may minimize these risks. Operative correction of the hips is similar to that of dysplasia, either unilateral or bilateral, and depending on severity. Surgical and rehabilitation goals are generally standing, walking, and transfers as possible, using assistive devices as needed. Functional expectations are also limited by hypotonia and weakness.

Wilms' tumor, or nephroblastoma, may be associated with hemihypertrophy, differential leg length, and secondary metastases to the skeleton. Renal ultrasound may be diagnostic in this regard. Additional metastatic tumors to the lower extremities include neuroblastoma and lymphomas of various types. Primary bone tumors to the lower extremities include those of the long bones, such as Ewing's sarcoma and histiocytosis X in the diaphysis, eosinophilic granuloma in the epiphysis, and osteogenic sarcoma in the metaphysis of the knee. Tumors more common in the area of the pelvis include osteoblastoma, aneurysmal bone cyst, and fibrous dysplasia. As with any diagnosis of skeletal neoplasia in children, referral to a cancer treatment center is mandatory.

Constitutional or Intrinsic Bone Conditions

Constitutional conditions of bone may be separated into five categories:

Category 1—defects of tubular bone or spinal growth, either present at birth or manifested later in life: achondroplasia and the various types of dwarfism, chondrodysplasias, epiphyseal and later-in-life spondyloepiphyseal dysplasias

Category 2—disorganized cartilage and fibrous components: fibrodysplasia and the multiple cartilaginous exostoses

Category 3—abnormal bony density or structure: osteopetrosis and osteogenesis imperfecta

Category 4—metabolic conditions usually affecting calcium or phosphorus metabolism: various types of rickets and mucopolysaccharidoses

Category 5—extraskeletal disorders: sickle cell anemia, renal osteodystrophy and hyperparathyroidism

More than 100 conditions may be placed into these categories, most with some heritable cause.[157,158] Many of these conditions are associated with short trunk and variant body proportions, including head size and short limbs.

Cervical spine involvement is frequent, particularly atlantoaxial instability. This involvement may consist of maldevelopment of the odontoid and excessive laxity of the transverse ligament or abnormalities of the longitudinal ligaments. Kyphoscoliosis is common. In achondroplasia, symptomatic spinal stenosis may be seen particularly in the lumbar region. Progressive spinal stenosis and disc herniation have been associated with weightlifting and unrelated conditions.[159] Hydrocephalus, if present in achondroplasia, usually requires no treatment.

Multiple epiphyseal dysplasia involves the capital femoral epiphysis and is usually bilateral. Because of similar involvement, differentiation from Legg-Calvé-Perthes disease is a common problem. In multiple epiphyseal dysplasia, nuclear medicine scans are normal, showing good uptake of tracer, and there is no true avascular necrosis as seen in Legg-Calvé-Perthes disease. In addition, with Legg-Calvé-Perthes disease the degree and stage of involvement may vary from one side to the other, and the acetabula are generally normal. In multiple epiphyseal dysplasia, the acetabula have lost definition with scalloping of subchondral bone. Multiple epiphyseal dysplasia is distinguished from spondyloepiphyseal dysplasia by the absence of severe vertebral changes. Both of these conditions may have involvement of the atlantoaxial articulations.

Fibrous dysplasia is a condition characterized by the presence of expanding fibro-osseous tissue in the interior of affected bones. It is primarily a lesion of the growing skeleton but may be associated with endocrine abnormalities. Precocious puberty, premature skeletal maturation, or hyperparathyroidism, which is more prevalent in girls, is commonly known as Albright's disease.[160] Osteogenesis imperfecta has been classified into four different types (Sillence) with some exceptions:[161,162]

Type 1—tarda form typically with a positive family history, blue sclerae, early-onset deafness, hypermobility, and bruising

Type 2—most severe with neonatal fractures, early death, or stillbirth; fractures may occur from simple infant handling

Type 3—progressive entity with bizarre skeletal deformity, scoliosis, sclerae whose blueness fades with age, extreme disability, and short stature

Type 4—more difficult to diagnose with normal sclerae, equivocal family history, and early radiographs that can be normal

The correct distinction between osteogenesis imperfecta and nonaccidental injury or child abuse is essential and has been the subject of many papers.[163,164] Expandable intramedullary rodding help in the preschool years to correct existing deformity or maintain alignment of long bones. Fractures may recur at the rod ends with or without dislodgment of the rods themselves. A focus on wheelchair mobility, safe transfers, and limited weight bearing throughout the early years is essential.[165,166] Fractures tend to be less common later in life.

Clinical features of nutritional rickets include progressive bowing of the legs; poor linear growth; a diet deficient in vitamin D; seizures; and abnormal serum calcium, phosphate, and alkaline phosphatase levels. Wrist radiographs showing metaphyseal flaring, cupping, and decreased mineralization of the distal metaphysis along with increased levels of alkaline phosphatase in the serum appear to be the most useful confirmatory tests. Breast milk itself may not contain enough vitamin D alone to protect infants from rickets after 6 months of age, particularly those with darker skins and living in cloudy northern climates.[167] With the introduction of vitamin D–supplemented infant formulas,[168,169] nutritional rickets has become rare in the United States.

The mucopolysaccharidoses are classified into various types by the deficiency of specific liposomal enzymes.[170,171] Patients with Morquio's disease (mucopolysaccharidosis type 4) are often of normal intelligence and achieve normal motor milestones in early life.[172-174] Gait may become progressively worse over time with severe genu valgum, ligamentous laxity, increased sternal protrusion, and severe pes planus. Chest deformities can cause cardiorespiratory symptoms secondary to restricted thoracic movement. Atlantoaxial instability is a major complication of this condition, frequently requiring fusion. Pediatric athletes with skeletal dysplasias and ligamentous laxity, particularly associated with spinal subluxations or stenoses, should be diverted from contact sports or other high-risk activities.

Most individuals with constitutional bone conditions are of normal intelligence, but because of their appearance are often perceived not to be so and as younger than their chronologic age. For this reason, proper measures should be taken to ensure that the child's maturity and cognitive and emotional abilities are recognized fairly by professionals, family, school, and community.

Musculoskeletal Pain and Trauma

Musculoskeletal pain in children varies with the individual and family. If there is a history of chronic pain in parents or other close relatives,

often this history repeats itself in the child. Pain may be difficult for children under the age of 5 years to describe, but with encouragement some localization can occur. At around 6 years, children can score pain generally on a scale of 0–10 by increasing severity.[175] Musculoskeletal pain that may be difficult to diagnose includes sickle cell bony infarcts, reflex sympathetic dystrophy after minor injury, growing pains in the lower extremities that are mostly nocturnal, fibromyalgia and morning stiffness, tension myalgia from ligamentous laxities, and episodic activity-related arthritis. Conversion symptoms producing pain in nonanatomic distributions always need to be considered.

The incidence of reflex sympathetic dystrophy in children is not known, but the condition is probably underdiagnosed.[176] The symptoms are generally the same for adults and children, but the presentations may be different. In children, it is more common in athletic girls, with 6:1 ratio in some reports. The average age of presentation is around 12 years. Clinical findings are erythema, warmth, moisture, puffy edema, and hyperesthesia. If identified and treated early, more rapid recovery is possible. Late diagnosis and progression of symptoms to contractures, atrophy, and severe osteoporosis can have disastrous sequelae. The diagnosis should always be considered with trauma and pain that is out of proportion to the stimulus and worsened with immobility. Treatment is directed at the relief of pain, including sympathetic blocks, mobilization, and psychosocial support.[177] Calcium channel blockers and β-blockers (propranolol) are advocated by some. In addition, tricyclic antidepressants such as amitriptyline may be helpful.

Trauma may be either microtrauma or macrotrauma. Microtrauma, or overuse syndromes, has been discussed in some detail earlier. Macrotrauma generally results in upper and lower extremity fractures. Salter's classification of epiphyseal injuries in children, types I through V, is shown in Figure 19–9. Growth plates or physes in children are the weakest link in the musculoskeletal chain. The physes separate or slide before a ligament tears or a bone breaks.

The most frequent bone fractured in children is the clavicle and may be associated with a brachial plexus injury, particularly in neonates. Supracondylar fractures of the distal humerus account for 50% of elbow injuries and may be associated with neurovascular insult. Pain, pallor, pulselessness, and paresthesia are the cardinal signs of impending Volkman's ischemia, which can occur even in the presence of a radial pulse.[178] Once casted, the extremity should feel

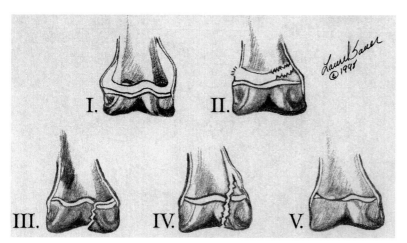

FIGURE 19–9. Salter's classification of epiphyseal injuries in children. Type I, epiphyseal separation without displacement. Type II, metaphyseal fragment, usually stable, easily reducible, and without growth impairment. Type III, epiphyseal fragment, and type IV, metaphyseal and epiphyseal fragments, are intra-articular usually requiring open reduction and associated with growth impairment and joint incongruities. Type V, axial compression, may also disturb growth.

relatively comfortable. Persistent restlessness and pain are indications to remove the cast rather than sedate the child. The classic gatekeeper's thumb in children also involves the ulnar collateral ligament. This injury is generally a Salter type III fracture because the proximal phalanx of the thumb has the collateral ligament attached to the epiphyseal fragment.[179] Open reduction and internal fixation may be necessary if the step-off or displacement is greater than 2 mm.

Midshaft femoral fractures are common in children, particularly with motor vehicle accidents. Immediate hip spica casting remains a primary method of treatment for most children, 6 years of age and younger.[180] Intramedullary rodding in older children and adolescents has the risk of avascular necrosis of the femoral head. Ninety/ninety traction of the hip and knee in flexion may be used with a pin inserted through the distal end of the femoral fracture. The child often has to remain in traction for a number of weeks until satisfactory alignment has been achieved, making overall care more difficult.[181]

Compartment syndromes are less common in children and, when they occur, are mostly associated with proximal tibial fractures. Presentations include diffuse anterior leg pain, decreased pedal pulses, dorsal foot paresthesias, and edema. The tibia, second and third metatarsals, and lateral malleolus also may be involved with stress fractures. Radionucleotide scanning can be diagnostic with the type of fractures and also may help to identify many prestress reactions. A stress fracture always should be considered with focal bone pain, particularly outside the joint space and associated with strenuous activity. Callus generally forms within 3–4 weeks, and weight bearing as tolerated is allowed after 6–8 weeks. A shoe lift helps on the weight-bearing

side by assisting the immobilized leg to swing forward. The family and child should be forewarned that limping may continue for several weeks after cast removal. Isometric exercises within the cast may help to facilitate a speedy recovery.

Child abuse or nonaccidental trauma continues to be a significant problem. The number of children in the United States with reports of alleged maltreatment increased from 2.6 million in 1990 to 2.9 million in 1994.[182] Multiple fractures in different stages of healing on radiographs are suspicious for child abuse. Fractures considered to have a high specificity for child abuse include those that are bilateral and involve the metaphyses, ribs, scapula, lateral clavicle, vertebrae with or without subluxation, fingers in nonambulatory children, and skull, complex type.[183,184] In contrast, fractures that are frequent in children but have a low specificity for child abuse include midclavicular, simple linear skull, and single diaphyseal fractures. Inappropriate clinical history, failure to seek medical attention, and discovery of an old fracture in a healing stage increase the suspicion of child abuse. Other clinical features with high specificity for this condition include bruising, burns, strap marks, and genital distortions. Parents who are at risk to become abusers often have histories of abuse themselves and are frequently young, single, and chemically dependent. The problem cuts across all socioeconomic classes and is more common in children with physical disability. If nonaccidental trauma is suspected, the physician is legally obligated to file a report with the appropriate child protective agency. Adequate supportive measures and counseling should be in place before returning any abused child to the home. When in doubt, temporary foster placement should be seriously considered.

References

1. Moore KL, Persaud TVN (eds): The Developing Human: Clinically Oriented Embryology, 5th ed. Philadelphia, WB Saunders, 1993.
2. Carlson BM: Human Embryology and Developmental Biology. St. Louis, Mosby, 1994.
3. Ros MA: Apical ridge dependent and independent mesodermal domains of G Hox-8 expression in chick limb buds. Development 1992;116:811.
4. Sassoon D: Hox genes: A role for tissue development. Am J Respir Cell Mol Biol 1992;7:1.
5. Behrman RE (ed): Nelson Textbook of Pediatrics, 14th ed. Philadelphia, WB Saunders, 1992.
6. Moore KL: Clinically Oriented Anatomy, 3rd ed. Baltimore, Williams & Wilkins, 1992.
7. Tachdjian MO: Pediatric Orthopedics, 2nd ed. Philadelphia, WB Saunders, 1990.
8. Caffey J: Pediatric X-Ray Diagnosis, 7th ed. Chicago, Year Book Medical Publishers, 1978.
9. Downey JA, Low NL (eds): The Child with Disabling Illness: Principles of Rehabilitation, 2nd ed. New York, Raven Press, 1982.
10. Kyzer SP, Stark SL: Congenital idiopathic clubfoot deformities. AORN 1995;61:492.
11. Highgenboten CL: Children's Knee Problems. Orthop Rev 1981;10:37.
12. Molnar GE: Pediatric Rehabilitation, 2nd ed. Baltimore, Williams & Wilkins, 1992.
13. Jones KL: Smith's Recognizable Patterns of Human Malformation, 5th ed. Philadelphia, WB Saunders, 1997.
14. Quan L, Smith DW: The Vater association: A spectrum of associated defects. J Pediatr 1973;82;104.
15. Schydlower M, Fuller PG, Heyman RB, et al: Fetal alcohol syndrome and fetal alcohol effects: American Academy of Pediatrics Committee on Substance Abuse. J Pediatr 1993;91:1004.
16. Duerbeck NB: Fetal alcohol syndrome. Compr Ther 1997;23:179.
17. Chung MK, Nissenbaum MM: Congenital and developmental defects of the shoulder. Orthop Clin North Am 1975;6:381.
18. Hollinshead WH: Anatomy for Surgeons, 3rd ed. Philadelphia, Harper & Row, 1982.
19. Rowland TW: Overtraining hazards in prepubertal athletes. J Musculoskeletal Med 1990;7:52.
20. Kannus P: Overuse problems in children. Clin Pediatr 1988;27:333.
21. Bright RW, Burstein AH, Elmore SM: Hypophyseal plate cartilage: A biomechanical and histological analysis of failure modes. J Bone Joint Surg 1974;56A:668.
22. Micheli LJ: Pediatric and adolescent sports injuries: Recent trends. Exerc Sports Sci Rev 1986;14:359.
23. Adams IE: Injury to the throwing arm: A study of traumatic changes in the elbow joints of boy baseball players. Calif Med 1965;102:127.
24. Albright JA, Torl P, Shaw R, et al: Clinical study of baseball pitchers: Correlation of injury to the throwing arm with method of delivery. Am J Sports Med 1978;6:15.
25. An KN, Morrey BF: Biomechanics of the elbow. In Morrey BF (ed): The Elbow and Its Disorders. Philadelphia, WB Saunders, 1985.
26. Caine D, Roy S, Singer KM, et al: Stress changes of the distal radial growth plate. Am J Sports Med 1992;20:290.
27. Albanese SA, Palmer AK, Kerr DR, et al: Wrist pain and distal growth plate closure of the radius in gymnasts. J Pediatr Orthop 1989;9:23.
28. Carter SR, Aldridge MJ, Fitzgerald R, et al: Stress changes of the wrist in adolescent gymnasts. Br J Radiol 1988;61:109.

29. Konig F: Uber freie Korper in den Gelenken. Dtsch C Chir 1988;27:90.
30. Blount WP: Fractures in Children. Baltimore, Williams & Wilkins, 1955.
31. Osborne G, Cotteril P: Recurrent dislocation of the elbow. J Bone Joint Surg 1986;48B:340.
32. Letts M: Dislocations of the child's elbow. In Morrey BF (ed): The Elbow and Its Disorders, 2nd ed. Philadelphia, WB Saunders, 1993.
33. Linscheid RL, O'Driscoll SW: Elbow dislocations. In Morrey BF (ed): The Elbow and Its Disorders, 2nd ed. Philadelphia, WB Saunders, 1993.
34. Linscheid RL, Wheeler DK: Elbow dislocations. JAMA 1965;194:1171.
35. Nevasier JS, Wickstrom JK: Dislocation of the elbow: A retrospective study of 115 patients. South Med J 1977;70:172.
36. Wilkins KE: Fractures and dislocations of the elbow region. In Rockwood CA, Wilkins KE, King RE (eds): Fractures in Children. Philadelphia, JB Lippincott, 1984.
37. Wilkins KE: Shoulder injuries. In Stanitski CL, DeLee JC, Drez D (eds): Pediatric and Adolescent Sports Medicine. Philadelphia, WB Saunders, 1994.
38. Ireland ML, Andrews JR: Shoulder and elbow injuries in the young athlete. Clin Sports Med 1988;7:473.
39. Dubey SP, Ghosh LM: Klippel-Feil syndrome with congenital conductive deafness: Report of a case and review of literature. Int J Pediatr Otorhinolaryngol 1993;25:201.
40. Pueschel SM, Annerén G, Durlach R, et al: Guidelines for optimal medical care of persons with Down's syndrome: Committee report. Acta Paediatr 1995;84:823.
41. AAP issues guidelines on supervision for children with Down's syndrome: Special medical report. Am Fam Physician 1994;50:695.
42. Hayes A, Batshaw ML: Down's syndrome. Pediatr Clin North Am 1993;40:523.
43. Harley EH, Collins MD: Neurologic sequelae secondary to atlantoaxial instability in Down's syndrome. Arch Otolaryngol Head Neck Surg 1994;120:159.
44. Hensinger RN: Acute back pain in children. Instructional Course Lectures 1995;44:111.
45. Calderone RR, Larson JM: Overview and classification of spinal infections. Orthop Clin North Am 1996;27:1.
46. Cushing AH: Diskitis in children: State of the art clinical article. Clin Infect Dis 1993;17:1.
47. Atar D, Lehman WB, Grant AD: Discitis in children: A review paper. Orthop Rev 1992;21:931.
48. Naim-Ur-Rahman, Jamjoom A, Jamjoon ZA, et al: Neural arch tuberculosis: Radiologic features and their correlation with surgical findings. Br J Neurosurg 1997;11:32.
49. Wynne Davies R: Familial (idiopathic) scoliosis: A family survey. J Bone Joint Surg 1968;50B:24.
50. Keim HA: Scoliosis. Clin Symp 1979;30:1.
51. Olafsson Y, Saraste H, Söderlund V, et al: Boston brace in the treatment of idiopathic scoliosis. J Pediatr Orthop 1995;15:524.
52. Nachemson AL, Peterson LE: Effectiveness of treatment with a brace in girls who have adolescent idiopathic scoliosis. J Bone Joint Surg 1995;77A:815.
53. Winter RB, Lonstein JE, Boachie-Adjei O: Congenital spinal deformity. Instructional Course Lectures. AAOS 1996;45:117.
54. Luque ER: Anatomy of scoliosis and its correction. Clin Orthop 1984;105:198.
55. Massoud WZ: Laparoscopic management of superior mesenteric artery syndrome. Int Surg 1995;80:322.
56. Risser JC: The iliac apophysis: An invaluable sign in the management of scoliosis. Clin Orthop 1958;2:111.

57. Bradford DS, Moe JH, Montalvo FJ, et al: Scheuermann's kyphosis and round back deformity, results of Milwaukee brace treatment in 22 patients. J Bone Joint Surg 1975;56A:749.

58. Murphy KP: Sports injuries in children. Phys Med Rehabil State Art Rev 1991;5:351.

59. Scheuermann HW: Kyphosis dorsalis juvenilis. Ugeskr Laeger 1920;82:385.

60. Commandre FA, Gagnerie G, Zakarian M, et al: The child, the spine and sport. J Sports Med Phys Fit 1988; 28:11.

61. O'Neill DD, Micheli LJ: Overuse injuries in the young athlete. Clin Sports Med 1988;7:591.

62. Sorenson HK: Scheuermann's Juvenile Kyphosis. Copenhagen, Munksgaard, 1964.

63. Keene JS, Drummond DS: Mechanical back pain in the athlete. Compr Ther 1985;11:7.

64. Epstein JA, Epstein NE, Marc J, et al: Lumbar intervertebral disk herniation in teenage children: Recognition and management of associated anomalies. Spine 1984;9:427.

65. DeOrio JK, Bianco AJ: Lumbar disk excision in children and adolescents. J Bone Joint Surg 1982;64A:991.

66. Jackson DW, Rettig A, Wiltse LL: Epidural cortisone injections in the young athletic adult. Am J Sports Med 1980;8:239.

67. Swärd L, Hellström M, Jacobsson B, et al: Acute injury of the vertebral ring apophysis and intervertebral disk in adolescent gymnasts. Spine 1990;15:144.

68. Gerbino PG, Micheli LJ: Back injuries in the young athlete. Clin Sports Med 1995;14:571.

69. Weir MR, Smith DS: Stress reaction of the pars interarticularis leading to spondylolysis: A cause of adolescent low back pain. J Adolesc Health Care 1989;10:573.

70. Weiss GB: Stresses at the lumbosacral junction. Orthop Clin North Am 1975;6:83.

71. Bellah RD, Summerville DA, Treves ST, et al: Low back pain in adolescent athletes: Detection of stress injury to the pars interarticularis with SPECT. Radiology 1991;180:509.

72. Meyerding HW: Spondylolisthesis. Surg Gynecol Obstet 1932;54:371.

73. Lippitt AB: Fracture of a vertebral body endplate and disk protrusion causing subarachnoid block in an adolescent. Clin Orthop 1976;116:112.

74. Techakapuch S: Rupture of the lumbar cartilage plate into the spinal canal in an adolescent: A case report. J Bone Joint Surg Am 1981;63:481.

75. Herzog RJ, Wiens JJ, Dillingham MS, et al: Normal cervical spine morphometry and cervical spine stenosis in asymptomatic professional football players. Spine 1991;16:S178.

76. Torg JS: Epidemiology pathogenesis and prevention of football induced cervical spinal cord trauma. Exerc Sport Sci Rev 1992;20:321.

77. Torg JS, Pavlov H, Genuario SE, et al: Neuropraxia of the spinal cord with transient quadriplegia. J Bone Joint Surg Am 1986;68:1354.

78. Clark A, Stanish WD: An unusual cause of back pain in a young athlete: A case report. Am J Sports Med 1985;13:51.

79. Charif P, Reichelderfer TE: Genu recurvatum congenitum in a newborn: Its incidence, course, treatment, prognosis. Clin Pediatr 1965;4:587.

80. Clayburg BJ, Henderson ED: Congenital dislocation of the knee. Proc Mayo Clin 1955;30:396.

81. Green JP, Waugh W: Congenital lateral dislocation of the patella. J Bone Joint Surg Br 1968;50:285.

82. Stanisavljevic S, Zemenick G, Miller D: Congenital irreducible permanent lateral dislocation of the patella. Clin Orthop 1976;116:190.

83. Stern M: Persistent congenital dislocation of the patella. Int Coll Surg J 1964;41:654.

84. Bernhang AM, Levine SA: Familial absence of the patella. J Bone Joint Surg 1973;55A:1088.

85. George R: Bilateral bipartite patellae. Br J Surg 1935;22:555.

86. Bourne MH: Bipartite patellae in the adolescent: Results of surgical excision. J Pediatr Orthop 1990; 10:255.

87. Lawson JP: Symptomatic radiographic variants in extremities. Radiology 1985;157:625.

88. Ogden JA, McCarthy SM, Jabl P: The painful bipartite patellae. J Pediatr Orthop 1982;2:263.

89. Keats TE (ed): Atlas of Normal Roentgen Variants that May Simulate Disease, 6th ed. St. Louis, Mosby, 1996.

90. Hubbard AM, Dormans JP: Evaluation of developmental dysplasia, Perthes disease, and neuromuscular dysplasia of the hip in children before and after surgery: An imaging update. Am J Roentgenol 1995;164: 1067.

91. Ozonoff MB: Pediatric Orthopedic Radiology, 2nd ed. Philadelphia, WB Saunders, 1992.

92. Graf R: The diagnosis of congenital hip dislocation by ultrasonic compound treatment. Arch Orthop Trauma Surg 1980;97:117.

93. Harcke TH: Hip in infants and children. Clin Diagn Ultrasound 1995;30:179.

94. Snider RK (ed): Essentials of Musculoskeletal Care. Rosemont, IL, American Academy of Orthopedic Surgeons, 1997.

95. Ortolani M: Un segno poco noto e sue importanza per la diagnosi precoce di preussasione congenita dellíanca. Pediatria 1937;45:129.

96. Barlo TG: Early diagnosis and treatment of congenital dislocation of the hip. J Bone Joint Surg 1962;44B:292.

97. Hensinger RN: Congenital dislocation of the hip. Clin Symp 1979;31:1.

98. McCluslkey WP, Bassett GS, Mora-Garcia G, et al: Treatment of failed open reduction for congenital dislocation of the hip. J Pediatr Orthop 1989;9:633.

99. Waters P, Kurica K, Hall J, et al: Salter innominate osteotomy in congenital dislocation of the hip. J Pediatr Orthop 1988;8:650.

100. Robinson HJ, Shannon MA: Avascular necrosis in congenital hip dysplasia: The effect of treatment. J Pediatr Orthop 1989;9:293.

101. Scarpa A: A memoir on the congenital clubfeet of children and the mode of correcting that deformity: The classic. Clin Orthop 1994;308:4.

102. Dias LS, Stern LS: Talectomy in the treatment of resistant talipes equinovarus deformity in myelomeningocele and arthrogryposis. J Pediatr Orthop 1987;7:39.

103. Koop S, Quanbeck D: Three common causes of childhood hip pain. Pediatr Clin North Am 1996;43:1053.

104. Hart JJ: Transient synovitis of the hip in children. Am Fam Physician 1996;54:1587.

105. Waters E: Toxic synovitis of the hip in children. Nurse Practitioner 1995;20:44.

106. Skaggs DL, Tolo VT: Legg-Calve-Perthes disease. J Am Acad Orthop Surg 1996;4:9.

107. McCoy RL, Dec KL, McKeag DB, et al: Common injuries in the child or adolescent athlete. Prim Care 1995;22:117.

108. McKeag DB, Hough DO: Primary Care Sports Medicine. Dubuque, Brown & Benchmark, 1993.

109. Stulberg SD, Cooperman DR, Wallensten R: The natural history of Legg-Calve-Perthes disease. J Bone Joint Surg 1981;63A:1095.

110. Carney B, Noble J, Weinstein S: Long-term follow-up of slipped capital femoral epiphysis. J Bone Joint Surg 1991;73A:667.

111. Jensen H, Mikkelsen S, Steinke M, et al: Hip physioly-sis: Bilaterality of 62 cases followed for 20 years. Acta Orthop Scand 1990;61:419.

112. Gelberman R, Kasser J, Siegel D, et al: Slipped capital femoral epiphysis: A quantitative analysis of motion, gait and femoral remodeling after in situ fixation. J Bone Joint Surg 1991;73A:659.

113. Goldman AB, Schneider R, Martel W: Acute chondroly-sis complicating slipped capital femoral epiphysis. Am J Roentgenol 1978;130:945.

114. Offrieski C: Traumatic dislocation of the hip in chil-dren. J Bone Joint Surg 1981;63B:194.

115. Waters BM, Millis MB: Hip and pelvic injuries in the young athlete. Clin Sports Med 1988;7:513.

116. Koch R, Jackson D: Pubic symphysitis in runners. Am J Sports Med 1981;9:62.

117. Singer IJ: Sports related knee injuries in the pediatric and adolescent athlete. Rhode Island Med J 1987; 70:255.

118. Micheli LJ, Foster TE: Acute knee injuries in the imma-ture athlete. Instructional Course Lectures 1993;42:473.

119. Reider B (ed): Sports Medicine: The School Age Athlete. Philadelphia, WB Saunders, 1996.

120. McCarroll JR, Rettig AC, Shelbourne KD: Anterior cru-ciate ligament injuries in the young athlete with open physis. Am J Sports Med 1988;16:44.

121. DeHaven KE, Lintner DM: Athletic injuries: Compari-son by age, sport and gender. Am J Sports Med 1986;14:218.

122. Young RT: The external semilunar cartilage as a com-plete disk. In Cleland J, Mackay JY, Young RB (eds): Memoirs and Memoranda in Anatomy. London, Williams & Norgate, 1889.

123. Cave RF, Staples OS: Congenital discoid meniscus: A cause of internal derangement of the knee. Am J Surg 1941;54:371.

124. Dickhaut SC, DeLee JC: The discoid lateral meniscus syndrome. J Bone Joint Surg 1982;64A:1068.

125. Middleton DS: Congenital disk shaped lateral menis-cus with snapping knee. Br J Surg 1936;24:246.

126. Smillie IS: The congenital discoid meniscus. J Bone Joint Surg 1948;30B:671.

127. Amako T: On the injuries of the menisci in the knee joint of Japanese. J Jpn Orthop Surg Soc 1960;33:1289.

128. Krause BL, Williams JP, Katterall A: Natural history of Osgood Schlatter disease. J Pediatr Orthop 1990;10:65.

129. Micheli LJ: The traction apophysitis. Clin Sports Med 1987;6:389.

130. Stanitski CL: Knee overuse disorders in the pediatric and adolescent athlete. Instructional Course Lectures 1993;42:483.

131. Peck DM: Apophyseal injuries in the young athlete. Am Fam Physician 1995;51:1891.

132. Klenerman L: Musculoskeletal injuries in child ath-letes. BMJ 1994;308:1556.

133. Griffin LY: Common sports injuries of the foot and ankle seen in children and adolescents. Orthop Clin North Am 1994;25:83.

134. Pizzutillo P: Osteochondroses. In Sullivan J, Grana W (eds): The Pediatric Athlete. Park Ridge, IL, American Academy of Orthopedic Surgeons, 1990.

135. Binek R, Levisohn E, Bersani F, et al: Freiberg disease complicating unrelated trauma. Orthopedics 1988; 11:753.

136. Manusov EG, Lillegard WA, Raspa RF, et al: Evaluation of pediatric foot problems: Part II. The hind foot and ankle. Am Fam Physician 1996;54:1012.

137. Borderlon RJ: Flatfoot in children and young adults. In Mann RA, Coughlin MJ (eds): Surgery of the Foot and Ankle, 6th ed. St. Louis, Mosby, 1993.

138. Skoals PV (ed): Pediatric Orthopedics in Clinical Practice, 2nd ed. Chicago, Year Book Medical Publishers, 1988.

139. O'Neill D, Micheli L: Tarsal coalition. Am J Sports Med 1989;17:544.

140. Gregg J, Das M: Foot and ankle problems in the preado-lescent and adolescent athlete. Clin Sports Med 1982; 1:131.

141. Sullivan JA: Ankle and foot injuries in the pediatric athlete. Instructional Course Lectures 1993;42:545.

142. Bleck E: Developmental orthopedics: III. Toddlers. Dev Med Child Neurol 1982;24:533.

143. Staheli LT: Medial femoral torsion. Orthop Clin North Am 1980;11:39.

144. Gage JR (ed): Gait Analysis in Cerebral Palsy: Clinics in Developmental Medicine. London, MacKeith Press, 1991.

145. Greene WB: Genu varum and genu valgum in children: Differential diagnosis and guidelines for evaluation. Compr Ther 1996;22:22.

146. Greene WB: Genu varum and genu valgum in children. In Schafer M (ed): Instructional Course Lectures 43. Rosemont, IL, American Academy of Orthopedic Surgeons, 1994.

147. Heath CH, Staheli LT: Normal limits of knee angle in white children genu varum and genu valgum. J Pediatr Orthop 1994;13:259.

148. Bowen JR, Torres RR, Forlin E: Partial epiphysiodesis to address genu varum or genu valgum. J Pediatr Orthop 1992;12:359.

149. Levine AM, Drennan JC: Physiological bowing and tibia vara: The metaphyseal-diaphyseal angle in the measurement of bowleg deformities. J Bone Joint Surg 1982;64A:1158.

150. Greene WB: Infantile tibia vara. Instr Course Lect 1993;42:525.

151. Olney BW, Cole WG, Menelaus MB: Three additional cases of focal fibrocartilaginous dysplasia causing tibia vara. J Pediatr Orthop 1990;10:405.

152. Shapiro F, Specht L: The diagnosis and orthopedic treatment of childhood spinal muscular atrophy, pe-ripheral neuropathy, Friedreich ataxia and arthrogry-posis: Current concepts review. J Bone Joint Surg 1993;75A:1699.

153. Hall JG: Genetic aspects of arthrogryposis. Clin Orthop 1985;194:44.

154. Banker BQ: Neuropathologic aspects of arthrogryposis multiplex congenita. Clin Orthop 1985;194:30.

155. Banker BQ: Arthrogryposis multiplex congenita. In Engel AG, Banker BQ (eds): Myology: Basic and Clinical. New York, McGraw-Hill, 1986.

156. Diamond LS, Alegado R: Perinatal fractures in arthrogry-posis multiplex congenita. J Pediatr Orthop 1981;1:189.

157. Wilson GN: Pediatric approach to the skeletal dyspla-sia. Pediatr Ann 1990;19:141.

158. Beighton P, Giedion A, Gorlin R, et al: International Classification of Osteochondrodysplasias: International Working Group on Constitutional Diseases of Bone. Am J Med Genet 1992;44:223.

159. Letts M, MacDonald P: Sports injuries to the pediatric spine. Spine State Art Rev 1990;4:49.

160. Warrick CK: Polyostotic fibrous dysplasia—Albright's syndrome. J Bone Joint Surg 1949;31B:175.

161. Smith R: Osteogenesis imperfecta nonaccidental injury and temporary brittle bone disease. Arch Dis Childhood 1995;72:169.

162. Brenner RE, Schiller B, Pontz BF, et al: Osteogenesis imperfecta in kindheit und adoleszenz. Monatsschr Kinderheilkd 1993;141:940.

163. Smith R: Osteogenesis imperfecta: From phenotype to genotype and back again. Int J Exp Pathol 1994;75:233.

164. Smith R: Osteogenesis imperfecta. Clin Rheum Dis 1986;12:655.

165. Binder H, Conway A, Hason S, et al: Comprehensive rehabilitation of the child with osteogenesis imperfecta. Am J Med Genet 1993;45:265.

166. Binder H, Hawks L, Graybill G, et al: Osteogenesis imperfecta: Rehabilitation approach with infants and young children. Arch Phys Med Rehabil 1984;65:537.

167. Feldman KW, Marcuse EK, Springer DA: Nutritional rickets. Am Fam Physician 1990;42:1311.

168. Martinez GA, Krieger FW: 1984 milk feeding patterns in the United States. Pediatrics 1985;76:1004.

169. Pitt MJ: Rickets and osteomalacia are still around. Radiol Clin North Am 1991;29:97.

170. Wraith JE: The mucopolysaccharidoses: A clinical review and guide to management. Arch Dis Childhood 1995;72:263.

171. Diaz JH, Belani KG: Perioperative management of children with mucopolysaccaridoses. Anesth Analg 1993;77:1261.

172. Ransford AO, Crockard HA, Stevens JM, et al: Occipito-atlanto-axial fusion in Morquio-Brailsford: A ten-year experience. J Bone Joint Surg 1996;78B:307.

173. Hughes DG, Chadderton RD, Cowie RA: MRI of the brain and cranial cervical junction in Morquio's disease. Neuroradiology 1997;39:381.

174. Gulati MS, Agin MA: Morquio's syndrome: A rehabilitation perspective. J Spinal Cord Med 1996;19:12.

175. Tyler DC, Smith M, Womack W, et al: Pain management in infants, children and adolescents. In Loeser JD, Egan KJ (eds): Managing the Chronic Pain Patient. New York, Raven Press, 1989.

176. Lloyd-Thomas AR, Lauder G: Reflex sympathetic dystrophy in children. BMJ 1995;310:1648.

177. Inhofe PD, Garcia-Moral CA: Reflex sympathetic dystrophy: A review of the literature and a long-term outcome study. Orthop Rev 1994;23:655.

178. Mubaraj SJ, Carroll MC: Volkmann's contracture in children: Etiology and prevention. J Bone Joint Surg 1979;61B:285.

179. Mass DP, Raasch WG: Hand and wrist injuries. In Rider B (ed): Sports Medicine: The School Age Athlete. Philadelphia, WB Saunders, 1991.

180. Buckley SL: Current trends in the treatment of femoral shaft fractures in children and adolescents. Clin Orthop Rel Res 1997;338:60.

181. Houston MS: Care of the school-aged child in 90/90 traction. Orthop Nurs 1996;15:57.

182. Church C, Botash AS, Blatt SD, et al: Autism, child abuse and sudden infant death syndrome. Curr Opin Pediatr 1997;9:189.

183. Carty HM: Fractures caused by child abuse. J Bone Joint Surg 1993;75B:849.

184. Alexander RC: Current and emerging concepts in child abuse. Compr Ther 1995;21:726.

Index

Page numbers in **boldface type** indicate complete chapters; *f* indicates a figure; *t* indicates a table.